Helicobacter pylori

Basic Mechanisms to Clinical Cure

Helicobacter pylori

Basic Mechanisms to Clinical Cure

Edited by

Richard H. Hunt
Professor of Medicine
Director, Division of Gastroenterology
McMaster University Medical Centre
1200 Main Street West
Hamilton, Ontario L8N 3Z5
Canada

Guido N.J. Tytgat
Professor, Department of
Gastroenterology and Hepatology
Academic Medical Centre
9 Meibergdreef
1105 AZ Amsterdam
The Netherlands

Proceedings of the International Symposium held at Amelia Island, Florida, USA, November 3–6, 1993

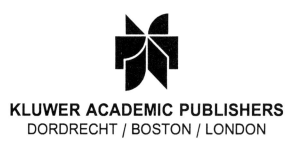

KLUWER ACADEMIC PUBLISHERS
DORDRECHT / BOSTON / LONDON

Distributors

for the United States and Canada: Kluwer Academic Publishers, PO Box 358, Accord
Station, Hingham, MA 02018-0358, USA
for all other countries: Kluwer Academic Publishers Group, Distribution Center, PO Box
322, 3300 AH Dordecht, The Netherlands

A catalogue record for this book is available from the British Library

ISBN 0-7923-8838-0

Published in the United Kingdom by Kluwer Academic Publishers,
PO Box 55, Lancaster, UK.

Kluwer Academic Publishers BV incorporates the publishing programmes of
D. Reidel, Martinus Nijhoff, Dr W. Junk and MTP Press.

Typeset by Lasertext Ltd, Stretford, Manchester, UK.

Printed in Great Britain by Hartnolls Ltd., Bodmin, Cornwall.

Contents

SECTION III. MECHANISMS OF *H. pylori* INDUCED DAMAGE

CONTENTS

CONTENTS

List of Principal Authors

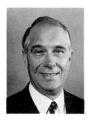

A. T. R. AXON
Centre for Digestive Diseases
The General Infirmary
Great George Street
Leeds LS1 3EX
UK

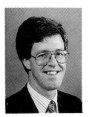

J. CALAM
Department of Medicine
Royal Postgraduate Medical School
Hammersmith Hospital
London W12 0NN
UK

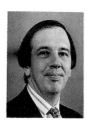

D. R. CAVE
Section of Gastroenterology
St Elizabeth's Medical Center
736 Cambridge Street, Box 43D
Boston, MA 02135
USA

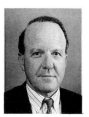

V. S. CHADWICK
Department of Experimental Medicine
University of Otago Medical School
Great King Street
Dunedin
New Zealand

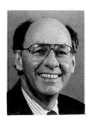

R. L. CLANCY
Department of Pathology
David Maddison Clinical Sciences Bldg.
Royal Newcastle Hospital
Newcastle, NSW 2300,
Australia

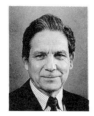

P. CORREA
LSU Medical Center
Department of Pathology
1901 Perdido Street
New Orleans, LA 70112
USA

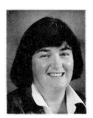

J. E. CRABTREE
Clinical Sciences Bldg., Level 7
Department of Medicine
St James' University Hospital
Leeds LS9 7TF
UK

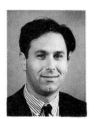

K. CROITORU
Intestinal Disease Research Program
McMaster University Health Sciences Centre
1200 Main Street West, Rm 4H17
Hamilton, Ontario L8N 3Z5
Canada

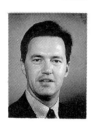

K. DEUSCH
II. Department of Medicine
Technical University
Ismaninger Str. 22
W-8000 Munich 80
Germany

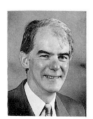

M. F. DIXON
Centre for Digestive Diseases
The General Infirmary
Leeds LS2 9JT
UK

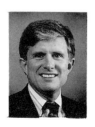

B. E. DUNN
Pathology and Laboratory Medicine Service (113)
Clement J Zablocki VA Hospital
5000 West National Avenue
Milwaukee, WI 53295
USA

LIST OF PRINCIPAL AUTHORS

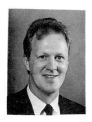

P. B. ERNST
Department of Pediatrics
Children's Hospital
Galveston, TX 77555-0366
USA

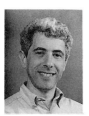

D. FORMAN
Imperial Cancer Research Fund
Cancer Epidemiology Unit
Gibson Bldg, Radcliffe Infirmary
Oxford OX2 6HE
UK

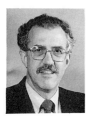

J. G. FOX
Division of Comparative Medicine
Massachusetts Institute of Technology
37 Vassar Street 45-104
Cambridge, MA 02139
USA

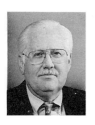

D. Y. GRAHAM
VA Medical Center (111D)
2002 Holcombe Blvd
Houston, TX 77030
USA

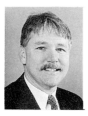

S. L. HAZELL
School of Microbiology/Immunology
University of New South Wales
PO Box 1, Kensington
Sydney, NSW 2033
Australia

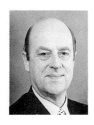

R. H. HUNT
Division of Gastroenterology
McMaster University Medical Centre
1200 Main Street West
Hamilton, Ontario L8N 3Z5
Canada

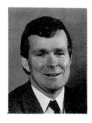

J. R. LAMBERT
Division of Medicine
Mornington Peninsula Hospital
Hastings Road
Frankston, Victoria 3120
Australia

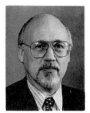

J. LECHAGO
Department of Pathology (MS 205)
The Methodist Hospital
6565 Fannin Street
Houston, TX 77030
USA

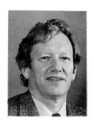

A. LEE
School of Microbiology and Immunology
University of NSW
PO Box 1
Kensingston, NSW 2033
Australia

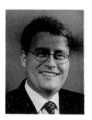

U. E. H. MAI
Arbeitsgruppe Gastrointestinale Infektionen
Institut für Medizinische Mikrobiologie
Medizinische Hochschule Hannover
Konstanty-Gutschow-Str.8
D-30625 Hannover
Germany

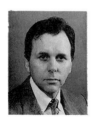

B. J. MARSHALL
940 Stanley Drive
Earlysville, VA 22936,
USA

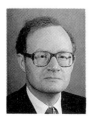

K. E. L. McCOLL
University Department of Medicine and Therapeutics
Western Infirmary
Glasgow G11 6NT
UK

LIST OF PRINCIPAL AUTHORS

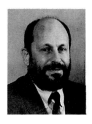

F. MÉGRAUD
Laboratoire de Bacteriologie
Hopital Pellegrin et Université de Bordeaux 2
F-33076 Bordeaux Cedex
France

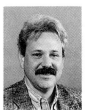

H. L. T. MOBLEY
Division of Infectious Diseases
University of Maryland School of Medicine
10 South Pine Street
Baltimore, MD 21201
USA

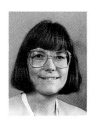

D. G. NEWELL
Central Veterinary Laboratory
New Haw
Weybridge
Surrey KT15 3NB
UK

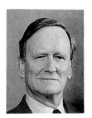

T. C. NORTHFIELD
Department of Medicine
St George's Hospital Medical School
Cranmer Terrace
Blackshaw Road
London SW17 0RE
UK

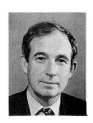

C. A. O'MORAIN
Department of Gastroenterology
Meath/Adelaide Hospitals
Dublin 8
Ireland

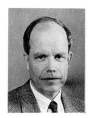

M. SALASPURO
Research Unit of Alcohol Disease
University of Helsinki
Tukholmankatu 8F
00290 Helsinki
Finland

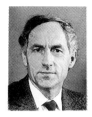

J. SAROSIEK
University of Virginia
Health Sciences Center
School of Medicine
Charlottesville, Virginia
USA

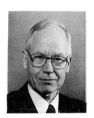

K. SEPPÄLÄ
Gastroenterology Unit
Department of Internal Medicine II
University Hospital of Helsinki
SF-00290 Helsinki
Finland

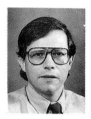

P. M. SHERMAN
Division of Gastroenterology (Rm 1448)
Hospital for Sick Children
555 University Avenue
Toronto, Ontario, M5G 1X8
Canada

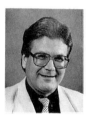

P. SIPPONEN
Department of Pathology
Jorvi Hospital
02740 Espoo
Finland

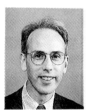

R. H. STEAD
Department of Pathology
McMaster University Health Sciences Centre
1200 Main Street West
Hamilton, Ontario L8N 3Z5
Canada

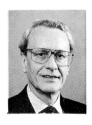

M. STOLTE
Institute of Pathology
Klinikum Bayreuth
Preuschwitzer Strasse 101
D-95445 Bayreuth,
Germany

LIST OF PRINCIPAL AUTHORS

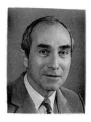

S. SZABO
Department of Pathology
Brigham & Women's Hospital
75 Francis Street
Boston, MA 02115
USA

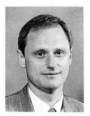

N. J. TALLEY
University of Sydney
Clinical Sciences Building
Nepean Hospital, PO Box 63
Penrith, NSW 2751
Australia

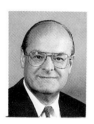

G. N. J. TYTGAT
Department of Gastroenterology-Hepatology
Academic Medical Centre
Meibergdreef 9
1105 AZ Amsterdam
The Netherlands

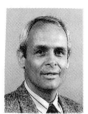

B. J. UNDERDOWN
Department of Pathology
Molecular Virology & Immunology Program
1200 Main Street West, Room 3N7
Hamilton, Ontario L8N 3Z5
Canada

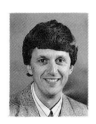

S. J. O. VELDHUYZEN VAN ZANTEN
Division of Gastroenterology
Victoria General Hospital
RC Dickson Centre, RM 4087
Halifax, NS, B3H 2Y9
Canada

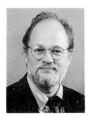

T. WADSTRÖM
Department of Medical Microbiology
University of Lund
S-223 62 Lund
Sweden

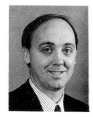

J. L. WALLACE
Gastrointestinal Research Group
Faculty of Medicine
University of Calgary
Calgary, Alberta, T2N 4N1
Canada

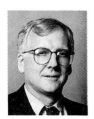

J. H. WALSH
UCLA School of Medicine
CURE Gastroenteric Biology Center
VA Wadsworth Medical Center
Los Angeles, CA 90073
USA

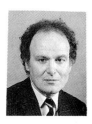

N. A. WRIGHT
ICRF/RCS Histopathology Unit
35-43 Lincoln's Inn Fields
London WC2A 3PN
UK

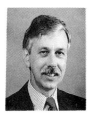

N. D. YEOMANS
Department of Medicine
Western Hospital, Gordon Street
Footscray
Victoria 3011
Australia

Preface

Helicobacter pylori infection has transformed our concepts of the pathophysiology of upper gastrointestinal disease and has stimulated much interest in research into the mechanisms and consequences of inflammation in the mucosa. In November 1993 a meeting was held at Amelia Island in Florida, which focused upon all aspects of *H. pylori*. A large faculty of internationally renowned basic and clinical scientists set out to explore the rapidly advancing knowledge of the basic mechanisms involved in acute and chronic *H. pylori* infection and the way in which this can lead to gastritis, duodenal and gastric ulcer and gastric cancer. The immunological mechanisms of the stomach are complex and important in regulating the factors which influence the progression of gastritis. Knowledge coming from this area of research will have important implications for the treatment and prevention of upper gastrointestinal disease.

H. *pylori* has proved to be especially difficult to eradicate and triple drug regimens containing bismuth have become the gold standard. The incorporation of effective acid suppression with antibiotics, a better understanding of the pharmacology of existing drugs, and the introduction of viable animal models to investigate them are all helping to identify optimal directions for future therapeutic research.

The meeting, entitled *Helicobacter pylori: Basic Mechanisms to Clinical Cure*, restricted the speakers to 15-minute presentations allowing an extensive discussion period after each section. It was not possible to include the discussion in the publication of the proceedings due to their length. However, the comprehensive manuscripts provided by each speaker reflect the state of the art in our knowledge of *H. pylori* at this time and make a timely summary and invaluable reference source for all those interested in this fascinating organism and its consequences. This meeting was supported by Mr Léon Gosselin of Axcan Pharma (Interfalk Canada Inc.) in Montreal, Canada, to whom we owe much gratitude for making it possible.

Richard H. Hunt
McMaster University Medical Centre
Hamilton, Ontario, Canada

Guido N. J. Tytgat
Academic Medical Centre
Amsterdam, The Netherlands

Scientific Organizers and Co-Chairmen, Amelia Island, November 1993

Section I
Basic bacteriology of
H. pylori

1
In vivo models of gastric *Helicobacter* infections

J. G. FOX

INTRODUCTION

Though it has been only a decade since the discovery of *Helicobacter pylori*, the organism is now known to be associated with three significant human diseases: active chronic gastritis, peptic ulcer disease and gastric adenocarcinoma[1-4]. Most recently, *H. pylori* has been incriminated in the aetiology of a fourth gastric disease, malignant lymphoma of mucosa-associated lymphoid tissue of the stomach[5]. Thus, the study of naturally occurring infections with gastric *Helicobacter* species in laboratory animals, as well as the use of selected animals experimentally infected with gastric helicobacters, have been increasingly used to dissect the role of this genus of bacteria in eliciting gastroduodenal disease.

It is important to remember basic tenets, established over the past several decades by investigators, in selection of the proper animal model to probe questions regarding pathogenesis and epidemiology of a particular human disease[6,7]. Criteria enumerated often include: (1) it is readily available commercially in sufficient numbers; (2) the species is amenable to transportation; (3) it is well adapted to the laboratory and has sufficient life span for the study in question; (4) its biology and genetics have been characterized; (5) its microbial flora, particularly pathogens, have been delineated, and if necessary specific pathogen-free (SPF) animals are available; (6) it reproduces the pathology and immune response of the human disease being studied; (7) the impact of cost, animal welfare, and restrictive legislation is considered. The issue of re-creating the disease syndrome with the aetiological agent of the human disease has particular relevance in the study of *H. pylori*-induced gastroin- testinal disease. Unfortunately, because of the restricted host range of *H. pylori*, development and refinement of the ideal animal model has remained elusive. However, despite this limitation, significant insights have been achieved in studies on pathogenesis, epidemiology and immunization using appropriate animal models.

This brief overview will highlight the attributes and limitations ascribed to particular models being used in this fascinating new area of clinical and basic research.

IN VIVO H. PYLORI MODELS

THE GERM-FREE ANIMAL

By definition, the germ-free animal must be maintained in rigid gnotobiotic conditions. This can be done only by using animals that have been Caesarean delivered and maintained in germ-free isolators. Rodents are much more amenable to these housing conditions because of their size, and the technology for achieving and maintaining germ-free rodents has been well developed and can be incorporated into a research laboratory without excessive costs and inordinate training of research personnel. Additionally, germ-free mice and rats can be purchased commercially. Unfortunately, to date *H. pylori* has not been successfully colonized in germ-free mice, germ-free rats, guinea pigs or ferrets[8-11]. However, both the germ-free pig and the germ-free dog have been experimentally infected with *H. pylori*[11-13]. The former has been more extensively used, particularly in short-term studies elucidating potential virulence factors of *H. pylori*. The gnotobiotic piglet is also being used to develop vaccines to protect against *H. pylori* gastritis. These models are limited because of their size, cost and specialized facilities required to perform the experiments germ-free. Furthermore, it is extremely difficult to endoscope animals being maintained in a germ-free isolator.

Pigs

The germ-free pig was the first animal model that was successfully colonized with *H. pylori*[11,12] (Table 1). Gnotobiotic piglets were pretreated with ranitidine or cimetidine prior to oral inoculation of *H. pylori*; in one study the pigs received 10^6 c.f.u. and two pigs received a second dose of *H. pylori*, 3 days after initial inoculation; in the second study, animals were dosed with 10^9 c.f.u. In the first study, culture samples were taken from one test and one control animal during intervals up to 24 days post-dosing. *H. pylori* was isolated from the antrum of all six experimentally infected piglets, the fundus in five of six and the duodenum in two of six. In the second study, consisting of 17 piglets from two litters, by weeks 2–4 all piglets were culture-positive. In both studies, *H. pylori* was not isolated from control animals maintained in separate isolators, nor was the organism cultured from the lower intestinal tract of experimentally infected animals[11].

Infected piglets had a chronic antral gastritis with lymphoid follicles and a diffuse mononuclear infiltrate of the mucosa. After 2–4 weeks of infection, elevated serum *H. pylori* IgG antibodies were also noted. Adherent bacteria, similar to those observed in human patients, with cup-like invaginations and adherence pedestals, and changes in microvilli and cell membrane morphology, were observed by electron microscopy[14].

Table 1 In vivo experimental infection with H. pylori

Animal	Age at dosing	Dose	Predose treatment	Histological findings	Length of study	Immune response	% Infected and period of infection	Reference
Gnotobiotic pig	3 days	10^9	Cimetidine	Acute gastritis (2 weeks), chronic thereafter	30 days	IgG	100% 30 days	11
SPF pig	8 weeks	5×10^8 2×1 week interval	Oral omeprazole 40 mg; 50 ml of fat per os	Chronic	6.5 months	NR	75% 6 months	21
Barrier maintained gnotobiotic pig, conventionalized at 24 days	3 days	10^9	None	Chronic	40 days	IgG ↑ IgA ↑	75% 45 days 100% 60 days 100% 90 days	20
Gnotobiotic dogs	7 days	3×10^8	None	Chronic	30 days	IgG ↑	30 days	13
Rhesus macaque	10 years	7 ml 10^9/ml	None	Acute (2 weeks) chronic	64 weeks	IgG 1–5 months ↑	25% 10 weeks 0% 14 weeks	26
Japanese macaque	Adult	5 ml, 10^9 c.f.u./ml	Na bicarbonate famphotidine 20 mg/kg	Chronic	28 days 2 years	IgG ↑	58% 28 days 100% 2 years	23,24

NR = not reported

5

Virulence studies

The gnotobiotic pig, despite the limited time the animals can be studied, has provided valuable *in vivo* data related to putative virulence factors of *H. pylori*. Motility of enteric bacteria is important for colonization, particularly for organisms that must penetrate the mucus layer of the gut. A highly motile strain 26695 proved to be an effective colonizer of gnotobiotic pigs; 100% of pigs dosed became infected, whereas TX30a, the least of the motile strains tested, successfully colonized only 17% (one of seven) piglets[15]. The strains were also analysed for cytotoxin production, another proposed virulence factor. Strain 26695 had high cytotoxin activity, whereas TX30a did not. Strain 60190 had the highest cytotoxin production, but low motility, and colonized only 40% of the germ-free piglets. The degree of gastritis and the infection rate was also greater with strain 26695. Vacuolation of gastric epithelial cells was observed in infected as well as uninoculated control pigs; however, the mean number of vacuoles per millimetre of mucosa was greater with strain 26695. Bacterial urease is known to augment vacuolization *in vitro*, but levels produced by each strain were not reported[16].

Urease activity of *H. pylori* with production of ammonia may provide a microbarrier around the organism during initial colonization in the hostile acidic gastric milieu. To test the hypothesis, a chemically created mutant strain was used[17]. The urease-negative mutant strain, when inoculated into gnotobiotic piglets, was unable to colonize, whereas the parent strain did. In addition, the parent strain produced a gastritis. These results suggest that urease is essential for colonization and survival in the gastric acidic environment.

Immunization trials

Oral and parenteral vaccination with formalin-killed *H. pylori* in the germ-free pig induced *H. pylori*-specific serum IgG and IgM and IgA, but did not prevent colonization by subsequent challenge with viable *H. pylori*[18]. Piglets immunized parenterally and then challenged with oral *H. pylori* developed a more severe lymphoplasmacytic gastritis and, in addition, an appreciable neutrophilic response in the gastric mucosa. This acute inflammatory response was not noted in *H. pylori*-infected pigs previously immunized with oral killed *H. pylori*, nor was this observed in *H. pylori*-infected piglets without prior immunization with *H. pylori*. These findings pose intriguing questions regarding immunization regimens and the direct effect these vaccines have on gastric mucosal integrity.

Dogs

H. pylori colonized the gastrointestinal tract of five gnotobiotic dogs orally challenged with 3×10^8 *H. pylori* at 7 days of age[13]. When necropsied 30 days later the dogs were colonized with *H. pylori* in the cardia, fundus, antrum and pyloric antrum. Although the fundus was the area most heavily colonized, urease mapping of multiple stomach sites indicated that the density of colonization was less than that observed in human tissue colonized with *H. pylori*. Microscopically, focal to diffuse lymphoplasmacytic infiltrates with follicle formation and focal infiltration of neutrophils and eosinophils in the gastric lamina propria were observed. *H. pylori* were present in the gastric epithelial cells beneath the mucus layer. Serum IgG was present in the infected beagles after 30 days. Both control dogs became infected with *H. pylori* after the 7-day contact period indicating, like humans, that *H. pylori* is transmissible by direct contact. *H. pylori* was cultured from the pharynx, oesophagus, duodenum and rectum, and in part explained the transmission but did not provide definitive proof of whether oral–oral or faecal–oral transmission occurred[13].

CONVENTIONAL (NON GERM-FREE) EXPERIMENTAL MODELS OF *H. PYLORI*

Pigs

Barrier-born, specific pathogen-free pigs (SPF) have also been used to investigate *H. pylori* pathogenesis (Table 1). Barrier-born pigs at 8 weeks of age were transferred to ordinary 'experimental sites', isolated from other pigs and fed conventional pig feed[19]. Fifteen animals were pretreated with omeprazole and orally dosed, with different regimens with 10^7 to 10^9 c.f.u. of a human strain of *H. pylori*. Endoscopy and gastric biopsies were performed weekly for the first 3 weeks and then every other week for up to 12 weeks. In 11 of the 15 pigs, *H. pylori* (based on Gram strain and growth in selective media) was cultured. Use of *H. pylori*-specific monoclonal antibody helped confirm the presence of *H. pylori* from gastric biopsies throughout the experiment varying from 6 to 12 weeks post-inoculation (p.i.). Higher doses of inoculum, plus repeated doses, appeared to enhance the infection. In *H. pylori*-infected pigs, the mononuclear cell infiltrate in mucosa and lamina propria increased 2–6 weeks p.i. but was most pronounced 4–8 weeks p.i. However, after 8 weeks the inflammatory response began to subside and by 12 weeks p.i. the mucosa appeared nearly identical to that observed prior to the experimental infection, thus posing the question whether colonization was persisting. Using monoclonal antibody, lymphocytes expressing Class II antigens were observed in the lamina propria. Ten weeks p.i. the pigs were treated orally by syringe with triple therapy, bismuth subsalicylate (500 mg), metronidazole (750 mg), and ampicillin (800 mg), BID for 2 weeks. This treatment successfully cleared *H. pylori* from gastric biopsies obtained shortly after the pigs were taken off treatment. True eradication of the organism (i.e. negative culture from biopsies taken 4 weeks after cessation of therapy) was not determined. Using an ELISA, antibody titres to *H. pylori* remained high in the four treated pigs, as did IgG titres in the other seven *H. pylori*-infected pigs[19]. Two other short-term studies using Caesarean-obtained, barrier-reared pigs or SPF barrier-maintained pigs, indicated that *H. pylori* also colonized the stomach of these animals[20,21].

Table 2 In vivo experimental infection with other gastric Helicobacter species

Animal	Organism	Histological findings	Predose treatment	Length of infection in study	Immune response	Chronic infection established	Reference
Ferret	H. mustelae 2×3 ml 1.5×10^8 c.f.u./ml	Chronic, MAG	Cimetidine 10 mg/kg	6 months–3 years*	IgG ↑	100% 3 years	10, 36
Gnotobiotic mouse (Swiss Webster)	H. felis 3×2 day interval 0.5 ml ~ 10^{10} c.f.u./ml	Active chronic	None	50 weeks	Early ↑ IgM IgG ↑	100% 50 weeks	37, 38
SPF mouse (Swiss Webster)	H. felis 3×2 day interval 0.5 ml ~ 10^{10} c.f.u./ml	Active chronic	None	50 weeks	Early ↑ IgM IgG ↑	100% 50 weeks	37, 38
Gnotobiotic rat	H. felis 0.5 ml ~ 10^{10} c.f.u./ml	Chronic	None	10 weeks	↑ IgG Early ↑ IgM	100% 10 weeks	44
Gnotobiotic dog	H. felis 2 ml ~ 10^9 c.f.u./2 ml	Chronic	None	30 days	↑ IgG	100% 28 days	51
Conventional mouse	H. heilmanni + H. muridarum	Chronic, MAG Epithelial and MALT hyperplasia	None	72 weeks	NR†	100% 72 weeks	83

MAG = multifocal atrophic gastritis; NR = not reported; MALT = mucosal-associated lymphoid tissue
*Fox et al., unpublished observation, 1993

Other laboratories have attempted to evaluate either conventional or gnotobiotic pigs experimentally infected with *H. pylori* on a long-term basis by placing them in conventional housing. Investigators from two separate laboratories, when attempting to reisolate *H. pylori* from gastric mucosa, were instead culturing a urease-positive *Campylobacter* sp.[22] (W. Bar, unpublished observations). Before the proper taxonomic characterization of the bacteria was determined by ribosomal RNA sequencing, urease-positive Gram-negative curved rods isolated from biopsies were presumptively assumed to be *H. pylori* strains experimentally inoculated into the pigs. Further studies are necessary before the SPF barrier pig can be used routinely to assess *in vivo* properties of *H. pylori*.

Non-human primates

Japanese macaques

The most recent studies involving experimentally infecting non-human primates consisted of dosing Japanese macaques (*M. fuscata*) with 5 ml suspension of *H. pylori* (10^9 c.f.u./ml). The animals had been pretreated with oral Na bicarbonate (1 g/day) and injections of famotidine 20 mg/kg i.m. for 3 days to raise gastric pH[23]. In seven of 12 (58%) animals, *H. pylori* was recovered up to 28 days post-inoculation and an active, chronic gastritis was observed histologically. In five *H. pylori*-infected monkeys treated with ampicillin for 21 days at a dose of 30 mg/kg BID, *H. pylori* was no longer cultured from antral gastric mucosa and the gastric ammonia concentration dropped, as did the gastritis score. However, the serum *H. pylori* IgG titres tended to increase in the five animals after treatment. The remaining two macaques remained positive at 6 months p.i.[23]. The same researchers, using another set of six Japanese macaques, demonstrated long-term *H. pylori* colonization and gastritis in all six monkeys for 2 years p.i.[24]. Thus, the Japanese macaque appears to offer considerable potential in following long-term progression of *H. pylori*-associated gastritis. Unfortunately, breeding colonies and availability of this macaque species are limited outside of Japan, and the status of infection with '*Gastrospirillum hominis*' in these animals must be clarified.

Rhesus macaques

Ten rhesus monkeys, culture-negative for *H. pylori*, were utilized, with one group being inoculated with 2×10^8 c.f.u. of a human strain of *H. pylori*, and the second group being orally dosed with 2×10^6 c.f.u. of *H. pylori* from a rhesus monkey[25]. Four of five rhesus inoculated with the human *H. pylori* were negative on culture during the 8-week study period; the fifth was colonized, but without gastritis. These results could have been influenced by the fact that the infecting strain had been attenuated by serial passage *in vitro*. In contrast, all five monkeys challenged with the rhesus strain not only became colonized with the organism by 14 days after inoculation, but also had a gastritis after 28 days p.i. The infection appeared focal, based on inconsistent positive isolation of *H. pylori* from three antral biopsies. One monkey had an antral ulcer after 4 weeks, which healed by the end of the 8-week study. Restriction enzyme analysis indicated that four of five *H. pylori* had identical patterns with Bam HI and the remaining one was only slightly different from the infecting *H. pylori* strain. Immune responses were not included in the study, but it raises important questions regarding the infectivity of human *H. pylori* in non-human primates. Similarly, investigators in Japan successfully colonized all four rhesus monkeys after experimental challenge with *H. pylori* (7 ml of broth containing 10^9 c.f.u./ml). Unfortunately, two of the four rhesus cleared the infection at 3 weeks p.i., while the other two monkeys cleared the *H. pylori* by 14 weeks p.i.[26]. Sera IgG *H. pylori* antibodies in the four rhesus increased at 1 month p.i., peaked at 4 months, then declined by 8 months p.i.

The non-human primate has the advantages of being infected with *H. pylori*, presumably the same organism infecting humans, the macaque stomach closely mimics that of humans, and the model is also amenable to long-term studies with frequent endoscopies if necessary. The disadvantages of the model are availability of the species, housing requirements, excessive costs, and the presence of *Gastrospirillum hominis* in many species.

Chimpanzee

A small group of chimpanzees identified by several diagnostic criteria to be free of *H. pylori* have been experimentally infected with *H. pylori* by oral challenge[27]. Interestingly, in the five animals challenged with *H. pylori*, only one became infected initially, whereas a secondary challenge 15 weeks after the first *H. pylori* dose was necessary to infect two of the other chimps. Mild gastric inflammation, and a systemic immune response, was noted in the three infected animals. Although the expense and limited availability of the chimpanzee severely restrict their use, the chimpanzee or other primate species may provide valuable information in efficacy and safety of *H. pylori* vaccines prior to initiating field trials when and if vaccines for *H. pylori* appear clinically feasible.

Athymic and euthymic mice

An interesting preliminary report also indicates that fresh clinical isolates of *H. pylori*, but not isolates maintained in stock culture, can colonize the stomach of athymic and euthymic mice for a much shorter time interval. This experiment needs to be verified and, if reproducible, can help elucidate the role of T lymphocytes in colonization of *H. pylori*[28].

NATURAL COLONIZATION AND PREVALENCE OF *H. PYLORI* IN LABORATORY ANIMALS

Because of the restricted host range of *H. pylori*, the non-human primate, particularly macaque species, are the only well-characterized naturally infected host other than humans.

Macaque species

Gastric spiral organisms were first noted in macaques in 1939[29]. Since then several authors have documented the gastric spiral organism '*G. hominis*' as well as *H. pylori* in several species of macaques; rhesus (*Macaca mulatta*) pig-tailed macaques (*M. nemistrina*), and cynomolgus (*M. fascicularis*). *H. pylori* colonization was documented in six of 11 colony-bred rhesus and none of five cynomolgus in one study in England[30]. *H. pylori* was cultured (two of seven tested) and/or detected by immunocytochemistry (four of six). In a subsequent report, *H. pylori* isolated from rhesus monkeys were further characterized by biochemical and antigenic criteria[31]. In the United States, *H. pylori* was cultured from stomach biopsies of 12 of 35 colony-reared rhesus, whereas none of the 21 cynomolgus monkeys surveyed in the United States had the organism cultured[25]. Lymphocytic infiltration of superficial layers of lamina propria in both antrum and fundus was seen in 10 of 12 (83%) of *H. pylori*-positive rhesus but in only four of 23 (17%) culture-negative animals[25]. However, *H. pylori* was not visualized in histological evaluation of the tissue. Though a urease assay was done on the animals, the authors did not use it as a predictive test for *H. pylori* colonization because of a high percentage of false-positive results they obtained[25]. Though no further explanation was provided, it is possible that the monkeys could have been infected with '*G. hominis*', a strongly urease-positive organism, or alternatively, due to coprophagy or bile reflux, other urease-positive bacteria could have contaminated the gastric biopsy tissue. Other studies indicated that rhesus monkeys colonized with *H. pylori* had a mild to heavy infiltration of the gastric lamina propria by lymphocytes, plasma cells and macrophages, but not PMN, located primarily in the antrum, but also present in fundus and pylorus[31]. Electron microscopy indicated that *H. pylori* heavily colonized epithelial surfaces, gastric pits and lumen of antral glands. The microvilli were also ablated. The presence of the organisms was demonstrated indirectly by serum IgG antibodies to *H. pylori* as measured by an ELISA, which was present in 13 of 23 rhesus tested. A 120-kDa protein, perhaps indicating an antibody response to the cytotoxin-associated gene, was consistently observed with a Western blot on all positive sera[30,31]. No discussion is presented on whether either the rhesus or cynomolgus monkeys were infected with '*G. hominis*'[25,31]. In another survey of 29 colony-bred rhesus monkeys, eight had bacteria in gastric mucus and on gastric epithelia that were morphologically compatible with *H. pylori*. Biopsies from three monkeys had urease-positive bacteria isolated that were identical to *H. pylori* when comparing SDS PAGE profile and antigenic profiles using antisera directed against *H. pylori* urease[32]. The eight rhesus with *H. pylori*-like organisms had gastritis, whereas only two of 14 monkeys with '*G. hominis*'-like organisms (GHLO) had gastritis. The '*G. hominis*' by electron microscopy were found in intact as well as damaged parietal cells. The invasion of parietal cells was associated with a significant increase of gastric acid output in rhesus infected with GHLO compared to non-infected and *H. pylori*-infected animals. Although the '*G. hominis*' infection may have been responsible for the hypersecretion of acid, further studies are needed to confirm this interesting observation[32]. Others also observed similar GHLO in parietal cells of stomachs in a large group of 45 rhesus monkeys[33]. Although 100% of the rhesus had GHLOs concentrated in the glands of the corpus, but not in the antrum or cardia, none had gastritis[33].

   H. pylori was also cultivated from six of 24 pig-tailed macaques[34]. Characterization of the organism was based on phenotypic, biochemical and DNA–DNA hybridization to the *H. pylori*-type strain, using whole genomic DNA probes[34]. Preliminary histological examination revealed plasma cell infiltration of gastric tissue and mucus depletion. Colonized animals were hypochlorhydric (pH 6.8–8.0) facilitating culture of *C. jejuni*, *C. coli* and *C. fetus* subsp. *fetus* from gastric biopsies of three monkeys. None of the *H. pylori*-negative macaques had a positive urease on gastric tissue, inferring they were not colonized with *H. pylori* or '*G. hominis*'. More recently, a new *Helicobacter* species, *H. nemistrina*, was isolated from gastric tissue of pig-tailed macaques. The ability of this organism to induce gastric disease requires further study[35].

EXPERIMENTAL INFECTION WITH OTHER GASTRIC *HELICOBACTER* SP.

H. mustelae in ferrets

Koch's postulates have been fulfilled establishing *H. mustelae* as a gastric pathogen in ferrets[36]. *H. mustelae*-negative ferrets treated with cimetidine and inoculated orally on two successive days with 3 ml (1.5×10^8 c.f.u.) of *H. mustelae* became colonized through week 24 of the experiment (Table 2). All infected ferrets had positive gastric culture, tissue urease, and Warthin-Starry staining of gastric biopsy tissue[36]. Superficial gastritis developed in the oxyntic gastric mucosa, and a full-thickness gastritis, composed primarily of lymphocytes and plasma cells plus small numbers of neutrophils and eosinophils, was present in the antrum. The inflammation was accompanied by an elevation of IgG antibody to *H. mustelae*. The stomach lesions, consisting of focal chronic antral gastritis induced by the experimental infection with *H. mustelae*, is similar to the gastritis observed in young ferrets that have been naturally colonized with the organism for a limited time period[36]. Since the completion of the study the four ferrets have remained colonized for 3 years p.i. and have a chronic gastritis as well as sustained IgG *H. mustelae* antibody response (J.G. Fox, unpublished observation).

   Another intriguing finding in the study was the transient hypochlorhydria

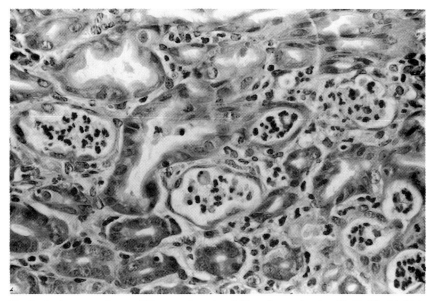

Fig. 1 Body mucosa from a GF mouse inoculated 10 weeks previously with *H. felis*. Multiple microabscesses and leukocytic infiltration of the lamina propria are depicted. H&E strain; bar, 25 μm. From ref. 38

observed approximately 4 weeks after the infection[36]. According to the urease tissue assay this period coincided with heavy *H. mustelae* colonization of the fundus. In the experimentally infected ferrets over time (>8 weeks), the organism, as in most naturally infected ferrets, colonizes the antrum in greater numbers[36].

H. FELIS IN MICE

Experimental infection with *H. felis* in germ-free and specific pathogen-free mouse stomachs resulted in a persistent chronic gastritis of 1 year duration[37,38]. The bacteria did not colonize the lower gastrointestinal tract. Gastric colonization was accompanied by an extensive infiltration of polymorphonuclear cells at 4 weeks p.i., including the presence of microabscesses. At 8 weeks p.i. the number of mononuclear inflammatory cells was sufficient to classify the lesion as active chronic gastritis (Fig. 1). Lymphoid nodules were also noted in the submucosa, indicating the chronic nature of the lesion. Interestingly, after 8 weeks p.i., hyperplastic changes of the mucosal epithelia were noted. Similar histological changes were also observed in specific pathogen-free mice inoculated with *H. felis*[39] (Figs 2–4). Thus, even though *H. felis* does not adhere to the gastric epithelia, it induced a significant inflammatory response. Recent immunohistochemical analysis using specific monoclonal antibodies revealed the presence of mucosal B220+ cells coalescing into lymphoid follicles surrounded by aggregates of Thy-

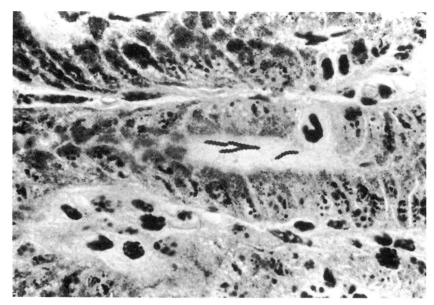

Fig. 2 Antral mucosa from a specific-pathogen-free mouse 30 weeks postinfection with *H. felis*. Spiral organisms characteristic of *H. felis* are noted within the lumen of a gland. Warthin-Starry stain; bar, 10 μm. From ref. 38

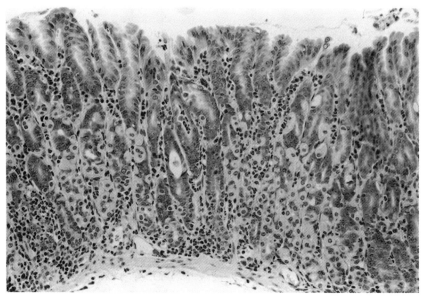

Fig. 3 Antral mucosa from a GF mouse 20 weeks postinfection with *H. felis*. Figure shows a leukocytic infiltrate in the lamina propria composed of lymphocytes and PMN leukocytes, a microabscess, and aggregates of lymphocytes and plasma cells at the level of the gastric pits. H&E stain; bar, 35 μm. From ref. 38

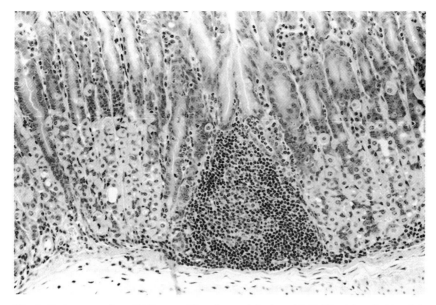

Fig. 4 Body mucosa from VAF mouse 20 weeks postinfection with *H. felis*. A lymphoid nodule is displacing glands, and a mild diffuse subglandular leukocytic infiltrate is noted. Small aggregates of lymphocytes and plasma cells in the lamina propria at the level of the gastric pits are also present. H&E stain; bar, 40 μm. From ref. 38

1.2[+] T cells, CD4[+], CD5[+] and $\alpha\beta$ T cells predominated in organized gastric mucosal and submucosal lymphoid tissue, and CD11b[+] cells occurred frequently in the mucosa[38]. Follicular B cells were composed of IgM[+] and IgA[+] cells. Numerous IgA-producing B cells were present in the gastric glands, the lamina propria, and gastric epithelium[38]. Infected animals developed anti-*H. felis* serum IgM antibody responses up to 8 weeks p.i., and significant serum IgG anti-*H. felis* antibody levels, which remained elevated throughout the 50-week course of the study[38] (Fig. 5).

Immunization trials

Because *H. pylori* is a persistent infection, difficult to eradicate by antimicrobial therapy, and approaches 95% infection rates in some underdeveloped populations, making eradication by antibiotics unfeasible, an immunological approach to prevent infection by *H. pylori* using oral vaccines has been suggested[40]. Czinn and Nedrud tested the feasibility of this approach by orally immunizing mice and ferrets with killed *H. pylori*[40]. Oral immunization induced IgG and IgA in gastrointestinal secretions and sera of both species. These antibody responses were substantially enhanced by addition of cholera toxin as a mucosal adjuvant. This initial observation was expanded by experiments utilizing the *H. felis*-infected mouse model[41]. Three groups of SPF mice were immunized on days 1, 3, 6, 30 and 54 with 0.5 ml PBS, 1 mg

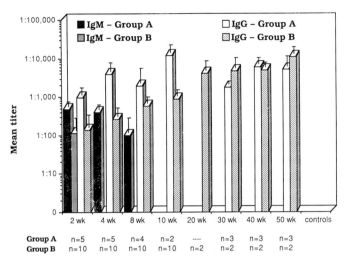

Fig. 5 Antibody response (IgG and IgM) in *H. felis*-infected GF (group A) and VAF (group B) mice. Uninoculated control mice served as baseline controls at each time point. From ref. 38

H. felis sonicate or 1 mg sonicate plus 10 µg cholera toxin (Sigma). Three days after completing the immunization protocol, all three groups of mice were challenged with 10^8 c.f.u. *H. felis*. All mice were killed and stomachs harvested for analysis 3 weeks post-challenge. All control mice were infected with *H. felis*, as were the mice immunized with bacterial sonicate only. However, only one of 19 mice immunized with sonicate plus cholera toxin became infected. The mice protected from experimental infection had increased IgA and IgM antibody response when compared to baseline levels[41]. Further studies including protection against *H. felis* in mice immunized with *H. pylori* sonicate, plus cholera toxin, suggest that a *H. pylori* oral vaccine to prevent infection offers promise.

EPIDEMIOLOGY OF *H. FELIS* INFECTION IN RODENTS

To understand the epidemiology of an infectious disease it is important to document route of transmission. The *H. felis*-infected mouse model has been used for this purpose. Though there are proponents to the theory that *H. pylori* is spread via the faecal–oral route, to date only selected laboratories have successfully cultured *H. pylori* from faeces, and a related organism, *H. mustelae*, has been isolated from ferret faeces. Lack of routine faecal culture of *H. pylori* but transmission via the faecal route is explained by the hypothesis that *H. pylori*, like *C. jejuni*, can enter a coccoid form that is non-culturable but still viable[42,43]. A series of experiments were designed to test whether *H. felis* (which also has coccoid forms) could be transmitted from mouse to mouse because of their copraphagic habits. In germ-free rodent experiments, *H. felis* was not transmitted to cage contact controls, nor could

H. felis be isolated from the intestine of germ-free mice or rats infected with the organism[37,44]. These experiments were also performed in SPF mice[45]. Specific pathogen-free mice infected with *H. felis* housed with control mice, either in small or large groups, did not transmit the organism to uninfected animals. Furthermore, females infected with *H. felis* did not transmit the gastric bacteria to their litters or to the males used to impregnate them. Rectal contents from an animal infected with both 'G. hominis' and *H. felis*, as well as gastric mucus containing these organisms, were fed to two separate groups of mice. The gastric mucus successfully colonized all mice, whereas the rectal homogenate did not colonize any of the experimentally challenged mice.

ANTIMICROBIAL SCREENING

The SPF mouse infected with *H. felis* has been assessed as an *in vivo* screening model to test the efficacy of potential therapeutic regimens to eradicate *H. pylori* in infected humans[46]. In *H. felis*-infected mice, 4 weeks after cessation of treatment, a 25% eradication rate was achieved with monotherapy with either erythromycin or bismuth subcitrate, whereas none of the *H. felis*-infected mice were cleared of infection with monotherapy with tetracycline. A high rate of eradication (67%) was achieved with amoxicillin therapy. Triple therapy with metronidazole, tetracycline and bismuth subcitrate eradicated the organism from 100% of the mice; if amoxicillin was substituted an 80% eradication rate was observed. The treatment regimen consisted of 14 daily doses of the antibiotics plus bismuth, followed by another 14 days of bismuth therapy alone[46]. When the compounds were given orally in three divided doses for a 14-day period, a different eradication rate was noted. There was a marked increase in eradication after a 4-week cessation of therapy for metronidazole alone (47% to 90%) and amoxicillin trihydrate (67% to 100%); eradication was less variable in triple therapy with amoxicillin metronidazole–bismuth (80% to 100%). Few differences were noted when comparing the dosing regimens for erythromycin alone, tetracycline alone, and bismuth subcitrate alone[46]. The model has the advantage in that previous transmission studies have shown that *H. felis* does not spread from mouse to mouse[45]. Therefore, positive *H. felis* mice after cessation of therapy are due to treatment failure rather than reinfection from cage-mates. The model is useful for screening of compounds, but because *H. felis* does not adhere to gastric mucosa, in a manner similar to *H. pylori* and *H. mustelae*, eradication for *H. felis*-colonized mice may be achieved more easily than hosts infected with *Helicobacter* species having adherent properties. Treatment regimens that appear promising should be tested further in the *H. pylori* pig model or the *H. mustelae*-infected ferret model[46].

Thus, the mouse model not only offers a practical screening model for therapeutic agents, but also offers tremendous potential to study immunology and pathogenesis of *Helicobacter*-induced gastric disease. This is due to its detailed genetic characterization, ability to manipulate genotype, and the diversity and specificity of immune reagents available for the mouse after antimicrobial therapy.

H. FELIS IN RATS

Experiments have also been done in gnotobiotic rats. Rats given 0.5 ml (10^{10} c.f.u./ml) of *H. felis* given per os on two successive days developed gastritis[44]. At 2 weeks, small numbers of lymphocytes and eosinophils were present in the subglandular portion of the antral mucosa that focally extended to the luminal portion of the antral mucosa that focally extended to the luminal surface. By 8 weeks p.i. the gastritis was confined to the antrum with increased numbers of lymphocytes and eosinophils in the subglandular mucosa and focal aggregates of lymphocytes in the submucosa extending through the mucosa and lamina propria to the luminal surface. *H. felis* in the rat localized in greater numbers in the antrum, the site of the most severe inflammation, and also produced an appreciable IgG antibody titre at 2, 4, and 8 weeks p.i., as well as a transitory IgM response[44].

PROPOSED RAT MODEL OF *H. PYLORI* ON GASTRIC ULCER HEALING

Experimental production of 4 mm diameter gastric ulcers in Sprague-Dawley rats was accomplished by applying 100% acetic acid to serosal surface of the fundus[47]. Thirty rats were then administered 2 ml *H. pylori* (10^8 c.f.u/ml) in normal saline BID for 7 days, and 20 rats were orally dosed with saline BID for 7 days. Three days later (10 days after ulcer production) all 50 rats were killed and examined. All 30 rats dosed with *H. pylori* had persistent chronic, active ulcers; ulcers had polymorphonuclear and mononuclear cell infiltrates, abundant fibrosis and capillary networks. The ulcer borders had dilated glands, lined by mature surface epithelium. Special silver stains and monoclonal antibody to *H. pylori* 'demonstrated' the presence of *H. pylori* in surface mucus and within fundic crypts. Ninety per cent of the control rats had healed ulcers and the other 10% had partially re-epithelialized ulcers. Though the results imply that *H. pylori* (or its products) delayed healing of the experimental ulcers, the investigators did not attempt to culture *H. pylori* from the stomach of rats, nor did they measure antibody response to the organism. Furthermore, the microbial status of the rats was not specified. It is possible that the *H. pylori* transient colonization with attendant local pH change (due to NH^3) allowed resident *H. muridarum* in the ileum and caeca to subsequently colonize the fundus and ulcers[48,49]. Dual colonization with *H. muridarum* and *H. felis* has been clearly demonstrated in the mouse, and may also selectively colonize the stomach of rats[50]. Cross-reaction of *H. muridarum* with *H. pylori* monoclonal antibody is also possible. Future experiments testing this hypothesis should verify that the rats used do not have *H. muridarum* in their ileum or caecum, and colonization of *H. pylori* must be verified by isolation of the organism from the ulcer's border and adjacent gastric mucosa.

CANINE MODEL

Because of the suspected role of *H. felis* as a cause of gastritis in dogs, five gnotobiotic beagle dogs were orally inoculated with a pure culture of *H. felis*[51]. The remaining two littermates served as contact controls. Thirty days after infection all animals were killed and specimens collected for evaluation. In infected dogs, *H. felis* was recovered from all areas of the stomach, with colonization being heaviest in the body and antrum. *H. felis* was not cultured from any segment of the gastrointestinal tract distal to the duodenum. Two weeks after infection all five infected dogs had detectable IgM and IgG serum antibody to *H. felis*, whereas control dogs had no measurable *H. felis* serum antibody throughout the study. Histopathological changes in the stomachs of infected dogs included large numbers of lymphoid nodules throughout all regions of the gastric mucosa, being most numerous in the fundus and body. A mild, diffuse lymphocytic infiltrate with small numbers of plasma cells and eosinophils was also present in the subglandular region of all portions of the gastric mucosa. Large numbers of spiral-shaped *H. felis* were noted in gastric mucus adjacent to, or superimposed over, the areas of inflammation. Occasionally, *H. felis* was observed within the canaliculi of gastric parietal cells. Thus, infection with *H. felis*, along with *G. hominis*, is likely to cause naturally occurring lymphofollicular gastritis seen commonly in laboratory-reared beagles[52,53].

NATURAL INFECTION IN ANIMALS WITH OTHER GASTRIC *HELICOBACTER* SPECIES

Ferret model

Fox *et al.*, in 1985, were the first to isolate a GCLO other than humans from a gastric ulcer of a mammalian host, the ferret (*Mustela putorius furo*)[54]. The authors subsequently named the organism *Helicobacter mustelae*[55,56]. Gastritis and gastric ulcers have been routinely reported in ferrets, colonized with *H. mustelae*, which live in the United States[10]. In our experience every ferret we have examined with chronic gastritis was infected with *H. mustelae*, while specific pathogen-free ferrets not infected with *H. mustelae* do not have gastritis, nor detectable IgG antibody to the organism[36,57]. Since the original report of *H. mustelae* isolation, the organism has been isolated from the stomachs of ferrets residing in Canada, England, and Australia, but not from ferrets in New Zealand[58,59].

In England, mature ferret stomachs have also been examined for the presence of gastric *Helicobacter*-like organisms (HLO)[58]. Although specific location of gastric sampling was not included, HLO were isolated from all of 17 gastric samples; morphologically and biochemically, the bacteria fulfilled the criteria for *H. mustelae*[58]. The mild lesions noted may indicate sparse colonization of *H. mustelae* strains in younger animals, or that the *H. mustelae* strains isolated in English ferrets are not as pathogenic as strains isolated from ferrets in the USA.

Detailed histological examination of commercially available ferrets in the

USA indicates that all ferrets examined had a gastritis coinciding with the presence of *H. mustelae*[57,59]. Superficial gastritis was noted in the oxyntic gastric mucosa, whereas in the distal antrum the chronic inflammatory response occupied the full thickness of the mucosa. In the proximal antrum and transitional mucosa, multifocal atrophic gastritis and regeneration were observed[57].

Ultrastructural examinations of ferret gastric tissue showed bacteria localized within the gastric pits with little evidence of bacteria on the external surface or in the overlying mucus layer[60]. Bacteria were very closely associated with the epithelial cells, being found alongside microvilli, aligning themselves along the surface of the epithelium, perpendicular to the surface of the epithelial cells and, in some instances, penetrating these cells. Extensive loss of microvilli was seen and, in such denuded areas, occasional adhesion pedestals were visible. Some organisms were undergoing endocytosis and localized within membrane-bound inclusions inside the epithelial cells. Bacterial cells were also noted infrequently in intercellular junctions; however, they did not appear to show a particular disposition for this site, as has been reported for *H. pylori*[61,62]. A fibre-like matrix or glyocalyx between the epithelial and bacterial cells formed a very dense matrix when the two surfaces were very close together, or showed more fibrous strands, especially when the bacterial cells were aligning with microvilli.

Epidemiology of natural infection

The faeces of weanling and adult ferrets have been screened for the presence of *H. mustelae* to determine whether faecal transmission could explain the 100% prevalence we observe in ferrets >6 weeks of age[63,64]. *H. mustelae* was isolated from the faeces of eight of 24 9-week-old and three of eight 8-month-old ferrets. These criteria were based on biochemical and phenotypic criteria as well as DNA probes and 16S RNA sequencing[64]. *H. mustelae* was not recovered from the faeces of 20-week-old ferrets which had been positive at weaning, or from the faeces of 1-year-old ferrets.

To test whether hypochlorhydria enhanced faecal recovery of *H. mustelae*, oral omeprazole, a proton pump inhibitor of the parietal cell, was administered to adult ferrets in two separate experiments to induce gastric hypochlorhydria pharmacologically[65]. The organisms were isolated on sequential faecal sampling in 23 of 55 (41.8%) of the ferrets during omeprazole therapy. *H. mustelae* identification was confirmed by using standard biochemical tests and reactivity to specific *H. mustelae* DNA probes[65]. Faeces from the same ferrets, when not on omeprazole treatment and with acidic gastric pH, were positive for *H. mustelae* faeces in only six of 62 (9.3%) of the ferrets. Gastric biopsy samples from all ferrets were positive for *H. mustelae* and in four of five ferrets, restriction enzyme patterns (using three restriction enzymes) of the gastric *H. mustelae* were identical to those of the faecal *H. mustelae* strains. These recent findings favour the hypothesis that hypochlorhydria promotes faecal–oral spread of *H. mustelae*. It also adds credence to our earlier argument that populations of hypochlorhydria patients, due to chronic atrophic gastritis or drug-induced pH elevation, could serve as reservoirs for faecal–oral spread of *H. pylori*. Additionally, these data support recent reports of *H. pylori* being recovered from human faeces.

Eradication of H. mustelae

H. mustelae, like *H. pylori* in humans, can be eradicated from gastric mucosa using triple antimicrobial therapy[66]. Treatment consisted of amoxicillin (10 mg/kg), metronidazole (20 mg/kg), and bismuth subsalicylate (17.5 mg/kg) dosed orally TID for 3 or 4 weeks, and was well tolerated. In five of seven (71%) adult ferrets the organisms were eradicated as determined by bacterial culture on gastric biopsies 1, 2, 3, 4, and 6 months post-therapy. We have subsequently achieved 100% eradication of *H. mustelae* in two separate trials. This may be due in part to raising the dose of amoxicillin to 20 mg/kg. This was in contrast to the the failure of monotherapy with chloramphenicol, or polytherapy with tetracycline, metronidazole, and bismuth subsalicylate, to eradicate *H. mustelae*. Several strains of *H. mustelae* isolated after unsuccessful polytherapy showed increased resistance to metronidazole, as in *H. pylori* patients.

The ferret possesses certain advantages for *in vivo Helicobacter* studies. The anatomical and physiological features of the ferret stomach are similar to those of humans[67,68] and the pathology with *H. mustelae* is similar to that produced by *H. pylori* in humans. Ferrets are readily available, easy to maintain, and relatively inexpensive. Oral dosing is straightforward, the animals tolerate anaesthesia and endoscopy well, and it is a relevant animal model of *H. pylori* chemotherapy. In addition, the ferret is currently being used to study the role of *Helicobacter* in gastric cancer.

Canine model

Because many of the bacteria observed in the stomachs of animals have not been cultured, or have been isolated only recently, the earlier descriptions of these gastric micro-organisms were morphological. This is particularly true for the spiral organisms found in the dog stomach. Lockard and Boler[69] observed three morphological forms of gastric spiral bacteria in dogs.

Lockard type 1 is a bacterium entwined with periplasmic fibrils which appear to cover the entire surface of the organism. Bryner *et al.* isolated a similar organism from aborted ovine fetuses and classified the organism as '*Flexispira rappini*'[70]. Recent molecular characterization of '*Flexispira rippini*' isolated from mouse colonic tissue indicates that this bacterium is also a *Helicobacter* species[71]. Because '*Flexispira rappini*' has not been cultured from the dog stomach, its status as a natural component of gastric flora versus a lower gastrointestinal tract colonizer in the dog (and other hosts) is unknown.

Lockard bacterium type 2 also has periplasmic fibrils, but they are more sparsely distributed on the organism and can appear singly or in groups of two, three or four. This organism has been cultured by Lee *et al.* from the cat and dog stomach, and has been named *H. felis*[72,73].

The third organism observed by Lockard and Boler is the bacterium most commonly seen in animal stomachs. This bacterium is also very tightly spiralled, but there are no periplasmic fibrils. This organism, though common in the dog and cat, has also been observed in the gastric tissue of non-human primates, and occasionally in humans. Though its natural host is either the dog or cat, the recent literature refers to the organism as '*Gastrospirillum hominis*'[74,75]. Although the bacterium has not been grown in culture, it can be maintained *in vivo* in the stomach of mice[76,77]. By using PCR and RNA ribosomal sequencing techniques it has been shown that '*Gastrospirillum hominis*' observed occasionally in human stomachs is also a *Helicobacter* species[78]. Because '*Gastrospirillum hominis*', *H. felis* and '*Flexispira rappini*' have been associated with naturally occurring gastritis in laboratory-reared dogs, the use of these naturally colonized animals for model development has been curtailed[51-53,69,76].

Cat

Gastric *Helicobacter*-like organisms historically have been commonly observed in cat stomachs[76,79]. Isolation of *H. felis* was first accomplished by culture of the organism from a cat stomach[51]. A study was recently performed to assess the prevalence of *Helicobacter* colonization in random-source cats based upon urease assay and histological examination. In 70% of the juveniles and 97% of the adult cats, chronic gastritis was associated with GHLOs. The high prevalence of infection is also important, because cats have recently been implicated as a potential reservoir for human infection by *Helicobacter*-like organisms, specifically *G. hominis*[80]. Further study is needed to determine what specific role GHLOs play in feline gastrointestinal disease, as well as their importance as a reservoir for human infection[74,75].

Rodents

In addition to *H. felis*, the mouse stomach is an efficient colonizer of *Gastrospirillum* (*Helicobacter*) *hominis*[76,77]. Indeed, this is the only mechanism to date that allows propagation of the organism in the laboratory. Like *H. felis*, '*G. hominis*' causes a chronic gastritis in mice[39]. Also of interest, when mice are colonized with either *H. felis* or '*G. hominis*', after an extended period of colonization, *H. muridarum*, which normally colonizes the ileum of mice, will also colonize gastric pits in significant numbers[81]. For example, when mice colonized with *H. muridarum* in their ileum were coinfected for 18 months with either *H. felis* or *G. hominis*, 77% and 100% of the mice, respectively, had their stomachs also colonized with *H. muridarum*[81]. In addition, in > 18-month-old control mice, 60% of their stomachs colonized with *H. muridarum*. Thus, changes in the gastric ecosystem appear to play an important role in gastric colonization with *Helicobacter* species. A gastritis associated with colonization of *H. muridarum* has also been noted by other investigators planning to use mice or rats for experimental gastric flora studies[50,82]. Of considerable interest is the observation that long-term colonization of mice with gastric spirals can elicit appreciable proliferation of gastric epithelia, as well as gastric mucosal-associated lymphoid tissue[83].

Cheetahs

Recently zoo-maintained cheetahs were evaluated because of chronic vomiting and weight loss. Biopsies submitted for culture and histology indicated that infected cheetahs had at least three identifiable gastric spiral organisms[84]. Two of these, *G. hominis* and *H. felis*, were diagnosed on morphological examination of their ultrastructure. The third organism, however, was cultured and appears unique based on 16S RNA sequencing data and SDS PAGE electrophoresis; it has been given the name *H. acinoynx*[85]. Histological examination of gastric tissue from cheetahs with the different species of *Helicobacter* revealed a chronic gastritis characterized by lymphocytes, numerous plasma cells, epithelial erosion and hyperplasia of gastric epithelium[84]. Experimental transmission of the gastric helicobacters from cheetahs to mice and domestic kittens resulted in lesions consistent with chronic gastritis[86]. Interestingly the large gastric spiral organisms, but not *H. acinoyx*, colonized the mouse.

CONCLUSION

In a short span of 10 years a great deal has been learned about the pathogenic potential of a new bacterial genus, *Helicobacter*. As the genus expands in number (currently there are nine recognized species) we can continue to study how these closely related microbes establish particular niches and interact with the various animal hosts. Hopefully, these *in vivo* studies will further our understanding of the mechanisms responsible for the organism's ability to persist in its host, and in some cases cause serious clinical disease.

References

1. Lee A, Fox JG, Hazell S. The pathogenicity of *Helicobacter pylori*: a perspective. Infect Immun. 1993;61:1601–10.
2. Fox JG, Correa P, Taylor NS *et al. Campylobacter pylori* associated gastritis and immune response in a population at increased risk of gastric carcinoma. Am J Gastroenterol. 1989;89:775–81.
3. Parsonnet J, Friedman GD, Vandersteen DP *et al. Helicobacter pylori* infection and the risk of gastric adenocarcinoma. N Engl J Med. 1991;325:1127–31.
4. Nomura A, Stemmermann GN, Chyou P, Kato I, Perez-Perez GE, Blaser MJ. *Helicobacter* infection and gastric adenocarcinoma among Japanese Americans in Hawaii. N Engl J Med. 1991;325:1132–6.
5. Wotherspoon AC, Doglioni C, Diss TC *et al.* Regression of primary low-grade B-cell gastric lymphoma of mucosa-associated lymphoid tissue type after eradication of *Helicobacter pylori*. Lancet. 1993;342:575–7.
6. Fox JG. *In vivo* models of enteric campylobacteriosis: natural and experimental infections. In: Nachamkin I *et al.*, editors. *Campylobacter jejuni*: current status and future trends. Washington, DC: American Society for Microbiology; 1992:131–8.

7. Migaaki G, Capen CC. Animal models in biomedical research. In: Fox JG, Cohen GJ, Loew FM, editors. Laboratory animal medicine. Orlando, FL: Academic Press; 1984:667–95.

8. Yoshihiro F, Yamamoto I, Tonokatsu Y, Tamura K, Shimoyama T. Inoculation of animals with human *Helicobacter pylori* and long-term investigation of *Helicobacter pylori*-associated gastritis. Eur J Gastroenterol Hepatol. 1992;4:S39–S44.

9. Cantorna MT, Balish E. Inability of human clinical isolates of *Helicobacter pylori* to colonize the alimentary tract of germ-free rodents. Can J Microbiol. 1990;36:237–41.

10. Fox JG, Otto G, Murphy JC, Taylor NS, Lee A. Gastric colonization of the ferret with *Helicobacter* species: natural and experimental infections. Rev Infect Dis. 1991;13:S671–S680.

11. Krakowka S, Morgan DR, Kraft WG, Leunk RD. Establishment of gastric *Campylobacter pylori* infection in the neonatal gnotobiotic piglet. Infect Immun. 1987;55:2789–96.

12. Lambert JR, Borromeo M, Pinkard KJ, Turner H, Chapman CB, Smith ML. Colonization of gnotobiotic piglets with *Campylobacter pyloridis* — an animal model? [Letter] J Infect Dis. 1987;155:1344.

13. Radin JM, Eaton KA, Krakowka S *et al. Helicobacter pylori* infection in gnotobiotic beagle dogs. Infect Immun. 1990;58:2606–12.

14. Rudmann DG, Eaton KA, Krakowka S. Ultrastructural study of *Helicobacter pylori* adherence properties in gnotobiotic piglets. Infect Immun. 1992;60:2121–4.

15. Eaton KA, Morgan DR, Krakowka S. *Campylobacter pylori* virulence factors in gnotobiotic piglets. Infect Immun. 1989;57:1119–25.

16. Cover TL, Puryear W, Perez-Perez GI, Blaser MJ. Effect of urease on HeLa cell vacuolation induced by *Helicobacter pylori* cytotoxin. Infect Immun. 1991;59:1264–70.

17. Eaton KA, Morgan DR, Brooks CL, Krakowka S. Essential role of urease in the pathogenesis of gastritis induced by *Helicobacter pylori* in gnotobiotic piglets. Infect Immun. 1991;59:2470.

18. Eaton KA, Krakowka S. Chronic active gastritis due to *Helicobacter pylori* in immunized gnotobiotic piglets. Gastroenterology. 1992;103:1580–6.

19. Engstrand L, Gustavsson S, Jörgensen A, Schwan A, Scheynius A. Inoculation of barrier-born pigs with *Helicobacter pylori*: a useful animal model for gastritis type B. Infect Immun. 1990;58:1763–8.

20. Eaton KA, Morgan DR, Krakowka S. Persistence of *Helicobacter pylori* in conventionalized piglets. J Infect Dis. 1990;161:1299–1301.

21. Engstrand L, Rosberg K, Hubinette R, Berglindh T, Rolfsen W, Gustavsson S. Topographic mapping of *Helicobacter pylori* colonization in long-term infected pigs. Infect Immun. 1992;60:653–6.

22. Morgan D, Murray P, Paster B *et al.* Gastric *Campylobacter*-like organisms (GCLOs) from swine. Abstract presented at ASM Annual Meeting, Anaheim, CA, 1990.

23. Shuto R, Fujioka T, Kubota I, Nasu M. Experimental gastritis induced by *Helicobacter pylori* in Japanese monkeys. Infect Immun. 1993;61:933–9.

24. Fujioka T, Shuto R, Kodama R *et al.* Experimental model for chronic gastritis with *Helicobacter pylori*: long term follow up study in *H. pylori*-infected Japanese macaques. Eur J Gastroenterol Hepatol. 1993;S1:S73–7.

25. Euler AR, Zurenko GE, Moe JB, Ulrich RG, Yagi Y. Evaluation of two monkey species (*Macacca mulatta* and *Macaca fascicularis*) as possible models for human *Helicobacter pylori* disease. J Clin Microbiol. 1990;28:2285–90.

26. Fukuda Y, Yamamoto I, Tonokatsu Y, Tamura K, Shimoyama T. Inoculation of rhesus monkeys with human *Helicobacter pylori*: a long-term investigation on gastric mucosa by endoscopy. Dig Endosc. 1992;4:19–30.

27. Hazell SL, Eichberg JW, Lee RD *et al.* Selection of the chimpanzee over the baboon as a model for *Helicobacter pylori* infection. Gastroenterology. 1992;103:848–54.

28. Karita M, Kohiyama T, Okita K, Nakazawa T. New small animal model for human gastric *Helicobacter pylori* infection: success in both nude and euthymic mice. Am J Gastroenterol. 1991;86:1596–603.

29. Doenges JL. Spirochetes in the gastric glands of macacas rhesus and of man without related disease. Arch Pathol. 1939;27:469–77.

30. Baskerville A, Newell DG. Naturally occurring chronic gastritis and *C. pylori* infection in the Rhesus monkey: a potential model for gastritis in man. Gut. 1988;29:465–72.

31. Newell DG, Hudson MJ, Baskerville A. Isolation of a gastric *Campylobacter*-like organism from the stomach of four Rhesus monkeys, and identification as *Campylobacter pylori*. J Med Microbiol. 1988;27:41–4.

32. Dubois A, Tarnawski A, Newell DG *et al*. Gastric injury and invasion of parietal cells by spiral bacteria in rhesus monkeys: are gastritis and hyperchlorhydria infectious diseases? Gastroenterology. 1991;100:884–91.

33. Sato T, Takeuchi TA. Infection by spirilla in the stomach of the rhesus monkey. Vet Pathol. 1982;19(Suppl. 7):17–25.

34. Bronsdon MA, Schoenknecht FO. *Campylobacter pylori* isolated from the stomach of the monkey, *Macaca nemistrina*. J Clin Microbiol. 1988;26:1725–8.

35. Bronsdon MA, Goodwin CS, Sly LI, Chilvers T, Schoenknecht FD. *Helicobacter nemestrinae* sp. nov., a spiral bacterium found in the stomach of a pigtailed macaque (*Macaca nemestrina*). Int J Syst Bacteriol. 1991;41:148–53.

36. Fox JG, Otto G, Taylor NS, Rosenblad W, Murphy JC. *Helicobacter mustelae*-induced gastritis and elevated gastric pH in the ferret (*Mustela putorius furo*). Infect Immun. 1991;59:1875–80.

37. Lee A, Fox JG, Otto G, Murphy JC. A small animal model of human *Helicobacter pylori* active chronic gastritis. Gastroenterology. 1990;99:1315–23.

38. Fox JG, Blanco M, Murphy JC *et al*. Local and systemic immune response in murine *Helicobacter felis* active chronic gastritis. Infect Immun. 1993;51:2309–15.

39. Lee A. Spiral organisms: what are they? A microbiologic introduction to *Helicobacter pylori*. Scand J Gastroenterol. 1991;26(Suppl. 187):9–22.

40. Czinn SJ, Nedrud JG. Oral immunization against *Helicobacter pylori*. Infect Immun. 1991;59:2359–63.

41. Chen M, Lee A, Hazell S. Immunization against gastric *Helicobacter* infection in a mouse (*Helicobacter felis*) model. Lancet. 1992;339:1120–1.

42. Jones DM, Sutcliffe EM, Curry A. Recovery of viable but non-culturable *Campylobacter jejuni*. J Gen Microbiol. 1991;137:2477–82.

43. Catrenich CE, Makin KM. Characterization of the morphologic conversion of *Helicobacter pylori* from bacillary to coccoid forms. Scand J Gastroenterol. 1991;26(Suppl. 181):58–64.

44. Fox JG, Otto G, Lee A, Taylor NS, Murphy JC. *Helicobacter felis* gastritis in gnotobiotic rats: an animal model of *H. pylori* gastritis. Infect Immun. 1991;59:785–91.

45. Lee A, Fox JG, Otto G, Dick-Hegedus E, Krakowka S. Transmission of *Helicobacter* spp.: a challenge to the dogma of faecal–oral spread. Epidemiol Infect. 1991;107:99–109.

46. Dick-Hegedus E, Lee A. Use of mouse model to examine anti-*Helicobacter pylori* agents. Scand J Gastroenterol. 1991;26:909–15.

47. Ross JS, Bui HX, del Rosario A, Sonbati H, George M, Lee CY. *Helicobacter pylori*: its role in the pathogenesis of peptic ulcer disease in a new animal model. Am J Pathol. 1992;141:721–7.

48. Phillips MW, Lee A. Isolation and characterization of a spiral bacterium from the crypts of the rodent gastrointestinal tract. Appl Environ Microbiol. 1983;45:675–83.

49. Lee A, Phillips MW, O'Rourke JL *et al*. *Helicobacter muridarum* sp. nov., a microaerophilic helical bacterium with a novel ultrastructure isolated from the intestinal mucosa of rodents. Int J Syst Bacteriol. 1992;42:27–36.

50. Queiroz DMM, Martin PWL, Pimenta RO, Martins PF, Rocha GA, Mendes A. Spiral bacterium associated with the gastric and intestinal mucosa of Wistar and Holtman rats. Act Gastroenterol Belg. 1993(Suppl. 56):99(abstract).

51. Lee A, Krakowka S, Fox JG, Otto G, Murphy JC. *Helicobacter felis* as a cause of lymphoreticular hyperplasia in the dog stomach. Vet Pathol. 1992;29:487–94.

52. Henry GA, Long PH, Burnes JL *et al*. Gastric spirillosis in beagles. Am J Vet Res. 1987;48:831–6.

53. Fox JG, Blanco M, Polidoro D *et al*. High prevalence of *Helicobacter*-associated gastritis in purpose bred beagles. Lab Anim Sci. 1992;42:420–1[Abstract].

54. Fox JG, Edrise BM, Cabot EB *et al*. *Campylobacter*-like organisms isolated from gastric mucosa of ferrets. Am J Vet Res. 1986;47:236–9.

55. Fox JG, Taylor NS, Edmonds P, Brenner DJ. *Campylobacter pylori* subspecies *mustelae* subsp. nov. isolated from the gastric mucosa of ferrets (*Mustela putorius furo*), and an emended description of *Campylobacter pylori*. Int J Syst Bacteriol. 1988;38:367–70.

56. Fox JG, Chilvers T, Goodwin CS *et al.* *Campylobacter mustelae*, a new species resulting from the elevation of *Campylobacter pylori* subsp. *mustelae* to species status. Int J Syst Bacteriol. 1989;39:301–3.
57. Fox JG, Correa P, Taylor NS *et al.* *Helicobacter mustelae*-associated gastritis in ferrets: an animal model of *Helicobacter pylori* gastritis in humans. Gastroenterology. 1990;99:352–61.
58. Tompkins DS, Wyatt JI, Rathbone BJ, West AP. The characterization and pathological significance of gastric *Campylobacter*-like organisms in the ferret: a model for chronic gastritis? Epidemiol Infect. 1988;101:269–78.
59. Morris A, Thomasen L, Tasman-Jones C, Nicholson G, Heap M. Failure to detect gastric *Campylobacter*-like organisms in a group of ferrets in New Zealand [Letter]. NZ Med J. 1988;101:275.
59. Gottfried MR, Washington K, Harrell LJ. *Helicobacter pylori*-like microorganisms and chronic active gastritis in ferrets. Am J Gastroenterol. 1990;85:813–18.
60. O'Rourke J, Lee A, Fox JG. An ultrastructural study of *Helicobacter mustelae*: evidence of a specific association with gastric mucosa. J Med Microbiol. 1992;36:420–7.
61. Hazell SL, Lee A, Brady L, Hennessy W. *Campylobacter pyloridis* and gastritis: association with intercellular spaces and adaption to an environment of mucus as important factors in colonization of the gastric epithelium. J Infect Dis. 1986;153:658–63.
62. Chen XG, Correa P, Offerhaus J *et al.* Ultrastructure of the gastric mucosa harboring *Campylobacter*-like organisms. Am J Clin Pathol. 1986;86:575–82.
63. Fox JG, Cabot EB, Taylor NS, Laraway R. Gastric colonization by *Campylobacter pylori* subsp. *mustelae* in ferrets. Infect Immun. 1988;56:2994–6.
64. Fox JG, Paster BJ, Dewhirst FE *et al.* *Helicobacter mustelae* isolation feces of ferrets: evidence to support fecal–oral transmission of gastric *Helicobacter* spp. Infect Immun. 1992;60:606–11.
65. Fox JG, Blanco M, Polidoro D, Yan L-L, Dewhirst FE, Paster BJ. Isolation of *Helicobacter mustelae* from feces of hypochlorhydric ferrets: role of gastric pH in the epidemiology of *Helicobacter* infection. Gastroenterology. 1993;104:86–92.
66. Otto G, Fox JG, Wu P-Y, Taylor NS. Eradication of *Helicobacter mustelae* from the ferret stomach: an animal model of *Helicobacter* (*Campylobacter*) *pylori* chemotherapy. Antimicrobial Agents Chemother. 1990;34:1232–6.
67. Andrews PLR. The physiology of the ferret. In: Fox JG, editor. Biology and diseases of the ferret, Philadelphia: Lea & Febiger; 1988:100–34.
68. Pfeiffer C. Surface topology of the stomach in man and the laboratory ferret. J Ultrastruct Res. 1970;33:252–62.
69. Lockard VF, Boler RK. Ultrastructure of a spiraled microorganism in the gastric mucosa of dogs. Am J Vet Res. 1970;31:1453–62.
70. Bryner JH. *Flexispira rappini*, gen. nov., sp. nov. A motile, urease-producing rod similar to *Campylobacter pyloridis*. IV International Workshop on Campylobacter Infections, 1988, p. 1440 (abstract).
71. Schauer DB, Ghori N, Falkow S. Isolation and characterization of '*Flexispiri rappini*' from laboratory mice. J Clin Microbiol. 1993;31:2709–14.
72. Lee A, Hazell SL, O'Rourke J, Kouprach S. Isolation of a spiral-shaped bacterium from the cat stomach. Infect Immun. 1988;56:2843–50.
73. Paster BJ, Lee A, Fox JG *et al.* Phylogeny of *Helicobacter felis*, sp. nov., *Helicobacter mustelae*, and related bacteria. Int J Syst Bacteriol. 1991;41:31–8.
74. Lee A, Dent J, Hazell S, McNulty CA. Origin of spiral organisms in human gastric antrum. Lancet. 1988;1:300–1.
75. Heilmann KL, Borchard F. Gastritis due to spiral shaped bacteria other than *Helicobacter pylori*: clinical, histological, and ultrastructural findings. Gut. 1991;32:137–40.
76. Weber AF, Hasa O, Sautter JH. Some observations concerning the presence of spirilla in the fundic glands of dogs and cats. Am J Vet Res. 1958;19:677–80.
77. Dick E, Lee A, Watson G, O'Rourke J. Use of the mouse for the isolation and investigation of stomach-associated spiral/helical shaped bacteria from man and other animals. J Med Microbiol. 1989;29:55–62.
78. Solnick JV, O'Rourke J, Lee A, Paster BJ, Dewhirst FE, Tompkins LS. An uncultured gastric spiral organism is a newly identified species of *Helicobacter* in humans. J Infect Dis. 1993;168:379–85.

79. Lim RKS. A parasite spiral organism in the stomach of the cat. Parasitology. 1920;12:108.
80. Otto G, Hazell SH, Fox JG *et al*. Gastric colonization of cats by *Helicobacter*-like organisms: animal and public health implications. J Clin Microbiol. (in press).
81. Coltro N, Lee A, Ferrero R, Phillips M. '*Helicobacter muridae*' — a peripatetic gut coloniser. Challenge for the microbial ecologist. Microb Ecol Health Dis. 1991;4:S150 (abstract).
82. Queiroz DMM, Contigli C, Coimbra RS *et al*. Spiral bacterium associated with gastric, ileal and cecal mucosa of mice. Lab Anim Sci. 1992;26:288–94.
83. Lee A, O'Rourke J, Dixon M, Fox JG. *Helicobacter* induced gastritis: look to the host. Acta Gastroenterol. Belg. Suppl. 1993;56:61 (Abstract).
84. Eaton KA, Radin MJ, Kramer L *et al*. Epizootic gastritis in cheetahs associated with gastric spiral bacilli. Vet Pathol. 1992;30:55–63.
85. Eaton KA, Dewhirst FE, Radin MJ, Fox JG, Paster BJ, Krakowka S, Morgan DR. *Helicobacter acinonyx* sp. nov., a new species of *Helicobacter* isolated from cheetahs with gastritis. Int J Syst Bacteriol. 1993;43:99–106.
86. Eaton KA, Radin MJ, Krakowka S. Animal models of bacterial gastritis: the role of host, bacterial species and duration of infection on severity of gastritis. Zbl Bakteriol. 1993; 28–37.

2
H. pylori species heterogeneity

F. MÉGRAUD

INTRODUCTION

The genus *Helicobacter* has been recently defined on the basis of the composition of its 16S ribosomal RNA as studied by sequencing and hybridization[1-5]. This genus constitutes, with the genera *Campylobacter*, *Arcobacter* and *Wolinella*, the superfamily VI of Gram-negative bacteria as defined by Vandamme *et al.*[6].

This group of bacteria has unique features with regard to its morphology: spiral shape, flagellation; physiology: microaerophily, asaccharolytic metabolism; and ecology: aptitude for living in mucus. The genus *Helicobacter* is composed of at least nine species (Table 1) which share common properties, especially those related to life in the stomach, an ecological niche previously thought to be very hostile. These bacteria possess a strong urease and sheathed flagella, with a few exceptions.

A species is defined on the basis of its DNA homology. When two strains share more than 70% homology, studied by DNA–DNA hybridization they are included in the same species[7]. There are homogeneous species, i.e. in which all the strains within the species exhibit the same characteristics both phenotypically and genotypically as, for example, the well-known pathogens

Table 1 Species of the genus *Helicobacter*

Species	Ecological niche	Site	Genetic homology with H. pylori (%)
H. pylori	Human	Stomach	
H. cinaedi	Hamster, human	Intestine	ND
H. fennelliae	Human	Intestine	ND
H. mustelae	Ferret	Stomach	93.7
H. felis	Dog, cat	Stomach	94.5
H. muridarum	Mouse	Intestine	94
H. nemestrinae	Macacca monkey	Stomach	ND
H. acinonyx	Cheetah	Stomach	97.5
'H. heilmanni'	Dog, cat, human	Stomach	96

ND: Not done

Salmonella typhi and *Vibrio cholerae*. There are also heterogeneous species which show a wider range of properties and are mostly found in the group of environmental bacteria.

Helicobacter pylori has the peculiarity of being a homogeneous species when it is considered phenotypically while its genomic diversity is probably one of the widest ever found. This mystery remains unanswered. In this chapter we shall consider the common features and the variable characteristics of *H. pylori*.

LOW DIVERSITY FEATURES OF *H. PYLORI*

These concern most of the phenotypic characteristics: morphology, biochemical tests, antibiotic susceptibility patterns, pathogenic properties and some features linked to the DNA: genome size and GC percentage.

Morphology

The morphology of *H. pylori* observed both by optical microscopy and electron microscopy is homogeneous[8]. It is an S-shaped bacterium $3\,\mu m$ long, $0.5-1.0\,\mu m$ wide. The external wall is smooth. Multiple flagella (up to five) are present at one pole. These flagella are sheathed with a terminal bulb.

Heterogeneity can be observed within each strain according to the growth conditions. This is particularly true when the growth requirements are no longer fulfilled. The organisms rapidly evolve towards coccoidal forms considered to be degenerated non-culturable organisms[9].

The heterogeneity in terms of size observed *in vivo* when bacterial cells are isolated from the duodenal bulb compared to the antrum or fundus is probably due to the environmental conditions. Smaller colonies are observed with bacteria grown from monkeys. This characteristic has not been studied in detail, but could correspond to a closely related but different *Helicobacter* species.

Biochemical and cultural characteristics

H. pylori strains are homogeneous with regard to their cultural requirements: media, atmosphere and temperature.

In contrast to *Campylobacter* species. *H. pylori* has not yet been cultured on a minimal medium to determine exact growth requirements.

Some strains have been reported to be able to adapt themselves to growth in air after subculture[10]. It is also known that some stains can grow at 42°C while others cannot[11].

The identification of *H. pylori* species is based on the presence of several enzymes which are always present: urease, oxidase, catalase, alkaline phosphatase, γ-glutamyl transferase, DNase and various esterases (C4–C12)[11].

During subculture, urease-negative mutants of urease-positive parent strains can occur[11,12]. This is a rare event. It is most likely the consequence of a problem in regulation of the urease-encoding genes rather than a deletion of one of the genes controlling this characteristic.

Catalase-negative strains have also been described[12,13]. Their occurrence was related to particular culture conditions not documented since then.

When a wide range of arylamidases was tested, an important heterogeneity was noted. However, the enzymatic activity was low and the reproducibility unsatisfactory. Therefore, it is most likely that the enzymatic expression varies according to environmental conditions which may question the validity of biotyping schemas[14,15].

Antimicrobial agent susceptibility pattern

This pattern has been found to be quite similar between isolates.

H. pylori strains are susceptible to all compounds except glycopeptides, sulphamides, 2,4-diaminopyridines, first-generation quinolones, and cefsulodin.

However, acquired resistance has been documented (see Chapter 54) for nitroimidazoles, fluoroquinolones, macrolides and rifamycins. The genetic support has not been defined, but is most likely a chromosomal mutation since the acquired resistance is very stable.

Genome size and GC content

H. pylori genome size has recently been determined for 30 isolates by pulsed-field gel electrophoresis after digestion with *NotI* and *NruI*. The range of genome sizes was 1.60–1.72 Mb (average 1.67 Mb)[16]. These sizes are relatively homogeneous and small compared with most of the other pathogenic bacteria.

The same homogeneity was observed when the GC percentages of 32 *H. pylori* strains were determined by using the melting point of DNA. The values ranged from 34.1 to 37.5 mol% (average 35.2 mol%)[17].

Pathogenic properties

Most research efforts are presently concentrated in this field in order to link particular properties with specific diseases, i.e. to determine pathovars. A clear separation between ulcerogenic strains and non-ulcerogenic strains, however, has not been achieved.

In 1988, Leunk *et al.* reported that the filtrates of approximately half of the *H. pylori* strains tested were able to induce vacuolization of epithelial cells[18]. Subsequently, this observation was reproduced by other authors[19–21], linked to the presence of ulcer in patients[20], and of specific proteins as detected by immunoblotting[22].

The cytotoxin is known to correspond to a protein of 87 kDa[23] for which the gene has been cloned (*vacA*)[24–27] and may be present in all strains. There is also a cytotoxin-associated protein (120–128 kDa) for which the gene has also been cloned (*cagA*)[28,29] and is present in about 80% of the strains. This gene does not mediate directly toxin activity but it can be hypothesized that it is needed for the expression of the toxin.

In terms of heterogeneity, *cagA* is the first gene among the 12 or more cloned genes known, not to be present in all *H. pylori* strains; however, it is found in most strains.

MODERATE DIVERSITY FEATURES OF *H. PYLORI*

Protein profile

The protein profile of *H. pylori* strains (whole-cell protein extracts) after sodium dodecyl sulphate–polyacrylamide gel electrophoresis (SDS-PAGE) is quite similar between strains, with five to seven major protein bands[11,30–32].

Costas *et al.*, using high-resolution (laser densitometer) SDS-PAGE and a numerical analysis (Pearson correlation coefficient and unweighted pair group method with average) of one-dimensional protein patterns showed that the profiles were, in fact, not identical, and they were able to fingerprint *H. pylori* strains[33]. Qualitative differences in pattern were evident mainly in two regions: the first ranged from 68 to 100 kDa and the second from 42 to 53 kDa. There were, in addition, qualitative and quantitative differences in the major bands. The patterns were highly reproducible and stable in the eight cases tested.

Perez-Perez *et al.* also showed the conservation of major protein antigens of *H. pylori*, some being conserved even within the group of spiral bacteria. More variability was found among the outer membrane protein profiles. This variability can be detected by another approach: immunoblotting with a serum from a hyperimmunized rabbit. Perez-Perez *et al.* found four different antigenic profiles among the seven strains tested[31]. The 150 isolates tested by Burnie *et al.* fell into nine groups. However, this immunoblot fingerprinting method was not very discriminative since two groups accounted for two-thirds of the 150 isolates[32].

LPS and surface antigens

LPS from *H. pylori* strains resemble those of smooth-type Enterobacteriaceae. Most *H. pylori* strains share core antigens with one another, but there is a great deal of heterogeneity[31,34]. These findings have been confirmed by Mills *et al.* using rabbit immune sera. After removal of cross-reactive antibodies they were able to distinguish six out of seven isolates[35].

A common way of giving insight to the heterogeneity of bacterial surface receptors is to study haemagglutination patterns of the strains. Such an approach has been used by Lelwala-Guruge *et al.* They could differentiate three classes of haemagglutination patterns and show that the class I receptor was sialic acid-specific[36].

By using antisera obtained from rabbits immunized with whole-cell antigens and a co-agglutination technique, Danielsson *et al.* demonstrated the existence of strain-specific and type-specific surface antigens. However, all the tested strains contained cross-reactive antigens[37].

Lior developed a typing schema based on the heat-labile antigens of *H. pylori* on the model of typing schema existing for the thermophilic Campylobacters. Five groups were defined[38]. Unfortunately, most of these strains fell into the same group, serotype 1, and consequently the heterogeneity does not seem sufficient to be used for the strain differentiation.

Plasmids

Plasmids have been observed in *H. pylori*. Tija *et al.* reported that 58% of the strains tested contained one or more plasmids ranging in size from 1.8 kb to 40 kb[39]. In another study, Penfold *et al.* found that 48% of the strains tested yielded plasmids ranging in size from 3.7 kb to > 148 kb[40], while Owen *et al.* detected plasmid DNA in 32%[41], Majewski and Goodwin in 48%[12] and Leclerc *et al.* 50%[42] of the strains tested. One of these plasmids (1.5 kb) was cloned and sequenced, and can be detected by PCR. The authors propose that using IS_5-related inverted repeat sequences, unique patterns can be obtained differentiating the isolates[43].

DNA–DNA hybridization

Using a probe obtained from a patient with duodenal ulcer, Yoshimura *et al.* could differentiate two hybridization groups among 19 target DNAs[44]. The two groups corresponded to strains isolated from duodenal ulcer patients and from asymptomatic gastritis cases. These interesting preliminary results have not been confirmed.

HIGH DIVERSITY FEATURES OF *H. PYLORI*

These features concern the *H. pylori* genome exclusively, and have been brought to light by the new methods of molecular fingerprinting.

Methods

These methods can be divided in two groups:

1. Those using restriction enzymes to cut the genome at specific sites: using enzymes with a large number of restriction sites: restriction fragment length polymorphism (RFLP) and its derivative where a universal (16S + 23S ribosomal RNA) or specific (urease gene) labelled probe is used to hybridize the transfer fragments onto nitrocellulose: ribotyping[45];

using enzymes with a low number of restriction sites: pulsed-field gel electrophoresis (PFGE)[46]. In fact, all these methods use gel electrophoresis but in the latter a specific type of electrophoresis is needed because high molecular weight fragments are generated.

2. Those using amplification of DNA fragments: PCR-based typing methods. Again two different approaches may be used: amplification of a specific fragment of *H. pylori*, e.g. urease gene or another gene followed by the treatment of amplification products with restriction enzymes and electrophoresis: amplified fragment length polymorphism (AFLP); or random amplification using primers determined at random. The primers must be short (10 nucleotides) with a rate of GC depending on the organism tested. The bands generated are subsequently separated by gel electrophoresis and the profiles compared. The name of this method is randomly amplified polymorphic DNA (RAPD)[47] or arbitrary primer PCR (AP-PCR)[48]. Another recent technique is the use of oligonucleotides matching repetitive extragenic palindromic (REP) elements as primers. These repetitive DNA sequences probably have regulatory functions in the chromosome. They are used in a PCR procedure, REP-PCR, and measure the distribution of these sequences in the genome[49].

Application to *H. pylori*

The first technique to be used was RFLP following the work of Langenberg *et al.*[50]. They found that the isolates from 16 patients all produced different DNA digest patterns. The patterns were stable after subculturing 10 times as well as *in vivo* during a period of 2 years. The endonuclease commonly used is *HindIII*, but *HaeIII* also gives satisfactory results. The association of two enzymes, *HindIII* and *Bst EII*, has also been proposed[42]. However, the complexity of the patterns allowed the detection of minor differences which were not artifact, but probably originated from the coexistence in the stomach of strains with slightly different chromosomal DNA, plasmids or both. The presence of such populations could be caused by mutations *in vivo*. Oudbier *et al.* found them in one-third of the patients[51]. In fact, the interpretation of the DNA digest patterns is rather difficult because of the large number of bands present. The difficulty has been overcome by using ribotyping. Only a limited number of bands are present, and the technique is reproducible. Tee *et al.* applied this technique to isolates from 100 patients and found 77 distinct ribotypes using a cloned *E. coli* DNA complementary to a 5S, 16S and 23S ribosomal RNA digoxigenine-labelled probe[52]. Prewett *et al.*, with a biotinylated probe prepared from 16S and 23S ribosomal RNA from *H. pylori*, also differentiated the strains isolated from 15 patients[53] and Owen virtually all of the 122 strains from different origins[54].

AFLP has been used with primers amplifying the urease structural subunit genes *ureA* and *ureB*. The 2.4 kb PCR products amplified from 22 clinical isolates produced 10 distinct patterns on agarose gels after *Hae III* endonuclease digestion[55]. A similar approach was used by Tonokatsu *et al.*[56]. The 1.1 kb PCR amplified portion of the *ureC* gene from 21 isolates subsequently treated separately with *Hind III*, *Alu I* and *Pvu I* were placed in 15 groups[57]. Evans *et al.* have used the gene *hpaA* for an adhesin instead of urease[58]. Owen and Hurtado claim that they are able to differentiate mixed strains of different genotypes from the same biopsy using this method[59]. The optimal approach with this technique may be a multiple PCR (simultaneous PCR amplification of two gene fragments) followed by a double restriction analysis (simultaneous use of two restricted enzymes). This method was proposed by Clayton *et al.* They amplified a large fragment (933 bp) within the urease B gene and a large fragment (1145 bp) within the 48 kDa stress protein gene (*htr A*). The enzymes subsequently used were *Sau3A* and *HaeIII* or *HaeIII* and *AluI*[60]. The recently isolated gene *cagA* also displays heterogeneity when studied by AFLP.

Akopyanz *et al.* were the first to apply RAPD to *H. pylori* fingerprinting. Primers of 10 nucleotides and GC percentage of 50 to 60 distinguished all 64 strains from different locations. About 15 bands were present. They found the method reproducible and more discriminant than AFLP of the urease gene using a single restriction enzyme[61]. Using this primer we have also obtained reproducible band patterns allowing a high level of discrimination between strains.

The new approach of REP-PCR was applied by Go *et al.* to 80 strains isolated from patients with various diseases in the USA. They obtained complex, stable and reproducible band patterns which revealed 78 different profiles when studied by computer-assisted phylogenetic analysis[62].

The obvious advantage of AFLP and RAPD is that these techniques do not need laborious preparation and purification of genomic DNA which are required for the standard RFLP analysis and ribotyping and, therefore, are much less time-consuming and expensive. Furthermore, they give much simpler profiles than RFLP, allowing easy visual analysis.

These techniques correlate with the gene sequencing. A comparison of urease structural gene sequences obtained from two different isolates showed 97% DNA homology[60,63]. Single base changes were mainly found, and were the cause for restriction site differences. The urease activity does not seem to be affected by these substitutions.

Study of the genomic DNA by PFGE is not as rapid as PCR-based methods, but shows the same diversity. Taylor *et al.* differentiated almost all of the 30 *H. pylori* strains studied after digestion with *NotI* or *NruI*, and the patterns were stable and reproducible[16].

Another tool which allows the study of the genetic diversity without examining the DNA is the multilocus enzyme electrophoresis (MEE). Go *et al.* applied the technique and confirmed the species heterogeneity by studying the enzymes coded by 12 genes. Each isolate showed a unique multilocus enzyme genotype[64].

Causes of the genomic diversity

The *H. pylori* genome displays a considerable amount of genomic diversity and this is found consistently regardless of the technique used. This heterogeneity seems unique in the microbial world, since each strain can virtually be differentiated from the others.

The reason for this phenomenon is not known. *H. pylori* strains may undergo genomic rearrangements in response to stress after infecting a new host[16].

Five hypotheses have been proposed by D. Taylor *et al.* to account for the *H. pylori* species heterogeneity[16]; they are as follows:

1. Variability may be explained by movement of short repetitive DNA sequences as has been noted in a number of different species. There is no evidence for this possibility. When PCR is used with different primers for amplification in the urease region, amplified products exhibit the same size despite the diversity (A. Labigne, personal communication).
2. Another mechanism, which has been observed in *Streptomyces* spp., may involve the amplification of particular chromosomal DNA sequences, possibly accompanied by the deletion of adjacent DNA.
3. *H. pylori* DNA may undergo changes in nucleotide sequence which are not associated with phenotypic changes. Sequencing has shown that mutations occur at random, concern mainly the third nucleotide and, therefore, do not have a consequence on the coded amino acid in 70% of the cases.
4. Genomic rearrangements may be associated with uptake of DNA by natural transformation if a coinfection occurs. However, *C. jejuni* and *C. coli* also undergo natural transformation but show considerably less genomic diversity than *H. pylori*. Natural competence for transformation was first described in 1990 in 22 out of 25 clinical isolates for streptomycin resistance[65]. It was also documented by Taylor for rifampicin and metronidazole resistance except when the resistance determinant was on the plasmid. In these cases only *H. pylori* recipients which contained a homologous resident plasmid could be transformed[66].
5. DNA in some strains of *H. pylori* may be protected from restriction endonuclease digestion by the production of an endogenous methylase(s) which is able to methylate nucleotides within the recognition sequences of *NotI*, *NruI*, or other endonucleases.

Consequences of genomic diversity

This unusual genomic diversity has an important consequence for the epidemiology of *H. pylori* infection. Since it is possible to have a unique fingerprint for each strain, regardless of the method used, it should be possible to trace the route of infection and, after eradication attempts, to differentiate between recurrence and reinfection.

Heterogeneity of infection

H. pylori infection is supposed to last for decades. So it is conceivable that during this time period a given subject may become superinfected by other strains.

Table 2 Molecular fingerprinting of *Helicobacter pylori* strains isolated from patients before and after unsuccessful therapy or long-term follow-up

Authors/reference	Technique	No. of patients	No. of recrudescences	Treatment used
Langenberg et al.[50]	RFLP	4	4	2 Amoxicillin 2 CBS
Owen et al.[68]	Ribotyping	17	16	9 CBS-metronidazole 3 CBS 2 cimetidine 1 ranitidine
Clayton et al.[60]	AFLP	19	19	Erythromycin
Akopyanz et al.[61]	RAPD	3	3	BSS + clindomycin
Rautelin et al.[69]	Ribotyping	11	10	
Salama et al.[70]	PFGE	20	20	

RFLP: restriction fragment length polymorphism; AFLP: amplified fragment length polymorphism; RAPD: randomly amplified polymorphism DNA; PFGE: pulsed field gel electrophoresis.

Beji *et al.* were the first to describe a case where the strains isolated from the fundus and antrum were not identical[67].

This question has been addressed in two studies: one using ribotyping[52] and one using PFGE[16], and in both cases the strains isolated from antrum, body and duodenum or fundus were identical. Five patients and one patient were concerned, respectively. Prewett *et al.* increased the number of patients to 15, and by the ribotyping of antrum, body and duodenal strains, identical clones were documented in 13 of the 15 patients[53].

It is possible that such studies carried out in a country with a higher prevalence of the infection than the UK would lead to different results.

Labigne *et al.* studied nine cases with strains originating from the antrum, fundus and gastric juice. In the nine cases the three strains were identical (personal communication).

Recrudescence or reinfection

All the studies agree that after attempts to eradicate *H. pylori*, if there is a relapse, it is most likely to be recrudescence rather than reinfection (Table 2).

Relation between genovar and phenotypic characteristics

It has not yet been possible to relate a particular genovar to metronidazole resistance[12,68], or to toxin production[54].

Intrafamilial spread

Such a high diversity of genomic DNA allows one to trace the spread of the infection, for example, within families.

Shames *et al.*[71], and Majewski and Goodwin[12], reported the occurrence of different strains in a husband and his wife, supporting the hypothesis that most of the infections are acquired in childhood.

Tee *et al.* studied seven families (18 subjects) and showed identical strains in only two[52].

Intrafamilial spread has also been studied in Ireland. Seven out of eight parents of four *H. pylori*-positive children were themselves *H. pylori*-positive. In three of the four families the same strain was present in at least two family members[72].

CONCLUSION

The characteristics described in this chapter fit with the fact that *H. pylori* is not a clonal pathogen but a bacterium which is highly adapted to its ecological niche. It is therefore not surprising that a unique pathogenic pathway has not been found. However, it remains possible that some strains may have evolved in a certain direction which is more hazardous for their host. These last years have seen the beginning of the gene dissection of the *H. pylori* chromosome. Following years will see new approaches and the completion of the mapping work[73]. Maybe then *H. pylori* will have unveiled the secrets of its diversity.

Acknowledgements

We express our thanks to Agnès Labigne (Institut Pasteur, Paris, France) for stimulating discussions, and for reviewing the manuscript.

References

1. Romaniuk PJ, Zoltowska B, Trust TJ et al. Campylobacter pylori, the spiral bacterium associated with human gastritis, is not a true Campylobacter sp. J Bacteriol. 1987;169: 2137–41.
2. Lau PP, Debrunner-Vissbrink B, Dunn B et al. Phylogenetic diversity and position of the genus Campylobacter. Syst Appl Microbiol., 1987;9:231–8.
3. Paster BJ, Dewhirst FE. Phylogeny of Campylobacters, Wolinellas, Bacteroides gracilis, and Bacteroides ureolyticus by 16S ribosomal ribonucleic acid sequencing. Int J Syst Bacteriol. 1988;38:56–62.
4. Thompson LM III, Smibert RM, Johnson JL et al. Phylogenetic study of the genus Campylobacter. Int J Syst Bacteriol. 1988;38:190–200.
5. Goodwin CS, Armstrong JA, Chilvers T et al. Transfer of Campylobacter pylori and Campylobacter mustelae to Helicobacter gen. nov. as Helicobacter pylori comb. nov. and Helicobacter mustelae comb. nov. respectively. Int J Syst Bacteriol. 1989;39:397–405.
6. Vandamme P, Falsen E, Rossau R et al. Revision of Campylobacter, Helicobacter, and Wolinella taxonomy: emendation of generic descriptions and proposal of Arcobacter gen. nov. Int J Syst Bacteriol. 1991;41:88–103.
7. Wayne LG, Brenner DJ, Colwell RR et al. Report of the adhoc committee on reconciliation of approaches to bacterial systematics. Int J Syst Bacteriol. 1987;37:463–4.
8. Mégraud F. Morphological and biochemical characterization of Campylobacter pylori. In Menge H, Gregor M, Tytgat GNJ, Marshall BJ editors. Campylobacter pylori. Berlin: Springer; 1988:3–16.
9. Jones DM, Curry A. The genesis of coccal forms of Helicobacter pylori. In: Malfertheiner P, Ditschuneit H. editors. Helicobacter pylori, gastritis and peptic ulcer. Berlin: Springer; 1990:30–7.

10. Tompkins DS, Dave J, Mapstone NP. Some strains of *Helicobacter pylori* will grow on air. Acta Gastroenterol Belg. 1993;56(Suppl.):100.
11. Mégraud F, Bonnet F, Garnier M *et al.* Characterization of *Campylobacter pyloridis* by culture, enzymatic profile, and protein content. J Clin Microbiol. 1985;22:1007–10.
12. Majewski SI, Goodwin CS. Restriction endonuclease analysis of the genome of *Campylobacter pylori* with a rapid extraction method: evidence for considerable genomic variation. J Infect Dis. 1988;157:465–71.
13. Westblom TU, Phadnis S, Langenberg W *et al.* Catalase-negative mutants of *Helicobacter pylori*. Eur J Clin Microbiol Infect Dis. 1992;11:522–6.
14. Reina J, Alomar P. Biotypes of *Campylobacter pylori* isolated in gastroduodenal biopsies. Eur J Clin Microbiol Infect Dis. 1989;8:175–7.
15. Kung JS, Ho B, Chan SH. Biotyping of *Campylobacter pylori*. J Med Microbiol. 1989;29:203–6.
16. Taylor DE, Easton M, Chang N. Construction of a *Helicobacter pylori* genome map and demonstration of diversity at the genome level. J Bacteriol. 1992;21:6800–6.
17. Beji A, Mégraud F, Vincent P *et al.* GC content of DNA of *Campylobacter pylori* and other species belonging or related to the genus *Campylobacter*. Ann Inst Pasteur/Microbiol. 1988;139:527–34.
18. Leunk RD, Johnston PT, David BC *et al.* Cytotoxic activity in broth culture filtrates of *Campylobacter pylori*. J. Med Microbiol. 1988;26:93–9.
19. Cover TL, Dooley CP, Blaser MJ. Characterization of and human serologic response to proteins in *Helicobacter pylori* broth culture supernatants with vacuolating cytotoxin activity. Infect Immun. 1990;58:603–10.
20. Figura N, Guglielmetti P, Rossolini A *et al.* Cytotoxin production by *Campylobacter pylori* strains isolated from patients with peptic ulcers and from patients with chronic gastritis only. J. Clin Microbiol. 1989;27:225–6.
21. Goossens H, Glupczynski Y, Burette A *et al.* Role of the vacuolating toxin from *Helicobacter pylori* in the pathogenesis of duodenal and gastric ulcer. Med Microbiol Lett. 1992;1:153–9.
22. Crabtree JE, Taylor JD, Wyatt JI *et al.* Mucosal IgA recognition of *Helicobacter pylori* 120 kDa protein ulceration, and gastric pathology. Lancet. 1991;338:332–5.
23. Cover TL, Blaser MJ. Purification and characterization of the vacuolating toxin from *Helicobacter pylori*. J Biol Chem. 1992;267:10570–5.
24. Burroni D, Dell'orco M, Commanducci M *et al.* The *Helicobacter pylori* cytotoxin: gene structure and expression. Acta Gastroenterol Belg. 1993;56(Suppl.):62.
25. Cover TL, Tummuru MKR, Blaser MJ. Conservation of genetic sequences for the vacuolating toxin among all *Helicobacter pylori* strains. Acta Gastroenterol Belg. 1993;56(Suppl.):47.
26. Phadnis SH, Ilver D. Nucleotide sequence of the vacuolating cytotoxin gene of *Helicobacter pylori*. Acta Gastroenterol Belg. 1993;56(Suppl.):105.
27. Schmitt W, Haas R. Cloning and genetic characterization of the *Helicobacter pylori* vacuolating cytotoxin gene. Acta Gastroenterol Belg. 1993;(Suppl.):105.
28. Tummuru MKR, Cover TL, Blaser MJ. Cloning and expression of a high-molecular-mass major antigen of *Helicobacter pylori*: evidence of linkage to cytotoxin production. Infect Immun. 1993;61:1799–809.
29. Covacci A, Censini S, Bugnoli M *et al.* Molecular characterization of the 129-kDa immunodominant antigen of *Helicobacter pylori* associated with cytotoxicity and duodenal ulcer. Proc Natl Acad Sci USA. 1993;90:5791–5.
30. Pearson AD, Bamforth J, Booth L *et al.* Polyacrylamide gel electrophoresis of spiral bacteria from the gastric antrum. Lancet. 1988;1:1349–50.
31. Perez-Perez GI, Blaser MJ. Conservation and diversity of *Campylobacter pyloridis* major antigens. Infect Immun. 1987;55:1256–63.
32. Burnie JP, Lee W, Dent JC *et al.* Immunoblot fingerprint of *Campylobacter pylori*. J Med Microbiol. 1988;27:153–9.
33. Costas M, Morgan DD, Owen RJ *et al.* Differentiation of strains of *Helicobacter pylori* by numerical analysis of 1-D SDS-PAGE protein patterns: evidence for post-treatment recrudescence. Epidemiol Infect. 1991;107:607–17.
34. Moran AP, Helander IM, Kosunen TU. Compositional analysis of *Helicobacter pylori*

roughform lipopolysaccharides. J Bacteriol. 1992;174:1370–7.

35. Mills SD, Kurjanczyk LA, Penner JL. Antigenicity of *Helicobacter pylori* lipopolysaccharides. J Clin Microbiol. 1992;30:3175–80.

36. Lelwala-Guruge J, Ljungh A, Wadström T. Hemagglutination patterns of *Helicobacter pylori*. APMIS 1992;100:908–13.

37. Danielsson D, Blomberg B, Järnerot G et al. Heterogeneity of *Campylobacter pylori* as demonstrated by co-agglutination testing with rabbit antibodies. Scand J Gastroenterol. 1998;23(Suppl. 142):58–63.

38. Lior H. Serological identification of *Helicobacter pylori*. A provisional serotyping schema. It J Gastroenterol. 1991;23(Suppl. 2):42.

39. Tija TN, Harper WES, Goodwin CS et al. Plasmids in *Campylobacter pyloridis*. Microbiol Lett. 1987;36:7–11.

40. Penfold SS, Lastovica AJ, Elisha BJ. Demonstration of plasmids in *Campylobacter pyloridis*. J Infect Dis. 1988;157:850.

41. Owen RJ, Bell GD, Desai M et al. Biotype and molecular fingerprints of metronidazole-resistant strains of *Helicobacter pylori* from antral gastric mucosa. J Med Microbiol. 1993;38:6–12.

42. Leclerc H, Beji A, Vincent P. Marqueurs moléculaires et identification des souches de *Campylobacter pylori*. Gastroentrol Clin Biol. 1989;13:44–8B.

43. Kleanthous H, Clayton CL, Tabaqchali S. Characterisation of a plasmid from *Helicobacter pylori* encoding a replication protein common to plasmids in gram-positive bacteria. Mol Microbiol. 1991;5:2377–89.

44. Yoshimura HH, Evans DG, Graham DY. DNA–DNA hybridization demonstrates apparent genetic differences between *Helicobacter pylori* from patients with duodenal ulcer and asymptomatic gastritis. Dig Dis Sci. 1993;38:1128–31.

45. Grimont F, Grimont PAD. Ribosomal ribonucleic acid gene restriction patterns as potential taxonomic tools. Ann Inst Pasteur Microbiol. 1986;137:165–7.

46. Schwartz DC, Canto CR. Separation of yeast chromosome-sized DNAs by pulsed-field gradient gel electrophoresis. Cell. 1984;37:67–75.

47. Williams JGK, Kubelik AR, Livak KJ et al. DNA polymorphisms amplified by arbitrary primers are useful as genetic markers. Nucl Acids Res. 1990;18:6531–5.

48. Welsh J, McClelland M. Fingerprinting genomes using PCR with arbitrary primers. Nucl Acids Res. 1990;18:7213–24.

49. Versalovic J, Koeuth T, Lupski JR. Distribution of repetitive DNA sequences in eubacteria and application to fingerprinting of bacterial genomes. Nucl Acids Res. 1991;19:6823–31.

50. Langenberg W, Rauws E, Widjojokusumo A et al. Identification of *Campylobacter pyloridis* isolates by restriction endonuclease DNA analysis. J Clin Microbiol. 1986;24:414–17.

51. Oudbier JH, Langenberg W, Rauws EJ et al. Genotypical variation of *Campylobacter pylori* from gastric mucosa. J. Clin Microbiol. 1990;28:559–65.

52. Tee W, Lambert JR, Smallwood R et al. Ribotyping of *Helicobacter pylori* from clinical specimens. J Clin Microbiol. 1992;30:1562–7.

53. Prewett EJ, Bickley J, Owen RJ et al. DNA patterns of *Helicobacter pylori* isolated from gastric antrum, body and duodenum. Gastroenterology. 1992;102:829–33.

54. Owen RJ, Hunton C, Bickley J et al. Ribosomal RNA gene restriction patterns of *Helicobacter pylori*: analysis and appraisal of *Hae III* digests as a molecular typing system. Epidemiol Infect. 1992;109:35–47.

55. Foxall PA, Hu LT, Mobley HLT. Use of polymerase chain reaction-amplified *Helicobacter pylori* urease structural genes for differentiation of isolates. J Clin Microbiol. 1992;30:739–41.

56. Tonokatsu Y, Hayashi T, Fukuda Y et al. Heterogeneity of restriction fragment length polymorphism in the urease gene. Eur J Gastroenterol Hepatol. 1993;5:S57–62.

57. Moore RA, Kureishi A, Wong S et al. Categorization of clinical isolates of *Helicobacter pylori* on the basis of restriction digest analyses of polymerase chain reaction-amplified *ureC* genes. J Clin Microbiol. 1993;31:1334–5.

58. Evans DG, Asnicar MA, Lee CH. Restriction fragment length polymorphism of *hpaA*, an adhesin gene of *Helicobacter pylori*. Acta Gastroenterol Belg. 1993;56(Suppl.):110.

59. Owen RJ, Hurtado A. A PCR-based molecular assay to test biopsy cultures of *Helicobacter pylori* for mixed strains of differing genotypes. Acta Gastroenterol Belg. 1993;56(Suppl.):50.

60. Clayton CL, Kleanthous H, Morgan DD *et al*. Rapid fingerprinting of *Helicobacter pylori* by polymerase chain reaction and restriction fragment length polymorphism analysis. J Clin Microbiol. 1993;31:1420–5.
61. Akopyanz W, Bukanov NO, Westblom TU *et al*. DNA diversity among clinical isolates of *Helicobacter pylori* detected by PCR RAPD fingerprinting. Nucl Acids Res. 1992;20: 5137–42.
62. Go MF, Chan KY, Versalovic J *et al*. DNA fingerprinting of *Helicobacter pylori* genomes with repetitive DNA sequence-based PCR (RFP-PCR). Gastroenterology. 1993;104:707.
63. Labigne A, Cussac V, Courcoux P. Development of genetic and molecular approches for the diagnosis and study of the pathogenesis of *Helicobacter pylori*. In: Malfertheiner P, Ditschuneit H, editors. *Helicobacter pylori*, gastritis and peptic ulcer. Berlin: Springer;1990:19–22.
64. Go MF, Graham DY, Musser JM. Multilocus enzyme electrophoresis: approach to identify *Helicobacter pylori*-disease specific relationships. Gastroenterology. 1992;102:A268.
65. Nedenskov-Sorensen P, Bukholm G, Bovre K. Natural competence for genetic transformation in *Campylobacter pylori*. J. Infect Dis. 1990;161:365–6.
66. Taylor DE, Roos, KP, Wang Y. Transformation of *Helicobacter pylori* by chromosomal metronidazole resistance and by a plasmid with a chloramphenicol resistance marker. Acta Gastroenterol Belg. 1993;56(Suppl.):106.
67. Beji A, Vincent P, Darchis J *et al*. Evidence of gastritis with several *H. pylori* strains. Lancet. 1989;2:1402–3.
68. Owen RJ, Bell GD, Desai M *et al*. Biotype and molecular fingerprint of metronidazole-resistant strains of *Helicobacter pylori* from antral gastric mucosa. J Med Microbiol. 1993;38:6–12.
69. Rautelin H, Tee W, Seppälä K. Kosunen TU. Ribopatterns and metronidazole resistance in paired samples of *Helicobacter pylori*. Acta Gastroenterol Belg. 1993;56(Suppl.):127.
70. Salama SM, Taylor DE, Jiang Q *et al*. Diversity of genomic DNA and protein profiles of *Helicobacter pylori* strains *in vivo* and *in vitro*. Acta Gastroenterol Belg. 1993;56(Suppl.):50.
71. Shames B, Krajden S, Babida C *et al*. Investigation of *Campylobacter pylori* strains isolated from a husband and his wife. In: Mégraud F, Lamouliatte H, editors. Gastroduodenal pathology and *Campylobacter pylori*. ICS 847, Amsterdam: Elsevier; 1989:439–42.
72. Bamford KB, Collins JSA, Bickley J *et al*. *Helicobacter pylori*: comparison of DNA fingerprints provides evidence for intrafamilial infection. Ir J Med Sci. 1992;161(Suppl. 10):18.
73. Bukanov NO, Berg DE. Ordered cosmid library and fine structure map of chromosome of *Helicobacter pylori*. Acta Gastroenterol Belg. 1993;56(Suppl.):57.

3
H. pylori urease

H. L. T. MOBLEY and P. A. FOXALL

INTRODUCTION

Urease is a relatively common enzyme that is produced by over 100 bacterial species. In the past, the activity of this enzyme has been used in taxonomic identification systems for the speciation of bacteria in the clinical laboratory. Over the past decade, however, the role for this enzyme in pathogenesis of many bacterial infections has been recognized (for review see ref. 1).

Urease (urea amidohydrolase, EC 3.5.1.5) catalyses the hydrolysis of urea to yield ammonia and carbamate; the latter spontaneously hydrolyses to yield another molecule of ammonia and carbonic acid.

$$H_2N-\overset{\overset{\displaystyle O}{\|}}{C}-NH_2 + H_2O-\text{Urease} \rightarrow NH_3 + H_2N-\overset{\overset{\displaystyle O}{\|}}{C}-OH$$

$$H_2N-\overset{\overset{\displaystyle O}{\|}}{C}-OH + H_2O \rightarrow NH_3 + H_2CO_3$$

Subsequently, ammonia equilibrates with water, forming ammonium hydroxide which results in a rapid increase in pH.

$$H_2CO_3 \rightarrow H^+ + HCO_3^-$$

$$2NH_3 + 2H_2O \rightarrow 2NH_4^+ + 2OH^-$$

This reaction is of some importance because of the abundance of urea in nature; it is a principal nitrogenous waste product of mammals and is not further degraded by enzymes produced by members of this class. The principal roles of bacterial urease in nature involve: (a) the enzyme's capacity to serve as a virulence factor in human infections of the urinary and gastrointestinal tracts; (b) recycling of nitrogenous wastes in the rumen of domestic livestock by anaerobic bacteria; and (c) hydrolysis by soil bacteria of urea provided in fertilizer, making utilizable nitrogen available for agricultural applications.

Interestingly, both urea and urease represented landmark molecules in early scientific investigation. Urea was the first organic molecule synthesized, and urease was the first enzyme crystallized[2], in addition to being the first enzyme shown to contain nickel[3].

BIOCHEMISTRY

Purification

One of the most significant features of *Helicobacter pylori* is the extraordinary amount of urease produced by this organism. With the possible exception of *Ureaplasma urealyticum*, *H. pylori* produces more urease than any other bacterial species that has been examined thus far. The purified enzyme is not significantly more active than purified enzymes from other species, but simply represents a larger proportion of total cell protein in this species. When crude lysates are electrophoresed on SDS-polyacrylamide gels and stained with Coomassie Blue, the two urease subunits of apparent molecular size 66 and 29.5 kDa appear as extremely prominent bands[4] (Fig. 1, lane A). When other urease-positive bacterial species are examined in this manner, urease subunits are not produced in sufficient quantities to detect the bands on such gels.

The native protein has been purified from *H. pylori* by isolation from the cytosol[4] or by elution from the cell surface with low ionic strength solvents[5-7]. For purification from the cytosol, French press cell lysates were chromatographed on DEAE-Sepharose, phenyl-Sepharose, Mono-Q, and Sepharose 6 resins (Fig. 1). In this purification scheme, purified urease represented 6% of the soluble protein of crude extract and was estimated to have a native molecular size of 550 kDa. On the basis of subunit size, a 1:1 subunit ratio as measured by scanning densitometry of Coomassie Blue stained SDS-polyacrylamide gels, and estimated native molecular weight, the data are consistent with the stoichiometry of $(29.5\,kDa–66\,kDa)_6$ for the structure of the native enzyme. The enzyme has an isoelectric point between 5.90 and 5.99[5-7].

Nickel metalloenzyme

Like all other ureases studied to date, nickel ions are present in the protein structure, probably as a component of the active site of the enzyme. The nickel content of *H. pylori* urease has been measured using atomic adsorption spectroscopy[8]. Nickel was detected only in the larger subunit (UreB) polypeptide and in the ratio of five to six atoms to one enzyme molecule.

Active site

The primary amino acid sequences of all ureases are fairly well conserved, but the region from amino acid residue 310–329 in the large subunit (UreB) is nearly invariant among *H. pylori*, *P. mirabilis*, *P. vulgaris*, *U. urealyticum*,

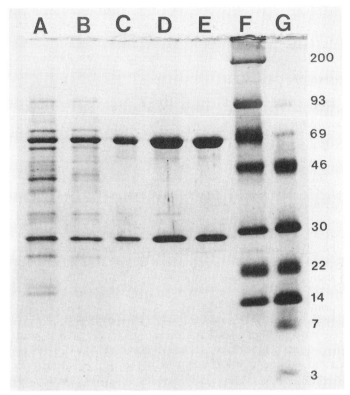

Fig. 1 Purified urease electrophoresed on an SDS-polyacrylamide gel. Protein (10 μg) from each purification step was electrophoresed on a 10–20% polyacrylamide gradient gel and stained with Coomassie Blue. Lane **A**, cell extract; **B**, DEAE-Sepharose; **C**, phenyl-Sepharose; **D**, Mono-Q; **E**, Superose 6; **F**, **G**, protein standards with molecular masses given in kilodaltons. Reprinted with permission from Hu and Mobley, 1990[4]

Klebsiella aerogenes, and jack bean[9] (Fig. 2). Site-directed mutagenesis studies in *P. mirabilis*[9] and *K. aerogenes*[10] have identified certain residues that, on the basis of the very high degree of homology, must play a critical role in catalysis by *H. pylori* urease. Three histidine residues (corresponding to His-314, His-322, and His-323 of *H. pylori* UreB) and one cysteine residue (Cys-321) were found critical for urea hydrolysis. Each histidine mutation reduced the amount of radiolabelled Ni^{2+} ions incorporated into the recombinant enzyme, suggesting that these residues coordinate the metal ion in the enzyme active site.

Kinetics

Enzyme activity of purified *H. pylori* urease has been quantitated at urea concentrations from 0 to 5 mmol/l at 23°C. Reciprocal plots of $1/V$ versus $1/S$ have revealed K_m values from 0.17 to 0.48 mmol/l urea[4–6]. Under

P. mirabilis	308	TVDEHLDMLMVCHHLDPSIP	327
Jack bean	581	:I:::::::::::::RE::	600
P. vulgaris	308	::::::::::::::::::::	327
H. pylori	310	:EA::M::::::::::K::K	329
U. urealyticum	314	:IA:::::::::::N:KV:	333
K. aerogenes	310	:I:::::::::::::D:A	329

Fig. 2 Conserved amino acid sequences within the large subunit of ureases that putatively reside within the active site. For bacterial ureases, numbers refer to the residue number within the large subunit UreB of *H. pylori*; UreC for other species. For jack bean urease, numbers refer to the residue number within the unique subunit. Amino acids identical to the *P. mirabilis* sequence are indicated (:) Reprinted with permission from Sriwanthana and Mobley, 1993[9]

saturating conditions, freshly purified enzyme had specific activities ranging from 1100 to 1700 μmol of urea hydrolysed per min per mg of protein[4,5].

The kinetic properties of the *H. pylori* urease are distinct from those of the ureases of other species. With a K_m of 0.17 mmol/l, this enzyme recognizes substrate with much higher affinity than the enzymes produced by *Proteus* or *Providencia* species. This observation is physiologically consistent with the respective niches of these organisms. *H. pylori*, after making its way to the gastric mucosa, must scavenge urea from serum, and at physiological blood urea concentrations of 10 to 20 mg/dl (1.7–3.4 mmol/l), urease is saturated and working at maximum rate. In the urinary tract urea is plentiful (about 400 mmol/l), so enzymes with lower affinity for urea are nevertheless saturated and working at maximum velocity. Therefore, high affinity for urea may be a selective advantage in the gastric mucosa, but unnecessary in the urinary tract. In addition to higher affinity, *H. pylori* isolates hydrolyse urea at more than twice the rate of the very active species *P. mirabilis*, and about 10 times the rate of other common urinary tract isolates. When substrate concentration is low, this high rate of hydrolysis may be necessary to achieve sufficient ammonia concentration to protect the bacteria from the nearby acid environment.

Localization within the bacteria

Individuals infected with *H. pylori* mount a strong serum IgG response against a number of antigens including urease. This response can easily be tested using Western blot of crude whole-cell lysate, developed with serum antibody from infected patients. The strong response against urease suggests that the urease of *H. pylori* is easily accessible to the immune system for processing. Ureases of other bacteria, principally uropathogenic species such as *P. mirabilis*[11], *Providencia stuartii*[12], and *Morganella morganii*[13], have been shown unambiguously to reside in the cytosolic fractions of the cells. DNA sequence analysis of urease genes predicts no signal sequences for the export of a multimeric enzyme by these species or *H. pylori*. We have

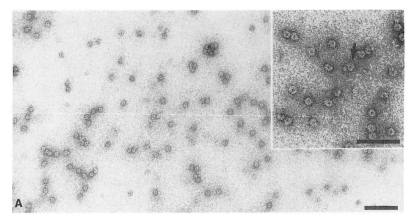

Fig. 3 Transmission electron micrograph of purified *H. pylori* urease. Purified *H. pylori* urease was fixed and negatively stained with 2% uranyl acetate. The bar represents 100 μm and 50 μm in the inset. Reprinted with permission from Austin *et al.*, 1992[16]

demonstrated that at least half of the activity is found in cytosol, yet other investigators are able to elute the urease from the surface of whole-cell suspensions at low ionic strength. Moreover, monoclonal antibodies specific for urease bind to the cell surface[14]. These data suggest that urease is exported to the surface of the cell by some mechanism. The cell surface urease and the cytosolic urease are identical, and are encoded by the single chromosomal urease gene cluster.

Appearance by EM

Purified native urease has been examined by transmission electron microscopy[7,15,16] and appears as a round, doughnut-shaped, hexagonal particle with a darkly staining core (Fig. 3). Proteins are 13 nm in diameter and display threefold rotational symmetry.

Urease, eluted from the bacterial cell surface, copurifies with a 60 kDa chaperonin heat-shock protein. When assembled, the heat-shock protein displays a very high native molecular weight similar to urease[16-18] and assembles into a macromolecular structure that is also similar in appearance to urease. This heat-shock protein was earlier thought to be a subunit of urease[19].

GENETICS

Genetic organization

The genes encoding the urease of *H. pylori* have been cloned[20-24] and sequenced[22,23,25] and reveal a genetic organization that is similar to urease gene clusters of other species (Fig. 4). Nine genes have been identified in the urease gene cluster. These include *ureC*, *D*, *A*, *B*, *I*, *F*, *G*, and *H*. UreA and

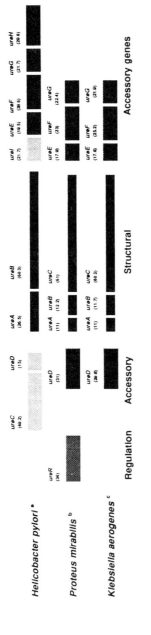

Fig. 4 Genetic organization of the *H. pylori* urease gene cluster. The positions of genes associated with urease activity for three bacterial species are shown. Structural genes encoding the enzyme are shown as black rectangles. Accessory genes that encode proteins that contribute to synthesis of an active enzyme or are associated with the gene cluster are shown as stippled rectangles. The number under each gene represents the molecular size (kDa) for each subunit. In the *H. pylori* urease operon, four genes (*ureE, ureF, ureG* and *UreH*) downstream of the two structural genes (*ureA* and *ureB*) are required for enzyme activity in *E. coli*. One additional open reading frame (*ureI*) is required for urease activity in wild-type *H. pylori*, but not in *E. coli*. *K. aerogenes* and *P. mirabilis* have three structural genes and four accessory genes (*ureD, ureE, ureF,* and *ureG*) that are also required for enzyme activity in *E. coli*. One gene (*ureR*), 1 kb upstream of *P. mirabilis* urease operon, regulates the gene expression of urease. References are shown in the figure. Reprinted with permission from Hu, L-T. (dissertation). Baltimore (MD): University of Maryland at Baltimore, 1993

UreB represent the structural subunits of the enzyme. *ureI, E, F, G,* and *H* have been termed accessory genes. Structural genes, *ureA* and *ureB,* and accessory genes *ureF, ureG,* and *ureH* have been shown to be essential for activity. By analogy to studies of homologous genes in *K. aerogenes* and *P. mirabilis*[9,10], some of the accessory genes play a role in activation of the apoenzyme. Ni^{2+} ions are necessary for activity, and it is believed that accessory proteins function to insert Ni^{2+} ions into the active site of the newly synthesized enzyme during assembly.

Conservation of genes

The first published nucleotide sequence of any urease gene, which appeared in 1989, was that of *Proteus mirabilis*[26]. The sequence predicted that the structural subunits of the enzyme were encoded by three contiguous genes, *ureA, ureB,* and *ureC* (Fig. 4). When the deduced amino acid sequences of the *P. mirabilis* urease subunits were compared with the amino acid sequence of the jack bean urease subunit[27], significant amino acid similarity was observed (58% exact matches; 73% exact plus conservative replacements). The 11.0 kDa polypeptide aligned with the N-terminal residues of the plant enzyme, the 12.2 kDa polypeptide lined up with internal residues, and 61 kDa polypeptide matched with the C-terminal residues, suggesting an evolutionary relationship of the urease genes of jack bean and *P. mirabilis.*

When the *H. pylori* urease sequence first appeared[25], as well as those of subsequent species, it became clear that all ureases are probably related and may share a common ancestral gene (Fig. 4). In addition to the structural genes, the urease accessory genes were often found to share homology among species. Regulatory genes, however, such as *ureR* of *P. mirabilis,* do not have a homologue in *H. pylori* or *K. aerogenes.*

Expression of recombinant urease

The genes encoding *H. pylori* urease, a nickel metalloenzyme, have been cloned and expressed in *E. coli.* Enzymatic activity, however, has been very weak compared to that of clinical isolates of *H. pylori*[22,28]. Conditions have been developed under which near wild-type urease activity is achieved. *E. coli* SE5000 containing recombinant *H. pylori* urease genes can be grown in minimal medium containing no amino acids, $NiCl_2$ is added to 0.75 μmol/l and structural genes *ureA* and *ureB* are over-expressed *in trans* to the complete urease gene cluster. Under these conditions, *E. coli* SE5000 (pHP808/pHP902) expresses a urease activity up to 87 μmol urea/min per mg protein (87 U/mg protein) a level approaching that of the wild-type *H. pylori* strain (100 U/mg protein), from which the genes were cloned. Poor catalytic activity of recombinant clones grown in Luria broth or M9 medium containing 0.5% casamino acids was due to chelation of nickel ions by medium components, particularly histidine and cysteine. In cultures containing these amino acids, $^{63}Ni^{2+}$ is prevented from being transported into the cell, and is not incorporated into urease protein. As a consequence, M9 minimal medium cultures containing histidine or cysteine produce only 0.05% and 0.9%, respectively, of active urease produced by control cultures containing no amino acids. Therefore, expression of active recombinant *H. pylori* urease is increased when Ni^{2+} transport is not inhibited, and when sufficient synthesis of urease subunits UreA and UreB is achieved (Fig. 5).

Production of the intact but inactive apoenzyme can be expressed from clones containing only *ureA* and *ureB*[24]. The apoenzyme produced from these clones is indistinguishable from native enzyme except that is has no detectable activity. This lack of catalytic activity correlates with the lack of Ni^{2+} ions inserted into the active site of the enzyme. This confirms the role of accessory polypeptides in activation of the enzyme.

ROLE IN PATHOGENESIS

Urease as antigen

As described above, the urease is the most prominent component of *H. pylori*. Not surprisingly, this protein, expressed on the surface, serves as a powerful immunogen for this organism[19,29–33]. Patients with active gastritis due to *H. pylori* show significantly elevated serum IgG and IgA titres to the urease when compared to preinfection levels. ELISA systems have been developed by using partially purified or purified urease as antigen to measure these immune responses (Fig. 6). Other outer membrane proteins have been used as well to measure elevated immune responses. Such tests are useful for diagnosis of acute infection, following eradication of *H. pylori* during antibiotic therapy, and conducting large-scale epidemiological studies.

Protective effect for the organism

Urease is critical for *H. pylori* colonization of a human gastric mucosa. *In vitro* the bacterium is quite sensitive to the effect of low pH[34] unless urea is present[35]. The initial colonization of the stomach with a pH of 3 or less would be difficult unless the organism could protect itself from exposure to acid. It is postulated that the organism hydrolyses urea, releasing ammonia, which neutralizes acid enabling survival and initial colonization. Urease-negative mutants of *H. pylori* have been generated by non-specific chemical mutagenesis[36,37], selection of naturally occurring mutants[38], or constructed by allelic exchange of *in vitro* constructed deletion mutations[39]. Representative mutants have demonstrated that urease is necessary for colonization in the gnotobiotic piglet model[40].

Direct toxicity to the host

In addition to the survival benefit of urease, there is evidence that ammonium hydroxide, generated by urea hydrolysis, contributes significantly to histologi-

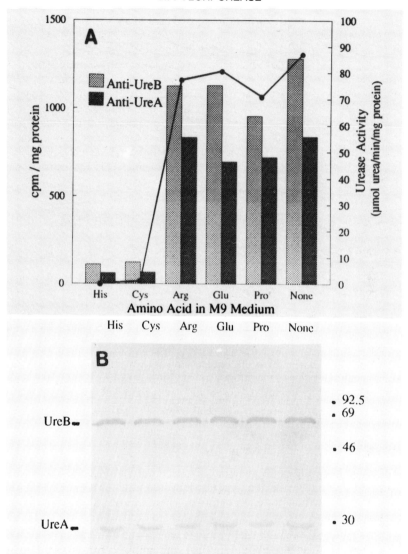

Fig. 5 Incorporation of $^{63}Ni^{2+}$ into urease after culture in the presence of various amino acids. *E. coli* containing cloned *H. pylori* urease genes was grown for 18 h in M9 medium with one of five different amino acids (listed on figure) or no amino acid. Each culture also contained 1 μmol/l NiCl$_2$ (250 nmol/l ^{63}NiCl$_2$ and 750 nmol/l unlabelled NiCl$_2$. **A:** Urease activity (●); $^{63}Ni^{2+}$ cpm immunoprecipitated by anti-UreA and anti-UreB antisera are shown as bars. **B:** Western blotting. Soluble protein (100 μg) derived from each culture was electrophoresed on an SDS-15% polyacrylamide gel, transferred to nitrocellulose, and reacted with antisera directed against both the large (UreB) and the small (UreA) subunits of *H. pylori* urease. The migration of protein standards is shown on the right in kilodaltons. Reprinted with permission from Hu and Mobley, 1993[28]

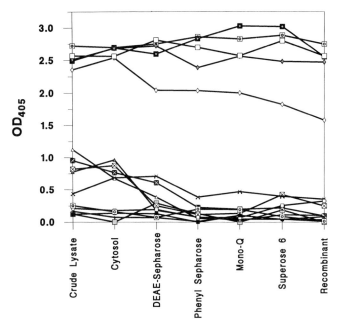

Fig. 6 ELISA of human serum samples using protein fractions from *H. pylori* urease purification as the substrates. Purified native urease (Superose 6 fraction) and purified recombinant *H. pylori* ureases were used as antigens in an ELISA against a standardized panel of sera from individuals with either high, intermediate, or low immunoglobulin titres to an *H. pylori* cell lysate antigen preparation. For comparison, antigen preparations obtained during purification of native enzyme (crude lysate, cytosol, DEAE-Sepharose, phenyl-Sepharose, and Mono-Q) were also included. Unique symbols represent the serum samples from 15 different individuals. Lines are used for the comparison of native and recombinant enzymes with the other antigen preparations for a given serum sample. Reprinted with permission from Hu *et al.*, 1992[24]

cal damage. It should be emphasized that ammonium ion *per se* is not toxic, but rather the hydroxide ion generated by the equilibration of ammonia with water. To demonstrate the cytotoxic effect of urease, cell cultures of a human gastric adenocarcinoma cell line were seeded with *H. pylori* and supplemented with various concentrations of urea[41]. Cell viability was found to be inversely proportional to ammonia concentrations generated by urea hydrolysis (Fig. 7). Viability was improved when the urease inhibitor, acetohydroxamic acid (AHA) was added to the culture before the exposure to *H. pylori*. AHA slowed the liberation of ammonia and reduced the cytotoxic effect.

Similar effects have been shown on Vero cells overlaid with filtrates of *H. pylori*[42]. Cell rounding and loss of viability were observed in cultures to which 30 mmol/l urea had been added. These changes were associated with a rise in pH. Further work with *H. pylori* supernatents used 4 mmol/l urea, duplicating urea concentrations found in the human stomach[43]. At this concentration, 10% of Vero cells showed intracellular vacuolization after 24 h of exposure to *H. pylori* supernatants. AHA reduced this effect by 75%.

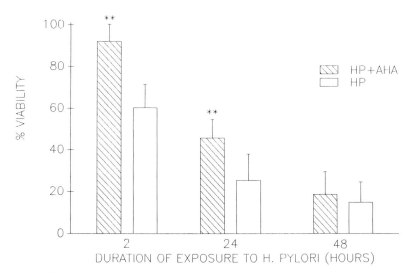

Fig. 7 Viability of gastric cells exposed to *H. pylori*. Monolayers of a human gastric adenocarcinoma cell line (CRL 1739) were overlaid with suspensions of *H. pylori* (5×10^6 c.f.u./ml). Bacterial suspensions were either not preincubated or were preincubated with 500 μg of acetohydroxamic acid (AHA) per ml. At 2, 24 and 48 h the viability of monolayers was assessed by incorporation of neutral red dye and expressed as a percentage of the control value. Cells exposed to *H. pylori* and AHA were significantly ($p < 0.0001$) more viable than cells exposed to *H. pylori* alone (**). Data are mean + standard deviation. Reprinted with permission from Smoot *et al.*, 1990[41]

These data suggested that histological damage may result directly from the localized generation of ammonia due to the hydrolysis of urea.

It has also been postulated that ammonia produced by urea hydrolysis had an additional effect[44]. Ammonia interfered with normal hydrogen ion back-diffusion across gastric mucosa, resulting in cytotoxicity to the underlying epithelium.

Induced immune response damage to the host

Urease activity is responsible for damage to the gastric epithelium via its interaction with the immune system. *H. pylori* whole cells can stimulate an oxidative burst in human neutrophils[45]. When neutrophils, *H. pylori*, and urea were incubated with rabbit fetal gastric mucosal cells, cytotoxicity was seen as evidenced by shrunken gastric cells. This cytotoxicity was not observed with urea-free medium, the addition of acetohydroxamic acid, or by incubation with inhibitors of the oxidative burst. It was suggested that hydrogen peroxide, from the oxidative burst, oxidizes chlorine ions, which react with ammonia liberated by *H. pylori* urease to give the highly toxic product monochloramine. The cytotoxic activity could be mimicked by the addition of monochloramine to the gastric cells.

The urease enzyme itself can also cause activation of monocytes and polymorphonuclear leukocytes, and recruitment of inflammatory response cells, resulting in indirect damage to the gastric epithelium. Water extracts of *H. pylori*, known to contain urease, can activate monocytes by an LPS-independent pathway[46]. *In vitro* stimulation of human monocytes led to secretion of inflammatory cytokines and reactive oxygen intermediates, all of which may be involved in mediating the inflammatory response in the gastric epithelium. Further investigation has shown that sonicates of *H. pylori* strains could prime, and also caused direct activation of the oxidative burst, in human polymorphonuclear leukocytes and monocytes[47]. Both properties were present in two separate molecular weight size ranges, which did not preclude the UreA subunit of urease. In contrast, it was reported that purified urease could not stimulate natural killer cell activity of isolated granular lymphocytes directly, unlike complete cells of *H. pylori*[48]. This suggests that such damage caused by urease is due to its interaction with cells responsible for cellular inflammatory signalling, rather than with the cytotoxic cells themselves.

There is also evidence of urease or urease-containing fractions from *H. pylori* acting as chemotactic factors for leukocytes, causing further local inflammation[49,50]. Such chemotactic activity for human monocytes and neutrophils was present in purified urease samples, and could be inhibited by specific antibody to the UreB urease subunit. Further, a 20 amino acid peptide based on the amino terminus of the UreB subunit protein also exhibited similar levels of chemotaxis in a microchamber test system. Immunocytochemical staining showed urease to be closely associated to the crypt cells in the lamina propria of patients with duodenal ulcers. It is postulated that urease is absorbed into the mucosa where it attracts leukocytes and causes mucosal inflammation.

Urease, by a variety of mechanisms, is at least partly responsible for the initial recruitment of monocytes and neutrophils, and further activation and stimulation of the immune system to produce the local inflammatory lesion associated with *H. pylori* infection. Further elucidation of urease's multifactorial role in causing potential damage to the gastric epithelium and its contribution to the variety of disease states associated with the bacterium is awaited.

DETECTION OF *H. PYLORI* USING UREASE

Urease biopsy test

The urease reaction can be exploited in the endoscopy suite by obtaining an endoscopic biopsy and placing the biopsy directly in a small volume of Christensen's urea broth or various modifications of this recipe[51]. If *H. pylori* is present in significant numbers, urea will be hydrolysed by urease, the pH will rise, and phenol red will turn from light orange to red, usually within 5 min. Since the reaction is due to preformed enzymes, the reaction can be carried out at 45°C to increase the speed of reaction[52]. Various modifications of the test exist, and the reactions can be carried out in a commercially available urea-containing gel. All of the biopsy urease tests have specificities approaching 100% and sensitivities of at least 90%[51].

Urease-positive colonies after culture

H. pylori can be cultured from these biopsies on blood-based media including Skirrow's or Dent's media at 37°C in an anaerobic jar with an activated Campy Pak, which supplies the proper microaerobic environment. After 3 to 5 days of culture, pinpoint colonies can be observed and tested for urease activity. *H. pylori* cultured directly from endoscopic biopsies always gives a strong urease reaction which, in the presence of positive oxidative and catalase reactions, is diagnostic for this species.

Urea breath test

Although the biopsy urease test reaction is simple, it does require biopsy by endoscopy, an invasive procedure. A non-invasive procedure, the urease breath test, has been developed that serves as a sensitive and specific, although qualitative, indicator of infection. The patient is given an oral dose of labelled urea, either $[^{13}C]$urea[53], or $[^{14}C]$urea[54]. If the organism is present, urea will be hydrolysed and $^{13}CO_2$ or $^{14}CO_2$ will be liberated, enter the blood stream, exchange in the lungs, and be exhaled. Exhaled CO_2 is trapped and quantitated in a mass spectrometer for $^{13}CO_2$ or a scintillation counter for $^{14}CO_2$. Since a mass spectrometer may be prohibitively expensive for most institutions, the $[^{14}C]$urea test used with a liquid scintillation counter may be preferred. Alternatively, samples can be collected in sealed tubes and processed in a central laboratory. While a number of normal anaerobic gut flora are urease-positive, and potentially could interfere with this test, the data collected thus far indicate that false-positive reactions are rare.

PCR identification

The use of the polymerase chain reaction (PCR) to detect specific DNA sequences has been particularly applicable to the identification of slow-growing bacterial pathogens. As urease production is ubiquitous in *H. pylori*, urease gene sequences are a suitable identifying target.

PCR amplification of a 411 bp fragment from the *ureA* gene has been used in identification of *H. pylori* strains[55,56]. The PCR fragment was amplified in a 26 cycle amplification from boiled supernatants of 50 strains of *H. pylori*. No amplification product was produced from 60 other strains, including *H. mustelae* and other urease-producing bacterial species. These primers were 100% specific and sensitive, and had a limit of detection of 10 to 100 bacterial cells. The primers were also able to amplify the 411 bp fragment from gastric biopsy supernatants, after vortexing the sample and boiling for 10 min, using a 35 cycle amplification. These studies were extended using the same PCR primers but with a more complex lysis of the biopsy material using SDS and proteinase K digestion, followed by phenol-chloroform extraction[57]. After 35 amplification cycles, 25 of 26 culture-positive samples produced the 411 bp amplification product, with one of 40 culture-negative samples being PCR-positive. The difference in rate of PCR detection of culture-negative samples may have been a reflection on the sensitivity of the culture protocol rather than the PCR assay. PCR amplification of a 365 bp product from an adjacent area of the 5' end of the *ureA* gene sequence has been reported using a pair of PCR primers, one of which was degenerate[58]. This PCR primer pair was also 100% sensitive and specific for *H. pylori*, with a reported limit of detection of 17 bacterial cells. Amplification from gastric juice samples using these primers resulted in 25 of 26 culture-positive samples producing the expected 365 bp PCR product, with eight culture-negative patients also being negative by PCR.

PCR amplification from regions of the *ureB* gene has also been used to detect *H. pylori* in paraffin-embedded biopsy samples[58]. Two PCR primer pairs were used to amplify a 132 bp product and a 115 bp product. Microtome sections were boiled for 15 min and subjected to two rounds of amplification, each of 25 cycles. In four of five samples tested, both *ureB* PCR primer pairs amplified the expected product, whereas no product was obtained from the larger *ureA* primer pair. This may reflect the poor quality of DNA obtained from paraffin-embedded samples and the greater efficiency of amplification of smaller PCR products.

Both the *H. pylori* urease subunit structural genes, *ureA* and *ureB*, have been demonstrated to be useful targets for PCR detection of *H. pylori* from culture supernatants, fresh and paraffin-embedded biopsy tissue, and gastric juice aspirates. These PCR detection systems can be applied to epidemiological and transmission studies, monitoring of treatment regimes, and diagnostic testing of *H. pylori*.

PCR TYPING SYSTEMS BASED ON UREASE GENES

It has been noted that there is a great deal of diversity between *H. pylori* strains with respect to restriction endonuclease sites within chromosomal DNA[59]. Indeed, there was so much diversity that nearly every strain revealed a new pattern. Previous studies have used gross differences in the restriction digest patterns of *H. pylori* chromosomal DNAs to differentiate strains. However, interpretation of these results is difficult because of the complexity of the restriction digest patterns, even with densitometric analysis of one signature area of the pattern.

To simplify comparison this microdiversity can be examined using PCR products of specific genes from the *H. pylori* chromosome. The first systems that were developed were based on PCR amplification of urease genes[60,61]. PCR-amplified urease structural subunit genes *ureA* and *ureB*, when digested with appropriate restriction endonucleases, produced different digest patterns in agarose gels (Fig. 8). The substrate for PCR amplification was DNA extracted from *H. pylori* by alkaline lysis and phenol-chloroform. The 2.4 kb

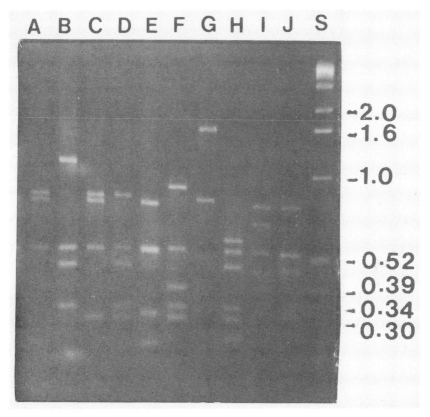

Fig. 8 A PCR typing technique for differentiation of *H. pylori* isolates. *Hae*III restriction digest patterns of the amplified urease genes on a 2409 bp PCR product from representative *H. pylori* clinical isolates. Amplified DNA was digested with *Hae*III and electrophoresed on a 3.5% Nusieve GTG agarose gel. Lanes A–J depict distinct *H. pylori* isolates; lane S: 1 kb ladder, sizes in kilobases. Reprinted with permission from Foxall *et al.*, 1992[61]

PCR products, amplified from 22 clinical isolates and subjected to *Hae*III digestion, produced 10 distinct patterns on agarose gels, with two patterns being shared between five and six strains. These patterns allowed easy differentiation between strains. Comparison of strains taken from one patient before and after a 6-month interval revealed the same restriction pattern of the PCR product, suggesting that the same strain was present in both biopsies. Another method amplified the *ureC* gene followed by direct DNA sequencing of the PCR product to distinguish between strains of *H. pylori*[62]. Numerous base-pair changes were detected and strains were easily differentiated. Again, strains taken from the same individual over various time periods demonstrated the stability of this sequence over time, allowing this method to confirm the presence of the same strain or a different strain.

Four subsequent reports[63-66] have confirmed that urease genes (*ureA*, *ureB*, and *ureC*) can be PCR amplified, subjected to restriction endonuclease digestion, and used to differentiate strains on the basis of patterns on agarose gels. It is probable that, for *H. pylori*, any PCR-amplified fragment will allow this type of differentiation. Indeed, this diversity is observed for the flagellin gene (*flaA*)[61], the 48 kDa stress protein (*htrA*) and a 26 kDa antigen-encoding gene[64] or by ribotyping[65].

References

1. Mobley HLT, Hausinger RP. Microbial urease: significance, regulation, and molecular characterization. Microbiol Rev. 1989;53:85–108.
2. Sumner JB. The isolation and crystallization of the enzyme urease. J Biol Chem. 1926;69: 435–41.
3. Dixon NE, Gazzola C, Blakeley RL, Zerner B. Jack bean urease (EC 3.5.1.5). A metallo-enzyme. A simple biological role for nickel? J Am Chem Soc. 1975;97:4131–3.
4. Hu L-T, Mobley HLT. Purification and N-terminal analysis of urease from *Helicobacter pylori*. Infect Immun. 1990;58:992–8.
5. Dunn BE, Campbell GP, Perez-Perez GI, Blaser MJ. Purification and characterization of urease from *Helicobacter pylori*. J Biol Chem. 1990;265:9464–9.
6. Evans Jr DJ, Evans DG, Kirkpatrick SS, Graham DS. Characterization of the *Helicobacter pylori* urease and purification of its subunits. Microbial Pathol. 1991;10:15–26.
7. Turbett GR, Hoj PB, Horne R, Mee BJ. Purification and characterization of the urease enzymes of *Helicobacter* species from humans and animals. Infect Immun. 1992;60: 5259–66.
8. Hawtin PR, Delves HT, Newell DG. The demonstration of nickel in the urease of *Helicobacter pylori* by atomic absorption spectroscopy. FEMS Microbiol Lett. 1991;77: 51–4.
9. Sriwanthana B, Mobley HLT. *Proteus mirabilis* urease: histidine 320 of UreC is essential for urea hydrolysis and nickel ion binding within the native enzyme. Infect Immun. 1993;61:2570–7.
10. Park I-S, Hausinger RP. Site-directed mutagenesis of *Klebsiella aerogenes* urease: identi-fication of histidine residues that appear to function in nickel ligation, substrate binding, and catalysis. Protein Sci. 1993;2:1034–41.
11. Jones BD, Mobley HLT. *Proteus mirabilis* urease: genetic organization, regulation, and expression of structural genes. J Bacteriol. 1988;170:3342–9.
12. Mobley HLT, Jones BD, Jerse AE. Cloning of urease gene sequences from *Providencia stuartii*. Infect Immun. 1986;54:161–9.
13. Hu L-T, Nicholson EB, Jones BD, Lynch MJ, Mobley HLT. *Morganella morganii* urease: purification, characterization, and isolation of gene sequences. J Bacteriol. 1990;172: 3073–80.
14. Hawtin PR, Stacey AR, Newell DG. Investigation of the structure and localization of the urease of *Helicobacter pylori* using monoclonal antibodies. J Gen Microbiol. 1990;136: 1995–2000.
15. Austin JW, Doig P, Stewart M, Trust TJ. Macromolecular structure and aggregation states of *Helicobacter pylori* urease. J Bacteriol. 1991;173:5663–7.
16. Austin JW, Doig P, Stewart M, Trust TJ. Structural comparison of urease and a GroEL analog from *Helicobacter pylori*. J Bacteriol. 1992;174:7470–3.
17. Dunn BE, Martin Roop II R, Sung C-C, Sharma SA, Perez-Perez GI, Blaser MJ. Identification and purification of a cpn60 heat shock protein homolog from *Helicobacter pylori*. Infect Immun. 1992;60:1946–51.
18. Evans Jr DJ, Evans DG, Engstrand L, Graham DY. Urease-associated heat shock protein of *Helicobacter pylori*. Infect Immun. 1992:60:2125–7.
19. Newell DG, Stacey A. Antigens for the serodiagnosis of *Campylobacter pylori*. Gastroenterol Clin Biol. 1989;13:37B–41B.
20. Labigne-Roussel A, Courcoux P. Cloning and expression of the urease genes of *Campylo-bacter pylori*. In: Megraud F, Lamouliatte H, editors. Gastroduodenal pathology and *Campylobacter pylori*. Amsterdam: Elsevier Science Publishers; 1989;119–23.

21. Clayton CL, Wren BW, Mullany P, Topping A, Tabaqchali S. Molecular cloning and expression of *Campylobacter pylori* species-specific antigens in *Escherichia coli* K-12. Infect Immun. 1989;57:623–9.
22. Cussac V, Ferrero RL, Labigne A. Expression of *Helicobacter pylori* urease genes in *Escherichia coli* grown under nitrogen-limiting conditions. J. Bacteriol. 1992;174:2466–73.
23. Labigne A, Cussac V, Courcoux P. Shuttle cloning and nucleotide sequence of *Helicobacter pylori* genes responsible for urease activity. J Bacteriol. 1991;173:1920–31.
24. Hu L-T, Foxall PA, Russell R, Mobley HLT. Purification of recombinant *Helicobacter pylori* urease apoenzyme encoded by *ureA* and *ureB*. Infect Immun. 1992;60:2657–66.
25. Clayton CL, Pallen MJ, Kleanthous H, Wren BW, Tabaqchali S. Nucleotide sequence of two genes from *Helicobacter pylori* encoding for urease subunits. Nucl Acids Res. 1990;18:362.
26. Jones BD, Mobley HLT. *Proteus mirabilis* urease: nucleotide sequence determination and comparison with jack bean urease. J Bacteriol. 1989;171:6414–22.
27. Mamiya G, Takishima K, Masakuni M, Kayumi T, Ogawa K, Sekita T. Complete amino acid sequence of jack bean urease. Proc Jpn Acad. 1985;61:395–8.
28. Hu L-T, Mobley HLT. Expression of catalytically active recombinant *Helicobacter pylori* urease at wild type levels in *Escherichia coli*. Infect Immun. 1993;61:2563–9.
29. Dent JG, McNulty CAM, Uff JS, Gear MWL, Wilkinson SP. *Campylobacter pylori* urease: a new serological test. Lancet. 1988;1:1002.
30. Newell DG. Identification of the outer membrane proteins of *Campylobacter pyloridis* and antigenic cross-reactivity between *C. pyloridis* and *C. jejuni*. J Gen Microbiol. 1987;133:163–70.
31. Jones DM, Eldridge J, Fox AJ, Sethi P, Whorwell PJ. Antibody to the gastric campylobacter-like organism ('*Campylobacter pyloridis*' – clinical correlations and distribution in the normal population. J Med Microbiol. 1986;22:57–62.
32. Czinn S, Can H, Sheffler L, Aronoff S. Serum IgG antibody to the outer membrane proteins of *Campylobacter pylori* in children with gastroduodenal disease. J Infect Dis. 1989;159:586–9.
33. Perez-Perez GI, Blaser MJ. Conservation and diversity of *Campylobacter pyloridis* major antigens. Infect Immun. 1987;55:1256–63.
34. Hazell SL, Lee A. The adaptation of motile strains of *Campylobacter pyloridis* to gastric mucus and their association with gastric epithelial intercellular spaces. In: Pearson AD, Skirrow MB, Lion H, Rowe B, editors. *Campylobacter* III. Proceedings of the Third International Workshop on *Campylobacter* Infections. Ottawa. London: Public Health Laboratory Service; 1985;189–91.
35. Marshall BJ, Barrett LJ, Prakesh C, McCallum RW, Guerrant RL. Protection of *Campylobacter pyloridis* but not *Campylobacter jejuni* against acid susceptibility by urea. In: Kaijser B, Falsen E, editors. *Campylobacter* IV. Goteborg: University of Goteborg (Sweden); 1988;402–3.
36. Blaser MJ, Cover TL, Steele R, Eaton K, Perez-Perez G, Labigne A. Characteristics of a urease-negative *H. pylori* mutant strain. Rev Esp Eng Digest. 1990;78(Suppl 1):26.
37. Segal ED, Shon J, Tompkins LS. Characterization of *Helicobacter pylori* urease mutants. Infect Immun. 1992;60:1883–9.
38. Cox DM, McLaren A, Snowden MA. The isolation and characteristics of urease-negative variants of *Helicobacter pylori*. Rev Esp Enf Digest. 1990;78(Suppl. 1):29.
39. Ferrero RL, Cussac V, Courcoux P, Labigne A. Construction of isogenic urease-negative mutants of *Helicobacter pylori* by allelic exchange. J Bacteriol. 1992;174:4212–17.
40. Eaton KA, Brooks CL, Morgan DR, Krakowka S. Essential role of urease in pathogenesis of gastritis induced by *Helicobacter pylori* in gnotobiotic piglets. Infect Immun. 1991;59:2470–5.
41. Smoot DT, Mobley HLT, Chippendale GR, Lewison JF, Resau JH. *Helicobacter pylori* urease activity is toxic to human gastric epithelial cells. Infect Immun. 1990;58:1992–4.
42. Barer MR, Elliott TSJ, Berkeley D, Thomas JE, Eastham EJ. Cytopathic effects of *Campylobacter pylori* urease. J Clin Pathol. 1988;41:597.
43. Xu J-K, Goodwin CS, Cooper M, Robinson J. Intracellular vacuolization caused by the urease of *Helicobacter pylori*. J Infect Dis. 1990;161:1302–4.
44. Hazell SL, Lee A. *Campylobacter pyloridis*, urease, hydrogen ion back diffusion, and gastric ulcers. Lancet. 1986;2:15–17.
45. Suzuki M, Miura S, Suematsu M et al. *Helicobacter pylori*-associated ammonia production

enhances neutrophil-dependent gastric mucosal cell injury. Am J Physiol. 1992;263(Gastrointest. Liver Physiol. 26):G719–G725.

46. Mai UEH, Perez-Perez GI, Wahl LM, Wahl SM, Blaser MJ, Smith PD. Soluble surface proteins from *Helicobacter pylori* activate monocytes/macrophages by lipopolysaccharide-independent mechanism. J Clin Invest. 1991;87:894–900.

47. Nielsen P, Anderson LP. Activation of human phagocyte oxidative metabolism by *Helicobacter pylori*. Gastroenterology. 1992;103:1747–53.

48. Tarkkanen J, Kosunen TU, Saksela E. Contact of lymphocytes with *Helicobacter pylori* augments natural killer cell activity and induces production of gamma interferon. Infect Immun. 1993;61:3012–16.

49. Mai UEH, Perez-Perez GI, Allen JB, Wahl SM, Blaser MJ, Smith PD. Surface proteins from *Helicobacter pylori* exhibit chemotactic activity for human leukocytes and are present in gastric mucosa. J Exp Med. 1992;175:517–25.

50. Craig PM, Territo MC, Karnes WE, Walsh JH. *Helicobacter pylori* secretes a chemotactic factor for monocytes and neutrophils. Gut. 1992;33:1020–3.

51. McNulty CAM. Detection of *Campylobacter pylori* by the biopsy urease test. In: Rathbone BJ, Heatley RV, editors. *Campylobacter pylori* and gastroduodenal disease. Oxford: Blackwell Scientific Publications; 1989:69–73.

52. Mobley HLT, Cortesia MJ, Rosenthal LE, Jones BD. Characterization of urease from *Campylobacter pylori*. J Clin Microbiol. 1988;26:831–6.

53. Graham DY, Klein PD, Evans DJ, Alpert LC, Opekun AR, Boutton TW. *Campylobacter pyloridis* detected by the ^{13}C-urea test. Lancet. 1987;1:1174–7.

54. Bell BD, Weil J, Harrison G *et al.* ^{14}C-urea breath analysis, a non-invasive test for *Campylobacter pylori* in the stomach. Lancet. 1987;1:1367–8.

55. Clayton C, Kleanthous K, Tabaqchali S. Detection and identification of *Helicobacter pylori* by the polymerase chain reaction. J Clin Pathol. 1991;44:515–16.

56. Clayton CL, Kleanthous H, Coates PJ, Morgan DD, Tabaqchali S. Sensitive detection of *Helicobacter pylori* by using polymerase chain reaction. J Clin Microbiol. 1992;30:192–200.

57. van Zwet AA, Thijs JC, Kooistra-Smid AMD, Schirm J, Snijder JAM. Sensitivity of culture compared with that of polymerase chain reaction for detection of *Helicobacter pylori* from antral biopsy specimens. J Clin Microbiol. 1993;31:1918–20.

58. Westblom TU, Phadnis S, Yang P, Czinn SJ. Diagnosis of *Helicobacter pylori* infection by means of a polymerase chain reaction assay for gastric juice aspirates. Clin Infect Dis. 1993;16:367–71.

59. Majewski SIH, Goodwin CS. Restriction endonuclease analysis of the genome of *Campylobacter pylori* with a rapid extraction method: evidence for considerable genomic variation. J Infect Dis. 1988;157:465–71.

60. Foxall PA, Hu L-T, Mobley HLT. Amplification of the complete urease structural genes from *Helicobacter pylori* clinical isolates and cosmid gene bank clones. Rev Esp Enf Digest. 1990;78(Suppl. 1):128–9.

61. Foxall PA, Hu L-T, Mobley HLT. Use of polymerase chain reaction-amplified *Helicobacter pylori* urease structural genes for differentiation of isolates. J Clin Microbiol. 1992;30:739–41.

62. Courcoux P, Freuland C, Piemont Y, Fauchere JL, Labigne A. Polymerase chain reaction and direct DNA sequencing as a method for distinguishing between different strains of *Helicobacter pylori*. Rev Esp Enf Digest. 1990;78(Suppl. 1):29–30.

63. Akopyanz N, Bukanov NO, Westblom TU, Berg DE. PCR-based RFLP analysis of DNA sequence diversity in the gastric pathogen *Helicobacter pylori*. Nucl Acids Res. 1992;20:6221–5.

64. Clayton CL, Kleanthous H, Morgan DD, Puckey L, Tabaqchali S. Rapid fingerprinting of *Helicobacter pylori* by polymerase chain reaction and restriction fragment length polymorphism analysis. J Clin Microbiol. 1993;31:1420–5.

65. Lopez CR, Owen RJ, Desai M. Differentiation between isolates of *Helicobacter pylori* by PCR-RFLP analysis of urease A and B genes and comparison with ribosomal RNA gene patterns. FEMS Microbiol Lett. 1993;110:37–44.

66. Moore RA, Kureishi A, Wong S, Bryan LE. Categorization of clinical isolates of *Helicobacter pylori* on the basis of restriction digest analysis of PCR-amplified *ureC* genes. J Clin Microbiol. 1993;31:1334–5.

4
Basic bacteriology of *H. pylori*: *H. pylori* colonization factors

A. LEE and H. MITCHELL

THE NEED TO UNDERSTAND COLONIZATION

Helicobacter pylori is an unusual bacterial pathogen. This organism infects its host most probably in childhood and remains in most persons for life unless there has been specific *H. pylori* antimicrobial therapy or the stomach becomes an inhospitable environment due to such events as changes in the stomach due to long-term gastritis or surgery. Most pathogenic bacteria either infect the host transiently until they are eradicated due to the non-specific and specific immune system, or they completely overwhelm the host, resulting in death. In a small number of chronic diseases such as tuberculosis or syphilis the organism may remain for long periods, but the numbers are greatly reduced, are difficult to find and are sequestered away in some inaccessible site. With respect to life in its chosen host *H. pylori* behaves more like a parasite. A characteristic of good parasites is that they are excellent colonizers.

Eradication of *H. pylori* has proved unexpectedly difficult; hence there is a need to understand the way *H. pylori* colonizes the stomach in order to devise a more rational approach to therapy and prophylaxis.

H. PYLORI AS AN EVOLVED PARASITE: ADAPTATION TO COLONIZATION OF THE GASTRIC MUCOSA

H. pylori is an extremely good colonizer because it is a highly evolved parasite. This bacterium has evolved with its human host just as a range of other different but related helicobacters have evolved to their own particular host, i.e. *H. felis* in the cat[1] and *H. mustelae* in the ferret[2].

The mammalian stomach itself has evolved so that it most efficiently serves a number of functions, the most essential being the preparation of foodstuffs for efficient utilization further down the bowel. However, the stomach also provides an extremely hostile environment for microorganisms which prevent the passage of ingested, potential pathogens into the gut. The increased susceptibility to bacterial infection when gastric function is impaired is evidence of the effectiveness of this defence mechanism[3,4].

To succeed in this hostile gastric environment where so many others have failed has meant the acquisition of some remarkable and still incompletely understood adaptations. Understanding these acquired traits is the key to understanding the colonization of *H. pylori*.

ADAPTATION TO OVERCOME BARRIERS TO GASTRIC COLONIZATION

Urease and gastric acidity

The most powerful of the gastric barriers is the production of copious amounts of hydrochloric acid and the maintenance of a pH of <2. The majority of bacteria cannot withstand such a low pH. Acidophilic bacteria do exist that can better cope with acidity, e.g. the lactobacilli of the human vagina, such organisms having acquired enzymes that function adequately at pH 4–5. In the mouse stomach, which is not as acidic as the human, acidophilic yeasts and lactobacilli have evolved which can also grow at a reduced pH[5]. However for *H. pylori* to withstand a pH as low as 2 a novel strategy had to be acquired. We believe that this is due to generation of a novel urease[6], i.e. modification of an enzyme system, which in the lower bowel serves a completely different function.

Many bacteria have a urease enzyme that catalyses the breakdown of urea into carbon dioxide and ammonia. In the lower bowel of humans and the rumen of ruminants this enzyme has a strictly physiological function, namely the utilization of urea nitrogen[7]. In high urea locations, such as the urinary tract, some urease-positive bacteria are clearly at an advantage[8]. Characteristics of this enzyme have been covered in the previous chapter. What is relevant to the current theme are two properties of the enzyme that we believe have been specifically acquired to allow the enzyme to be protective in an acid environment. Firstly, although there is some debate on this, the enzyme appears to be transported outside the cell, possibly with the help of the HSP 60-like heat shock protein acting as a chaperonin[9,10]. This is different from other urease-positive bacteria. Also unlike other ureases, the *H. pylori* enzyme appears to have two pH optima; one of which is at a low pH[6]. Thus as *H. pylori* enters the gastric lumen it is immersed in the very acidic gastric juice where small amounts of urea are present. The external enzyme is able to break down this substrate due to its ability to act at a lower pH. Ammonia is produced in 'a cloud' around the bacterium, thus protecting it from the acid. Two sets of *in vitro* experimental data are consistent with this hypothesis. Firstly, if *H. pylori* is placed in a test tube at pH 2 it is rapidly killed. However, if urea at the concentration found in the stomach is added then the organism is protected[6,11,12]. Significantly, the non-gastric bacteria such as *Proteus* spp. are not protected; also, all the *Helicobacter* species that can colonize a gastric surface in animals have a similar enzyme and are protected from acid in *in vitro* experiments[6]. A number of new *Helicobacter* spp. have recently been discovered that are not gastric colonizers, but normally inhabit the lower bowel of animals. These bacteria either have no urease, i.e. *H. fennelliae* or *H. cinaedi*[13] or the urease is different and does not protect them in a low pH in the presence of urea, i.e. *H. muridarum*[6].

Evidence that the possession of urease is essential for initial colonization of the gastric mucosa comes from the importamt work of Eaton and Krakowka, where urease-negative mutants of *H. pylori* were shown to lose their ability to colonize the stomach of gnotobiotic piglets in contrast to the urease-positive wild-type which colonizes in this animal model very well[14]. A similar result has been shown in a primate model by Japanese workers[15]. Also, in a series of preliminary experiments, immunization of mice with a purified recombinant *H. pylori* urease has been shown to protect mice from challenge with *H. felis*[16].

Whereas urease is essential for initiating an infection in the stomach, activity of this enzyme is not essential for colonization once established. Two different sets of animal experiments show that administration of potent urease inhibitors such as acetohydroxymate or fluorofamide will protect from gastric *Helicobacter* infection, but has absolutely no effect on already-established infection. These results were disappointing, as they showed that anti-urease drugs were not likely to be useful in the treatment of *H. pylori*-associated disease[6,17].

Motility and gastric mucus

Many years ago we postulated that it was no coincidence that the bacteria dominating the populations naturally colonizing the mucus lining of intestinal surfaces were spiral-shaped. We suggested that this shape, and their peculiar motility, gave them an advantage in the viscous mucus[18]. *In vitro* experiments showed that these bacteria coped much better in viscous solutions of methylcellulose than conventional rod-shaped motile bacteria[19]. We proposed that mucus colonization was an important property of many gut bacteria, including the gut pathogen *Campylobacter jejuni*[20]. When we first started work on *H. pylori* we were struck by its spiral/helical morphology, and suggested that this could be another mucus-associated spiral bacterium. Similar experiments in methylcellulose showed that *H. pylori* moved very rapidly in a viscous environment[21]. Examination of motile bacteria under the microscope revealed that the helical shape was actually accentuated as the organism 'bored' its way through the medium. We have also noted that those organisms seen in gastric mucus in human biopsies are the ones with the most pronounced helical morphology.

Thus, once in the stomach, *H. pylori* scurries away from the gastric acidity where its specialized motility allows it to move from the lumen down through the mucus onto the gastric cell surface. Many organisms remain free in the mucus and presumably are rapidly moving about the gastric surface. We are used to looking at fixed specimens where we solely see immobilized organisms.

It is very revealing, however, to look at specimens of fresh squashed *Helicobacter*-infected gastric scrapings under the phase contrast microscope, where the very impressive and very active motility of these bacteria is revealed.

Once again, as with urease, proof of the importance of motility in colonization came from experiments in gnotobiotic piglets with non-motile variants and mutants of *H. pylori*[22]. In these studies it was shown that a non-motile variant of a clinical isolate of *H. pylori* showed poor colonization in the gnotobiotic piglet which was in contrast with that of a motile strain. Confirmation of these studies in the gnotobiotic piglet model using the *H. pylori fla* A and *fla* B mutants constructed by Suerbaum *et al.* should further clarify the role of flagella and motility in the pathogenesis of *H. pylori*[23].

ADAPTATION TO SPECIFIC LOCATIONS IN THE HUMAN STOMACH

Urease activity and motility are the only proven factors in colonization. However, *H. pylori* shows very definite specificity of colonization for the stomach that cannot be explained by these properties. Thus if one gives *Helicobacter* spp. to germ-free piglets, dogs or mice there is remarkable localization in the stomach with very few bacteria elsewhere in the intestinal tract[24–26]. *H. pylori* has only been consistently found in the human stomach apart from the special case of duodenal-associated infection. Also, within the stomach there appears to be a specificity of colonization, e.g. antral predominance. We have to be able to explain these colonizing specificities. What follows are the speculations and hypotheses that have been proposed to be responsible for the patterns of colonization of *H. pylori*.

Gastric tissue

Evidence

In the very first papers on *H. pylori* coming out from Perth, the elegant micrographs of Armstrong demonstrated a firm attachment of the bacterium to the gastric mucosa and a number of what appeared to be 'adherence pedestals' equivalent to those seen with the enterotoxigenic *Escherichia coli*[27,28]. This suggested a specific association with the gastric epithelium. In the gnotobiotic piglet Rudmann *et al.* have shown the patterns of adherence of *H. pylori* to be similar to that seen in the gastric mucosa of humans colonized with this organism[29]. As had been reported in humans[30] organisms were frequently observed near the parietal cells, and Rudmann *et al.* suggested that *H. pylori* may inhibit normal functioning of parietal cells resulting in achlorhydria which may create an environment more conducive to *H. pylori* colonization.

Specificity of adhesion *in vivo* was confirmed by Carrick *et al.* and Wyatt *et al.*, who in some photographs of *H. pylori* in the duodenum, showed that the bacteria were only associated with gastric type cells in islets of gastric metaplasia. At the edge of the infected tissue, bacteria were seen adherent to all the gastric-type cells on the epithelium, whereas the first neighbouring cell of a small bowel morphology was free of organisms[31,32]. This would indicate considerable specificity of colonization.

Adhesins

Based on experience with other bacterial pathogens, tissue tropism is usually explained by the presence of specific 'adhesins', molecules that have complementarity with receptor sites in the tissues with the bacteria binding by specific ligand interaction. Thus there was a flurry of activity in the early days of *H. pylori* research to try to identify the adhesins.

The problem has been that *H. pylori* sticks to many cell types *in vitro*, and so it is difficult to make a judgement as to whether the putative adhesins responsible for *in vitro* adhesion are the same as those responsible for the specificity shown for gastric cells shown *in vivo*.

One of the first cell types examined were erythrocytes. *H. pylori* adheres very well to red cells from a number of different animal species[33-37]. The first *H. pylori* haemagglutinin to be extensively characterized was identified as a *N*-acetylneuraminyl-lactose binding fibrillar-like protein[34]. Many others suggested a range of haemagglutinins with different specificities[33,35,36,38,39]. Indeed, Wadstrom *et al.*[40] divided *H. pylori* into nine major different haemagglutinin groups. Lingwood *et al.* have suggested that a factor related to the exoenzyme S of *Pseudomonas aeruginosa* binds specifically to the *Helicobacter* glycerolipid receptor isolated from human stomach or human red blood cells[41], while Doig *et al.* have purified a 19.6-kDa protein which had some N-terminal sequence homology with the TcpA pilus protein of *Vibrio cholera*[42]. Other adhesins have been isolated in water washes of *H. pylori*[43], and Fauchere and Blaser have described loosely bound surface material with both urease and binding capabilities[44]. Ascencio *et al.* describe binding of *H. pylori* to heparin sulphate, and speculate that this could be involved *in vivo*[45]. Thus there are a myriad of described adhesins, many of which could be the same, but no clues as to which are important. With these studies there is no indication as to how these adhesins relate to specific association with gastric cells. The ability to genetically manipulate *H. pylori* now gives us an opportunity to resolve this issue.

For example, the gene for the receptor binding subunit of the *N*-acetylneuraminyl-lactose-binding haemagglutinin has recently been cloned and sequenced[46]. This gene *HpaA* contains a short sequence of amino acids (KRTIDK) which is equivalent to the sialic binding motif of the adhesins SfaS, K99 and CFA/I of *Escherichia coli*. Relevant to the debate on whether these adhesins play any role in specific adhesion to gastric epithelial cells is the observation that antibody to a 12-residue synthetic peptide including this sequence not only blocked the haemagglutinin activity of *E. coli*, but also bound to the surface of thin sections of human gastric biopsies. As *H. pylori* will adhere to gastric cell lines this antibody needs to be used in comparative studies with these cells, or better still in passively immunized animals such as gnotobiotic piglets. Recently Janzon *et al.* have constructed deletion mutants in the *Hpa* gene encoding for the binding subunit of fibrillar adhesin of *H. pylori*[47]. Such mutants will be important tools with which to examine the importance of the N-acetylneuraminyl-lactose-binding haemagglutinin.

A final note of warning to those intent on unravelling the adhesin quagmire is the comment by Figueroa *et al.*[48] that the relevant specific adhesins may only be expressed *in vivo*, and that an adherence mechanism, not depending on the expression of specific haemagglutinin antigen, operates for *H. pylori*. In part this comment was prompted by the observation that the haemagglutinins are present only on *H. pylori* cells grown in semi-solid medium and not if grown in liquid culture, whereas *H. pylori* adhered to HEp-2 cells irrespective of how the bacterial cells were grown.

RECEPTORS

The receptors for the adhesins that *H. pylori* acquired via adaptation obviously would need an affinity for structures that are exposed on the gastric cell surface. The majority of bacteria/receptor interactions are mediated by carbohydrate residues on the host cell. Often the carbohydrate is linked to lipid (glycerolipid) rather than to protein (glyceroprotein). Large varieties of linkage positions, sugar types and possible branching makes cell surface carbohydrates ideal information molecules[49]. More than 250 different glycerolipids have been identified.

Thus, it was not surprising when Lingwood *et al.* demonstrated in gastric tissue a *H. pylori* receptor glycerolipid[50]. More of this receptor was found to be present in antral tissue, and there was less found in the infant stomach. Pig gastric mucosa contained the same glycerolipid type. Subsequently, this glycerolipid has been shown to be a form of phosphatidyl ethanolamine[41]. The adhesin reported by Evans *et al.* has a specificity for sialic acid-rich macromolecules, and is probably the molecule involved in the inhibition of *in vitro* adhesion by GM3 ganglioside as noted by Slomiany *et al.*[39]. The existence of two different *H. pylori* receptors, one containing the neuraminyl-lactose moiety (GM3-ceramide) and the other sulphated lactosylceramide in human gastric mucosa[51], supports the concept of two different *H. pylori* ligands complementary to the receptors.

Lingwood has noted similarities between the lipid-binding specificity of *H. pylori* and purified *Pseudomonas aeruginosa* exoenzyme S. He suggests that this may be the basis of a new family of surface adhesins conferring gangliotetraosyl and gangliotetraosyl ceramide (Gg_3/Gg_4) and phosphatidyl ethanolamine binding specificity[49].

Thus, slowly, a basis for the specificity of adherence to gastric cells is emerging. Once again a note of caution as to the importance of adhesion in *H. pylori* colonization is needed. Many, indeed perhaps the majority, of *H. pylori* cells in the gastric mucosa are not attached but are swimming freely in the mucus. Two other gastric helicobacters, *H. felis* and 'H. heilmanii', specifically colonize the stomachs of animal hosts and are predominantly antral-located. Yet these bacteria show no adherence to gastric epithelial cells, and the former does not haemagglutinate red blood cells[52–54]. Clearly, the possession of adhesins is not essential for colonization of the gastric mucosa. However, close association with the gastric cell may play some role in the severity of the disease.

Mucus

Mucus is the natural habitat of *H. pylori*. While many cells ultimately closely associate with the epithelial surface by adhesion to cells, these cells are rapidly turning over and are regularly ejected and flushed down into the lower bowel. Presumably, the newly synthesized gastric cells become colonized by other bacteria that are existing in the mucus. What other characteristics have these bacteria acquired to ensure they flourish in the mucus other than the specialized motility mentioned above? Many claim that the enzymes of *H. pylori* degrade the mucus, and this contributes to a weakening of the barrier and increased chance of an acid-damaged mucosa[55,56]. This simple concept does have some flaws. Why does not everyone get ulcers if they are infected? Would a bacterium destroy the very environment that it has evolved to colonize? We think not. However, there is mucus depletion associated with *H. pylori* infection[57]. Could this not simply be that mucus is turned over more rapidly in an *H. pylori*-infected stomach? Certainly, there is a logic to the organism stimulating more of its preferred environment. There do, however, appear to be mucus changes following *H. pylori* infections. It has been noted in the early literature that ulcer patients have a modified mucus. There is an urgent need for more systematic study on the actual composition of *H. pylori*-infected mucus collected from infected persons compared to non-infected persons. *In vitro* investigations are so difficult to interpret, and are probably often meaningless. If *H. pylori* does modify mucus to its advantage then interference with this change may make the gastric environment inhospitable and so reduce colonization. Does *H. pylori* behave differently in antral mucus compared to mucus covering the body of the stomach?

The intercellular junctions

In his classic paper on the ultrastructure of the gastric mucosa when Steer so beautifully illustrated *H. pylori* infection, but missed the culture of the organism[58], spiral/helical cells could be seen to fill the crevices between gastric cells. Hazell also noted this association with the intercellular junctions, and postulated that this was a preferred site for the organism and so is thus a factor in colonization. It was suggested that possible nutrients such as urea could come through these junctions[21]. This localization was later challenged as an artefact[59]; however, many studies since have shown intercellular localization, and reveal that in many cases the bacterium actually penetrates a significant distance down this junction and may indeed be disrupting it[21,30,60–63]. So this is a real phenomenon, and any thesis on colonization would need to explain the mechanism and purpose of the congregation around, and migration down into, these junctions.

Microaerophilicity

H. pylori is a microaerophile. It likes a little oxygen, but not too much, and so grows neither aerobically at atmospheric oxygen tensions nor anaerobically in the absence of oxygen. Bacteria evolve optimum gaseous requirements similar to that in the environment in which they live. In the case of *H. pylori* certainly this will be between the highly aerated tissue and the relatively reduced gastric lumen. Could it be that at the intercellular junctions the correct balance of gases is available? There are no answers to these questions as microaerophilism has been a completely ignored area of *H. pylori* research. Could changing the local gaseous environment reduce *H. pylori* colonization?

Laminin receptors

Slomiany *et al.* have made the interesting but unsubstantiated suggestion that it is interference with laminin binding that leads to a loosening of the intercellular bonding, thus allowing *H. pylori* to penetrate to a limited degree[64]. Lipopolysaccharide appears to be involved in laminin binding, and is discussed in Chapter 13.

Antrum versus body

Antral dominance of gastritis was reported in duodenal ulcer patients long before *H. pylori* was suspected[65]. Close inspection of patterns of bacterial colonization in the *H. pylori*-infected stomach seems to confirm that the organism appears to prefer the antrum of the stomach, and we have claimed before that the antrum is the preferred niche of this bacterium and that major symptomatic disease appears to be associated with areas outside this normal niche[66]. There is some conflict in reports on *H. pylori* distribution. Thus Genta and Graham submit that the organism is evenly distributed throughout the stomach[67], while the Leeds group[68] suggest there are more bacteria in the antrum of ulcer patients, and the associated inflammation is more severe.

There is a priority to understand antral versus body colonization. The following hypothesis is based on observations in the early literature that procedures which result in a diminution of acid output result in differences in the patterns of gastritis[69], and the observations of Danon *et al.* that colonization of rodents with *H. felis* is also antral-restricted and correlates with the number of parietal cells per gastric gland[70]. It is an hypothesis that is open to test both in animal models and humans. Investigations aimed at proving or refuting the hypothesis will not only provide an understanding of *H. pylori* colonization but may offer insights as to success and failures of current therapeutic regimens.

Local acid output as a major factor in *H. pylori* colonization – an hypothesis

The acquisition of an ability to survive transient gastric acidity allows *H. pylori* to reach the mucus and rapidly move to the acid-free location of the antral mucosa. However, the bacterium is still relatively acid-sensitive and so cannot thrive in those areas of gastric mucosa where acid is being actively generated, i.e. the gastric body. The organism can survive in the body by rapid movement through the overlying neutral mucus, but it cannot penetrate into the gastric pit and colonize in large numbers. Colonization to some extent correlates with local acid output, i.e. the number of parietal cells in that local area. Thus, *H. pylori* can colonize the gastric cardia, an area devoid of parietal cells[67]. Colonization will be influenced by differences in local output; thus vagotomy or acid-suppressive therapy will lead to changes in the distribution of the organism and so the associated gastritis[69,71,72]. In populations with a lower acid output due to malnutrition and accompanying infection, the distribution of colonization and gastritis is different, as seen in gastric cancer-prone peoples such as Colombia and Japan when compared to those where antral gastritis and duodenal ulcer are the norm, e.g. the USA. A recent influential commentary in the *Lancet* is in agreement with the above hypothesis, and so the challenge is on for proof or disproof[73].

OTHER FACTORS IN COLONIZATION

The topics covered above are those that are traditionally discussed in articles on colonization, but there are other possibilities which have to date been ignored, but which need to be addressed if we are to achieve complete understanding of this fascinating host–parasite relationship.

A PROTECTED NICHE: THE INFLUENCE OF OVERGROWTH

A feature of ecosystems in harsh environments is low species diversity[74], i.e. not many organisms are able to acquire the specialized traits necessary for survival. Thus, *H. pylori* is the only bacterium that normally colonizes the human gastric mucosa. It does not need to compete with others as it has the gastric niches all to itself. However, should the harsh environmental factor, i.e. the acidity, be completely removed, then *H. pylori* no longer has the advantage. For this reason in achlorhydric stomachs, where bacterial overgrowth is present, *H. pylori* colonization is likely to be very different due to competition.

Specialized physiology

H. pylori makes a remarkable amount of the enzyme urease. If this were only required for acid survival then it is likely that enzyme production would be down-regulated once the bacterium was safely in the mucus or attached to a gastric cell. This clearly does not happen; hence the success of many of the commercial diagnostic biopsy urease tests. There must be another reason for this specialized physiology. Hazell and Mendz have suggested that, because of the microaerophilic nature of *H. pylori* and the organism's requirement for CO_2/HCO_3^- in the stomach and at other mucosal surfaces (e.g. the caecal crypts of rodents colonized by *H. muridarum*), *Helicobacter* urease could act to maintain an environment with a high partial pressure of CO_2. Mendz and Hazell suggested that this activity may denote a common function for urease in gastric and non-gastric *Helicobacter* spp.[75]. This conclusion was based on some fundamental experiments into the basic physiology of *H. pylori*. Such studies are scarce. Another attribute to successful colonization is that the bacterium can grow well in its chosen site. We do not know why *H. pylori* grows so well on the gastric mucosa. The elegant nuclear magnetic resonance studies of Mendz and Hazell are starting to reveal the possible biochemical pathways that the organism could use, but we do not know those that are essential for survival. As stated above, urease activity is not essential despite its high activity[75-78]. There must be essential pathways. Identify them and we can prevent colonization by blocking the pathway. Yet another research priority.

Evasion of host defences

The host has a highly evolved series of non-specific and specific defence mechanisms that usually allow it to successfully repel most bacterial invaders. The best parasites can completely evade these mechanisms; *H. pylori* certainly does. In a consideration of phagocyte evasion or immunoregulation it needs to be remembered that these too are characteristics acquired by adaptation over the millennia, and so we should never be surprised at their sophistication. In this area of understanding we are also only at the beginning.

A change in the niche: intestinalization

Much has been made above of the specificity of *H. pylori* for gastric tissue. Ironically, in a grossly damaged stomach resulting from decades of *H. pylori*-induced immunopathology, one tissue response is to change the tissue architecture, intestinalization of the mucosa occurs with antral tissue being replaced by a primitive lower bowel-type epithelium. *H. pylori* is not adapted to this changed environment and so the organism is slowly lost. Did the host win in the end?

CONCLUSION

Ten years after the discovery of *H. pylori* we know some of the factors that allow this clever parasite to succeed in the stomach where others fail. But much of our understanding is speculation and false interpretation of laboratory epiphenomena. Above are the conjecture, the hypotheses and the challenges. Better understanding of colonization of the gastric mucosa by us is needed if we are to attain our goal of safe, effective therapeutic and prophylactic regimens.

Acknowledgements

The support of the National Health and Medical Research Council of Australia to Professor Adrian Lee is gratefully acknowledged.

References

1. Lee A, Hazell SL, O'Rourke J, Kourpach S. Isolation of a spiral-shaped bacterium from the cat stomach. Infect Immun. 1988;56:2843–50.
2. Fox JG, Cabot EB, Taylor NS, Laraway R. Gastric colonization by *Campylobacter pylori* subsp. *mustelae* in ferrets. Infect Immun. 1988;56:2994–6.
3. Belitsos PC, Greenson JK, Yardley JK, Sisler JR, Bartlett JG. Association of gastric hypoacidity with opportunistic enteric infections in patients with AIDS. J Infect Dis. 1992;166:277–84.
4. Wildersmith CH. Bacterial overgrowth and gastric dysfunction. Br J Anaesth. 1992;69:545.
5. Savage DC. Microbial ecology of the gastrointestinal tract. Annu Rev Microbiol. 1977;31:107–33.
6. Ferrero RL, Lee A. The importance of urease in acid protection for the gastric-colonising bacteria *Helicobacter pylori* and *Helicobacter felis* sp. nov. Microbiol Ecol Health Dis. 1991;4:121–34.
7. Hungate RE. Symbiotic associations: the rumen bacteria. In: Symbiotic associations. Thirteenth symposium of the Society of General Microbiology. New York: Cambridge University Press; 1963:266–97.
8. Mobley HLT, Hausinger RP. Microbial urease: significance, regulation and molecular characterisation. Microbiol Rev. 1989;53:85–108.
9. Bode G, Malfertheiner P, Nilius M, Lehnhardt G. Ultrastructural localisation of urease in outer membrane and periplasm of *Campylobacter pylori*. J Clin Pathol. 1989;42:778–79.
10. Evans DJ, Evans DG, Engstrand L, Graham DY. Urease-associated heat shock protein of *Helicobacter pylori*. Infect Immun. 1992;60:2125–7.
11. Marshall BJ, Barrett LJ, Prakash C, McCallum RW, Guerrant RL. Urea protects *Helicobacter* (*Campylobacter*) *pylori* from the bactericidal effect of acid. Gastroenterology. 1990;99:697–702.
12. Mobley HLT, Hu L-T, Foxall PA. *Helicobacter pylori* urease: properties and role in pathogenesis. Scand J Gastroenterol. 1991;Suppl. 187:39–46.
13. Vandamme P, Falsen E, Rossau R *et al*. Revision of *Campylobacter*, *Helicobacter* and *Wolinella* taxonomy: emendation of generic descriptions and proposal of *Arcobacter* gen. nov. Int J Syst Bacteriol. 1991;41:88–103.
14. Eaton KA, Brooks CL, Morgan DR, Krakowka S. Essential role of urease in pathogenesis of gastritis induced by *Helicobacter pylori* in gnotobiotic piglets. Infect Immun. 1991;59: 2470–5.
15. Hirata I, Itoh T, Suzuki K *et al*. Colonisation of urease positive and negative strains of *Helicobacter pylori* in gastric mucosa of cynomolgus monkeys. Acta Gastroenterol Belg. 1993;56(S):112.
16. Corthesy-Theulaz I, Haas R, Davin C *et al*. *Helicobacter pylori* urease elicits protection against *Helicobacter felis* infection in mice. Acta Gastroenterol Belg. 1993;56(S):64.
17. McColm AA, Bagshaw J, O'Malley CO, McLaren A. Is urease a lethal target for therapy of *Helicobacter pylori*? Microbial Ecol Health Dis. 1991;4(S):S145.
18. Lee A. Neglected niches: the microbial ecology of the gastrointestinal tract. In: Marshall KC, editor. Advances in microbial ecology, vol. 8. New York: Plenum Press; 1985:115–62.
19. Ferrero RL, Lee A. Motility of *Campylobacter jejuni* in a viscous environment: comparison

with conventional rod-shaped bacteria. J Gen Microbiol. 1988;134:53–9.

20. Lee A, O'Rourke JL, Barrington PJ, Trust TJ. Mucus colonization as a determinant of pathogenicity in intestinal infection by *Campylobacter jejuni*: a mouse cecal model. Infect Immun. 1986;51:536–46.

21. Hazell SL, Lee A, Brady L, Hennessy W. *Campylobacter pyloridis* and gastritis: association with intercellular spaces and adaptation to an environment of mucus as important factors in colonization of the gastric epithelium. J Infect Dis. 1986;153:658–63.

22. Eaton KA, Morgan DR, Krakowka S. Motility as a factor in the colonisation of gnotobiotic piglets by *Helicobacter pylori*. J Med Microbiol. 1992;37:123–7.

23. Suerbaum S, Josenhans C, Labigne A. Cloning and genetic characterization of the *Helicobacter pylori* and *Helicobacter mustelae flaB* flagellin genes and construction of *H. pylori flaA*-negative and *flaB*-negative mutants by electroporation-mediated allelic exchange. J Bacteriol. 1993;175:3278–88.

24. Krakowka S, Morgan DR, Kraft WG, Leunk RD. Establishment of gastric *Campylobacter pylori* infection in the neonatal gnotobiotic piglet. Infect Immun. 1987;55:2789–96.

25. Radin MJ, Eaton KA, Krakowka S *et al. Helicobacter pylori* gastric infection in gnotobiotic beagle dogs. Infect Immun. 1990;58:2606–12.

26. Lee A, Fox JG, Otto G, Murphy J. A small animal model of human *Helicobacter pylori* active chronic gastritis. Gastroenterology. 1990;99:1315–23.

27. Goodwin CS, Armstrong JA, Marshall BJ. *Campylobacter pyloridis*, gastritis, and peptic ulceration. J Clin Pathol. 1986;39:353–65.

28. Goodwin CS, Armstrong JA, Peters M. Microbiology of *C. pylori*. In: Blaser MJ, editor. *Campylobacter pylori* in gastritis and peptic ulcer disease. New York: Igaku-Shoin; 1989: 25–49.

29. Rudmann DG, Eaton KA, Krakowka S. Ultrastructural study of *Helicobacter pylori* adherence properties in gnotobiotic piglets. Infect Immun. 1992;60:2121–4.

30. Chen XG, Correa P, Offerhaus J *et al.* Ultrastructure of the gastric mucosa harbouring *Campylobacter*-like organisms. Am J Clin Pathol. 1986;86:575–82.

31. Carrick J, Lee A, Hazell S, Ralston M, Daskalopoulos G. *Campylobacter pylori* duodenal ulcer, and gastric metaplasia: possible role of functional heterotopic tissue in ulcerogenesis. Gut. 1989;30:790–7.

32. Wyatt JI, Rathbone BJ, Dixon MF, Heatley RV. *Campylobacter pyloridis* and acid induced gastric metaplasia in the pathogenesis of duodenitis. J Clin Pathol. 1987;40:841–8.

33. Emody L, Carlsson A, Ljungh A, Wadstrom T. Mannose-resistant haemagglutination by *Campylobacter pylori*. Scand J Infect Dis. 1988;20:353–4.

34. Evans DG, Evans DJ, Moulds JJ, Graham DY. *N*-acetylneuraminyl-lactose-binding fibrillar hemagglutinin of *Campylobacter pylori*: a putative colonization factor antigen. Infect Immun. 1988;56:2896–906.

35. Wadstrom T. *Helicobacter pylori* haemagglutinins. In: Menge H, Gregor M, Tytgat GNJ, Marshall BJ, McNulty CAM, editors. *Helicobacter pylori* 1990. Berlin, Heidelberg: Springer-Verlag; 1990:19–26.

36. Robinson J, Goodwin CS, Cooper M, Burke V, Mee BJ. Soluble and cell-associated haemagglutinins of *Helicobacter* (*Campylobacter*) *pylori*. J Med Microbiol. 1990;33:277–84.

37. Huang J, Smyth CJ, Kennedy NP, Arbuthnott JP, Keeling PWN. Haemagglutination activity of *Campylobacter pylori*. FEMS Microbiol Lett. 1988;56:109–12.

38. Huang JZ, Keeling PWN, Smyth CJ. Identification of erythrocyte-binding antigens in *Helicobacter pylori*. J Gen Microbiol. 1992;138:1503–13.

39. Slomiany BL, Piotrowski J, Samanta A, VanHorn K, Murty VL, Slomiany A. *Campylobacter pylori* colonization factor shows specificity for lactosylceramide sulfate and GM3 ganglioside. Biochem Int. 1989;19:929–36.

40. Wadström T, Guruge JL, Wei S, Aleljung P, Ljungh A. *Helicobacter pylori* hemagglutinins – possible gut mucosa adhesions. In: Malfertheiner P, Ditschuneit H, editors. *Helicobacter pylori*, gastritis and peptic ulcer. Berlin: Springer-Verlag; 1990:96–103.

41. Lingwood CA, Huesca M, Kuksis A. The glycerolipid receptor for *Helicobacter pylori* (and exoenzyme-S) is phosphatidylethanolamine. Infect Immun. 1992;60:2470–4.

42. Doig P, Austin JW, Kostrzynska M, Trust T. Production of a conserved adhesin by the human gastroduodenal pathogen *Helicobacter pylori*. J Bacteriol. 1992;174:2539–47.

43. Lelwala-Guruge J, Ascencio F, Kreger AS, Ljungh A, Wadstrom T. Isolation of a sialic

acid-specific surface haemagglutinin of *Helicobacter pylori* strain NCTC 11637. Zbl Bakt. 1993;280:93–106.

44. Fauchere JL, Blaser MJ. Adherence of *Helicobacter pylori* cells and their surface components to HeLa cell membranes. Microb Pathog. 1990;9:427–39.
45. Ascencio F, Fransson LA, Wadstrom T. Affinity of the gastric pathogen *Helicobacter pylori* for the N-sulphated glycosaminoglycan heparin sulphate. J Med Microbiol. 1993;38:240–4.
46. Evans DG, Karjalainen TK, Evans DJ, Graham DY, Lee CH. Cloning, nucleotide sequence, and expression of a gene encoding an adhesin subunit protein of *Helicobacter pylori*. J Bacteriol. 1993;175:674–83.
47. Janzon L, Wickman M. Construction of deletion mutants in the *hpaA* gene encoding the binding subunit of fibrillar adhesion of *Helicobacter pylori*. Acta Gastroenterol Belg. 1993;56(S):103.
48. Figueroa G, Portell DP, Soto V, Troncoso M. Adherence of *Helicobacter pylori* to HEp-2 cells. J Infect. 1992;24:263–7.
49. Lingwood CA. *Helicobacter pylori*: receptors and adhesins. In: Goodwin CS, Worsley BW, eds. *Helicobacter pylori*: biology and clinical practice. Boca Raton: CRC Press; 1993:209–22.
50. Lingwood CA, Law H, Pellizzari A, Sherman P, Drumm B. Gastric glycerolipid as a receptor for *Campylobacter pylori*. Lancet. 1989;2:238–41.
51. Saitoh T, Natomi H, Zhao WL et al. Identification of glycolipid receptors for *Helicobacter pylori* by TLC-immunostaining. FEBS. 1991;282:385–7.
52. Lee A, O'Rourke J. Gastric bacteria other than *Helicobacter pylori*. Gastroenterol Clin N Am. 1993;22:21–42.
53. O'Rourke JL, Lee A, Fox JG. *Helicobacter* infection in animals: a clue to the role of adhesion in the pathogenesis of gastroduodenal disease. Eur J Gastroenterol Hepatol. 1992;4:S31–7.
54. Taylor NS, Hasubski AT, Fox JG, Lee A. Haemagglutination profiles of *Helicobacter* species that cause gastritis in man and animals. J Med Microbiol. 1992;37:299–303.
55. Slomiany BL, Bilski J, Sarosiek J et al. *Campylobacter pyloridis* degrades mucin and undermines gastric mucosal integrity. Biochem Biophys Res Commun. 1987;144:307–14.
56. Sidebotham RL, Batten JJ, Karim QN, Spencer J, Baron JH. Breakdown of gastric mucus in presence of *Helicobacter pylori*. J Clin Pathol. 1991;44:52–7.
57. Sarosiek J, Marshall B, Peura DA, Hoffman S, Feng T, McCallum RW. Gastroduodenal mucus gel thickness in patients with *Helicobacter pylori*: a method for assessment of biopsy specimens. Am J Gastroenterol. 1991;86:729–34.
58. Steer HW. Ultrastructure of cell migration through the gastric epithelium and its relationship to bacteria. J Clin Pathol. 1975;28:639–46.
59. Thomsen LL, Gavin JB, Tasman Jones C. Relation of *Helicobacter pylori* to the human gastric mucosa in chronic gastritis of the antrum. Gut. 1990;31:1230–6.
60. Chan WY, Hui PK, Leung KM, Thomas TMM. Modes of *Helicobacter* colonization and gastric epithelial damage. Histopathology. 1992;21:521–8.
61. Hessey SJ, Spencer J, Wyatt JI et al. Bacterial adhesion and disease activity in *Helicobacter* associated chronic gastritis. Gut. 1990;31:134–8.
62. Wyle FA, Tarnawski A, Schulman D, Dabros W. Evidence for gastric mucosal cell invasion by *C. pylori*: an ultrastructural study. J Clin Gastroenterol. 1990;12(Suppl. 1):S92–8.
63. Bode G, Malfertheiner P, Ditschuneit H. Pathogenetic implications of ultrastructural findings in *Campylobacter pylori* related gastroduodenal disease. Scand J Gastroenterol. 1988;23:25–39.
64. Slomiany A, Piotrowski J, Yotsumoto F, Czajkowski A, Slomiany BL. *H. pylori* lipopolysaccharide inhibition of gastric mucosal laminin receptor: effect of sulglycotide. Acta Gastroenterol Belg. 1993;56(S):120.
65. Earlam RJ, Amerigo J, Kakavoulis T, Pollock DJ. Histological appearances of oesophagus, antrum and their correlation with symptoms in patients with a duodenal ulcer. Gut. 1985;26:95–100.
66. Lee A, Fox J, Hazell S. Pathogenicity of *Helicobacter pylori* – a perspective. Infect Immun. 1993;61:1601–10.
67. Genta RM, Graham DY. The gastric cardia in *Helicobacter pylori* infection. Gastroenterology. 1993;104:A86.

68. Lynch DAF, Mapstone NP, Clarke AMT *et al.* Correlation between cell proliferation in *H. pylori* associated gastritis and histological scoring using the Sydney system. Acta Gastroenterol Belg. 1993;56(S):54.
69. Jonsson KA, Strom M, Bodemar G, Norrby K. Histological changes in the gastroduodenal mucosa after long-term medical treatment with cimetidine or parietal cell vagotomy in patients with juxtapyloric ulcer disease. Scand J Gastroenterol. 1988;23:433–41.
70. Danon SJ, O'Rourke JL, Lee A. The importance of local acid production on the distribution of *Helicobacter* spp. in the gastric mucosa. Acta Gastroenterol Belg. 1993;56(Suppl.):109.
71. Dixon MF. Reflux gastritis. Acta Gastroenterol Belg. 1989;52:292–6.
72. O'Connor HJ, Dixon MF, Wyatt JI *et al.* Effect of duodenal ulcer surgery and enterogastric reflux on *Campylobacter pyloridis*. Lancet. 1986;2:1178–81.
73. Dixon M. Acid, ulcers, and *H. pylori*. Lancet. 1993;342:384–5.
74. Alexander M. Introduction to soil microbiology. New York: John Wiley & Sons; 1961:472.
75. Mendz GL, Hazell SL. Pathways of glucose metabolism in *Helicobacter pylori*. Acta Gastroenterol Belg. 1993;56(S):44.
76. Mendz GL, Hazell SL. Glucose phosphorylation in *Helicobacter pylori*. Arch Biochem Biophys. 1993;300:522–5.
77. Mendz GL, Hazell SL, Burns BP. Glucose utilisation by *Helicobacter pylori*. J Gen Microbiol. 1993 (in press).
78. Mendz GL, Hazell SL. Evidence for a pentose phosphate pathway in *Helicobacter pylori*. FEMS Lett. 1991;84:331–6.

Section II
Prevalence and mechanisms of spread of *H. pylori*

5
Epidemiology of *H. pylori* in Western countries

B. J. MARSHALL

INTRODUCTION

Before discussing the epidemiology of *Helicobacter pylori* infection the methodology for cited studies needs to be examined. Ideally, the detection of *H. pylori* should be by a harmless, non-invasive method which does not bias the selection of those being tested. At present the best method appears to be the $[^{13}C]$urea breath test, which also has the advantage of being given with food so that even small children can be easily tested. The disadvantage of the test is that it takes 60 min, so that persons tested are likely to be those with time to spare, possibly leading to an over-representation of unemployed persons, a lower socioeconomic group. The $[^{13}C]$urea breath test gives a sensitivity and specificity of at least 95%, and has been used in epidemiological studies of the southern USA by Graham *et al.* in Texas[1].

Serological testing can be done on large numbers of persons, with far less effort. The disadvantage is that a needlestick is involved. Serological studies therefore might select a group of persons who are willing to assist medical research, or who volunteer as blood donors. Thus serological studies might sample a higher socioeconomic group. Serological tests which detect specific IgG directed towards *H. pylori* have been shown to be highly accurate in volunteers and patients, with a sensitivity and specificity of around 95%[2].

PREVALENCE OF *H. PYLORI* IN WESTERN COUNTRIES

Figure 1 shows the seroprevalence of *H. pylori* in several Western countries, including Australia[3], the USA[2,4,5], the UK[6], Netherlands[7], Austria[8], France[9], Japan[10], the UK[11], Italy[12], Finland[13], New Zealand[14], Ireland[15], Israel[16] and Greece[17].

The most obvious feature of the prevalence curves is that *H. pylori* is more common in older persons. Note also that some of the curves run parallel to the X-axis below the age of 40 years, then rise between 40 and 60 years, but

75

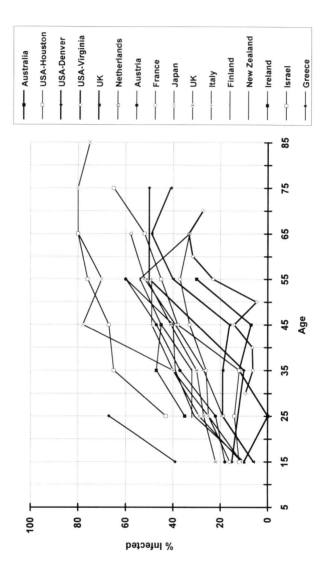

Fig. 1 Prevalence of *H. pylori* in Western countries

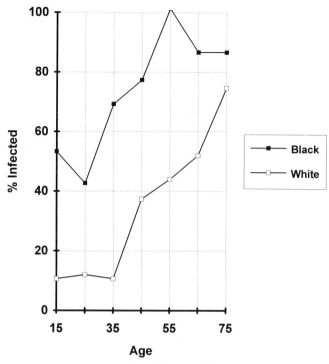

Fig. 2 Relationship between age and *H. pylori* according to race

level out again after 60. In a few studies prevalence has even decreased slightly after age 60. An apparent increasing prevalence with age led many to believe that *H. pylori* was commonly acquired in adulthood with an acquisition rate of 1–2% per annum. As discussed below, however, this may not actually be so.

The truth behind the rising prevalence of *H. pylori* with age may be seen in Figs 2 and 3. In the study descibed in Fig. 2, black volunteers in Houston were more than twice as likely to be infected with *H. pylori* than whites. This increased prevalence could have been either racial or socioeconomic. Figure 3, however, shows that even whites have a high prevalence of *H. pylori* infection when they are poor. Figure 3 can be used to predict *H. pylori* prevalence in whites throughout the USA. Referring to Fig. 1, for example, in Charlottesville, Virginia, where average family income is \$40 000 per annum, only 15% of white blood donors have *H. pylori*[5]. In Houston blacks, however, no good correlation between *H. pylori* prevalence and income was seen. This may be because improved living conditions take at least one generation to affect prevalence in the population. For example, even affluent blacks in Houston may have had a poorer childhood socioeconomic status.

Further light has been thrown on this point by a study reported by Mendall *et al.*[18]. They looked at *H. pylori* serological status and tried to correlate it with various socioeconomic indicators. The most outstanding

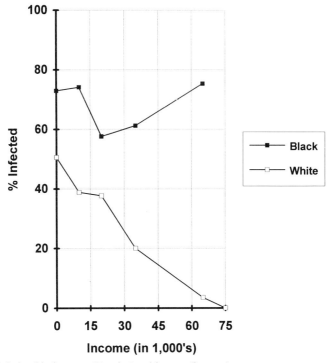

Fig. 3 Relationship between *H. pylori* and income (by race)

predictors of infection were related to childhood socioeconomic status. The presence of hot running water in the family home, and the number of persons per room in the house, were the most important predictors of *H. pylori*. *H. pylori* was particularly common in adults who had more than one person per room in their home during childhood.

In general, the following statements can be made to summarize prevalence of *H. pylori* in Western countries:

1. *H. pylori* affects about 20% of persons below the age of 40 years, and 50% of those above the age of 60 years.
2. *H. pylori* is uncommon in young children.
3. Low socioeconomic status predicts *H. pylori* infection.
4. Immigration is responsible for isolated areas of high prevalence in some Western countries.

SOURCE AND MODE OF TRANSMISSION

Faecal–oral spread

H. pylori has not been detected to any extent in the environment, so transmission is probably from close contact between humans. In the Gambia,

Thomas was able to isolate *H. pylori* from the stools of nine of 23 children below the age of 2 years[19]. The high prevalence of *H. pylori* in young Gambian children suggests that faecal–oral spread is the main route of infection. In Western countries, faecal–oral spread is less common in early life because families are smaller, there is less crowding, and the background prevalence of infection is far lower.

Faecal–oral spread may be an important source of infection for nursing staff or sanitation workers exposed to faecal matter. Wilhoite *et al.*[20] found a higher serological prevalence of *H. pylori* in nurses. Age and duration of nursing career were determinants of *H. pylori* prevalence, with approximately 50% of nurses infected compared to 30% of age-matched controls.

Oral–oral spread and contaminated secretions

The importance of an *H. pylori* reservoir in the oropharynx is undecided at present. Investigators have been able to detect the *Helicobacter genus* 16S-RNA urease gene by polymerase chain reaction (PCR)[21] and some have even been able to culture *H. pylori* from dental plaque[22]. However, even with PCR, the prevalence of plaque infection in infected patients has not exceeded 40% and the viability of this *Helicobacter* genetic material is uncertain. It is known, however, that *H. pylori* can be cultured from gastric juice, so viable organisms certainly do reflux up to the oropharynx. Dentists have not been found to have a higher prevalence of *H. pylori* than controls, although some dental hygienists may have an increased prevalence[23].

Oral–oral spread of *H. pylori* may be of relevance in some occupational groups. Mitchell *et al.*[24] demonstrated that Australian gastroenterologists have a clearly increased prevalence of *H. pylori* infection consistent with the known fact that gastroenterologists did not routinely wear gloves for endoscopy prior to 1983, and the biopsy channel of endoscopes at that time was located very near the endoscopist's mouth. In Mitchell's study, 52% of senior gastroenterologists were infected; exactly twice that of the control group.

INCIDENCE OF NEW INFECTION, SPONTANEOUS CURE AND REINFECTION

The ultimate prevalence of any infectious disease in the community is related to the incidence of new infections, the duration of the infection and the rate at which the infection is cured. The incidence of new *H. pylori* infection has been studied by only a few investigators, who have been able to obtain serial serum samples from large population groups over at least a 10-year period.

Parsonnet *et al.*[25] studied serum samples from doctors recruited to the Centers for Disease Control in Atlanta. These recruits had serum stored from before 1970 with further samples taken 10 and up to 20 years later. It was thus possible to estimate the seroconversion rate over an average 12-year follow-up period. The incidence of new infection was low, less than 1%

Table 1   *H. pylori* seroconversion rate in the USA[25]

Initial status	No. of subjects	No. who changed status over 12 years	Change per annum (%)	Net change per annum (%)
H. pylori-negative	278	11 (neg. to pos.)	+0.3	
H. pylori-positive	63	6 (pos. to neg.)	−0.7	1.2

per annum, and was partially neutralized by a similar incidence of spontaneous cure. The incidence of new infection was not enough to explain the rising prevalence of *H. pylori* seen with age in most Western countries and led the authors to suggest that incidence is less today than it was before 1970. This declining incidence was reflected in the prevalence of *H. pylori* in 30-year-old CDC recruits in 1968 (42%) versus those recruited after 1974 (20%).

The net change in prevalence over time is also related to the net rate of spontaneous cure. In Parsonnet's study spontaneous cure was reported in less than 1% of persons. In an earlier longitudinal study done between 1975 and 1980, Ormiston, Gear and Codling[26] reported a 5-year follow-up of gastritis in 50 patients rebiopsied after 5 years. Of these, 37 had gastritis on initial biopsy. Gastritis healed in only two, but improved in five others. If we say that between two and seven of these had reversion from *H. pylori*-positive to *H. pylori*-negative, then the spontaneous cure rate was between 1% and 3.7% per annum. In the Ormiston *et al.* study two of 11 normal patients developed gastritis in the 5-year follow-up period, an incidence rate of 3.6% per annum. Thus it appears that the net prevalence of *H. pylori* in Western countries has been static, and may even have decreased, in recent decades.

Reinfection is uncommon in Western countries; usually less than 1% per annum. Data to support this come from a study by Forbes *et al.*[27], in which patients in Perth, Australia, were followed up 7 years after *H. pylori* eradication. Reinfection rate was less than 1% per annum, similar to that reported earlier by Borody *et al.*[28]. Since spouses are often infected with *H. pylori*, one might ask whether or not infected spouses need to be treated to prevent reinfection of the patient. Cutler and Schubert[29] noted that the presence of an infected spouse does not affect cure rate. Thus early reinfection (before 1 month) seems to be rare.

In Virginia we have followed 300 patients at least 3 months and have seen only three reinfections after proven cure. These three persons all had infected spouses. Allowing for an average infection prevalence of 50% in spouses, it appears that the reinfection rate for a person with an infected spouse is only 2–5% per annum. Therefore, at this time it is not essential routinely to screen for *H. pylori* in asymptomatic spouses of infected patients.

Reinfection in children may be more common according to data reported by Oderda *et al.*[30]. In that report the reinfection rate was 18% after 1 year. Thus eradication therapy may not provide a permanent cure in children where infected siblings provide an easy source of reinfection[31]. It might be useful, therefore, to screen for, and treat, all *H. pylori* cases in the family when the index case is a child.

COMPUTER MODELLING OF PREVALENCE AND INCIDENCE

Data on infection and spontaneous cure rates can be used to predict the epidemiology of *H. pylori* in various populations. An attempt to generate known prevalence curves using constant infection rates is shown in Fig. 4a. The spontaneous remission rate of 1% per annum is used in all the shown curves. It can be seen that an infection rate of 8% per annum approximates the curve seen for some Third World countries. In contrast, however, a 1% infection rate does not completely explain the low prevalence of *H. pylori* in young whites in the USA, or the far greater proportion of infected persons seen after the age of 50 years.

If a changing incidence is allowed, however, the curve shown in Fig. 4b can be developed. This shows a constant (Third World) infection rate of 8% per annum for persons born before 1943, with a rate which halved in each of the subsequent 5 years until 1963 when a stable incidence rate of 0.5% per annum was achieved. This curve can be seen to approximate that of the epidemiology of *H. pylori* in the USA and other Western countries where the current incidence of *H. pylori* is low.

One other observation which has puzzled some authors is an apparent decline of *H. pylori* in persons above the age of 60. In a study of New Zealand endoscopy patients the prevalence was 64% at 65 years, but declined to less than 40% by age 90[32]. This can also be explained by the computer model. In any population with an initial prevalence of 65% an incidence of 0.5% or less per annum and spontaneous cure rate of at least 1% per annum will cause the prevalence to decrease towards 33%. Thus elderly patients will, on average, have a declining prevalence of *H. pylori* over time.

CONCLUSION: A DECLINING DISEASE IN WESTERN COUNTRIES

The epidemiological data indicate that *H. pylori* epidemiology is compatible with a cohort effect, in that cohorts born before 1940 have a far greater incidence of infection than subsequent cohorts. It appears that *H. pylori* was a declining disease in Western countries, even before it was rediscovered in 1981. The high prevalence of *H. pylori* in persons older than 60 years of age reflects the conditions present when they were children. Before 1940, average socioeconomic status and public health standards were poor, even in the USA. In European countries, social dislocation after the Second World War (1940–1955) probably maintained these poor conditions so that an observed decrease in *H. pylori* prevalence was delayed. Where living standards have improved rapidly, such as Japan and emerging Asian nations, we may expect a precipitous decline in the prevalence of *H. pylori* in younger persons.

SUMMARY

The epidemiology of *H. pylori* in Western countries shows a consistent pattern, with the disease being uncommon in persons below the age of 40 years but rising in prevalence after that to reach approximately 50% in most

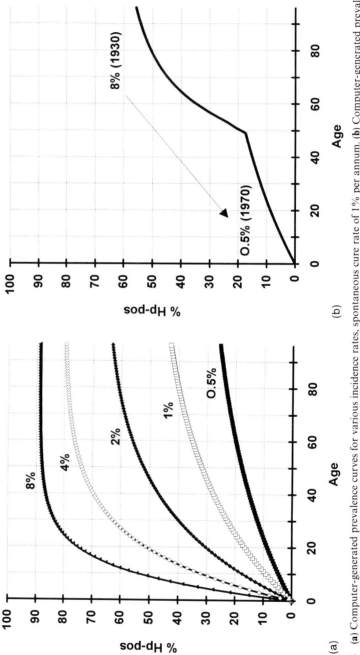

Fig. 4 (a) Computer-generated prevalence curves for various incidence rates, spontaneous cure rate of 1% per annum. (b) Computer-generated prevalence curve for changing incidence (see text)

groups of elderly persons. Since there is no evidence for increasing infection rates during life, the apparent 1% increase per annum must be explained in other ways. Data from several studies show that the prevalence of *H. pylori* changes very little over the lifetime of any studied group, and that *H. pylori* has been decreasing in prevalence with a 50% reduction in the past 25 years. This can all be explained by the concept of birth cohorts. *H. pylori* was far more common in the environment of persons born before the Second World War (1940–45) but has decreased greatly since then. In computer models the epidemiological data can best be reproduced by a cohort effect with a rapid decline in incidence between 1940 and 1960.

References

1. Graham DY, Klein PD, Evans DJ Jr *et al. Campylobacter pylori* detected noninvasively by the ^{13}C-urea breath test. Lancet. 1987;1:1174–7.
2. Perez Perez GI, Dworkin BM, Chodos JE, Blaser MJ. *Campylobacter pylori* antibodies in humans. Ann Intern Med. 1988;109:11–17.
3. Dwyer B, Kaldor J, Tee W, Marakowski E, Raios K. Antibody response to *Campylobacter pylori* in diverse ethnic groups. Scand J Infect Dis. 1988;20:349–50.
4. Graham DY, Malaty HM, Evans DG, Evans DJ, Klein PD, Adam E. Epidemiology of *H. pylori* in an asymptomatic population in the United States. Effect of age, race and socioeconomic status. Gastroenterology. 1991;100:1495–501.
5. Marshall BJ, Caldwell SH, Yu ZJ, Darr F, Chang T, McCallum RW. Prevalence of *C. pylori* and history of upper GI investigation in healthy Virginians. Gastroenterology. 1989;96(Suppl.2):A321(abstract).
6. Jones DM, Eldridge J, Fox AJ *et al.* Antibody to gastric *Campylobacter*-like organism ('*Campylobacter pyloridis*') – clinical correlations and distribution in the normal population. J Med Microbiol. 1986;22:57.
7. Loffeld RJ, Stobberingh E, van Spreeuwel JP, Flendrig JA, Arends JW. The prevalence of anti-*Helicobacter* (*Campylobacter*) *pylori* antibodies in patients and healthy blood donors. J Med Microbiol. 1990;32:105–9.
8. Hirschl AM. Frequency of occurrence of *Campylobacter pylori* and analysis of the systemic and local immune response. Zentralbl Bakteriol Mikrobiol Hyg. 1987[A];266:526.
9. Megraud F, Brassens Rabbe MP, Denis F, Belbouri A, Hoa DQ. Seroepidemiology of *Campylobacter pylori* infection in various populations. J Clin Microbiol. 1989;27:1870–3.
10. Asaka M, Kimura T, Kudo M *et al.* Relationship of *H. pylori* to serum pepsinogens in an asymptomatic Japanese population. Gastroenterology. 1992;102:760–6.
11. Newell DG, Claygill CPJ, Stacey AR *et al.* The distribution of anti-*C. pylori* antibodies in patients undergoing endoscopy and in the normal population relative to age and geographical distribution. In Takemoto T, Kawai K, Shimoyama T, editors. *Campylobacter pylori* and gastroduodenal diseases, Vol. 2. Tokyo, Taisho; 1990:54.
12. Vaira D, Miglioi M, Holton J *et al.* Prevalence of IgG antibodies to *H. pylori* in Italian blood donors. Rev Esp Enferm Dig. 1990;78(Suppl.1):46.
13. Kosunen TU, Hook J, Rautelin HI, Myllyla G. Age-dependent increase of *Campylobacter pylori* antibodies in blood donors. Scand J Gastroenterol. 1989;24:110–14.
14. Morris A, Nicholson G, Lloyd G, Haines D, Rogers A, Taylor D. Seroepidemiology of *Campylobacter pyloridis*. NZ Med J. 1986;99:657–9.
15. Basso L, Clune J, Beattie S *et al.* Epidemiology of *H. pylori* infection. Rev Esp Enferm Dig. 19990;78(Suppl.I):40.
16. Fich A, Carel R, Keret D *et al.* Seroepidemiology of *H. pylori* in the Israeli population. Gastroenterology. 1992;102:A68.
17. Pateraki E, Mentis A, Spiliadis C *et al.* Seroepidemiology of *H. pylori* infection in Greece. FEMS Microbiol Immunol. 1990;2:129–36.
18. Mendall MA, Goggin PM, Molineaux N *et al.* Childhood living conditions and *H. pylori* seropositivity in adult life. Lancet. 1992;339:896–7.

19. Thomas JE, Gibson GR, Darboe MK, Dale A, Weaver LT. Isolation of *H. pylori* from human faeces. Lancet. 1993;340:1194–5.
20. Wilhoite SL, Ferguson DA Jr, Soike DR, Kalbfleisch JH, Thomas E. Increased prevalence of *H. pylori* antibodies among nurses. Arch Intern Med. 1993;153:708–12.
21. Nguyen AM, Engstrand L, Genta RM, Graham DY, el Zaatari FA. Detection of *H. pylori* in dental plaque by reverse transcription–polymerase chain reaction. J Clin Microbiol. 1993;31:783–7.
22. Shames B, Krajden S, Fuksa M, Babida C, Penner JL. Evidence for the occurrence of the same strain of *Campylobacter pylori* in the stomach and dental plaque. J Clin Microbiol. 1989;27:2849–50.
23. Malaty HM, Evans DJ Jr, Abramovitch K, Evans DG, Graham DY. *H. pylori* infection in dental workers: a seroepidemiology study. Am J Gastroenterol. 1992;87:1728–31.
24. Mitchell HM, Lee A, Carrick J. Increased incidence of *Campylobacter pylori* infection in gastroenterologists: further evidence to support person-to-person transmission of *C. pylori*. Scand J Gastroenterol. 1989;24:396–400.
25. Parsonnet J, Blaser MJ, Perez Perez GI, Hargrett Bean N, Tauxe RV. Symptoms and risk factors of *H. pylori* infection in a cohort of epidemiologists. Gastroenterology. 1992;102:41–6.
26. Ormiston MC, Gear MWL, Codling BW. Five year follow-up study of gastritis. J Clin Pathol. 1982;35:757–60.
27. Forbes GM, Glaser ME, Cullen DJE, Warren JR, Marshall BJ, Collins BJ. Seven year follow-up of duodenal ulcer treated with *H. pylori* eradication therapy (Submitted).
28. Borody TJ, Cole P, Noonan S *et al.* Recurrence of duodenal ulcer and *Campylobacter pylori* infection after eradication. Med J Aust. 1989;151:431–5.
29. Cutler AF, Schubert TT. Patient factors affecting *H. pylori* eradication with triple therapy. Am J Gastroenterol. 1993;88:505–9.
30. Oderda G, Vaira D, Ainley C *et al.* Eighteen month follow up of *H. pylori* positive children treated with amoxycillin and tinidazole. Gut. 1992;33:1328–30.
31. Oderda G, Vaira D, Holton J *et al. H. pylori* in children with peptic ulcer and their families. Dig Dis Sci. 1991;36:572–6.
32. Bateson MC. *H. pylori* infection with age. Lancet. 1992;339:1121.

6
H. pylori in developing countries

S. L. HAZELL

Discussion of *Helicobacter pylori* infection in developing countries represents a fascinating challenge, as it cannot be assumed that populations living in diverse countries designed 'developing' share sufficient habits, traditions or social identity to be treated as a single group. Despite this potential complication we may be able to learn from studies of health and disease within such societies much about the transmission of *H. pylori* and the precise role this organism plays in upper gastrointestinal disease.

It has been suggested that in developing countries infection with *H. pylori* induces more gastric cancer than peptic ulcer disease, whereas in the developed world the reverse is true[1-4]. This view, however, is not consistent with our group's findings in China, nor with the findings of other groups throughout the world[5,6] (Table 1). Thus, although in general *H. pylori* infection is more prevalent in developing countries than developed countries, the designation of a country as either 'developed' or 'developing' appears insufficient to predict the profile of upper gastrointestinal disease. Furthermore, even within 'developed' countries there are populations that could be said to have *H. pylori* infection patterns not unlike those seen in developing countries[7,8]. Indeed, the apparent *H. pylori* infection rates in Japanese, both in Japan and elsewhere, have characteristics more in common with some populations found in the developing world than with their economic counterparts in Europe and America[9,10].

Table 1 Comparison of the incidence of gastrointestinal disease in dyspeptic patients from developed and developing countries

Study locations	Number of patients	Percentage incidence of disease		Ratio of duodeal ulcer to gastric ulcer
		Duodenal ulcer	Gastric cancer	
U.K./Norway[4]	2883	11.6	1.0	2:1
Peru[4]	1796	5.2	4.5	1.2:1
Southern China[5]	1006	35.6	2.4	10.2:1
Northern China*	199	17.6	9.1	3.2:1

*Unpublished data

So where does this leave our understanding of the role of *H. pylori* in upper gastrointestinal disease in the 'developing' world? We have suggested that a higher prevalance of *H. pylori* infection will lead to a higher overall prevalence of upper gastrointestinal disease; however, the form of such disease may be dictated by the habits and traditions of the people as well as socioeconomic and environmental factors[5]. To prove this is so, our task is to determine the infection patterns in different populations and to look for the factors that influence the development of particular disease profiles. In short, we need good epidemiological studies. Once we have these data it may be possible to identify triggers that are responsible for the diverse disease processes associated with *H. pylori* infection.

In undertaking the above, we need to avoid small, poorly planned studies; for while such studies have given us some direction in the past, in the future they will only serve to cloud our understanding of disease processes. Fortunately we can now work from a base of an established aetiological relationship between *H. pylori*, gastritis and peptic ulcer disease[11-14]. Also, there is now a *prima-facie* case establishing a link between infection with *H. pylori* and the development of gastric cancer[10,15-17].

PREVALENCE OF *H. PYLORI* IN DEVELOPING NATIONS

To understand the significance of *H. pylori* in the developing world, data on the current rate of infection within regions are required. A brief review of the present knowledge regarding the prevalence of *H. pylori* in developing countries will be presented below.

Latin America has been the location of some of the earliest studies looking at the epidemiology of *H. pylori* infection. In Peru a high prevalence of *H. pylori* infection has been reported[18,19]. In Lima, Klein *et al.*[19] found the prevalence of *H. pylori* infection in 407 children aged 2 months to 12 years to be 48%. Within this group the number of infected individuals increased rapidly with age. Although *H. pylori* infection was found in both wealthy and poor families, the prevalence of infection was shown to be higher among children from low-income families compared to that in high-income families (56% vs 32%). In a large serological study based in Chile, it was also found that *H. pylori* infection was more prevalent in people of lower socioeconomic status[20]. Interestingly, the investigators in the Chilean study noted that the differences among socioeconomic groups could be detected only at and after the age of 4 years.

Studies in patient groups in Peru support the perception that there is a high prevalence of *H. pylori* infection in that country[4,21]. In coastal Peru, the Amazon jungle and the Andes Mountains, the prevalence of *H. pylori* infection in symptomatic patients was reported by Ramirez-Ramos *et al.* to be greater than 80%[22], a figure significantly higher than that found in symptomatic patients from developed countries ($\sim 50\%$)[23-25]. In their study, Ramirez-Ramos *et al.*[22] noted that people from the non-coastal regions of Peru had significantly higher rates of infection than did those living on the coast. Whereas the findings within these communities (coastal, high-altitude and jungle) may be related to ethnic and social differences, investigators from the same group[26] found that in dyspeptic patients in Lima, socioeconomic status was not an important factor in the prevalence of *H. pylori* infection. While this finding appears in conflict with the prevalence data of Klein *et al.* cited earlier[19], the disparity may relate to a higher rate of infection in symptomatic individuals irrespective of social order.

In addition to the impact of socioeconomic status on the prevalence of *H. pylori* in parts of Latin America, a slight gender bias has also been noted by some groups. In a study by the Gastrointestinal Physiology Working Group it was noted that women from higher socioeconomic groups had a lower age-specific rate of *H. pylori* infection than women from lower socioeconomic groups and men from all groups[18]. This finding is to a degree in accord with the observations of Ramirez-Ramos *et al.*[22], who found that, in the regions of Peru they studied, the *H. pylori* infection rates for men were in the order of 10% higher than for women. The significance of these observations remains to be determined; however, close examination of the lifestyle of females from higher socioeconomic groups in Peru may give some suggestion as to the usual route of transmission of *H. pylori*.

Studies in other Latin American populations also display a similarly high prevalence of *H. pylori* infection, although again many such studies are based on symptomatic patient populations. High prevalence rates of *H. pylori* infection have been reported in Mexico where Guarner *et al.*[27] found 183 (75%) of 245 symptomatic patients to be seropositive for *H. pylori*. In an area of high gastric cancer mortality in Colombia, Correa *et al.* found an extremely high prevalence of *H. pylori* infection (93%)[7]. Yet in this same report we find that in the United States of America, in an area where gastric cancer rates are high in black persons, the prevalence of *H. pylori* infection in black adults was 70% versus 43% in white adults[7]. Thus within the black population within this region of the United States, the infection profile is similar to that of a developing nation.

Within Asia the prevalence of infection appears, as within Latin America, to be high. In a study of the seroprevalence of *H. pylori* infection in India, Graham *et al.*[28] examined people drawn from the lower socioeconomic classes. The results of this study showed that the frequency of serologically determined *H. pylori* infection rose rapidly in children to around a prevalence of 80% by the age of 20 years. In another study in India, Katelaris *et al.*[29] examined the prevalence of *H. pylori* infection in male Tibetan monks (median age 28 years) and found it to be just under 80%. An interesting finding from this study was the lack of correlation between upper abdominal symptoms and infection with *H. pylori*. Despite the high prevalence of *H. pylori* the point prevalence of peptic ulcer disease was relatively low (6.6%); this finding may be partly attributed to the fact that these men do not smoke or ingest non-steroidal anti-inflammatory drugs (NSAID). It should also be noted that, despite the apparent high prevalence of *H. pylori* infection in India, the incidence of gastric cancer is only moderate by world standards[30].

Kolt *et al.*[31] noted a high prevalence of duodenal ulcer disease in Indochinese migrants to Australia; suggestive of a high prevalence of *H.*

pylori within the Indochinese population. Yet Dwyer and associates reported that the seroprevalence of *H. pylori* in Indochinese living in Australia was no different from that in Australian blood donors of European ancestry[32]. Is there something unique about the Indochinese? Megraud *et al.*[33] examined the seroprevalence of *H. pylori* in four countries (France, Vietnam, Algeria and the Ivory Coast). In Vietnam, in marked contrast to Algeria and the Ivory Coast, they found that few children were infected, even though there were very high infection rates in adults. This is an interesting observation; however, this population requires further study and independent confirmation. If verified, re-examination of populations in Vietnam may provide interesting comparative data regarding the transmission of *H. pylori*.

Although there have been a number of studies into the prevalence of *H. pylori* in developing countries, many of these have used small sample numbers and therefore meaningful interpretation of their data is difficult. In our studies in China, adequate sample size from a representative population sample was a major consideration. We conducted a cross-sectional serologically based study involving 1727 people in Guangdong province in southern China as part of an on-going programme to examine the transmission of *H. pylori* and its relationship to disease[34]. The long-term aim of this programme is to develop intervention strategies for the prevention of disease. The overall prevalence of *H. pylori* infection within this sample was 44.2%. A significantly higher prevalence of *H. pylori* was found in the city of Guangzhou (52.4%) compared with that in the rural areas of Guangdong province (38.6%). Comparison of the seroprevalence of *H. pylori* and the data from a questionnaire completed by each individual, indicated that high density of living conditions was related to the acquisition of *H. pylori*. Infection with *H. pylori* was evident from an early age, with 23% of the sample from the children under 5 years of age being seropositive. After 5 years of age the rate of increase in the seroprevalence of *H. pylori* was about 1% per year. This was noted as being similar to the rate of increase in the seroprevalence seen in adults from developed nations. This could suggest that factors that are important in the transmission of infection in children may be different from the factors that are important in adults.

Although the latter study has not answered the question as to how *H. pylori* is transmitted, it has helped us to define the questions that need to be addressed. When in the first 5 years of life are children in southern China, and other developing areas, at greatest risk of infection? What factors, customs or events are associated with infection within the under-5 age group? Which groups in the under-5-year population are at greatest risk of infection? In what way does the transmission in adults differ from that in children? We are currently analysing data from approximately 3000 individuals, including 600 children under 5 years of age, from northern China (an area with a high incidence of gastric cancer) with the hope that some of these questions can be answered. Serological data from this subsequent study show a higher prevalence of infection in young children living in this region than those living in Guangdong province; although there are marked variations within the sample areas from the north region.

TRANSMISSION OF *H. PYLORI*

The major message that comes through most of the epidemiological studies so far conducted in the 'developed' and 'developing' world is that there is a higher incidence of *H. pylori* infection among children in the 'developing' world than in the 'developed'. This in part appears to relate to density of living and socioeconomic factors, as well as the prevalence of infection in the parents of these children. Indeed, if one was looking for the single characteristic that separates the discussion of *H. pylori* infection in developed and developing countries, infection in children would be the issue. Yet it may be argued that in developed nations this a new phenomenon. A recent study by Banatvala *et al.*[35], using sera collected in the United Kingdom between 1969 and 1989, suggests that the incidence of *H. pylori* is falling in developed nations and that a high proportion of current adult infections may be attributed to acquisition of *H. pylori* at or below 15 years of age. That a large proportion of adult infections in developing nations can be attributed to acquisition of infection in childhood is evident. However, is the increasing seroprevalence with age in adults we and others have noted in populations from developing nations the product of a cohort effect, and hence a declining incidence of *H. pylori* infection, or true adult acquisition?

There have been numerous proposals as to the mechanisms of transmission of *H. pylori*. Both the faecal–oral and oral–oral route have been proposed[8,36–40]. Data obtained using techniques for the detection of *H. pylori* DNA (polymerase chain reaction: PCR), indicate that both faeces and saliva/dental plaque contain specific *H. pylori* gene fragments[41–43]. These data alone cannot establish a pattern for the spread of infection, as DNA from non-viable or non-infectious cells could be detected by PCR.

Culture of faeces, saliva and dental plaque in different hands has resulted in the reported isolation of *H. pylori* in a number of cases[39,40,44–48]. The presence of *H. pylori* in the mouth, particularly in saliva[47], supports the argument for oral–oral transmission of the organism by exchange of oral secretions. The use of chopsticks and communal eating habits have been implicated in the transmission of *H. pylori* within Chinese communities outside of China[40,49]. We have also suggested that parents masticating the food of children at weaning could be a vehicle for transmission of infection if the bacterium is present in the mouth. Practices such as communal eating are so widespread in China, that there is probably insufficient power in any analysis to detect significant effects of this and other practices upon the rate of transmission of *H. pylori*.

The recent reports in the *Lancet* of the isolation of *H. pylori* from the faeces of nine of 23 (39%) children in Gambia, where infection rates reach 90% by the age of 5 years, argues in favour of faecal–oral transmission[39], without necessarily eliminating the possibility of oral–oral spread. Because of the potential significance of these reports it is important that molecular studies be used to confirm the identity of the isolates as *H. pylori*. If the faecal–oral route is an important means of transmission of *H. pylori*, special circumstances may be necessary for this to occur. *H. pylori* has been noted to be sensitive to bile salts which would hinder the passage of the organism through the gut[50-53], and some animal studies suggest that faecal–oral transmission is unlikely[36]. However, other animal studies demonstrate that under specific circumstances faecal–oral spread may occur[38]. Fox and associates were able to isolate *H. mustelae* from the faeces of young ferrets but not older animals with established infection by *H. mustelae*[38]. They postulated that this may have been associated with the transient hypochlorhydria that occcurred early in the infection of their study animals[38]. Despite the data summarized above, there appears no clear resolution of the issue of how *H. pylori* is disseminated. Indeed we cannot determine if there is only one mode of transmission. As noted previously, there may be two patterns of infection within populations from developing countries, with a high incidence of infection in young children and a possible 'steady-state' acquisition in adults and different transmission mechanisms.

If faeces are a vehicle for the transmission of *H. pylori*, is it important on a community basis or only in the setting of the family? Familial clustering of infection and the potential for direct person-to-person spread has been noted by several groups[54,58]. A large epidemiological study by Hopkins *et al.* involving children and young adults in Chile, found that infection with *H. pylori* correlated in part with the consumption of uncooked vegetables[20]. The authors of this report considered that contamination of vegetables by water containing raw sewage, and their subsequent consumption without cooking, could be a key factor in the transmission of *H. pylori*. However, as the authors noted, this factor was associated more with older children (>5 years) and unknown confounding factors need to be considered. It should also be noted that there was a weighting given to faecal transmission in the study by Hopkins and associates, as their study was also directed towards understanding the faecal transmission of hepatitis A virus.

Because of the potential association of *H. pylori* infection with particular sources of water[19], in our studies in China we questioned our subjects on their water source and utilization habits. We found no association between water and infection in southern China, and noted that it was a common practice in China to boil drinking water[34].

We have attempted to address the issue of faecal contamination and the transmission of *H. pylori* in China by looking at the prevalence of antibody to hepatitis A in habitants of Guangdong province and correlating this with the seroprevalence of *H. pylori* (manuscript submitted). We selected hepatitis A because it represents a sensitive marker of faecal–oral exposure. Similar comparisons between *H. pylori* infection and the prevalence of hepatitis A antibody have been undertaken in India by Graham *et al.*[28]. When we looked at the data from rural communities in southern China we found a high prevalence of antibody to hepatitis A and a correlation between hepatitis A antibody and the seroprevalence of *H. pylori*. This finding is within broad agreement with the findings of Graham's group[28]. In contrast, when we examined the sera obtained from residents of Guangzhou city a surprising pattern emerged. Again we found a high seroprevalence of hepatitis A; however, whereas in the order of 31% of children under 5 years of age in Guangzhou were infected with *H. pylori*, none of the sera from individuals under the age of 17 years from the same sample had antibody to hepatitis

A. After 17 years of age there was a dramatic increase in the seroprevalence of hepatitis A. Dramatic improvements in hepatitis A infection patterns occur with the introduction of improved sanitation; such as the establishment of sewage treatment facilities[59]. These data suggest that, in Guangzhou, community exposure to faecal contamination does not represent a risk factor for the acquisition of H. pylori.

Most of the debate about the transmission of H. pylori has centred upon mechanisms of horizontal transmission (adult-to-adult, adult-to-child, child-to-child and even child-to-adult). In a number of the larger studies cited above, high rates of infection have been reported in young children (under 5 years). We have argued previously that because infection with H. pylori prevails in most populations, this organism may be considered to be 'almost normal microbiota (flora)'[60]. In China we have shown that there is a correlation between the rate of infection in adults of childbearing age and the rate of infection in children[34]. This suggests adult-to-child horizontal transmission in the early years of life is common, and that infection with H. pylori may be analogous to the normal process by which the autochthonous microbiota of the gut is established.

Acknowledgements

Our team's original research in China was supported by a grant from the International Development Program of Australian Colleges and Universities. The studies in China would not have been possible without the cooperation of a number of individuals. I would like to acknowledge in particular Drs HU Pinjin and LI Yuyuan from Guangzhou, whose knowledge and organizational skills have been the major driving force within China, and Dr Hazel Mitchell who has contributed significantly to the planning and operation of the programme. Professor Adrian Lees is thanked for his encouragement and support over many years.

References

1. Sipponen P, Hyvarinen H. Role of *Helicobacter pylori* in the pathogenesis of gastritis, peptic ulcer and gastric cancer. Scand J Gastroenterol. 1993;28 (Suppl. 196):3–6.
2. Sitas F, Forman D, Yarnell JW et al. *Helicobacter pylori* infection rates in relation to age and social class in a population of Welsh men. Gut. 1991;32:25–8.
3. Graham DY. *Campylobacter pylori* and peptic ulcer disease. Gastroenterology. 1989;96: 615–25.
4. Burstein M, Monge E, Leon BR et al. Low peptic ulcer and high gastric cancer prevalence in a developing country with a high prevalence of infection by *Helicobacter pylori*. J Clin Gastroenterol. 1991;13:154–6.
5. Hu PJ, Li YY, Zhou MH et al. *Helicobacter pylori* and upper gastrointestinal disease. No direct correlation between the incidence of disease and the prevalence of infection. Gut (Submitted).
6. Lam SK. Peptic ulcer: from epidemiology to cause. J Gastroenterol Hepatol. 1989;2:1–6.
7. Correa P, Fox J, Fontham E et al. *Helicobacter pylori* and gastric carcinoma. Serum antibody prevalence in populations with contrasting cancer risks. Cancer. 1990;66: 2569–74.

8. Graham DY, Malaty HM, Evans DG, Evans DJJ, Klein PD, Adam E. Epidemiology of *Helicobacter pylori* in an asymptomatic population in the United States. Effect of age, race, and socioeconomic status. Gastroenterology. 1991;100:1495–501.
9. Inouye H, Yamamoto I, Tanida N *et al. Campylobacter pylori* in Japan: bacteriological feature and prevalence in healthy subjects and patients with gastroduodenal disorders. Gastroenterol Jpn. 1989;24:494–504.
10. Nomura A. Stemmermann GN. *Helicobacter pylori* and gastric cancer. J Gastroenterol Hepataol. 1993;8:294–303.
11. Coghlan J, Hutchinson L, Giligan D *et al.* Dosage of colloidal bismuth subcitrate in duodenal ulcer healing and clearance of *Campylobacter pylori*. Aliment Pharmacol Ther. 1990;4:49–54.
12. Marshall BJ, Goodwin CS, Warren JR *et al.* Prospective double-blind trial of duodenal ulcer relapse after eradication of *Campylobacter pylori*. Lancet. 1998;2:1437–42.
13. Bayerdörffer E, Mannes GA, Sommer A *et al.* Long-term follow-up after eradication of *Helicobacter pylori* with a combination of omeprazole and amoxycillin. Scand J Gastroenterol. 1993;28 (Supl. 196):19–25.
14. Graham DY, Lew GM, Klein PD *et al.* Effect of treatment of *Helicobacter pylori* infection on the long-term recurrence of gastric or duodenal ulcer, a randomized, controlled study. Ann Intern Med. 1992;116:705–8.
15. Parsonnet J, Friendman GD, Vandersteen DP *et al. Helicobacter pylori* infection and the risk of gastric carcinoma. N Engl J Med. 1991;325:1127–31.
16. Forman D. *Helicobacter pylori* infection: a novel risk factor in the etiology of gastric cancer. J. Natl Cancer Inst. 1991;83:1702–3.
17. Forman D, Coleman M, Debacker G *et al.* An international association between *Helicobacter pylori* infection and gastric cancer. Lancet. 1993;341:1359–62.
18. Gastrointestinal Physiology Working Group. *Helicobacter pylori* and gastritis in Peruvian patients: relationship to socioeconomic level, age and sex. Am J Gastroenterol. 1990;85:819–23.
19. Klein PD, Gastrointestinal Physiology Working Group, Graham DY, Gaillour A, Opckun AR, Smith EO. Water source as risk factor for *Helicobacter pylori* infection in Peruvian children. Lancet. 1991;337:1503–6.
20. Hopkins RJ, Vial PA, Ferreccio C *et al.* Seroprevalence of *Helicobacter pylori* in Chile – vegetables may serve as one route of transmission. J Infect Dis. 1993;168:222–6.
21. Gastrointestinal Physiology Working Group. *Helicobacter pylori* and gastritis in Peruvian patients: relationship to socioeconomic level, age and sex. Am J Gastroenterol. 1990;85:819–23.
22. Ramirez-Ramos A, Gilman R, Spira W *et al.* Ecology of *Helicobacter pylori* in Peru – infection rates in coastal, high altitude, and jungle communities. Gut. 1992;33:604–5.
23. Hazell SL, Hennessy WB, Borody TJ *et al. Campylobacter pyloridis* gastritis. II: Distribution of bacteria and associated inflammation in the gastroduodenal environment. Am J Gastroenterol. 1987;82:297–301.
24. Hazell SL, Borody TJ, Gal A, Lee A. *Campylobacter pyloridis* gastritis. I: Detection of urease as a marker of bacterial colonization and gastritis. Am J Gastroenterol. 1987;82:292–6.
25. Bayerdörffer E, Oertel H, Lehn N *et al.* Topographic association between active gastritis and *Campylobacter pylori* colonisation. J Clin Pathol. 1989;42:834–9.
26. Ramirez-Ramos A, Hurtado-Munoz O, Rodriguez-Ulloa C *et al. Campylobacter pyloridis* and socioeconomic levels. Acta Gastroenterol Latinoam. 1987;17:35–42.
27. Guarner J, Mohar A, Parsonnet J, Halperin D. The association of *Helicobacter pylori* with gastric cancer and preneoplastic gastric lesions in Chiapas, Mexico. Cancer. 1993;71:297–301.
28. Graham DY, Adam E, Reddy GT *et al.* Seroepidemiology of *Helicobacter pylori* infection in India. Comparison of developing and developed countries. Dig Dis Sci. 1991;36:1084–8.
29. Katclaris PH, Tippett HK, Norbu P, Lower DG, Brennan R, Farthing MJG. Dyspepsia, *Helicobacter pylori*, and peptic ulcer in a randomly selected population in India. Gut. 1992;33:1462–6.
30. Whelan SL, Parkin DM, Masuyer E (Eds). Patterns of Cancer in Five Continents, World Health Organization. Lyon: International Agency for Research on Cancer; 1990.

31. Kolt SD, Kronborg IJ, Yeomans ND. High prevalence of duodenal ulcer in Indochinese immigrants attending an Australian university hospital. J Gastroenterol Hepatol. 1993;8:128–32.

32. Dwyer B, Kaldor J, Tee W, Marakowski E, Raios K. Antibody response to *Campylobacter pylori* in diverse ethnic groups. Scand J Infect Dis. 1988;20:349–50.

33. Megraud F, Brassens Rabbe MP, Denis F, Belbouri A, Hoa DQ. Seroepidemiology of *Campylobacter pylori* infection in various populations. J Clin Microbiol. 1989;27:1870–3.

34. Mitchell HM, Li YY, Hu PJ *et al.* Epidemiology of *Helicobacter pylori* in Southern China – identification of early childhood as the critical period for acquisition. J Infect Dis. 1992;166:149–53.

35. Banatvala N, Mayo K, Megraud F, Jennings R, Deeks JJ, Feldman RA. The cohort effect and *Helicobacter pylori*. J Infect Dis. 1993;168:219–21.

36. Fox JG, Lee A, Otto G, Taylor NS, Murphy JC. *Helicobacter felis* gastritis in gnotobiotic rats: an animal model of *Helicobacter pylori* gastritis. Infect Immun. 1991;59:785–91.

37. Lee A, Fox JG, Otto G, Dick EH, Krakowka S. Transmission of *Helicobacter* spp.: a challenge to the dogma of faecal-oral spread. Epidemiol Infect. 1991;107:99–109.

38. Fox JG, Paster BJ, Dewhits FE *et al.* *Helicobacter mustelae* isolation for feces in ferrets: evidence to support fecal-oral transmission of a gastric helicobacter. Infect Immun. 1992;60:606–11.

39. Thomas JE, Gibson GR, Darboe MK, Dale A, Weaver LT. Isolation of *Helicobacter pylori* from human faeces. Lancet. 1992;340:1194–5.

40. Birac C, Traore A, Albenque M, Labigne A, Megraud F. Possible oral–oral transmission of *Helicobacter pylori* from mothers to children. V International Congress of Pediatric Laboratory Medicine – Bordeaux, France. 10–12 June 1992.

41. Banatvala N, Lopez CR, Owen R *et al.* *Helicobacter pylori* in dental plaque. Lancet. 1993;341:380.

42. Mapstone NP, Lynch DAF, Lewis FAC *et al.* Identification of *Helicobacter pylori* DNA in the mouths and stomachs of patients with gastritis using PCR. J Clin Pathol. 1993;46: 540–3.

43. Nguyen AMH, Engstrand L, Genta RM, Graham DY, Elzaatari FAK. Detection of *Helicobacter pylori* in dental plaque by reverse transcription polymerase chain reaction. J Clin Microbiol. 1993;31:783–7.

44. Shames B, Krajden S, Fuksa M, Babida C, Penner JL. Evidence for the occurrence of the same strain of *Campylobacter pylori* in the stomach and dental plaque. J Clin Microbiol. 1989;27:2849–50.

45. Krajden S, Fuksa M. Anderson J *et al.* Examination of human stomach biopsies, saliva, and dental plaque for *Campylobacter pylori*. J Clin Microbiol. 1989;27:1397–8.

46. Majmudar P, Shah SM, Dhunjibhoy KR, Desai HG. Isolation of *Helicobacter pylori* from dental plaques in healthy volunteers. Indian J Gastroenterol. 1990;9:271–2.

47. Ferguson DA Jr, Li C, Patel NR *et al.* Isolation of *Helicobacter pylori* from saliva. J Clin Microbiol. 1993;31:2802–4.

48. Desai HG, Gill HH, Shankaran K *et al.* Dental plaque: a permanent reservoir of *Helicobacter pylori*. Scand J Gastroenterol. 1991;26:1205–8.

49. Chow THF, Lambert JR, Wahlquist ML, Hage BH. The influence of chopstick culture on the epidemiology of *Helicobacter pylori* – a study of two representative populations in Melbourne. Gastroenterology. 1992;120(abstract).

50. Arnaout AH, Abbas SH, Shousha S. *Helicobacter pylori* is not identified in areas of gastric metaplasia of gall bladder. J Pathol. 1990;160:333–4.

51. Dixon MF. Reflux gastritis. Acta Gastroenterol Belg. 1989;52:292–6.

52. Hanninen ML. Sensitivity of *Helicobacter pylori* to different bile salts. Eur J Clin Microbiol Infect Dis. 1991;10:515–18.

53. Mitchell HM, Li YY, Hu P, Hazell SL *et al.* The susceptibility of *Helicobacter pylori* to bile may be an obstacle to faecal transmission. Eur J Gastroenterol Hepatol. 1992;4:79–84.

54. Drumm B, Perez PGI, Blaser MJ, Shermann PM. Intrafamilial clustering of *Helicobacter pylori* infection. N Engl J Med. 1990;322:359–63.

55. Nowottny U, Heilmann KL. Epidemiology of *Helicobacter pylori* infection. Leber Magen Darm. 1990;20:183–6.

56. Mitchell HM, Bohane T, Hawkes RA, Lee A. *Helicobacter pylori* infection within families.

Zentral Bakt (Int J Med Microbiol.) 1993;in press.

57. Mitchell JD, Mitchell HM, Tobias V. Acute *Helicobacter pylori* infection in an infant, associated with gastric ulceration and serological evidence of intra-familial transmission. Am J Gastroenterol. 1992;87:382–6.

58. Mitchell HM, Bohane TD, Berkowicz J, Hazell SL, Lee A. Antibody to *Campylobacter pylori* in families of index children with gastrointestinal illness due to *C pylori*. Lancet. 1987;2:681–2.

59. Boughton CR, Hawkes RA, Ferguson V. Viral hepatitis A and B. Med J Aust. 1980;1: 177–80.

60. Lee A, Hazell SL. *Campylobacter pylori* in health and disease: an ecological perspective. Microbial Ecol Health Dis. 1988;1:1–16.

7
Prevalence/disease correlates of *H. pylori*

J. R. LAMBERT and S.K. LIN

INTRODUCTION

Helicobacter pylori infects a high percentage of the world's adult population. Results from different countries, using endoscopic studies, have determined the prevalence of *H. pylori* in upper gastrointestinal tract disease. *H. pylori* is primarily found in the antrum and body of the stomach, but is also seen in the duodenum within areas of gastric metaplasia and in the fundus[1-3]. It does not colonize metaplastic intestinal epithelium in the stomach[4,5]. *H. pylori* infection causes histological chronic antral gastritis with activity. All diseases associated with antral gastritis are also associated with *H. pylori* infections, including duodenal ulcer, gastric ulcer, and gastric carcinoma. An aetiological role for this organism in duodenal ulcer, gastric ulcer and gastric carcinoma is still unclear, although evidence strongly supports a major role. This chapter will review the prevalence of *H. pylori* infection in human upper gastrointestinal diseases.

HISTOLOGICAL GASTRITIS

The strong association of *H. pylori* infection with chronic gastritis has been reported world-wide. The prevalence of *H. pylori* infection in active chronic gastritis has been reported from 70% to 92%, and is summarized in Table 1. The differences reported are due to different techniques and diagnostic criteria used. The frequency of *H. pylori* positivity in active chronic gastritis is much higher than with inactive gastritis. Epidemiological studies of different communities have shown that the prevalence of gastritis is similar to the prevalence of *H. pylori* infection[11-15]. The rate of acquisition of gastritis is approximately 1% per year[16]. This is similar to the acquisition of *H. pylori* in the normal population[12,17]. The prevalence of *H. pylori* in autoimmune gastritis[18], lymphocytic gastritis[19] and bile reflux gastritis found in postoperative stomachs[20] is low. In both NSAID-associated and non-

Table 1 *Helicobacter pylori* and chronic gastritis

		Active		Inactive	
Authors/reference	Country	n	Percentage H. pylori-*positive*	n	Percentage H. pylori-*positive*
Fiocca et al.[6]	Italy	239	89	124	73
Goodwin et al.[7]	Australia	51	92	23	35
Jiang et al.[8]	China	49	90	72	50
Morris et al.[9]	New Zealand	28	82	7	14
Rawles et al.[10]	USA	23	70	47	15
Wyatt et al.[5]	UK	109	87	35	37

Source: Dixon MF. *Campylobacter pylori* and chronic gastritis. In: Rathbone BJ, Heatly RV, editors. *Campylobacter pylori* and gastroduodenal disease. Oxford: Blackwell Scientific Publications; 1989:106

Table 2 Prevalence of *H. pylori* in atrophic gastritis

Author/reference	Country	No. studied	Percentage H. pylori-*positive*
Booth et al.[29]	USA	34	71
Correa et al.[30]	Colombia	66	97
Correa et al.[30]	USA	57	65
Fiocca et al.[6]	Italy	38	90
Guarner et al.[31]	Mexico	65	92
Jiang et al.[8]	China	64	81
Karnes et al.[32]	Finland	124	86
Le Bodic et al.[33]	France	12	75
Menge et al.[34]	Germany	31	68
Price et al.[35]	UK	13	62
Sethi et al.[36]	UK	23	44

NSAID-associated gastric ulcer patients, the gastritis is related to the *H. pylori* status[21–23]. Studies have shown that gastritis improves after eradication of *H. pylori*[24–26] and gastritis returns with relapse of the infection[24]. The activity of the gastritis is related to the number of organisms[27].

The role of *H. pylori* in chronic gastritis is further supported by studies in the paediatric population. *H. pylori* is present in more than 60% of children with gastritis. *H. pylori* colonization of the gastric mucosa is always associated with chronic gastritis in children. Clearing of *H. pylori* from the gastric mucosa is associated with healing of the antral gastritis[28].

Chronic active gastritis may progress to atrophic gastritis with intestinal metaplasia in a small number of subjects. The prevalence of *H. pylori* in these histopathological changes is summarized in Tables 2 and 3. Atrophic gastritis, intestinal metaplasia and dysplasia are discussed further with gastric cancer.

FUNCTIONAL DYSPEPSIA

In subjects with functional dyspepsia the role of *H. pylori* is still unclear[37]. *H. pylori* is found in 41% to 78% of subjects with functional dyspepsia (Table 4).

Table 3 Prevalence of *H. pylori* in intestinal metaplasia and dysplasia

Author/reference	Country	No. studied	Percentage H. pylori-positive
Intestinal metaplasia			
Correa et al.[30]	Colombia	28	93
Correa et al.[30]	USA	51	59
Guarner et al.[31]	Mexico	57	83
Dysplasia			
Correa et al.[30]	Colombia	6	100
Correa et al.[30]	USA	2	100
Guarner et al.[31]	Mexico	23	87

Table 4 *H. pylori* infection in functional dyspepsia subjects and population controls (when available)

Study/reference	Country	Percentage H. pylori-positive Functional dyspepsia subjects	Controls
Adults			
Pettross et al.[38]	USA	43	13
Rauws et al.[25]	Netherlands	70	20
Lambert et al.[39]	Australia	61	36
Marshall et al.[40]	Australia	66	–
Rokkas et al.[41]	England	45	13
Strauss et al.[42]	USA	63	25
Loffeld et al.[43]	Netherlands	56	–
Blomberg et al.[44]	Sweden	45	–
Collins et al.[45]	England	50	–
Rathbone et al.[46]	England	54	–
Sobala et al.[47]	England	41	–
Jiang et al.[8]	China	74	–
Vaira et al.[48]	England	58	–
Jeena et al.[49]	South Africa	78	–
Children			
Thomas et al.[50]	England	20	4
Cadranel et al.[51]	Belgium	73	25
Elderly			
O'Riordan et al.[52]	Ireland	78	–

The wide variation of the frequency of *H. pylori* in functional dyspepsia subjects reflects both differences in the criteria to diagnose functional dyspepsia and the different populations evaluated. Few studies have compared *H. pylori* prevalence in functional dyspepsia subjects with age-matched, sex-matched, and ethnically matched representative populations. In developed countries from which populations data are available, the prevalence of *H. pylori* infection in functional dyspepsia subjects is consistently higher than that in control subjects[25,38,39,41,42]. In children with chronic abdominal pain a higher rate of *H. pylori* infection is observed than in control children[50,51]. Elderly dyspeptic subjects without peptic ulcer disease commonly have *H.*

Table 5 Prevalence of *H. pylori* infection in duodenal ulcer patients

Author/reference	Country	No. studied	Percentage H. pylori-*positive*
Adults			
Booth et al.[29]	USA	32	78
Fiocca et al.[6]	Italy	34	88
Goodwin et al.[53]	Australia	107	93
Jiang et al.[8]	China	14	86
Marshall et al.[40]	Australia	70	90
O'Connor et al.[20]	UK	35	97
Price et al.[35]	UK	21	80
Rauws et al.[25]	Netherlands	36	100
Dooley et al.[54]	Ireland	64	90
Children			
Drumm et al.[55]	Canada	2	100
Hassall and Dimmick[58]	Canada	27	85
Kilbridge et al.[56]	USA	9	89

pylori infection, and it has been associated with 78% of the cases of symptomatic gastritis in these patients[52].

DUODENAL ULCER

Duodenal ulcer is a multifactorial disease with a lifetime prevalence of approximately 10% in developed countries. All studies indicate that *H. pylori* is closely associated with duodenal ulcer disease. The prevalence of *H. pylori* infection in duodenal ulcer (DU) patients is 80 to 100% and the studies are summarized in Table 5. *H. pylori*-associated gastritis was also found in 90–100% of children with duodenal ulcer disease[55-58]. Duodenal ulceration in adults with no *H. pylori*-associated gastritis is generally due to other aetiological factors such as Zollinger-Ellison syndrome, Crohn's disease or neoplasm[59].

The relationship of *H. pylori* to peptic ulcer disease is inferential and is largely based upon a plausible hypothesis, the strong association with *H. pylori*-induced gastritis, an improved rate of healing with *H. pylori* suppression[60-63] and the markedly decreased recurrence rates for DU disease after eradication of the bacteria[64]. This latter finding also occurs in children with DU after *H. pylori*-associated gastritis is treated[65,66]. The prevalence of *H. pylori* infection in DU patients is very high, however, but should be compared to the age-adjusted prevalence in a normal population.

GASTRIC ULCER

Compared to DU, the role of *H. pylori* in gastric ulcer is less clear. Gastric ulcer is less likely to be a direct consequence of *H. pylori* gastritis as other injurious factors such as gastric acid, NSAID, alcohol, duodenogastric bile reflux also are important factors in ulcer development.

Table 6 Prevalence of *H. pylori* in gastric ulcer patients

Author/reference	Country	No. studied	Percentage H. pylori-*positive*
Bedossa et al.[67]		71	70
Feng and Wang[68]	China	28	86
Fiocca et al.[6]	Italy	30	90
Jiang et al.[8]	China	21	86
Hui et al.[69]	Hong Kong	67	73
Marshall et al.[40]	Australia	40	68
Niemala et al.[70]	Finland	33	58
O'Connor et al.[71]	UK	54	72
Vorobjova et al.[72]	Finland	87	94

Idiopathic gastric ulcer

An increased frequency of *H. pylori* infection is identified in subjects with gastric ulcers compared with controls. The prevalence of *H. pylori* in subjects with gastric ulcer is 58–94% and the results of studies are summarized in Table 6. A study from Japan has shown that 96% (50/52) of gastric ulcers had *H. pylori* in the exudate[73].

Preliminary studies have suggested that eradication of *H. pylori* reduces the relapse tendency as well as enchancing ulcer healing[74].

NSAID-associated gastric ulcer

Gastric ulcers may result from NSAID use and bile reflux. The prevalence of gastric erosions in patients on long-term NSAID therapy is approximately 40–50% with gastric ulcers occurring in at least 15% of subjects[75,76]. The prevalence of *H. pylori* infection in patients taking NSAID has been reported to range from 22% to 63%[77,78]. Most studies have shown that the prevalence of *H. pylori* was not significantly different between NSAID users and non-users[23,78–81]. Thus subjects on chronic NSAID are not more susceptible to *H. pylori* infection.

It has been suggested that *H. pylori* infection increases the susceptibility of the mucosa to damage from NSAID[79,81,82]. The role of *H. pylori*-induced gastritis in enhancing the damage caused by these agents is unclear. Histological gastritis in patients taking NSAID is related to the *H. pylori* infection rather than the use of NSAID[21–23].

The prevalence of *H. pylori* in patients with NSAID-associated gastric ulcer has been reported to be similar to that of NSAID users without gastric ulcer, suggesting that ulcer development is independent of *H. pylori* status[21,23,77]. Katz et al.[81] however has suggested that the prevalence of *H. pylori* is similar in subjects with gastric ulcer from NSAID compared to those with no NSAID use. The role of *H. pylori* in NSAID-associated gastric lesions thus still remains controversial.

Table 7 Prevalence of *H. pylori* in gastric cancer subjects

Authors/reference	Country	H. pylori Diagnosis	No. studied	Percentage H. pylori-*positive*
Gastric adenocarcinoma				
Buruk et al.[86]	Turkey	Histology	46	75
Jaskiewicz et al.[87]	South Africa	Histology	6	100
Kuipers et al.[88]	Netherlands	ELISA	116	77
Lambert et al.[89]	Australia	Histology	24	63
Loffeld et al.[90]	Netherlands	ELISA	105	59
Sipponen et al.[91]	Finland	ELISA	54	70
Talley et al.[92]	USA	ELISA	37	65
Wee et al.[93]	Singapore	Histology	132	61
Gastric lymphoma *(MALT type):*				
Wotherspoon et al.[94]	UK	Histology	101	92

GASTRIC CANCER

Although stomach cancer has declined on an annual basis in most developed countries, its remains the most common malignancy among men and the second most common among women[83–85] in Asia and other developing countries.

Between 59% and 100% of subjects with adenocarcinoma are infected with *H. pylori* at diagnosis (Tables 7 and 8). In the Netherlands, 61% of cancer patients were found on biopsy or gastric resection to be infected with *H. pylori* compared with 34% of age-matched blood donor controls (risk ratio 4.2, $p < 0.001$)[90]. However, *H. pylori* is found in only 10% of patients with gastric cancer when malignant tissue only is examined[98]. Most studies relating *H. pylori* and gastric cancer use serological tests to determine *H. pylori* status. The ability to detect *H. pylori* in the mucosa from surgical specimens of subjects with gastric cancer is low. The reason for this is unclear, but may be due to fixative techniques, the presence of intestinal metaplasia or the development of coccoid (non-stainable) forms of *H. pylori*.

Infection with *H. pylori* has been linked with the later development of chronic atrophic gastritis. Gastric cancer is associated with atrophic gastritis and the further progression to intestinal metaplasia and dysplasia. The prevalence of *H. pylori* infection has been reported in 44–97% of subjects with atrophic gastritis, 59–93% with intestinal metaplasia and 87–100% with dysplasia (Tables 2 and 3). Early acquisition of *H. pylori* infection in childhood has been hypothesized as important in the development of precursors lesions of gastric cancer and in the impaired development of gastric acid secretion. Scott et al.[99] have reported a high prevalence of *H. pylori* infection and gastric intestinal metaplasia in members of a gastric cancer family.

A large epidemiological study from 49 rural Chineses counties has found a significant correlation between *H. pylori* seroprevalence and gastric cancer rates ($r = 0.34$, $p = 0.02$)[100]. *H. pylori* infection also correlates with gastric cancer incidence rates in various populations of Colombia and Louisiana[30,101].

Table 8 Prospective studies of *H. pylori* and gastric cancer

Study/reference	Population	Mean interval between seropositivity and cancer diagnosis	No. of cases infected (%)	No. of controls infected (%)	Matched odds ratio (95% CI)
Forman et al.[95]	British and Welsh males	6	10/29 (69)	54/116 (47)	2.8 (1.0, 8.0)
Parsonnet et al.[96]	California males and females	14	92/109 (84)	66/109 (66)	3.6 (1.8, 7.3)
Nomura et al.[97]	Japanese–American males	13	103/109 (94)	83/109 (76)	6.0 (2.1, 17.3)

Source: Parsonnet J. *Helicobacter pylori* and gastric cancer. Gastroenterol Clin N Am 1993;22:89–104

Table 9 Prevalence of *H. pylori* infection in chronic renal failure

Authors/reference	Diagnosis of H. pylori	Percentage H. pylori-*positive*	
		Renal failure	Control
Offerhaus et al.[103]	ELISA	44	45 (blood donor) 93 (duodenal ulcer)*
Shousha et al.[104]	Biopsy	24	42 (upper GI symptoms)*
Wee et al.[105]	Biopsy	31	–
Davenport et al.[106]	ELISA	29	–
Ala-Kaila et al.[107]	Biopsy	17	–
Rowe et al.[108]	Biopsy	46	–

*Significant difference

Three nested case–control studies[95–97] in different populations support an association between previous *H. pylori* infection and an increased risk for gastric cancer (Table 8).

Association of H. pylori *with different types of gastric tumour*

The intestinal type of gastric cancer is the result of chronic inflammation and is associated with a higher bacterial load than the diffuse type. Diffuse-type gastric cancer occurring in the proximal stomach is genetically linked. In California, 89.2% (32/37) with intestinal-type cancer were infected with *H. pylori* in non-cancerous tissue, compared with 31.8% (7/22) with diffuse-type cancer (odds ratio 17.7, $p < 0.001$). This association remained strong when controlled for age, sex and site and number of sections reviewed[102]. Other studies, however, have reported that *H. pylori* prevalence was similar in both types of cancer[91,93,97]. These differences may reflect different methods of detection of *H. pylori*. Gastric lymphoma of the MALT type is commonly associated with *H. pylori*-induced gastritis, and is present in up to 92% of cases[94].

OTHER DISEASES

H. pylori in chronic renal failure

Gastric symptoms and severe gastritis are frequent in uraemic patients. *H. pylori* has been reported to be present in 17–46% of subjects with chronic renal failure (Table 9). The prevalence of the *H. pylori* in patients with renal disease is similar to that reported in the normal population. Offerhaus *et al.*[103] found that patients with chronic renal failure had a similar prevalence of *H. pylori* antibodies in those with (45%) or without (44%) a previous history of peptic ulcer disease. Di Giorgio *et al.*[109] found that the prevalence of *H. pylori* in chronic renal failure patients was not significantly different between those who received no treatment and those who underwent regular haemodialysis. Similar rates of *H. pylori* infection have also been found between patients with end-stage renal failure who receive regular haemodialysis and patients with functioning renal transplants[106]. These studies suggest

Table 10 Summary of prevalence of *H. pylori* in HIV-infected patients

Authors/reference	Diagnosis of H. pylori	Percentage (n) of H. pylori-positive		
		HIV-positive	HIV-negative	p
Aceti et al.[111]	ELISA	64	29	<0.05
Marano et al.[115]	Histology	15 (11/73)		
Battan et al.[116]	Histology culture	40 (16/40)	39 (14/36)	NS
Edwards et al.[117]	Histology	3 (6/201)	59 (81/137)	0.009
Francis et al.[113]	Histology	14 (7/51)	47 (28/59)	<0.05
Logan et al.[114]	Histology	13 (2/15)	60 (18/30)	<0.01

that there is no predisposition of *H. pylori* infection among patients with chronic renal failure, and that *H. pylori* infection does not play a significant role in the ulcer diathesis in these patients. *H. pylori*-positive patients may, however, have significantly more frequent upper gastrointestinal symptoms than *H. pylori*-negative individuals[106,107]. The lower prevalence of *H. pylori* in chronic renal failure may be related to the wide variety of medications, including antibiotics, which these patients are prescribed during the course of their illness.

Human immunodeficiency virus (HIV)

Patients infected with the human immunodeficiency virus (HIV) with or without AIDS, have a high incidence (50–90%) of gastrointestinal symptoms. *H. pylori* causes a local and systemic immune response[110]. Studies of the relationship between HIV infection and *H. pylori* have produced conflicting results.

Aceti et al.[111] reported that the seroprevalence of *H. pylori* infection in HIV-positive individuals (64%) was significantly higher than in age-matched healthy controls (29%). In HIV-positive subjects a significant difference in seroprevalence was observed between symptom-free individuals (73%) and those with AIDS or AIDS-related complex (ARC) (53%). There was no difference in *H. pylori* seroprevalence between HIV-positive and HIV-negative at risk (homosexual and intravenous drug users) individuals. Polish et al.[112] studied the seroprevalence of antibodies to *H. pylori* in 370 men attending a sexually transmitted disease clinic and showed that race – and not HIV status, sexual preference, or age – was associated with *H. pylori* seropositivity.

Two groups[113,114] have shown that the prevalence of *H. pylori* in antral biopsies in HIV-seropositive patients was significantly lower than age-, sex- and symptom-matched HIV-negative controls. No subjects had received bismuth compounds or antibiotics known to be effective against *H. pylori* in the 1–2 months before endoscopy. The prevalence of *H. pylori* infection in HIV antibody-positive patients with or without AIDS was not significantly different[113]. Similar findings of a low prevalence of *H. pylori* in HIV-positive patients are summarized in Table 10.

The lower prevalence of *H. pylori* infection suggests that cell-mediated immune deficiency does not appear to increase the risk of infection with *H.*

Table 11 Summary of the prevalance of *H. pylori* in Zollinger–Ellison syndrome compare to duodenal ulcer patients

Authors	Zollinger–Ellison syndrome	Duodenal ulcer
Koop et al.[123]	35%	94%
Saeed et al.[124]	30%	100%
Fich et al.[125]	44%	89%

pylori. Another potential explanation is the frequent use of antimicrobial therapy in this group, which may impair successful colonization of *H. pylori*. Impaired acid secretion may also reduce colonization of gastric mucosa and explain the low rate of *H. pylori* observed.

In AIDS/ARC (AIDS-related complex) patients, chronic active gastritis is as common as in other patients referred for upper endoscopy[115,116]. The prevalence of *H. pylori* in AIDS patients with histological chronic active gastritis is much lower than the prevalence previously reported for HIV-negative patients with similar pathology[115,117]. However, Battan *et al.*[116] found that there was no significant difference between AIDS patients and controls. The lower frequency of *H. pylori* positivity in ARC and AIDS again might be attributable to the use of chemotherapeutic agents active against *H. pylori* or to impaired immune function.

Pernicious anaemia

The prevalence of *H. pylori* in pernicious anaemia subjects ranges from 0% to 21%[18,118–122]. Blaser *et al.*[121] found that *H. pylori* IgG antibody in patients with pernicious anaemia (0%) was significantly less than in age- and sex-matched healthy controls (40%). Similar results was reported by Fong *et al.*[120], using biopsy specimens. Hodenbro *et al.*[122] reported 27 patients with atrophic body gastritis diagnosed by histology. Past and/or present *H. pylori* infection was significantly higher in non-pernicious anaemia patients (73%) compared to those with pernicious anaemia (0%). These studies suggested *H. pylori* infection is negatively associated with pernicious anaemia.

Zollinger-Ellison syndrome

H. pylori has been implicated in the pathogenesis of duodenal ulcer disease. The relationship between *H. pylori* infection and duodenal ulcer in Zollinger-Ellison syndrome is unknown. Several studies have investigated the frequency of *H. pylori* infection in Zollinger-Ellison syndrome and compared it to duodenal ulcer disease without this syndrome. The results are summarized in Table 11.

These studies show that the frequency of *H. pylori* in patients with Zollinger-Ellison syndrome is lower than in those with duodenal ulcer disease. Koop *et al.*[123] suggested that the frequency was similar to age-matched controls (35%). *H. pylori* infection in Zollinger-Ellison syndrome may also be associated with decreased gastric acid secretion[124,125]. Fich *et al.*[125] also observed that chronic antral gastritis scores are significantly higher in patients with duodenal ulcer disease than those with Zollinger-Ellison syndrome.

The present results indicate that *H. pylori* is not a major contributing factor in duodenal ulcer associated with Zollinger-Ellison syndrome. Development of duodenal ulcer does not necessarily require *H. pylori*.

Colonic polyps

Previous studies have reported elevated plasma gastrin levels in subjects with colorectal adenocarcinoma and polyps. *H. pylori* infection is also associated with elevated meal-stimulated gastrin levels. Lambert *et al.*[126] recently reported that the prevalence of *H. pylori* in an Anglo-Celtic population with colonic polyps (56%) in Melbourne was significantly higher than control subjects (38%) after adjustment for age, sex, smoking habit and education levels (OR 1.89, 95% CI 1.29, 2.76). This association may relate to the increase in gastrin levels in *H. pylori*-infected subjects with a trophic effect on colonic mucosa. Further studies are required to confirm this finding, and to assess the interrelationship between food intake, gastrin and colonic mucosal change.

H. PYLORI AND ABO BLOOD GROUP

Duodenal ulcer is associated with genetic characteristics such as blood group O and non-secretor status. Individuals with blood group O have a 30–40% higher incidence of duodenal ulcer than those of the remaining blood groups, and non-secretors are 40–50% more likely to develop a duodenal ulcer than secretors[127–131]. *H. pylori* has been shown to be an important factor in the pathogenesis of duodenal ulcer. Several studies have reported the frequency of *H. pylori* antibodies in people with different blood group antigens. In healthy blood donors no significant differences between secretors and non-secretors were found when the frequencies of *H. pylori* antibodies in IgA, IgG and IgM classes were compared. Nor were there any significant differences when blood group O non-secretors were compared with A, B, and AB secretors for IgA, IgG and IgM antibodies against *H. pylori*[132,133].

Mentis *et al.*[134] studied 454 endoscopic patients and found that there was no association between ABO blood group and the prevalence of *H. pylori*. The prevalence of *H. pylori* among non-secretors with gastric ulcer (12.5%) was significantly lower than that for non-secretors with duodenal ulcer (100%). Recently, Dickey *et al.*[135] studied 101 patients with symptoms of dyspepsia undergoing endoscopy, and showed that the relative risk of gastroduodenal disease for non-secretors compared with secretors was 1.9. Non-secretor status of ABO blood group antigens is not related to *H. pylori* infection, but is independently and significantly associated with endoscopic gastroduodenal disease. This suggests that *H. pylori* and different blood group antigens may be independently linked to duodenal ulcer.

Table 12 Prevalence (percentages) of *H. pylori* in gastro-intestinal disease

Histological gastritis	
Chronic active gastritis	70–100
Atrophic gastritis	44–97
Intestinal metaplasia	59–93
Dysplasia	87–100
Non-ulcer dyspepsia	41–78
Duodenal ulcer	78–100
Gastric ulcer	58–96
Idiopathic	58–94
NSAID-associated	22–63
Gastric carcinoma	59–100
Chronic renal failure	17–46
HIV	3–64
Pernicious anaemia	0–21
Ulcerative oesophagitis	20–51
Zollinger-Ellison syndrome	30–44
Colonic polyps	56
Normal population	
Developing countries	60–80
Developed countries	25–50

SUMMARY

H. pylori infection is implicated as a major pathogenic factor in duodenal ulcer, gastric ulcer and gastric malignancy. The prevalence in diseases of the upper gastrointestinal tract is summarized in Table 12. Lower isolation rates of *H. pylori* in some diseases may be coupled with the considerable differences which are found in the prevalence rates of this organism between different age and ethnic groups. Difficulties experienced when attempting to culture this organism may account for different prevalence of *H. pylori* observed in upper gastrointestinal diseases. The mechanism(s) for development of different disease may relate to bacterial factors, age of acquisition, duration and extent of infection, environmental and other host factors including the gastric acid secretion.

References

1. Steer HW. Surface morphology of the gastroduodenal mucosa in duodenal ulceration. Gut. 1984;25:1203–10.
2. Wyatt JI, Rathbone BJ, Dixon MF, Heatley RV. *Campylobacter pyloridis* and acid induced gastric metaplasia in the pathogenesis of duodenitis. J Clin Pathol. 1987;40:841–8.
3. Caseli M, Bovolenta MR, Aleotti E. Epithelial morphology of duodenal bulb and *Campylobacter-like* organisms. J Submicrosc Cytol Pathol. 1998;20:237–42.
4. Meyrick-Thomas J. *Campylobacter*-like organisms in gastritis. Lancet. 1984;1:1217.
5. Wyatt JI, Rathbone BJ, Heatley RV. Local immune response to gastric *Campylobacter* in non-ulcer dyspepsia. J Clin Pathol. 1986;38:863–70.
6. Fiocca R, Villani L, Turpini R, Salcia E. High incidence of *campylobacter*-like organisms in endoscopic biopsies from patients with gastritis with or without peptic ulcer. Digestion. 1987;38:234–44.
7. Goodwin CS, Armstrong JA, Marshall BJ. *Campylobacter pyloridis* gastritis and peptic

ulceration. J Clin Pathol. 1986;39:353–65.

8. Jiang SJ, Liu WZ, Zhang DZ et al. *Campylobacter*-like organisms in chronic gastritis, peptic ulcer, and gastric carcinoma. Scand J Gastroenterol. 1987;22:553–8.
9. Morris A, Arthur J, Nicholson G. *Campylobacter pyloridis* infection in Auckland patients with gastritis. NZ Med J. 1986;99:353–5.
10. Rawles JW, Paull G, Yardley JH et al. Gastric *Campylobacter*-like organisms in a US hospital population. Gastroenterology. 1986;91:A1599.
11. Jones DM, Eldrige J, Fox AJ, Sethi P, Whorwell PJ. Antibody to the gastric *Campylobacter*-like organisms (*Campylobacter pyloridis*). Clinical correlations and distribution in the normal population. J Med Microbiol. 1986;22:57–62.
12. Graham DY, Malaty HM, Evans DG, Evans DJ Jr, Klein PD, Adam E. Epidemiology of *Helicobacter pylori* in an asymptomatic population in the United States. Effect of age, race, and socioeconomic status. Gastroenterology. 1991;100:1495–501.
13. Hazell SL, Hennessy WB, Borody TJ, Carrick J, Ralston M, Brady L, Lee A. *Campylobacter pyloridis* gastritis. II: Distribution of bacteria and associated inflammation in the gastroduodenal environment. Am J Gastroenterol. 1987;82:297–301.
14. Siurala M, Isokoski M, Varis K, Kekki M. Prevalence of gastritis in a rural population. Bioptic study of subjects selected at random. Scand J Gastroenterol. 1968;3:211–23.
15. Siurala M, Sipponen P, Kekki M. *Campylobacter pylori* in a sample of Finnish population: relations to morphology and functions of the gastric mucosa. Gut. 1988;29:909–15.
16. Siurala M, Sipponen P, Kekki M. Chronic gastritis: dynamic and clinical aspects. Scand J Gastroenterol. 1985 (Suppl 109);20:69–76.
17. Lin SK, Lambert JR, Wahlqvist ML, Schembri M, Lukito W, Nicholson L. Prevalence of *Helicobacter pylori* in a representative Anglo-Celtic population of urban Melbourne. Gastroenterology. 1993;104 (4):A135.
18. Flejou JF, Bahame P, Smith AC, Stockbrugger RW, Rode J, Price AB. Pernicious anaemia and *Campylobacter*-like organisms, is the gastric antrum resistant to colonisation. Gut. 1989;30:60–4.
19. Dixon MF, Wyatt JI, Burke DA, Rathbone BJ. Lymphocytic gastritis: relationship to *Campylobacter pylori* infection. J Pathol. 1988;154:125–32.
20. O'Connor HJ, Dixon MF, Wyatt JI, Axon AT, Dewar EP, Johnston D. Effect of duodenal ulcer surgery and enterogastric reflux on *Campylobacter pyloridis*. Lancet. 1986;2:1178–81.
21. Laine L, Marin-Sorensen M, Weinstein WM. *Helicobacter pylori* prevalence and mucosal injury in gastric ulcer. Relationship to chronic nonsteroidal antiinflammatory drug (NSAID) ingestion. Gastroenterology. 1991;100:A103.
22. Caselli M, Pazzi P, LaCorte R, Aleotti A, Trevisani L, Stabellini G. *Campylobacter*-like organisms, nonsteroidal anti-inflammatory drugs and gastric lesions in patients with rheumatoid arthritis. Digestion. 1989;44:101–4.
23. Shallcross TM, Rathbone BJ, Wyatt JI, Heatley RV. *Helicobacter pylori* associated chronic gastritis and peptic ulceration in patients taking non-steroidal anti-inflammatory drugs. Aliment Pharmacol Ther. 1990;4:515–22.
24. Patchett S, Beattie S, Leen E, Keane C, O'Morain C. *Helicobacter pylori* and duodenal ulcer recurrence. Am J Gastroenterol. 1992;87:24–7.
25. Rauws EA, Langenberg W, Houthoff HJ, Zanen HC, Tytgat GN. *Campylobacter pyloridis*-associated chronic active antral gastritis. A prospective study of its prevalence and the effects of antibacterial and antiulcer treatment. Gastroenterology. 1988;94:33–40.
26. Valle J, Seppala K, Sipponen P, Kosunen T. Disappearance of gastritis after eradication of *Helicobacter pylori*: a morphometric study. Scand J Gastroenterol. 1991;26:1057–65.
27. Pinkard KJ, Harrison B, Capstick JA, Medley G, Lambert JR. Detection of *Campylobacter pyloridis* in gastric mucosa by phase contrast microscopy. J Clin Pathol. 1986;39:112–13.
28. Drumm B. *Helicobacter pylori* in the pediatric patient. Gastroenterol Clin N Am. (*Helicobacter pylori* infection). 1993;22(1):169–82.
29. Booth L, Holdstock G, MacBride H et al. Clinical importance of *Campylobacter pyloridis* and associated serum IgG and IgA antibody responses in patients undergoing upper gastrointestinal endoscopy. J Clin Pathol. 1986:39:215–19.
30. Correa P, Fox J, Fontham E et al. *Helicobacter pylori* and gastric carcinoma: serum antibody prevalence in populations with contrasting cancer risks. Cancer 1990;66:2569–74.
31. Guarner J, Mohar A, Parsonnet J, Halperin D. The association of *Helicobacter pylori* with

gastric cancer and preneoplastic gastric lesions in Chiapas, Mexico. Cancer. 1993;71: 297–301.

32. Karnes WE Jr, Samloff IM, Siurala M *et al.* Positive serum antibody and negative tissue staining for *Helicobacter pylori* in subjects with atrophic body gastritis. Gastroenterology. 1991;101:167–74.

33. Le Bodic MF, Barre P, Freeland C. *Campylobacter pylori* et muqueuse gastrique: etude histologique, bacteriologique et resultats preliminaires d'une enquete epidemiologique dans la region nantaise. Gastroenterol Clin Biol. 1987;11:543–9.

34. Mengc H, Warrehman M, Joy W *et al. Campylobacter pylori* in Magen, Duodenum und Kolon Gastroenterologischer Patienten. Dtsch Med Wochenschr. 1987;112:1403–7.

35. Price AB, Levi J, Dolby JM *et al. Campylobacter pylori* in peptic ulcer disease: microbiology, pathology, and scanning electron microscopy. Gut. 1985;26:1183–8.

36. Sethi P, Banerjee AK, Jones DM. Gastritis and gastric *Campylobacter-like* organisms in patients without peptic ulcers. Postgrad Med J. 1987;63:543–5.

37. Lambert JR. The role of *Helicobacter pylori* in nonulcer dyspepsia: a debate – for. Gastroenterol Clin N Am. 1993;22(1):141–52.

38. Pettross CW, Appleman MD, Cohen H, Valenzvela JE, Chandrasona P, Laine LAS. Prevalence of *Campylobacter pylori* and association with antral mucosal histology in subjects with and without upper gastrointestinal symptoms. Dig Dis Sci. 1988;33:649–53.

39. Lambert JR, Dunn K, Borromeo M, Korman MG, Hansky J. *Campylobacter pylori* – a role in non-ulcer dyspepsia? Scand J Gastroenterol Suppl. 1989;1607–13.

40. Marshall BJ, McGechie DB, Rogers PA, Clancy RJ. Pyloric *Campylobacter* infection and gastroduodenal disease. Med J Aust. 1985;142:439–44.

41. Rokkas T, Pursey C, Uzoechina E *et al. Campylobacter pylori* and non-ulcer dyspepsia. Am J Gastroenterol. 1987;82:1149–52.

42. Strauss RM, Wang TC, Kelsey PB. Association of *Helicobacter pylori* infection with dyspeptic symptoms in patients undergoing gastroduodenoscopy. Am J Med. 1990;89:464.

43. Loffeld RJ, Potters HV, Arends JW, Stobberingh E, Flendrig JA, van Spreeuwel JP. *Campylobacter* associated gastritis in patients with non-ulcer dyspepsia. J Clin Pathol. 1998;41:85–8.

44. Blomberg B, Jarnerot G, Kjellander J, Kanielsson D, Kraaz W. Prevalence of *Campylobacter pylori* in an unselected Swedish population of patients referred for gastroscopy. Scand J Gastroenterol. 1988;23:358–62.

45. Collins JS, Knill-Jones RP, Sloan JM. Comparison of symptoms between nonulcer dyspepsia patients positive and negative for *C. pylori* using a single bias computer system for history taking. Klin Wochenschr. 1989;67(Suppl 18):11.

46. Rathbone BJ, Wyatt J, Heatley RU. Symptomatology in *C. pylori* positive and negative non-ulcer dyspepsia. Gut. 1988;29:A1473.

47. Sobala GM, Dixon MF, Axon ATR. Symptomatology of *Helicobacter pylori* associated dyspepsia. Eur J Gastroenterol Hepatol. 1990;2:445–9.

48. Vaira D, Holton J, Osborn J *et al.* Endoscopy in dyspeptic patients: Is gastric mucosal biopsy useful? Am J Gastroenterol. 1990;85:701–4.

49. Jenna CP, Simjee AE, Pettengell KE. Comparison of symptoms in *Campylobacter pylori* positive and negative patients presenting with dyspepsia for upper gastrointestinal endoscopy. S Afr Med J. 1988;73:659.

50. Thomas J, Eastham EJ, Elliot TSJ. *Campylobacter pylori* gastritis in children – a common cause of symptoms? Gut. 1988;29:A707.

51. Cadranel S, Goossens H, De Boeck M, Malengreav A, Rodesch P, Butzler JP. *Campylobacter pyloridis* in children [letter]. Lancet. 1986;1:735–6.

52. O'Riordan TG, Tobin A, O'Morain C: *Helicobacter pylori* infection in elderly dyspeptic patients. Age Ageing. 1991;20:189.

53. Goodwin CS, Marshall BJ, Blincow ED, Wilson DH, Blackbourn S, Phillips M. Prevention of nitroimidazole resistance in *Campylobacter pylori* by co-administration of colloidal bismuth subcitrate: clinical and in vitro studies. J Clin Pathol. 1988;41:207–10.

54. Dooley CP, McKenna D, Humphreys H *et al.* Histological gastritis in duodenal ulcer: relationship to *Campylobacter pylori* and effect of ulcer therapy. Am J Gastroenterol. 1988;83:278–82.

55. Drumm B, O'Brien A, Cutz E, Sherman P. *Campylobacter pyloridis* associated primary

gastritis in children. Pediatrics. 1987;80:192–5.

56. Kilbridge PM, Dahms BB, Czinn SJ. *Campylobacter pylori*-associated gastritis and peptic ulcer disease in children. Am J Dis Child. 1988;142:1149–52.

57. Drumm B, Perez-Perez GI, Blaser MJ, Sherman P. Intrafamilial clustering of *Helicobacter pylori* infection. N Engl J Med. 1990;322:359–63.

58. Hassall E, Dimmick JE. Unique features of *Helicobacter pylori* disease in children. Dig Dis Sci. 1991;36:417–23.

59. Nensey YM, Schubert TT, Bologna SD, Ma CK. *Helicobacter pylori*-negative duodenal ulcer. Am J Med. 1991;91:15–18.

60. Bayerdorffer E, Simon T, Bastlein C, Ottenjann R, Kasper G. Bismuth/ofloxacin combination for duodenal ulcer [letter] Lancet. 1987;2:1467–8.

61. Coughlan JG, Gilligan D, Humphries H *et al. Campylobacter pylori* and recurrence of duodenal ulcers – a 12-month follow-up study. Lancet. 1987;2:1109–11.

62. Marshall BJ, Goodwin CS, Warren JR *et al.* Prospective double-blind trial of duodenal ulcer relapse after eradication of *Campylobacter pylori.* Lancet. 1988;2:1439–42.

63. Graham DY, Opekun A, Lew GM, Evans DJ Jr, Klein PD, Evans DG. Ablation of exaggerated meal-stimulated gastrin release in duodenal ulcer patients after clearance of *Helicobacter (Campylobacter) pylori* infection. Am J Gastroenterol. 1990;85:394–8.

64. Tytgat GNJ, Noach LA, Rauws EAJ. *Helicobacter pylori* infection and duodenal ulcer disease. Gastroenterol Clin N Am. 1993;22(1):127–40.

65. Oderda G, Farina L, Ansaldi N. Peptic ulcer in children: 5 years follow-up after ranitidine therapy. Pediatr Res. 1988;24:417.

66. Yeung CK, Fu KH, Yuen KY. *Helicobacter pylori* and associated duodenal ulcer. Arch Dis Child. 1990;65:1212–16.

67. Bedossa P, Poynard T, Chaput JC, Martin E. A decade of *Campylobacter pylori.* Lancet. 1988;1:417–18.

68. Feng YY, Wang Y. *Campylobacter pylori* in patients with gastritis, peptic ulcer, and carcinoma of the stomach in Lanzhou, China [letter] Lancet. 1988;1:1055.

69. Hui WM, Lam SK, Chan PY. Pathogenetic role of *Campylobacter pyloridis* in gastric ulcer. J Gastroenterol Hepatol. 1987;2:309–16.

70. Niemala S, Karttunen T, Lehtola J. *Campylobacter*-like organisms in patients with gastric ulcer. Scand J Gastroenterol. 1987;22:487–90.

71. O'Connor HJ, Dixon MF, Wyatt JI, Axon AT, Dewar EP, Johnston D. *Campylobacter pylori* and peptic ulcer disease [letter]. Lancet. 1987;2:633–4.

72. Vorobjova T, Maaroos HI, Uibo R, Wadstrom T, Wood WG, Sipponen P. *Helicobacter pylori*: histological and serological study on gastric and duodenal ulcer patients in Estonia. Scand J Gastroenterol. 1991;26(Suppl 186):84–9.

73. Ohjusa T, Okayasu I, Yamada M *et al.* A high frequency of detection of *Helicobacter pylori* in whitish exudate of gastric ulcer. J Clin Gastroenterol. 1991;13:649–55.

74. Graham DY, Lew GM, Klein PD, Evans DG, Evans DJ Jr, Saeed ZA, Malatry HM. Effect of treatment of *Helicobacter pylori* infection on the long-term recurrence of gastric or duodenal ulcer. A randomized, controlled study [see comments]. Ann Intern Med. 1992;116:705–8.

75. Larkai EN, Smith JL, Lidsky MD, Graham DY. Gastroduodenal mucosa and dyspeptic symptoms in arthritis patients during chronic nonsteroidal anti-inflammatory drug use. Am J Gastroenterol. 1987;82:1153–9.

76. Silvos GR, Levy KJ, Butt JH. Incidence of gastric lesions in patients with rheumatic disease on chronic aspirin therapy. Ann Intern Med. 1979;91:517.

77. Loeb D, Ahlquist D, Carpenter H. Role of *Helicobacter pylori* in non-steroidal anti-inflammatory drug (NSAID) induced gastroduodenopathy. Am J Gastroenterol. 1990;85:1236.

78. Maxton DG, Srivastava ED, Whorwell PJ, Jones DM. Do non-steroidal anti-inflammatory drugs or smoking predispose to *Helicobacter pylori* infection? Postgrad Med J. 1990;66:717–19.

79. Martin DF, Montgomery C, Dobek AS, Patrissi GA, Peura DA. *Campylobacter pylori*, NSAIDs and smoking: risk factors for peptic ulcer disease. Am J Gastroenterol. 1989;84:1268–72.

80. Graham DY, Lidsky MD, Cox AM *et al.* Long-term non-steroidal antiinflammatory drug

use and *Helicobacter pylori* infection. Gastroenterology. 1991;100:1653–7.

81. Katz B, Lambert JR, Nicholson L *et al. H. pylori* infection, upper gastrointestinal (UGI) symptoms and blood loss in patients with rheumatoid arthritis on NSAID. Gastroenterology. 1991;100:A96.

82. Heresbach D, Raoul JL, Donniopy Y *et al. Helicobacter pylori*: a risk and severity factor in NSAID induced gastropathy. Gastroenterology. 1991;100:A82.

83. Parkin DM. Cancer occurrence in developing countries. IARC Scientific Publications No. 75, Lyon, France. International Agency for Research on Cancer, 1986.

84. Parking DM, Laara E, Muir CS. Estimates of the worldwide frequency of sixteen major cancers in 1980. Int J Cancer. 1988;41:184.

85. Waterhouse J, Muir C, Shanmugaratnam K. (editors). Cancer incidence in five continents. IARC Scientific Publications No. 42, Lyon, France. International Agency for Research on Cancer, 1986.

86. Buruk F, Berberoglu U, Pak I, Aksaz E, Celen O. Gastric cancer and *Helicobacter pylori* infection. Br J Surg. 1993;80:378–9.

87. Jaskeiwicz K, Louwrens HD, Woodroof CW, van Wyke MJ, Price SK. The association of *Campylobacter pylori* with mucosal pathological changes in a population at risk for gastric cancer. S Afr Med J. 1989;75:417–19.

88. Kuipers EJ, Gracia-Casanova M, Pena AS *et al. Helicobacter pylori* serology in patients with gastric carcinoma. Scand J Gastroenterol. 1993;28:433–7.

89. Lambert JR, Hansky J, Eaves EK. *Campylobacter*-like organisms in human stomach. Gastroenterology. 1985;88:1463.

90. Loffeld RJLF, Willems I, Flendring JA, Arends JW. *Helicobacter pylori* and gastric carcinoma. Histopathology. 1990;17:537–41.

91. Sipponen P, Kosunen TU, Valle J, Riihela M, Seppala K. *Helicobacter pylori* infection and chronic gastritis in gastric cancer. J Clin Pathol. 1992;45:319–23.

92. Talley NJ, Zinsmeister AR, Weaver A *et al.* Gastric adenocarinoma and *Helicobacter pylori* infection. J Natl Cancer Inst. 1991;83:1734–9.

93. Wee A, Kang JY, Teh M. *Helicobacter pylori* and gastric cancer: correlation with gastritis, intestinal metaplasia and tumour histology. Gut. 1992;33:1029–32.

94. Wotherspoon AC, Ortiz-Hidalgo C, Falzon MR, Isaacson PG. *Helicobacter pylori*-associated gastritis and primary B-cell gastric lymphoma. Lancet. 1991;338:1175–6.

95. Forman D, Newell DG, Fullerton F *et al.* Association between infection with *H. pylori* and risk of gastric cancer: evidence from a prospective investigation. BMJ. 1991;302:1302–5.

96. Parsonnet J. Friedman GD, Vandersteen DP *et al. Helicobacter pylori* infection and risk for gastric cancer. N Engl J Med. 1991;323:1127–31.

97. Nomura A, Stemmermann GN, Ghyou PH, Kato I, Perez-Perez GI, Blaser M. *Helicobacter pylori* infection and gastric carcinoma among Japanese Americans in Hawaii. N Engl J Med. 1991;325:1132–6.

98. Robey-Cafferty SS, Ro JY, Cleary KR. The prevalence of *Campylobacter pylori* in gastric biopsies from cancer patients. Med Pathol. 1989;2:473.

99. Scott N, Lansdown M, Diament R *et al. Helicobacter* gastritis and intestinal metaplasia in a gastric cancer family [letter]. Lancet. 1990;335:728.

100. Forman D, Sitas F, Newell DG *et al.* Geographic association of *Helicobacter pylori* antibody prevalence and gastric cancer mortality in rural China. Int J Cancer. 1990;46:608–11.

101. Fox JG, Correa P, Taylor NS *et al. Campylobacter pylori*-associated gastritis and immune response in a population at increased risk of gastric carcinoma. Am J Gastroenterol. 1989;84:775–81.

102. Parsonnet J, Vandersteen D, Goates J. *Helicobacter pylori* in intestinal- and diffuse-type gastric adenocarcinoma. J Natl Cancer Inst. 1991;83:640.

103. Offerhaus GJ, Kreuning J, Valentijn RM *et al. Campylobacter pylori*: prevalence and significance in patients with chronic renal failure. Clin Nephrol. 1989;32:239–41.

104. Shousha S, Arnaout AH, Abbas SH, Parkins RA. Antral *Helicobacter pylori* in patients with chronic renal failure. J Clin Pathol. 1990;43:397–9.

105. Wee A, Kang JY, Ho MS, Choong HL, Wu AY, Sutherland IH. Gastroduodenal mucosa in uraemia: endoscopic and histological correlation and prevalence of *Helicobacter*-like

organisms. Gut. 1990;31:1093–6.

106. Davenport A, Shallcross TM, Crabtree JE, Davison AM, Will EJ, Heatley RV. Prevalence of *Helicobacter pylori* in patients with end-stage renal failure and renal transplant recipients. Nephron. 1991;59:597–601.

107. Ala-Jaila K, Vaajalahti P, Karvonen AL, Kokki M. Gastric *Helicobacter* and upper gastrointestinal symptoms in chronic renal failure. Ann Med. 1991;23:403–6.

108. Rowe PA, el Nujumi AM, Williams C, Dahill S, Briggs JD, McColl KE. The diagnosis of *Helicobacter pylori* infection in uremic patients. Am J Kidney Dis. 1992;20:574–9.

109. Di Giorgio P, Rivellini G, D'Alessio L, Di Benedetto A, De Luca B. The influence of high blood levels of urea on the presence of *Campylobacter pylori* in the stomach: a clinical study. Ital J Gastroenterol. 1990;22:64–5.

110. Rathbone BJ, Wyatt JI, Worsley BW *et al.* Systemic and local antibody responses to gastric *Campylobacter pyloridis* in non-ulcer dyspepsia. Gut. 1986;27:642–7.

111. Aceti A, Celestino D, Pennica A, Leri O, Caferro M. Antibodies to *Helicobacter pylori* in HIV infection [letter]. Lancet. 1990;336:571.

112. Polish LB, Douglas JM Jr, Davidson AJ *et al.* Characterization of risk factors for *Helicobacter pylori* infection among men attending a sexually transmitted disease clinic: lack of evidence for sexual transmission. J Clin Microbiol. 1991;29:2139–43.

113. Francis NDS, Logan RPH, Walker MM *et al. Campylobacter pylori* organisms in the upper gastrointestinal tract of patients with HIV-1 infection. J Clin Pathol. 1990;43:60–2.

114. Logan RP, Polson RJ, Rao *et al. Helicobacter pylori* and HIV infection [letter]. Lancet. 1990;335:1456.

115. Marano BJ Jr, Smith F, Bonanno CA. *Helicobacter pylori* prevalence in acquired immunodeficiency syndrome. Am J Gastroenterol. 1993;88:687–90.

116. Battan R, Raviglione MC, Palagiano A *et al. Helicobacter pylori* infection in patients with acquired immune deficiency syndrome. Am J Gastroenterol. 1990;85:1576–9.

117. Edwards PD, Carrick J, Turner J, Lee A, Mitchell H, Cooper DA. *Helicobacter pylori*-associated gastritis is rare in AIDS: antibiotic effect or a consequence of immunodeficiency? Am J Gastroenterol. 1991;86:1761–4.

118. O'Connor HJ, Axon ATR, Dixon MF. *Campylobacter*-like organisms unusual in type A (pernicious anemia) gastritis [letter]. Lancet. 1984;1:57.

119. Gonzalez JD, Sancho FJ, Sainz S, Such J, Fernandez M, Mones Xiol J. *Campylobacter pylori* and pernicious anemia [letter]. Lancet. 1988;1:57.

120. Fong TL, Dooley CP, Dehesa M *et al. Helicobacter pylori* infection in pernicious anemia: a prospective controlled study. Gastroenterology. 1991;100:328–32.

121. Blaser MJ, Perez-Perez GI, Lindenbaum J *et al.* Association of infection due to *Helicobacter pylori* with specific upper gastrointestinal pathology. Rev Infect Dis. 1991;13(Suppl 8):S704–8.

122. Hedenbro JL, Benoni C, Schalen C *et al. Helicobacter pylori* and atrophic gastritis. Tokai J Exp Clin Med. 1992;17:1–4.

123. Koop H, Stumpf M, Eissele R *et al.* Antral *Helicobacter pylori*-like organisms in different states of gastric acid secretion. Digestion 1991;48:230–6.

124. Saeed ZA, Evans DJ Jr, Evans DG *et al. Helicobacter pylori* and Zollinger-Ellison syndrome. Dig Dis Sci. 1991;36:15–18.

125. Fich A, Talley NJ, Shorter RG, Phillips SF. Zollinger-Ellison syndrome. Relation to *Helicobacter pylori*-associated chronic gastritis and gastric acid secretion. Dig Dis Sci. 1991;36:10–14.

126. Lambert JR, Lin SK, Midolo P, Korman MG, MacLennan R. *Helicobacter pylori* infection is associated with colonic adenomas. Gastroenterology. 1993;104(4):A128.

127. Aird J, Bentall H, Mehigan JA. The blood groups in relation to peptic ulceration and Ca of the colon, rectum, breath and bronchus. BMJ. 1954;2:317–21.

128. Clarke CA, Edwards JW, Haddock DR, Howell-Evans AW, McLonnell RB, Sheppard PM. ABO blood groups and secretor character in duodenal ulcer. BMJ. 1956;2:725–31.

129. Lam SK, Sircus W. Studies on duodenal ulcer, the clinical evidence for the existence of two populations. Q J Med. 1975;44:369–87.

130. Langman MJS. Blood groups and alimentary disorders. Clin Gastroenterol. 1973;2:497–506.

131. McConnell RB. Peptic ulcer, early genetic evidence – families, twins and markers. In:

Rotter JI, Samloff IM, editors. The genetics and heterogeneity of common gastrointestinal disorders. New York: Academic Press; 1980;31–41.

132. Hook-Nikanne J, Sistonen P, Kosunen TU. Effect of ABO blood group and secretor status on the frequency of *Helicobacter pylori* antibodies. Scand J Gastroenterol. 1990;25: 815–18.

133. Loffeld RJ, Stobberingh E. *Helicobacter pylori* and ABO blood groups. J Clin Pathol. 1991;44:516–17.

134. Mentis A, Blackwell CC, Weir DM, Spiliadis C, Dailianas A, Skandalis N. ABO blood group, secretor status and detection of *Helicobacter pylori* among patients with gastric or duodenal ulcers. Epidemiol Infect. 1991;106:221–9.

135. Dickey W, Collins JS, Watson RG, Sloan JM, Porter KG. Secretor status and *Helicobacter pylori* infection are independent risk factors for gastroduodenal disease. Gut. 1993;34: 351–3.

8
Reinfection with *H. pylori*

D. Y. GRAHAM and R. M. GENTA

INTRODUCTION

Helicobacter pylori therapy can either succeed (cure the infection) or fail.
Failure is demonstrated by return of the original infecting organism soon
after ending antimicrobial therapy (recrudescence of the infection). Cure of
the infection does not guarantee that the individual will not be re-exposed
to the bacterium and become reinfected with either the same or a new strain
of *H. pylori*. Discovery of return of infection after a course or courses of
antimicrobial therapy can be the result of either reinfection or recrudescence.
It is not always easy to distinguish between them.

The concept of reinfection implies the ability to cure *H. pylori* infections
and reliably to recognize that cure has occurred. Before one can discuss
reinfection one must agree that the infection has been cured. The current
functional definition of cure is no evidence of *H. pylori* at 4 or more weeks
after ending antimicrobial therapy (the 4-week rule)[1]. This definition is
arbitrary and has not been prospectively evaluated for its predictive value.
The 4-week rule is a reasonable working definition because experience has
shown that, in the majority of cases, within 4 weeks of ending therapy the
infection will have returned to full vigour and is easy to demonstrate. The
general experience has been that at this time the proportion of false-negative
tests for *H. pylori* infection will be low, and the outcome of therapy will be
correctly categorized. The frequency of false-negative tests depends on which
test or group of tests is used to define absence of *H. pylori* and on the ability
of the laboratory to perform the test(s) accurately. The caveat that must
accompany any statement concerning 'experience' is that most published
reports come from units with a particular interest and expertise in *H. pylori*
disease. Whether similar results can be obtained easily in a busy community
hospital is unknown.

LIMITATIONS OF TESTS FOR PRESENCE OF *H. PYLORI*

All the available tests to determine the absence of *H. pylori* infection have
limitations[2]. Most published evaluations of the various tests have been

performed on patients with untreated infections where the infection is both widespread within the stomach and the number of bacteria is high and the histological response is florid. Results from untreated infections are unlikely to be completely applicable to the recent post-treatment situation. False-negative results are infrequent in untreated *H. pylori* infection but the rate is higher than in untreated patients as therapy may suppress the bacteria and the histological response rather than actually cure the disease. The rapid biopsy urease test (e.g. CLOtest, Delta West, Bentley, Western Australia) requires a high density of bacteria and thus has the highest likelihood of missing the presence of a low level of remaining infection (false-negative results). A negative rapid urease test should not be taken as the sole evidence for cure. Breath tests have an advantage over biopsy urease tests because they sample the entire gastric mucosa. Although urea breath tests share the limitations of the biopsy urease test in that they also measure urease activity and require a high density of bacteria, the rate of false-negative results from breath tests is less than with biopsy urease tests.

Culture is theoretically the most sensitive test; it is certainly the most specific. *H. pylori* is a fastidious micro-organism and many laboratories find it difficult to isolate. Culture also requires transport from the endoscopy laboratory to the microbiology laboratory and delay, drying, and poor choice of transport media all serve to reduce the value of culture as a clinically useful diagnostic test. Choice of culture media and culture conditions, as well as expertise and laboratory experience, also influence the results of culture. Serology can be used to follow the course of infection, but unless paired sera are used, accurate confirmation of cure by a fall in antibody levels for an individual patient may require as long as 1–2 years.

Histology is most often used as the gold standard for *H. pylori* infection as it is standardized and provides an objective and permanent record of whether the bacteria are present or absent. The histopathologist has an additional advantage because, even when the bacteria are sparse, the other features of *H. pylori* gastritis are usually evident. Despite these advantages, histopathology has serious potential and practical limitations.

The pathologist accepts whatever specimens are submitted and cannot dictate to the endoscopist requirements for biopsy size, number or handling. There are a number of potential pitfalls that may occur in the endoscopy unit that can reduce the diagnostic value of gastric mucosal biopsies. The three most important determinants of accurate results are biopsy size, number, and handling. The ecological niche for *H. pylori* is the surface of the stomach. A large biopsy offers a large surface area. Multiple biopsies further increase the surface area examined and partially avoid the potential for the infection being 'patchy'. Since *H. pylori* predominantly inhabits the mucous layer overlying the gastric epithelium, biopsies should be handled in such a manner as to minimize tissue distortion and to dislodge as little mucus as possible. Methods that involve placing the fresh biopsy on a supporting structure such as a piece of filter paper should be avoided. We believe that it is best not to touch the specimen, and to simply shake it off the forceps and into formalin. Although mucosal biopsies tend to curl due to contraction of the smooth muscle of the muscularis mucosae, optimal orientation of the tissue at the time of paraffin embedding is easily achieved by a trained technician.

The importance of specimen number has not been prospectively evaluated. Using jumbo biopsy forceps we found that any site in the stomach of an untreated *H. pylori*-infected patient has a yield of at least 91% in the body and 92.5% in the antrum[3]. This result was based on examination of large, well-oriented specimens with excellent staining and a pathologist both interested and experienced in *H. pylori* work. Whether the results would be as good in the post-therapy stomach is unknown. We have certainly seen examples of post-therapy evaluations where only one of many biopsies was positive, and even then only in one very small focus. We believe that, for results to approach 100% accuracy, three biopsy specimens should be taken; two from the gastric antrum (preferably one of the two from the angulus insuria) and one from the gastric body. The gastric corpus specimen is particularly important for patients with gastric ulcer because intestinal metaplasia is especially common in that group and *H. pylori*-containing mucosa may not be sampled if only antral biopsies are taken. This is less of a problem for patients with duodenal ulcer and possibly those with functional dyspepsia as the rate of intestinal metaplasia in the antrum is low. If only two specimens are taken, one should be taken from the antrum and the other from the corpus.

There are a number of additional potential problems which can occur within pathology laboratories that influence optimal specimen evaluation. Probably the most critical step is for the tissue to be well-oriented so that both the surface and pits can be examined. This requires extra care and training on the part of the technician responsible for embedding the tissue. The technician's job is made considerably easier if the specimens are large, and if no more than three are placed in any specimen bottle. The stain chosen by the laboratory will be largely a matter of personal preference of the pathologist. Whatever stain is used, it should provide information about the type and severity of the gastritis and the presence or absence of the bacteria. Special stains for the presence of *H. pylori* are useful, especially in clinical trials where as much accuracy as possible is desired. We routinely use the Genta stain which combines H&E (for detailed histology), the Steiner stain (an easy silver stain that highlights the bacteria), and Alcian blue at pH 2.5, which emphasizes the presence of intestinal metaplasia[4]. The advantage of this stain is that it provides all the desired information without the need for several separate stains. The ability to see the histology and the bacteria in the same slide is especially important when the number of *H. pylori* is low and the infection focal. For example, if one sees a focus of neutrophils, one can also see the bacteria (Fig. 1).

Newer tests such as those relying on molecular methods such as the polymerase chain reaction (PCR) are undergoing trial, but because of the added expense and the propensity for false-positive results due to contamination in the laboratory, we doubt whether they will soon replace what is currently available.

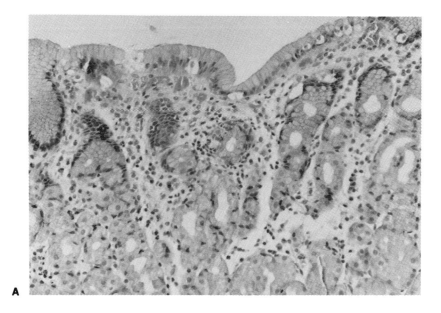

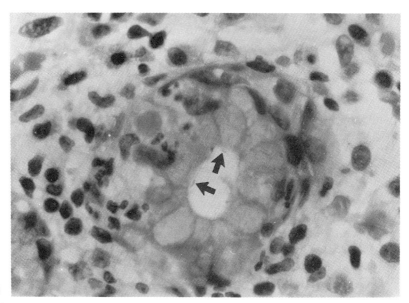

Fig. 1 **A**: example of a post-therapy biopsy in which only one of 11 biopsy specimens had a tiny focus of polymorphonuclear cells (Genta stain × 100). **B**: closer examination showed *H. pylori* (arrows). If the block had been recut to examine the same site with a special stain for *H. pylori*, the focus of polys might not have been found. (Genta stain × 1000)

REINFECTION VERSUS RECRUDESCENCE

When studies that provide data concerning recurrence rates are examined generally recurrence is rare[5–13]. When recurrence occurs it is usually diagnosed within 6 months of ending therapy. Such early recurrence has not been well studied, and we suspect that most cases reflect false-negative results and problems with interpretation of the test(s) responsible for defining cure. Most such cases are probably recrudescence and not reinfection.

Both the initial infection and reinfection require exposure to the bacteria. Transmission of H. pylori is still incompletely understood, but it seems likely that the most common sources of bacteria are the environment, the endoscopy laboratory, and the family. The rate of reinfection in developing countries is said to be much greater than in developed nations[14–16]. One possibility for an apparent increase in recurrence rate is reinfection at the time of endoscopy done to obtain specimens to confirm cure of the infection. Reinfection may occur at this time because of inadequate disinfection of endoscopes or endoscopic accessories, especially biopsy forceps[17,18]. Another possibility is heavy contamination of the environment with H. pylori. Poor sanitation practices as reflected by the frequent presence of other faecal–orally transmitted bacterial diarrhoeal diseases such as enterotoxigenic E. coli diarrhoea or cholera, probably are markers of a heavily H. pylori-contaminated environment[19]. Finally, there is good evidence for clustering of H. pylori infections within families, especially those with children[20–23]. It has also been suggested that infants may serve as a conduit for transmission of H. pylori[24]. If that proves correct, the presence of infants and young children in the home may identify a group at high risk for rapid recurrence.

Now that genetic techniques are available that can identify whether isolates are identical, it should be possible to ask whether rapid or frequent recurrence represents reinfection or recrudescence[25–32]. Repeat isolation of the same strain may result from recrudescence or from reinfection from a source that carries the same strain. It will be important to study the family members (e.g. PCR on H. pylori isolated from stool) to identify which strains are present within a family and who gives the infection to whom. Epidemiology studies are also needed to identify patterns of behaviour that may predispose to infection or reinfection. In addition, it is not known whether treatment of infected family members will reduce the rate of reinfection, especially in developing countries. Such studies are needed.

Reinfection may also be a reflection of increased susceptibility to H. pylori infection. Data from twin studies have shown that there are genetic differences in susceptibility to H. pylori infection[33]. Whether there are populations with increased susceptibility is unknown, but it is certainly not impossible. Similarly, although there are currently no studies demonstrating differences in virulence (e.g. minimal infectious dose) between H. pylori isolates, it is possible that such strains exist. If such strains do exist, it is likely that in some populations a high proportion of circulating H. pylori strains are of increased virulence.

In summary, current therapies are effective in curing H. pylori infection in the majority of cases. Because of the propensity of the organism rapidly to repopulate the stomach, identification of failure to cure is generally easy. The use of the 4-week rule to define cure, and the difficulties faced by pathologists in obtaining, processing, and evaluating gastric mucosal biopsies for histology and culture, inevitably lead to a percentage of false-negative results. The actual percentage observed probably relates to the type of therapy used, the test(s) employed and the interest, expertise, and communication between the medical practitioner and the pathologist. More and better communication is needed, as well as standardization of methods, to confirm cure of *H. pylori* infection. Studies are needed to examine recrudescence versus reinfection and to define whether a 12-week (or some other time) rule may be more appropriate. The large multicentre trials that are currently under way will provide prospective comparative data from a variety of practices and detection methods. Such data are needed to allow accurate assessment of the results of clinical trials, and to understand different cure rates obtained from different studies in different locales.

SUMMARY

The ability to recognize reinfection implies the ability reliably to recognize that cure of a *H. pylori* infection has occurred. The current functional definition of cure is no evidence of *H. pylori* at 4 or more weeks after ending antimicrobial therapy (the 4-week rule). Because of the propensity of the organism to repopulate the stomach rapidly, the rule has reasonable positive predictive and negative predictive value. False categorization is usually the result of poor test selection or test performance. Within the first 3 months to a year after ending therapy, recrudescence is more common than reinfection. Studies are needed to examine recrudescence versus reinfection and to define whether a 12-week (or some other time) rule may be more appropriate. The large multicentre trials that are currently under way will provide prospective comparative data from a variety of practices and detection methods. Such data are needed to allow accurate assessment of the results of clinical trials and to understand different cure rates obtained from different studies in different locales. Both the initial infection and reinfection require exposure to the bacteria; common sources of bacteria may be the environment, the endoscopy laboratory, and the family. Now that genetic techniques are available that can identify whether isolates are identical, it should be possible to ask whether rapid or frequent recurrence represents reinfection or recrudescence.

Acknowledgements

This work was supported by the Department of Veterans Affairs and by the generous support of Hilda Schwartz.

References

1. Borsch GM, Graham DY. *Helicobacter pylori.* In: Collen MJ, Benjamin SB, editors. Pharmacology of peptic ulcer disease. Handbook of experimental pharmacology, Vol. 99. Berlin: Springer-Verlag; 1991:107–48.
2. Alpert LC, Graham DY, Evans DJ Jr *et al.* Diagnostic possibilities for *Campylobacter pylori* infection. Eur J Gastroenterol Hepatol. 1989;1:17–26.
3. Genta RM, Graham DY. Where to biopsy for the histopathologic diagnosis of *Helicobacter pylori*: a topographic study of *H. pylori* density and distribution. Gastrointest Endosc. 1993:in press.
4. Genta RM, Robason GO, Graham DY. Simultaneous visualization of *Helicobacter pylori* and gastric morphology: a new stain. Hum Pathol. 1993:in press.
5. Borody T, Andrews P, Mancuso N, Jankiewicz E, Brandl S. *Helicobacter pylori* reinfection 4 years post-eradication [letter]. Lancet. 1992;339:1295.
6. Veenendaal RA, Peña AS, Meijer JL *et al.* Long term serological surveillance after treatment of *Helicobacter pylori* infection. Gut. 1991;32:1291–4.
7. Coelho LG, Passos MC, Chausson Y *et al.* Duodenal ulcer and eradication of *Helicobacter pylori* in a developing country. An 18-month follow-up study. Scand J Gastroenterol. 1992;27:362–6.
8. Schutze K, Hentschel E, Brandstatter G. More on the eradication of *Helicobacter pylori* and the recurrence of duodenal ulcer. N Engl J Med. 1993;328:1356.
9. Morris AJ, Ali MR, Nicholson GI, Perez-Perez GI, Blaser MJ. Long-term follow-up of voluntary ingestion of *Helicobacter pylori.* Ann Intern Med. 1991;114:662–3.
10. Seppala K, Farkkila M, Nuutinen H *et al.* Triple therapy of *Helicobacter pylori* infection in peptic ulcer. A 12-month follow-up study of 93 patients. Scand J Gastroenterol. 1992;27:973–6.
11. Oderda G, Vaira D, Ainley C *et al.* Eighteen month follow up of *Helicobacter pylori* positive children treated with amoxycillin and tinidazole. Gut. 1992;33:1328–30.
12. Patchett S, Beattie S, Leen E, Keane C, O'Morain C. *Helicobacter pylori* and duodenal ulcer recurrence. Am J Gastroenterol. 1992;87:24–7.
13. Culter AF, Schubert TT. Long-term *Helicobacter pylori* recurrence after successful eradication with triple therapy. Am J Gastroenterol. 1993;88:1359–61.
14. Graham DY. *Helicobacter pylori*: its epidemiology and its role in duodenal ulcer disease. J Gastroenterol Hepatol. 1991;6:105–13.
15. Graham DY, Adam E, Klein PD *et al.* Epidemiology of *Campylobacter pylori* infection. Gastroenterol Clin Biol. 1989;13:84–8B.
16. Graham DY, Adam E, Reddy GT *et al.* Seroepidemiology of *Helicobacter pylori* infection in India. Comparison of developing and developed countries. Dig Dis Sci. 1991;36:1084–8.
17. Graham DY, Alpert LC, Smith JL, Yoshimura HH. Iatrogenic *Campylobacter pylori* infection is a cause of epidemic achlorhydria. Am J Gastroenterol. 1988;83:974–80.
18. Langenberg W, Rauws EA, Oudbier JH, Tytgat GN. Patient-to-patient transmission of *Campylobacter pylori* infection by fiberoptic gastroduodenoscopy and biopsy. J. Infect Dis. 1990;161:507–11.
19. Klein PD, Graham DY, Gaillour A, Opekun AR, Smith EO. Water source as risk factor of *Helicobacter pylori* infection in Peruvian children. Gastrointestinal Physiology Working Group. Lancet. 1991;337:1503–6.
20. Drumm B, Perez-Perez GI, Blaser MJ, Sherman PM. Intrafamilial clustering of *Helicobacter pylori* infection. N Engl J Med. 1990;322:359–63.
21. Mitchell HM, Bohane TD, Berkowicz J, Hazell SL, Lee A. Antibody to *Campylobacter pylori* in families of index children with gastrointestinal illness due to *C. pylori* [letter]. Lancet. 1987;2:681–2.
22. Oderda G, Vaira D, Holton J *et al.* *Helicobacter pylori* in children with peptic ulcer and their families. Dig Dis Sci. 1991;36:572–6.
23. Malaty HM, Graham DY, Klein PD, Evans DG, Adam E, Evans DJ. Transmission of *Helicobacter pylori* infection. Studies in families of healthy individuals. Scand J Gastroenterol. 1991;26:927–32.
24. Graham DY, Klein PD, Evans DG *et al.* *Helicobacter pylori*: epidemiology, relationship to gastric cancer and the role of infants in transmission. Eur J Gastroenterol Hepatol.

1992;4(Suppl. 1):S1–6.

25. Morgan DR, Costas M, Owen RJ, Williams EA. Characterization of strains of *Helicobacter pylori*: one-dimensional SDS-PAGE as a molecular epidemiologic tool. Rev Infect Dis. 1991;13(Suppl. 8):S709–13.

26. Langenberg W, Rauws EA, Widjojokusumo A, Tytgat GN, Zanen HC. Identification of *Campylobacter pyloridis* isolates by restriction endonuclease DNA analysis. J Clin Microbiol. 1986;24:414–17.

27. Go MF, Chan KY, Versalovic J, Koeuth T, Graham DY, Lupski JR. DNA fingerprinting of *II. pylori* genomes with repetitive DNA sequence-based PCR (REP-PCR). Gastroenterology. 1993;104:A2401(abstract).

28. Akopyanz N, Bukanov NO, Westblom TU, Berg DE. PCR-based RFLP analysis of DNA sequence diversity in the gastric pathogen *Helicobacter pylori*. Nucl Acids Res. 1992;20: 6221–5.

29. Foxall PA, Hu LT, Mobley HL. Use of polymerase chain reaction-amplified *Helicobacter pylori* urease structural genes for differentiation of isolates. J Clin Microbiol. 1992;30: 739–41.

30. Lopez CR, Owen RJ, Desai M. Differentiation between isolates of *Helicobacter pylori* by PCR-RFLP analysis of urease A and B genes and comparison with ribosomal RNA gene patterns. FEMS Microbiol Lett. 1993;110:37–43.

31. Clayton CL, Kleanthous H, Morgan DD, Puckey L, Tabaqchali S. Rapid fingerprinting of *Helicobacter pylori* by polymerase chain reaction and restriction fragment length polymorphism analysis. J Clin Microbiol. 1993;31:1420–5.

32. Tee W, Lambert J, Smallwood R, Schembri M, Ross BC, Dwyer B. Ribotyping of *Helicobacter pylori* from clinical specimens. J Clin Microbiol. 1992;30:1562–7.

33. Malaty HM, Engstrand L, Pederson N, Graham DY. Is there a genetic influence in *Helicobacter pylori* susceptibility and transmission: the twin study. Am J Gastroenterol. 1992;399:1342(abstract).

Section III
Mechanisms of *H. pylori* induced damage

9
Breakdown of the mucus layer by *H. pylori*

J. SAROSIEK, Z. NAMIOT, B. J. MARSHALL, D. A. PEURA,
R. L. GUERRANT, D. HARLOW and R. W. McCALLUM

INTRODUCTION

Mucosal integrity in the gastrointestinal (GI) tract is preserved due to an equilibrium between exogenous and endogenous aggressive factors and protective mechanisms operating within pre-epithelial, epithelial and post-epithelial compartments. Since most aggressive factors operate within the lumen of the gastrointestinal tract, pre-epithelial defence seems to be a vanguard of mucosal protection and the target absorbing the major impetus of aggressive factors. The mucus layer, because of its ability to maintain a dynamic equilibrium between the rate of *de novo* synthesis and secretion, and luminal degradation due to proteolytic cleavage, is considered as a core component of pre-epithelial mucosal defence. Therefore, measurement of mucus components within gastric juice may provide direct information regarding the current status of the mucus layer, since it reflects the net results of mucosal secretory potential and degradative potency of luminal aggressive factors. Furthermore, the measurement of physical properties of the gastric juice may provide valuable information regarding the integrity of the pre-epithelial barrier.

BARRIER FUNCTION OF MUCUS

The GI tract mucosa is covered by an approximately $162 \pm 45 \, \mu m$ thick mucus layer[1] which provides a pH gradient that ensures the neutral pH at the luminal domain of the surface epithelium. In addition, the mucus layer remains a complete barrier for larger molecules such as pepsin, non-diffusible through the mucin polymer, whereas it maintains a concentration gradient for small molecules such as hydrogen ion and bicarbonate which diffuse at various rates through its unstirred layer[2-4]. Although the generation of a barrier for various chemical molecules seems to be a primary goal of the mucus layer, it may also absorb major physical forces generated during grinding of food particles and subsequent aboral passage within the lumen.

It is generally believed that the mucus layer provides a unique biological niche for colonization by *Helicobacter pylori*, one of the most enigmatic microorganisms within the alimentary tract. *H. pylori* elaborates various factors that give it an advantage over other potential competing microorganisms and significantly benefit its own survival, multiplication and transmission. This Chapter reviews protective aspects of some of the biochemical and physical properties of the gastric mucus and the damaging potential of various chemically active components elaborated by *H. pylori* with emphasis on the interaction and impact of this organism on the function of the gastric mucosal barrier. Such insight is essential to understanding the pathogenesis of *H. pylori*-related gastroduodenal disease.

COMPOSITION AND PROTECTIVE QUALITY OF GASTRIC MUCUS

Composition of mucus

Alimentary tract mucus is a viscoelastic gel that covers the epithelium and is a complex mixture of mucus glycoprotein (mucin), non-mucin proteins, lipids and electrolytes. It is synthesized and stored in the form of secretory granules and subsequently secreted from the mucous cells stimulated by both physical and chemical (secretagogues) factors[2-4].

Mucus gel comprises inorganic and organic components. Inorganic components, predominantly bicarbonate, are imbedded into an architectural framework provided by the major organic constituent, mucus glycoprotein polymer.

Since mucus gel covers the surface of the epithelium, its organic composition is affected both by luminal and mucosal factors. Among luminal factors that may influence its composition are components of salivary secretion, food ingredients, and solubilized mucus components adsorbed secondarily to the surface of the mucus gel. Components originating within the gastric mucosa can be divided into the three broad categories[2-4].

1. *Secretory components:* mucus glycoprotein (mucin), secretory IgA, IgM, vitamin B_{12}-binding proteins, pepsinogens, pepsins and gastricsins.
2. *Transudatory components:* serum albumin, serum glycoproteins, lipoproteins, serum IgG, IgM and IgA.
3. *Exfoliatory components:* plasma membrane glycoproteins, phospholipids, glycosphingolipids, nucleic acids, integrins and ligands for integrins.

The approximate composition of the mucus gel, adhering to the plasma membranes of the surface epithelium, is 70% proteins, 14% sugars and 16% lipids[5,6]. Mucus glycoprotein, so-called mucin, is a major constituent and a leading determinant of the chemical composition and physical properties of mucus. This glycoprotein consists of 60–80% carbohydrates, 20–40% protein and 0.3–0.4% covalently bound fatty acids[2-4]. Mucin exists as a polymer, with an approximate molecular weight of 2×10^6, formed of subunits covalently bound to a linking protein. To its protein core rich in threonine, serine, glycine, and proline are linked carbohydrate chains composed of N-acetylglucosamine, N-acetylgalactosamine, galactose, fucose and sialic (N-acetylneuraminic) acid[3,4]. Controversy exists regarding the spatial organization of mucus molecules. The 'coiled thread' model, 'windmill' organization with 'bottle brush' shape of subunits rotated 120° along the linking protein are the most widely accepted three-dimensional configurations[2–4]. Only the last conformation, however, considers the modulatory role of lipids in the maintenance of viscous and the permselective properties of mucus[4].

Protective function of mucus

The polymeric structure of mucin and its highly hydrophilic and expanded molecular configuration allow it to form a gel. This gel provides a viscoelastic, spinnable, and permselective layer, crucial for protection against exogenous or endogenous damaging luminal factors. In addition, mucus is the most physiological lubricant. It also agglutinates and aggregates microorganisms, binds bacterial toxins, and modifies the activity of pepsin[3,4,7–9]. Bicarbonate secreted by glandular mucosa is trapped in the mucus gel architectural network and helps the mucus layer maintain the pH gradient between the acidic gastric luminal milieu and the neutral epithelial cell surface[10].

Although one cannot overestimate the role of bicarbonate in the maintenance of the pH gradient within the mucus gel, mucin and non-mucin components also participate in the retardation of hydrogen ion diffusion. As we have demonstrated[11] the retardative capacity of purified gastric mucin was approximately 10-fold greater than control solutions. This ability of gastric mucin has also been confirmed by Bhaskar *et al.*[12] using viscous fingering methodology. A variety of factors, such as phospholipids, albumin, IgA and prostaglandins further enhance the protective physical properties (viscosity, retardation of hydrogen ion diffusion) of mucus[13–15]. These data support an active role of organic mucus components, mainly mucus glycoprotein, in the generation of a barrier to hydrogen ion diffusion. Both the viscosity and permselectivity of gastric mucus and mucin can be significantly compromised through interaction with damaging compounds such as acetylsalicylic acid, lysophosphatidylcholine (lysolecithin) or pepsin[11,16,17]. Various anti-ulcer drugs improve the physico-chemical properties of gastric mucus, therefore generating conditions favourable for the restoration *ad integrum* of the surface epithelium damaged during ulcerogenesis[18–21].

The luminal surface of the mucus gel is subject to continuous erosive activity from various agents and factors within the gastric luminal milieu. Pepsin, especially within the range of acidic pH, is the leading mucus-degrading factor. Since mucous cells actively secrete newly synthesized mucin after restoration of their intracellular mucin stores, equilibrium is maintained between the degradation and restoration of a mucus gel during physiological conditions. This balance, however, changes dynamically with the pace of continuously modifying stimuli and challengers and may reach a state of disequilibrium if aggressive forces overcome protective factors. One factor known to affect the balance within the mucous barrier is *H. pylori*.

CLINICAL CONSEQUENCES OF *H. PYLORI* COLONIZATION

H. pylori, a spiral-shaped Gram-negative microorganism, 2.5–3.5 μm long and 0.5–1.0 μm wide with unipolar flagella[22-27], is one of the most intriguing microorganisms in the alimentary tract of humans. Its causative role in the development of active inflammatory changes within the gastroduodenal mucosa and association with duodenal (95%) and gastric (50–65%) ulcer has been established[28-31]. Relapse of ulcer disease is uncommon after eradication of *H. pylori*[32-34] and it has been suggested that one should attempt to eradicate the *H. pylori* in all patients with peptic ulcer disease. Even in NSAID users with concomitant *H. pylori* infection, eradication may prevent ulcer recurrence and complications[34,35].

Recent evidence suggests that prolonged colonization of the gastric mucosa by this microorganism may also lead to chronic atrophic gastritis and subsequently adenocarcinoma[36-38]. Thus further research into the mechanism of *H. pylori*-mediated mucosal damage is justified. It may be possible to prevent the progress of gastritis by early eradication of the infection; however, any potential effect on carcinogenesis will take years to evaluate.

INTERACTION BETWEEN MUCUS AND *H. pylori*

Mucus-related factors potentially affecting *H. pylori*

Mucus, covering the surface epithelium, due to its multiple components and structural diversity may serve both as a repellent and attractant for various exposed surface structures of *H. pylori*. Since exfoliated epithelial cells with specific *H. pylori* receptors are continuously shed into the mucus layer, one would expect that some receptor molecules would be exposed on the surface of a mucus gel. Therefore, initial docking of *H. pylori* on the surface of the mucus gel could potentially be mediated by gel-embedded membrane fragments with intact receptor molecules for the organism. This initial stage could allow *H. pylori* to contact and anchor within the mucus gel. The difference in viscosity and permselectivity of gastric mucus and purified mucus glycoprotein among individuals (unpublished data) could have a potential impact on both an early stage of *H. pylori* colonization and its survival during eradication regimens. In addition, chemical and physical modification of the mucus layer could potentially enhance the pharmacological effects of antimicrobial agents by allowing them to achieve a high concentration within the pre-epithelial and epithelial compartments. Increased concentrations of lysolecithin in patients with gastric ulcer exhibit a close relationship with the rate of luminal release of glyceroglucolipid[39], a molecule considered to be a receptor for *H. pylori* adhesion[40]. Such free receptor molecules may bind to *H. pylori* adhesins and potentially prevent an attachment of this microorganism to the surface epithelium. Interestingly, we also found that 4 weeks of therapy with ranitidine significantly enhanced secretion of glyceroglucolipid in patients with peptic ulcer[41]. Potential inhibition of *H. pylori* attachment by 'false receptors' released into the mucus gel could eliminate a direct impact on the metabolism and survival of the surface epithelium. Such a phenomenon could potentially contribute to the healing effects of this H_2 receptor antagonist in addition to inhibition of acid and pepsin secretions. These issues, however, still require further investigation.

H. pylori-related factors potentially influencing mucus

H. pylori flourishes within a complex environment that is greatly influenced by various components of ingested food, the mucosal barrier constituents and factors elaborated by its own secretory potential. The organism's high metabolic activity and enormous mobility are presumably significant factors facilitating colonization. These factors may aid *H. pylori* in its continuous search for adhesion molecules. Short-range forces such as hydrogen bonding, ionic and hydrophobic binding may permit the microorganism initially to anchor within the mucus layer. Hydrophobic regions of *H. pylori*, recently described by two independent groups using hydrophobic interaction chromatography[42,43], may play an important role in such non-specific binding. Also strongly hydrophilic *H. pylori* surface structures have been described by salt aggregation testing, contact angle determination and adherence to sulphonated polystyrene[43]. Therefore, both hydrophilic and hydrophobic *H. pylori* membrane structures may play some role in adhesion of the microorganism to the mucus gel and in subsequent colonization of mucous cell membranes. Furthermore, dynamic changes in both the mucus layer and cell membrane milieu may favour hydrophilic or hydrophobic interaction at various stages of colonization.

The potential role of hydrophobic or lipophilic domains in *H. pylori* colonization has also been recently underscored by Goggin *et al.*[44,45] who demonstrated a decrease in hydrophobicity of the surface of the mucus layer in patients with *H. pylori*. This impairment in mucosal hydrophobicity normalized after eradication of the microorganism. Furthermore, we have recently found that the gastric juice of patients with dyspepsia, who are colonized with *H. pylori*, has a significantly higher ability to bind a hydrophobic probe when compared to dyspepsia patients without *H. pylori*[46]. Although our method measuring hydrophobicity is based on recording relative fluorescence generated by BIS-ANS bound to hydrophobic binding sites and is different from the method utilized by Goggin, both publications suggest excessive shedding of hydrophobic molecules from the mucus layer into the gastric lumen. This may be due to the enzymatic cleavage of mucus components by protease and phospholipase identified in some strains of *H. pylori*[47–52]. Therefore, perhaps *H. pylori* benefits from the presence of hydrophobic molecules within the mucus gel during the primary phase of colonization (docking in the mucus gel). However, mucus gel hydrophobic structures may impair the ability of *H. pylori* to attain its ultimate goal of colonization, an attachment to the cell surface receptor (secondary phase of

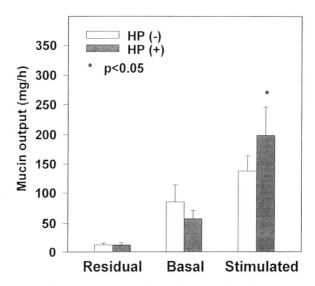

Fig. 1   Mucin output in gastric juice of patients with and without *H. pylori* colonization

colonization). Although excessive luminal release of hydrophobic molecules may benefit colonization, it would inevitably compromise the protective quality of the mucus gel as a barrier to hydrogen ion diffusion.

A detrimental impact of *H. pylori* on the mucous barrier has also been confirmed during our insight into the rate of secretion of mucin and protein within gastric juice in patients colonized by this organism. *H. pylori* positive individuals secreted an excessive amount of mucin (Fig. 1) and protein (Fig. 2) into the gastric juice especially after stimulation with pentagastrin. Such a phenomenon may result both from excessive degradation of the mucus components within the mucus gel and/or the augmented release of mucin depot from mucous cells due to their increased turnover accompanying inflammation. The former explanation is especially attractive, since we have found that the total output of all the components contributing to the viscosity of gastric juice in the same *H. pylori* colonized patients declined significantly (Fig. 3). These data confirm our earlier findings that there are differences in the viscosity of gastric mucus in patients with dyspepsia with and without *H. pylori* colonization[46]. Both groups of selected patients showed the same proteolytic profile of the gastric juice. However, in patients colonized by *H. pylori* the viscosity of mucus, isolated from the gastric juice, was significantly lower when compared to *H. pylori*-negative patients. It seems, therefore, that the gastric mucosal barrier in patients with *H. pylori* is physically compromised by bacterially-related factors. The decrease in the viscosity of gastric mucus may, at least partly, explain why gastroduodenal mucus gel thickness in *H. pylori*-positive patients with dyspepsia was significantly impaired as compared with *H. pylori*-negative dyspepsia patients. In those with confirmed *H. pylori* infection the thickness of the mucus layer

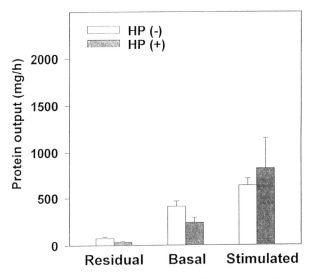

Fig. 2 Total protein output in gastric juice of patients with and without *H. pylori* colonization

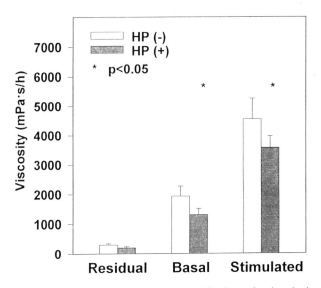

Fig. 3 Hourly output of gastric juice components contributing to its viscosity in patients with and without *H. pylori* colonization

(mean $\pm$ SD) was 0.093 $\pm$ 0.033 mm in duodenal, 0.085 $\pm$ 0.027 mm in antral, and 0.105 $\pm$ 0.033 mm in corpus mucosa. In those without concomitant *H. pylori* colonization the thickness of the mucus gel was 0.162 $\pm$ 0.045 mm; 0.175 $\pm$ 0.067 mm; 0.161 $\pm$ 0.064 mm in the duodenum, antrum and corpus respectively. These differences were statistically significant[53].

Finally, a link between excessive concentrations of lysolecithin in the gastric juice and the presence of active phospholipase in patients colonized by *H. pylori* has also been clearly demonstrated[54]. We showed significantly elevated levels of lysolecithin in patients with gastric ulcer in 1983, when the *H. pylori* saga was still in its early stage of conception. The detrimental impact of lysolecithin on the gastric mucosal barrier may, at least partly, be related to its profound negative impact on viscosity and permeability to hydrogen ion of gastric mucin and its susceptibility to proteolytic cleavage by pepsin[17]. The net result of these effects is to reduce the protective quality of the mucus gel. How this relates to gastritis and peptic ulcer still remains to be determined.

H. pylori appears to secrete glycosulphatase, which removes sulphate (SO_3^-) groups from the gastric mucus glycoprotein molecule. Sulphate groups within mucin enhance its protective quality by inhibiting the proteolytic activity of pepsin and interference with *H. pylori* binding to its epithelial receptor[55,56]. Therefore, desulphation may further diminish the protective quality of the mucus gel layer. Furthermore, *H. pylori* can elaborate toxins[57,58] and PAF-acether[59] which may in turn impair the rate of biosynthesis of mucus within mucous cells.

We have also demonstrated that ammonia, generated by *H. pylori* urease, diminishes the viscosity of the human gastric mucin, purified through equilibrium density-gradient centrifugation (Fig. 4). Ammonia significantly affected the ability of gastric mucin to withstand the higher shear rates, representing forces applied to the mucus layer *in vivo* during phase III of migrating motor complexes. Ammonia ion concentration during these measurements was maintained at levels comparable to the content of ammonia within the gastric compartment in patients colonized by *H. pylori*[60-62]. Changes in gastric mucin viscosity due to ammonia may partly explain its profound damaging effect on the gastric mucosa in an experimental setting[63,64] and offer insight to its pathogenetic effect on human gastric mucosa.

Since patients colonized by *H. pylori* exhibit a significantly higher proteolytic activity within gastric juice compared to healthy non-colonized individuals, one might wonder how *H. pylori* copes with the enormous destructive power of numerous gastric aspartic proteinase isozymes[65]. Furthermore, one should not underestimate the destructive potential of pepsin, which, although it requires low pH for maximal activity, still remains active when pH in *H. pylori* colonized areas drops below 4.0. Recently, we have demonstrated that gastric juice, aspirated from patients with *H. pylori*, inhibits proteolytic activity of pepsin in a dose-dependent fashion from 63% to 92% (Fig. 5). Interestingly, *H. pylori*-related pepsin inhibition was absent when *H. pylori* colonization was accompanied by severe atrophic changes and subsequent achlorhydria. So on the one hand *H. pylori* secretes its own protease, active at neutral pH, fully controlled by the microorganism and presumably helping to maintain an optimal viscosity of the mucus gel. On the other hand, in order to control a very strong endogenous proteinase such as pepsin, *H. pylori* secretes a pepsin inhibitor. Secretion of a pepsin

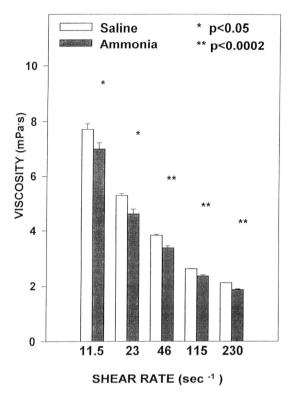

Fig. 4 Impact of ammonia on gastric mucin viscosity

inhibitor may protect *H. pylori* surface structures, presumably crucial for adhesion to cellular receptors. We cannot exclude, however, that human gastric mucosa could also potentially be the source of the pepsin inhibitor. Further investigations into this new and interesting area with respect to ulcer disease seem to be worthwhile.

   H. pylori-induced quantitative and qualitative changes within the gastro-duodenal mucus layer presumably provide optimal conditions for organisms residing in the mucus gel some distance from the surface epithelium and for those firmly attached to the mucosal cell membranes. We have recently shown that *H. pylori* exhibits either predominantly diffuse or predominantly focal type adherence to the surface of cultured human gastric epithelium isolated from patients with non-ulcer dyspepsia[66]. During physical contact between *H. pylori* and the surface of mucous cells, mucin granules were released and acted as a major repelling force on the surface of epithelium. Some *H. pylori* became entrapped by mucin granules. Final adhesion of *H. pylori* occurred only when cells were depleted of their mucin stores and reduced in size by approximately 40–50%[46,66]. Coaggregation where many *H. pylori* microorganisms bind to other *H. pylori* already attached to the epithelial cell surface in a focal pattern of adhesion was also seen[46,66].

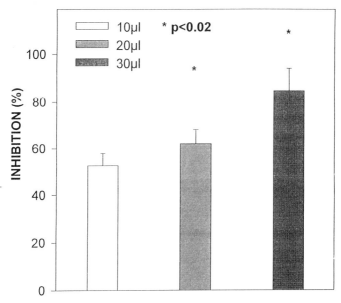

Fig. 5 Inhibitory effect of *H. pylori* (+) gastric juice on proteolytic activity of pepsin

Therefore, the mucus layer provides *H. pylori* with an ideal environment from which it initiates the pathogenic sequelae leading from mild and moderate inflammatory changes to severe gastritis accompanied by progressive atrophic changes, and ultimately the potential for adenocarcinoma.

In general, there are two categories of *H. pylori*-related biologically active factors in patients colonized by this microorganism (Fig. 6). One category includes substances directly released by the organism such as protease, glycosulphatase, phospholipase, urease, toxins and a possible pepsin inhibitor. The second category includes factors indirectly generated by bacterial activity such as ammonia (by urease) and lysolecithin (by phospholipase). Both ammonia and phospholipase are extensively generated *in vivo* and have a profound impact on the mucosal barrier. If the damaging potential of all these *H. pylori*-elaborated factors overlap with the aggressive power of luminal acid and pepsin, corrosion of the mucus gel resulting in a decline of the mucus thickness (Fig. 7) would inevitably occur.

Considering all the available data we would like to present a scheme by which *H. pylori* may mediate damage to the gastric mucosal barrier, especially to the mucus layer (Fig. 8). There are two types of *H. pylori*-related epithelial damage: (1) direct and (2) indirect. Both direct and indirect weakening of the mucosal barrier may generate the optimal conditions required for *H. pylori* colonization and replication. During direct contact between *H. pylori* and the cell, membrane structures are exposed to extremely high concentrations of potential cytotoxins, ammonia generated by *H. pylori* urease, proteases and phospholipases inevitably leading to cell damage. Injury may cause a total disruption of the mucosal barrier. This exaggerated damage may lead

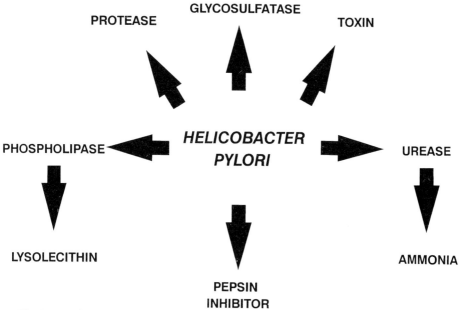

Fig. 6   *H. pylori*-related biologically active factors

to bacterial elimination or force *H. pylori* to move to surrounding less damaged areas to ensure its survival. Numerous *H. pylori*, however, reside in the mucus gel freely spread throughout the entire mucus layer. Damaging factors secreted by the organism into the surrounding milieu lead through proteolysis, desulphation and lipolysis to degradation of the mucus glycoprot-ein-lipid complex within the mucus gel resulting in a decrease of the mucus gel thickness. Quantitative changes of the mucus gel layer are accompanied by qualitative changes such as a decrease in viscosity, potentiation of permeability to hydrogen ion and impairment in hydrophobicity. Both quantitative and qualitative changes within the mucus gel would enhance back-diffusion of hydrogen ions leading to dissipation of the pH gradient in the mucus layer exposing the surface epithelium to an excessive amount of hydrogen ion. These effects in turn, may result in the metabolic impairment of mucus secreting surface epithelium leading to a decline in mucin secretion directly compromising the mucus layer thickness and facilitating any exposure of the mucous cells (affected by a direct impact of all *in situ* elaborated damaging factors by *H. pylori*) to luminal aggressive factors. Such a scenario would inevitably lead to the development of inflammation and perhaps, subsequently, ulcer.

FUTURE IMPLICATIONS

In summary: In patients with gastroduodenal colonization by *H. pylori* a variety of abnormalities within the mucus layer can be demonstrated. These

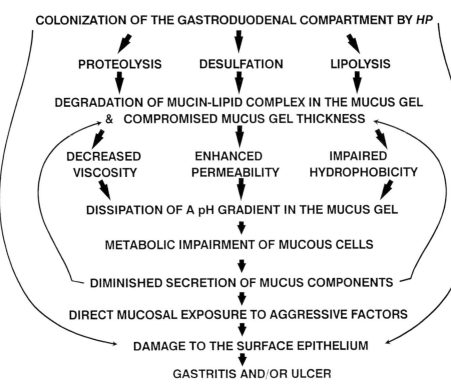

COLONIZATION OF THE GASTRODUODENAL COMPARTMENT BY *HP*

PROTEOLYSIS   DESULFATION   LIPOLYSIS

DEGRADATION OF MUCIN-LIPID COMPLEX IN THE MUCUS GEL
& COMPROMISED MUCUS GEL THICKNESS

DECREASED   ENHANCED   IMPAIRED
VISCOSITY   PERMEABILITY   HYDROPHOBICITY

DISSIPATION OF A pH GRADIENT IN THE MUCUS GEL

METABOLIC IMPAIRMENT OF MUCOUS CELLS

DIMINISHED SECRETION OF MUCUS COMPONENTS

DIRECT MUCOSAL EXPOSURE TO AGGRESSIVE FACTORS

DAMAGE TO THE SURFACE EPITHELIUM

GASTRITIS AND/OR ULCER

Fig. 7 Schematic outline of contribution of *H. pylori*-related damaging factors and luminal acid and pepsin in impairment of the mucous barrier

include (1) a decline of hydrophobicity with subsequent loss of hydrophobic components into the gastric juice; (2) a decrease of viscosity of gastric mucus accompanied by a significant reduction of the mucus layer thickness within the gastric body, antrum and proximal duodenum; and (3) a decline of gastric mucin viscosity. These changes within the mucus gel are accompanied by a decline of viscosity and an increase of hydrophobicity of gastric juice. The proteolytic activity of gastric juice depends upon the net result of a stimulatory impact on secretion of gastric acid and pepsin by the gastric mucosa and the content of pepsin inhibitor released into gastric milieu. The clinical importance of these interesting findings still needs to be defined. Targeting these abnormalities during therapy may not only facilitate healing of mucosal pathology but perhaps also eradication of the microorganisms.

References

1. Lee A, Carrick J, Borody TJ. Campylobacter pyloridis infection as possible complication of weight loss therapy [letter]. Lancet. 1986;2:1343.
2. Allen A. Structure and function of gastrointestinal mucus. In: Johnson LR, ed. Physiology of the gastrointestinal tract. New York: Raven Press; 1981:617–39.
3. Neutra MR, Forstner JF. Gastrointestinal mucus: synthesis, secretion, and function. In: Johnson LR, ed. Physiology of the gastrointestinal tract. New York: Raven Press; 1987:

Gastroduodenal Mucus Gel Milieu

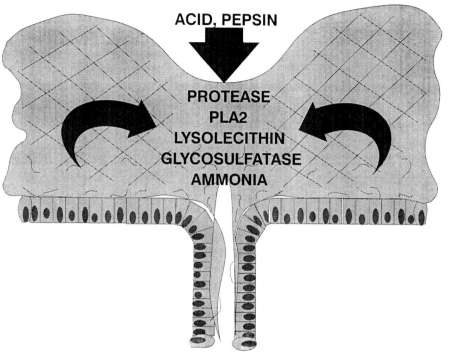

Fig. 8 The direct and indirect effects of *H. pylori* on the gastric mucosal barrier

975–1009.

4. Slomiany BL, Sarosik J, Slomiany A. Gastric mucus and the mucosal barrier. Dig Dis. 1987;5:125–45.

5. Slomiany BL, Piasek A, Sarosiek J, Slomiany A. The role of surface and intracellular mucus in gastric mucosal protection against hydrogen ion. Scand J Gastroenterol. 1985;20: 1191–6.

6. Slomiany BL, Sarosiek J, Slomiany A. Lipids of salivary and gastrointestinal mucus. NY Med Q. 1984;4:124–30.

7. Smart JD, Kellaway IW, Worthington HEC. An in vitro investigation of mucosa-adhesive materials for use in controlled drug delivery. J Pharm Pharmacol. 1984;36:295–9.

8. Cohen PS, Rossol A, Cabelli CJ, Yang SL, Laux DC. Relationships between thy mouse colonizing ability of a human fecal EC strains and its ability to bind a specific colonic mucus gel protein. Infect Immun. 1983;40:62–9.

9. Edwards PAW. Is mucus a selective barrier to macromolecules? Br Med Bull. 1978;34: 55–6.

10. Williams SE, Turnberg LA. Demonstration of a pH gradient across mucus adherent to rabbit gastric mucosa: Evidence for a mucus-bicarbonate barrier. Gut. 1981;22:94–6.

11. Sarosiek J, Slomiany A, Slomiany BL. Retardation of hydrogen ion diffusion by gastric mucus constituents: Effect of proteolysis. Biochem Biophys Res Commun. 1983;113: 1053–60.

12. Bhaskar KR, Garik P, Turner BS, Bradley JD, Bansil R, Stanley HE, LaMont JT. Viscous fingering of HCl through gastric mucin. Nature. 1992;360:458–61.

13. Sarosiek J, Slomiany A, Takagi T, Slomiany BL. Hydrogen ion diffusion in dog gastric mucus glycoprotein: Effect of associated lipids and covalently bound fatty acids. Biochem Biophys Res Commun. 1984;118:523–31.

14. Sarosiek J, Slomiany BL, Jozwiak Z, Liau UH, Slomiany A. Rheological properties of gastric

mucus glycoproteins: contribution of associated lipids. Ann NY Acad Sci. 1984;435:575–7.

15. Sarosiek J, Murty VLN, Nadziejko C, Slomiany A, Slomiany BL. Prostaglandin effect on the physical properties of gastric mucin and its susceptibility to pepsin. Prostaglandins. 1986;32:635–6.

16. Sarosiek J, Mizuta K, Slomiany A, Slomiany BL. Effect of acetylsalicylic acid on gastric mucin viscosity, permeability to hydrogen ion and susceptibility to pepsin. Biochem Pharmacol. 1986;35:4291–5.

17. Slomiany BL, Sarosiek J, Liau YH, Laszewicz W, Murty VLN, Slomiany A. Lysolecithin affects the viscosity, permeability and peptic susceptibility of gastric mucin. Scand J Gastroenterol. 1986;21:1073–9.

18. Gabryelewicz A, Sarosiek J, Laszewicz W. The effect of ranitidine on gastric mucus and pepsin secretion in patients with peptic ulcer. Acta Med Pol. 1981;16:226–34.

19. Sarosiek J, Bilski J, Tsukada H, Slomiany A, Slomiany BL. Effect of solon on gastric mucus viscosity, permeability to hydrogen ion and susceptibility to pepsin. Digestion. 1987;37: 238–46.

20. Bilski J, Sarosiek J, Murty VLN, Aono M, Moriga M, Slomiany A, Slomiany BL. Enhancement of the lipid content and physical properties of gastric mucus by geranylgeranyl-acetone. Biochem Pharmacol. 1987;36:4059–65.

21. Slomiany BL, Liau YH, Carter SR, Sarosiek J, Tsukada H, Slomiany A. Enzymatic sulfation of mucin in gastric mucosa: effect of solon, sucralfate and aspirin. Digestion. 1987;38: 178–86.

22. Jones DM, Curry A, Fox AJ. An ultrastructural study of the gastric campylobacter-like organism Campylobacter pyloridis. J Gen Microbiol. 1985;131:2335–41.

23. Chen XG, Correa P, Offerhaus J, Rodriguez E, Janney F, Hoffmann E, Fox J, Hunter F, Diavolitsis S. Ultrastructure of the gastric mucosa harboring Campylobacter-like organisms. Am J Clin Pathol. 1986;86:575–82.

24. Goodwin CS, McCulloch RK, Armstrong JA, Wee SH. Unusual cellular fatty acids and distinctive ultrastructure in a new spiral bacterium (Campylobacter pyloridis) from the human gastric mucosa. J Med Microbiol. 1985;19:257–67.

25. Fich A, Talley NJ, Shorter RG, Phillips SF. Histological evaluation of Campylobacter pylori from tissue specimens stored in formaldehyde can be misleading [letter]. J Clin Gastroenterol. 1989;11:585.

26. Brown KE, Peura DA. Diagnosis of Helicobacter pylori infection. Gastroenterol Clin N Am. 1993;22:105–15.

27. Chamberlain CE, Peura DA. Campylobacter (Helicobacter) pylori. Is peptic disease a bacterial infection? Arch Intern Med. 1990;150:951–5.

28. Marshall BJ, Warren JR, Goodwin CS. Duodenal ulcer relapse after eradication of Campylobacter pylori [letter]. Lancet. 1989;1:836–7.

29. Warren JR, Marshall B. Unidentified curved bacilli on gastric epithelium in active chronic gastritis [letter]. Lancet. 1983;1:1273–5.

30. Goodwin CS, Armstrong JA, Marshall BJ. Campylobacter pyloridis, gastritis, and peptic ulceration. J Clin Pathol. 1986;39:353–65.

31. Graham DY, Lew GM, Klein PD, Evans DG, Evans DJ, Jr, Saeed ZA, Malaty HM. Effect of treatment of helicobacter pylori infection on the long-term recurrence of gastric or duodenal ulcer. Ann Intern Med. 1992;116:705–8.

32. Marshall BJ, Goodwin CS, Warren JR, Murray R, Blincow ED, Blackbourn SJ, Phillips M, Waters TE, Sanderson CR. Prospective double-blind trial of duodenal ulcer relapse after eradication of Campylobacter pylori. Lancet. 1988;2:1439–42.

33. Hentschel E, Brandstatter G, Dragosics B, Hirschl AM, Nemec H, Schutze K, Taufer M, Wurzer H. Effect of ranitidine and amoxicillin plus metronidazole on the eradication of Helicobacter pylori and the recurrence of duodenal ulcer [see comments]. N Engl J Med. 1993;328:308–12.

34. Graham DY. Treatment of peptic ulcers caused by Helicobacter pylori [editorial; comment]. N Engl J Med. 1993;328:349–50.

35. Martin DF, Montgomery E, Dobek AS, Patrissi GA, Peura DA. Campylobacter pylori, NSAIDs, and smoking: risk factors for peptic ulcer disease. Am J Gastroenterol. 1989;84:1268–72.

36. Correa P. Chronic gastritis: a clinico-pathologic correlation. Am J Gastroenterol.

1988;83:504–9.

37. Correa P, Fox J, Fontham E *et al. Helicobacter pylori* and gastric carcinoma. Serum antibody prevalence in populations with contrasting cancer risks. Cancer. 1990;66:2569–74.

38. Correa P, Ruiz B. *Helicobacter pylori* and gastric cancer. In: Rathbone BJ, Heatley RV, eds. *Helicobacter pylori* and gastroduodenal disease. Oxford: Blackwell Scientific Publications; 1992:158–64.

39. Sarosiek J, Slomiany BL, Gabryelewicz A, Slomiany A. Lysolecithin and glyceroglucolipids in gastric secretion of patients with gastric and duodenal ulcers. Scand J Gastroenterol. 1983;18:935–8.

40. Lingwood CA, Law H, Pellizzari A, Sherman P, Drumm B. Gastric glycerolipid as a receptor for *Campylobacter pylori*. Lancet. 1989;2:238–41.

41. Sarosiek J, Slomiany BL, Slomiany A, Gabryelewicz A. Effect of ranitidine on the content of glyceroglucolipids in gastric secretion of patients with gastric and duodenal ulcer. Scand J Gastroenterol. 1984;19:650–4.

42. Pruul H, Goodwin CS, McDonald PJ, Lewis G, Pankhurst D. Hydrophobic characterisation of *Helicobacter (Campylobacter) pylori*. J Med Microbiol. 1990;32:93–100.

43. Smith JI, Drumm B, Neumann AW, Policova Z, Sherman PM. *In vitro* surface properties of the newly recognized gastric pathogen *Helicobacter pylori*. Infect Immun. 1990;58:3056–60.

44. Goggin PM, Northfield TC, Spychal RT. Factors affecting gastric mucosal hydrophobicity in man. Scand J Gastroenterol. Suppl. 1991;181:65–73.

45. Goggin PM, Marrero JM, Spychal RT, Jackson PA, Corbishley CM, Northfield TC. Surface hydrophobicity of gastric mucosa in *Helicobacter pylori* infection: effect of clearance and eradication. Gastroenterology. 1992;103:1486–90.

46. Sarosiek J, Peura DA, Guerrant RL, Marshall BJ, Laszewicz W, Gabryelewicz A, McCallum RW. Mucolytic effects of *Helicobacter pylori*. Scand J Gastroenterol. Suppl. 1991;187:47–55.

47. Baxter A, Campbell CJ, Cox DM, Grinham CJ, Pendlebury JE. Proteolytic activities of human *Campylobacter pylori* and ferret gastric *Campylobacter*-like organism. Biochem Biophys Res Commun. 1989;163:1–7.

48. Sarosiek J, Slomiany A, Slomiany BL. Evidence for weakening of gastric mucus integrity by *Campylobacter pylori*. Scand J Gastroenterol. 1988;23:585–90.

49. Slomiany BL, Sarosiek J, Bilski J, Slomiany A. Evidence for proteolytic disruption of gastric mucus coat by *Escherichia pylori*. S Afr Med J. 1988;74:40–1.

50. Slomiany BL, Bilski J, Sarosiek J, Murty VL, Dworkin B, VanHorn K, Zielenski J, Slomiany A. *Campylobacter pyloridis* degrades mucin and undermines gastric mucosal integrity. Biochem Biophys Res Commun. 1987;144:307–14.

51. Slomiany BL, Nishikawa H, Piotrowski J, Okazaki K, Slomiany A. Lipolytic activity of *Campylobacter pylori*: effect of sofalcone. Digestion. 1989;43:33–40.

52. Sarosiek J, Slomiany A, VanHorn K, Zalesna G, Slomiany BL. Lipolytic activity of *Campylobacter pylori*: effect of Sofalcone. Gastroenterology. 1988;88:A399.

53. Sarosiek J, Marshall BJ, Peura DA, Hoffman S, Feng T, McCallum RW. Gastroduodenal mucus gel thickness in patients with *Helicobacter pylori*: a method for assessment of biopsy specimens. Am J Gastroenterol. 1991;86:729–34.

54. Langton SR, Cesareo SD. *Helicobacter pylori* associated phospholipase A2 activity: a factor in peptic ulcer production? J Clin Pathol. 1992;45:221–4.

55. Slomiany BL, Murty VL, Piotrowski J, Liau YH, Sundaram P, Slomiany A. Glycosulfatase activity of *Helicobacter pylori* toward gastric mucin. Biochem Biophys Res Commun. 1992;183:506–13.

56. Piotrowski J, Slomiany A, Murty VL, Fekete Z, Slomiany BL. Inhibition of *Helicobacter pylori* colonization by sulfated gastric mucin. Biochem Int. 1991;24:749–56.

57. Hupertz V, Czinn S. Demonstration of a cytotoxin from *Campylobacter pylori*. Eur J Clin Microbiol Infect Dis. 1988;7:576–8.

58. Leunk RD, Johnson PT, David BC, Kraft WG, Morgan DR. Cytotoxic activity in broth-culture filtrates of *Campylobacter pylori*. J Med Microbiol. 1988;26:93–9.

59. Denizot Y, Sobhani I, Rambaud JC, Lewin M, Thomas Y, Benveniste J. Paf-acether synthesis by *Helicobacter pylori*. Gut. 1990;31:1242–5.

60. Marshall BJ, Langton SR. Urea hydrolysis in patients with *Campylobacter pyloridis* infection [letter]. Lancet. 1986;1:965–6.
61. Graham DY, Go MF, Evans DJ, Jr. Review article: urease, gastric ammonium/ammonia, and *Helicobacter pylori* – the past, the present, and recommendations for future research. Aliment Pharmacol Ther. 1992;6:659–69.
62. Langenberg ML, Tytgat GN, Schipper ME, Rietra PJ, Zanen HJ. Campylobacter-like organisms in the stomach of patients and healthy individuals [letter]. Lancet. 1984;1: 1348–9.
63. Murakami M, Yoo JK, Teramura S, Yamamoto K, Saita H, Matuo K, Asada T, Kita T. Generation of ammonia and mucosal lesion formation following hydrolysis of urea by urease in the rat stomach. J Clin Gastroenterol. 1990;12:S104–S109.
64. Kawano S, Tsujii M, Fusamoto H, Sato N, Kamada T. Chronic effect of intragastric ammonia on gastric mucosal structures in rats. Dig Dis Sci. 1991;36:33–8.
65. Taggart RT. Genetic variation of human aspartic proteinases. Scand J Gastroenterol. 1992;52(Suppl.210):111–19.
66. Sarosiek J, Marshall BJ, Hoffman S, Barrett L, Guerrant RL, Anderson H, Hamlin J, McCallum RW. The attachment of *Helicobacter pylori* to human gastric epithelium in vitro: A model for the study of the pathomechanism of colonization. Gastroenterology. 1991;100:A155(Abstract).

10
Decreased hydrophobicity of gastroduodenal mucosa due to *H. pylori* infection in humans

T. C. NORTHFIELD

INTRODUCTION

It is 80 years since Schwarz[1] first put forward the hypothesis that peptic ulcer is a product of self-digestion, due to an imbalance between aggressive factors in the lumen and mucosal defence. Since that time, research has concentrated on the aggressive factors, especially gastric acid, because this has been easier to measure. The emergence of *Helicobacter pylori* infection as the most important aetiological agent in peptic ulceration provides an opportunity and a stimulus to reassess the situation; but mucosal defence remains difficult to measure in clinical practice. Measurement of hydrophobicity on endoscopic biopsies provides a valid method of assessment[2] that can be applied to patients with peptic ulcer and to controls, and that can be repeated following treatment. It is also a rational method of assessment, since it reflects the ability of the mucosa to repel aqueous solutions including acid and pepsin.

MEASUREMENT OF HYDROPHOBICITY

We take endoscopic biopsy specimens and orient them on the specimen stage of a goniometer (Rame-Hart 100/00) by means of a dissecting microscope (Fig. 1). Hydrophobicity is assessed by measuring the advancing contact angle of a drop of saline applied to the biopsy specimen using a micro-syringe attachment[2]. On application of a drop, two cross-hairs fitted within the microscope of the goniometer are aligned to the tangent of the air–liquid-biopsy interface (Fig. 2) and the contact angle is read from a scale encircling the eyepiece. As the biopsy specimen dries at room temperature, the contact angle rises, to reach a plateau at about 30 min, and we express hydrophobicity in terms of this plateau contact angle (Fig. 3).

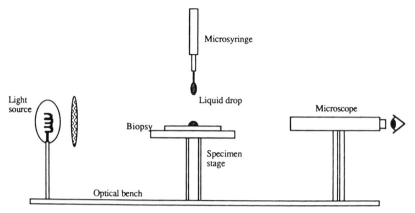

Fig. 1 Goniometer

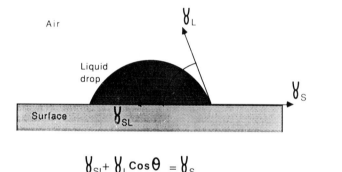

$$\gamma_{SL} + \gamma_L \cos\theta = \gamma_S$$

Fig. 2 Balance of surface forces[6] at the triple point is defined by Young's equation, $Y_{sl} + Y_l \cos\theta = Y_s$, where Y_s represents the solid surface free energy, θ is the contact angle of a liquid with surface tension Y_1, and Y_{sl} is the solid–liquid interfacial energy. (Reproduced from ref. 2 by permission of the publishers)

We found this plateau contact angle very reproducible (intra- and inter-observer variation both less than 4% in humans), whereas the contact angle after a set time interval was highly dependent on ambient conditions of temperature and humidity. The gastric mucosal surface had a significantly higher mean contact angle than the submucosal surface (69° versus 47°) using saline. Glycerol drops gave a lower contact angle than saline drops (55° versus 69°) but gave the same derived values for surface free energy (42 versus 41 mJ/m²), providing an internal validation of the method. In health the highest contact angle, and thus the most hydrophobic surface, was found in that part of the gastrointestinal tract exposed to the most acidic contents, the stomach. The mean contact angle[2] was the same for the antrum as for the body (70° for both), but was significantly lower in the duodenal bulb (62°), distal duodenum (50°) and rectum (57°). The comparison between body and stomach and distal duodenum is illustrated in Figs 3 and 4.

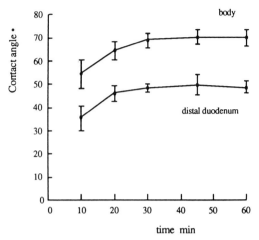

Fig. 3 Effect of air-drying on contact angle after washing: biopsy specimens from the body of stomach and distal duodenum (mean ± SEM of six biopsies). (Reproduced from ref. 2 by permission of the publishers)

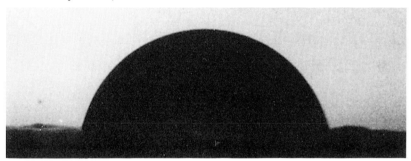

A

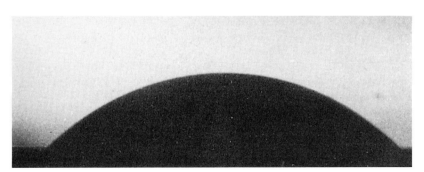

B

Fig. 4 Contact angles of saline drops applied to the gastric body (**A**) and distal duodenum (**B**) during the plateau phase. (Reproduced from ref. 2 by permission of the publishers)

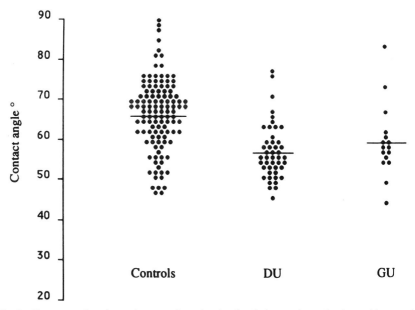

Fig. 5 Contact angles of antral mucosa in active duodenal ulcer and gastric ulcer subjects and in non-ulcer controls

RELATIONSHIP TO PEPTIC ULCER DISEASE AND *H. PYLORI* INFECTION

The mean value for plateau advancing contact angle of antral mucosa for duodenal ulcer subjects (57°) and for gastric ulcer subjects (59°) was significantly lower than for controls (66°, Fig. 5). The contact angle of duodenal bulb mucosa[3] was also reduced in patients with duodenal ulcer (51° versus 63°).

The effect of *H. pylori* infection cannot easily be assessed in patients with peptic ulceration, since there are very few who are *H. pylori*-negative for purposes of comparison. Figure 6 shows contact angles for patients with gastritis, dividing them into those who are positive and negative for *H. pylori*. There is a significant difference between the two groups[3]. The values for the *H. pylori*-positive gastritis subjects were similar to those for *H. pylori*-positive duodenal ulcer subjects, whereas those for *H. pylori*-negative gastritis were similar to those for *H. pylori*-negative controls without gastritis (Fig. 6).

We studied the effect of treatment with bismuth and antibiotics on contact angle[4]. There was a significant increase in contact angle towards normal values in patients who had eradicated *H. pylori* infection 1 month after the cessation of treatment, but not in those who did not achieve eradication (Fig. 7).

ANATOMICAL AND BIOCHEMICAL BASIS OF HYDROPHOBICITY

In order to clarify this, we have studied the gastric mucosa and mucus obtained from pigs immediately after slaughter in an abattoir[5]. The contact

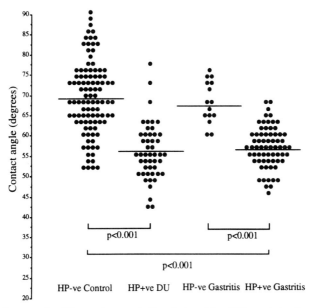

Fig. 6 *H. pylori*-negative (Hp − ve) control, *H. pylori*-positive (HP + ve) duodenal ulcer, *H. pylori*-negative gastritis and *H. pylori*-positive gastritis subjects

angle of mucus samples was the same on glass as on polypropylene, and the results correlated ($r = 0.97$, $p < 0.001$). Mucus samples of two different thicknesses (100 and 1000 μm) had similar contact angles and were correlated ($r = 0.90$, $p < 0.0001$). We compared the contact angle of mucus obtained from different areas with that of the corresponding mucosa with overlying mucus, and found that the results correlated ($r = 0.076$, $p < 0.001$). We also related the contact angle of mucus samples to their phospholipid content. The highest phospholipid concentrations in the mucus layer were those for lecithin and lysolecithin. Contact angle correlated positively with lecithin content ($r = 0.66$, $p < 0.01$) and negatively with lysolecithin content ($r = -0.58$, $p < 0.05$).

DISCUSSION

When a liquid drop is applied to a solid, it forms a contact angle that is a resultant of the equilibrium of surface forces at the triple point of the air–liquid–solid interface[6]. This contact angle (Fig. 2) has an inverse relationship with the surface free energy of the solid. When the same liquid is used on a variety of solid surfaces with different surface energies, the contact angle will increase as the solid surface energy decreases[6]. The surface energy of solids can be derived from contact angles in accordance with Young's equation[6], and this has been applied to a variety of biological tissues. It was first applied to gastric mucosa in the dog by Hills and colleagues[7,8], who reported that

143

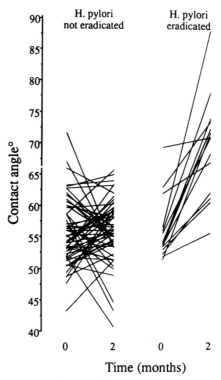

Fig. 7 Contact angle before and 1 month after cessation of treatment in patients in whom *H. pylori* was eradicated or failed to eradicate. (Reproduced from ref. 7 by permission of the publishers)

the stomach had a relatively hydrophobic luminal surface, with a large contact angle.

We have shown that contact angle can be measured on human endoscopic biopsies, and that the surface free energy is the same whether saline or glycerol is used. Others have shown that the surface free energy values obtained by this approach agree closely with those obtained by methods that do not rely on contact angles[9]. This validates the method of using contact angles as a means of assessing the biophysical properties of a tissue surface. We found that the plateau values for contact angle are very reproducible, whereas angles read at a fixed time interval after drying are not[2], probably due to variability in the initial amount of water present on the surface, and in the total surface area.

These measurements provide a unique quantitative method of assessing mucosal defence in the clinical situation, and of assessing the response to treatment. Sarosiek and colleagues[10] have shown that mucus gel thickness on fresh biopsy specimens obtained at endoscopy is reduced in patients with *H. pylori* infection. Although the effect of eradication has not been studied, it appears likely that this reduction in mucus gel thickness is an effect of *H.*

pylori infection. Mucus thickness is, however, a different property to hydrophobicity, since the contact angle is independent of mucus gel thickness, according to our pig mucus experiments. Mucus pH gradient has been investigated as a method of measuring mucosal defence at endoscopy, but the evidence that this is altered by *H. pylori* infection is contradictory[11,12]. This may reflect the large size of the pH electrode used, the diameter of which (1–1.3 mm) is more than three times the depth of the unstirred layer. To reach the juxtamucosal space the electrode must push the mucus out of the way, but once it is in place the electrode itself is a barrier to the diffusion of hydrogen ions from the lumen, so that the unopposed secretion of bicarbonate, or ammonia production by *H. pylori*, will raise the pH above that which is present in a static situation. There are thus serious doubts about the validity of these measurements in the *in vivo* situation. These problems do not arise with the microelectrodes used in animal and human *in vitro* studies.

Our *in vivo* measurements of hydrophobicity can be applied to large numbers of subjects, and can be repeated following treatment. Not only was gastric mucosal hydrophobicity reduced in peptic ulcer patients, but duodenal mucosal hydrophobicity also was reduced in duodenal ulcer patients, possibly reflecting the presence of gastric metaplasia in the duodenal bulb of these patients. Although the drying process necessary to achieve a reproducible plateau contact angle is not physiological, the relative differences found must reflect some underlying abnormality, because the conditions of measurement were the same for all subjects. This abnormality in hydrophobicity was associated with the presence of *H. pylori* infection in patients with gastritis, and was reversed by eradication of the infection, indicating a causal relationship. It was not reversed by healing achieved by acid-suppressing agents. It was not due to some effect of bismuth on gastric mucosa independent of its activity against *H. pylori*, because repeat measurements 1 month after stopping treatment only showed a continued reversal of the abnormality in those showing eradication of the *H. pylori* infection.

The mechanism by which *H. pylori* reduces gastric mucosal hydrophobicity is more difficult to determine, since contact angle measurement does not provide specific information about the molecular configuration at a tissue surface[13]. Furthermore, the physiological determinants of gastric mucosal hydrophobicity are not clear. Lichtenburger and his colleagues, in seeking to explain the hydrophobicity of canine gastric mucosa, suggested a layer of surface-active phospholipids with their hydrophilic heads adsorbed to the gastric mucosa and their hydrophobic tails pointing into the gastric lumen[7,8]. However, surface free energy is by definition the free energy at the surface of a solid, and the surface of the gastric mucosa is covered by a layer of mucus. Our studies on the pig have confirmed that gastric mucosal hydrophobicity is indeed a property of this mucus layer. The mucus layer does itself contain phospholipids, and an increase in lecithin content is associated with an increase in hydrophobicity. By contrast, an increase in lysolecithin content is associated with a decrease in hydrophobicity, as can be predicted from the fact that it has only one hydrophobic fatty acid tail, whereas lecithin has two. The significance of this finding is that lysolecithin is a degradation product of lecithin, due to the action of phospholipase A_2. This enzyme can be produced by *H. pylori*, either directly as shown in *in vitro* studies[14], or indirectly by activation of polymorphs, which also contain phospholipase A_2. Production of lysolecithin within the mucus layer, either directly or indirectly, may therefore be the mechanism by which *H. pylori* reduces mucosal hydrophobicity, thus predisposing to peptic ulceration.

SUMMARY

Valid measurements can be made of mucosal hydrophobicity on biopsies taken from patients undergoing endoscopy. These provide a unique quantitative method of assessing mucosal defence against acid in clinical practice in different groups of patients before and after treatment. Gastric ulcer patients have a reduced hydrophobicity of gastric mucosa, and duodenal ulcer patients have a reduced hydrophobicity of duodenal mucosa also. This abnormality is associated with *H. pylori* infection, and is reversed by eradication of *H. pylori* infection, whereas there is no change in hydrophobicity in patients whose ulcers heal on H_2 receptor antagonists. Hydrophobicity is a property of the overlying mucus layer. It is unrelated to the thickness of this layer, but is related to its phospholipid content, rising with an increase in lecithin content and falling with an increase in lysolecithin content. The *in vitro* finding that *H. pylori* releases phospholipase A_2 provides a plausible explanation for the presence of lysolecithin in the mucus layer *in vivo*, and thus for the mechanism whereby this organism reduces mucosal hydrophobicity and predisposes to peptic ulceration.

References

1. Schwarz Z. Ueber penetrierende Magen- und Jejunalgeschwure. Beitr Klin Chir. 1910;67: 96–128.
2. Spychal RT, Marrero JM, Saverymuttu SH, Northfield TC. Measurement of the surface hydrophobicity of human gastrointestinal mucosa. Gastroenterology. 1989;97:104–11.
3. Spychal RT, Goggin PM, Marrero JM *et al.* Surface hydrophobicity of gastric mucosa in peptic ulcer disease: relationship to gastritis and *Campylobacter pylori* infection. Gastroenterology. 1990;9:1250–4.
4. Goggin PM, Marrero JM, Spychal RT, Jackson PA, Corbishley CM, Northfield TC. Surface hydrophobicity of gastric mucosa in *Helicobacter pylori* infection: effect of clearance and eradication. Gastroenterology. 1992;103:1486–90.
5. Goggin PM, Northfield TC. Anatomical and biochemical basis of gastric mucosal hydrophobicity of isolated pig gastric mucosa. J Physiol. 1989;422:65P.
6. Adamson AW. Physical chemistry of surfaces, 4th edn. New York: Wiley; 1982.
7. Hills BA, Butler BD, Lichtenberger LM. Gastric mucosal barrier: hydrophobic lining to the lumen of the stomach. Am J Physiol. (Gastrointest Liver Physiol.) 1983;244:G561–8.
8. Hills BA. Gastric mucosal barrier: stabilisation of hydrophobic lining to the stomach by mucus. Am J Physiol. (Gastrointest Liver Physiol.) 1985;249:G342–9.
9. Neumann AW, Absolom DR, Francis DW *et al.* Measurement of surface tensions of blood cells and proteins. Ann NY Acad Sci. 1983;416:276–98.
10. Sarosiek J, Marshall BJ, Peura DA *et al.* Gastroduodenal mucus gel thickness in patient with *Helicobacter pylori*: a method for assessment of biopsy specimens. Am J Gastroenterol. 1991;86:729–34.

11. Talley NJ, Ormand JE, Frie CA *et al.* Stability of pH gradients *in vivo* across the stomach in *Helicobacter pylori* gastritis, dyspepsia, and health. Am J Gastroenterol. 1992;87:590–4.
12. Kelly SM, Crampton JR, Hunter JO. *Helicobacter pylori* increases gastric antral juxtamucosal pH. Dig Dis Sci. 1993;38:129–31.
13. Holly FJ, Refojo MF. Water wettability of hydrogels. In: Andrade JD, editor. Hydrogels for medical and related applications. Washington: American Chemical Society; 1976: 252–66.
14. Slomiany B, Nishikawa H, Piotrowski J, Okozaki K, Slomiany A. Lipolytic activity of *Campylobacter pylori*: effect of sofalcone. Digestion. 1989;43:33–40.

11
Adherence and internalization of *H. pylori* by epithelial cells

P. M. SHERMAN

INTRODUCTION

The Gram-negative bacterium, currently referred to as *Helicobacter pylori*[1], is now firmly established as a human pathogen causing chronic-active gastritis[2]. *H. pylori* infection fulfils each of Koch's postulates as a cause of chronic–active gastritis[3] since orogastric challenge of humans[4,5] and experimental animals[6] results in the development of gastritis. Therapy which clears the bacterial infection results in healing of the associated gastritis[7]. There is specificity to *H. pylori* infection because other causes of gastritis, including drug ingestion (i.e. non-steroidal anti-inflammatory agents and corticosteroids), gastroduodenal Crohn's disease, and eosinophilic gastro-enteritis are not correlated with *H. pylori* colonization of the gastric mucosa[8–10].

Accumulating evidence indicates that *H. pylori* infection also has an aetiological role in peptic ulcer disease. Relapse rates following healing of peptic ulcers are markedly reduced by using treatment regimens that eradicate associated *H. pylori* infection[11–13]. Epidemiological studies also provide evidence of a strong correlation between the presence of *H. pylori* infection in the gastric antrum and duodenal ulcer disease[14,15]. In addition, there are epidemiological data that support association between *H. pylori* infection and the development of a variety of types of gastric cancer[16–19]. Although epidemiological reports do not alone provide evidence of a cause-and-effect relationship, these studies suggest that long-standing *H. pylori* infection may be a risk factor for the development of gastric carcinomas and gastric lymphomas.

The pathogenetic mechanisms of *H. pylori*-induced gastroduodenal disease are not well established[20–24]. Factors involved in the pathogenesis of enteric diseases caused by other bacterial pathogens include oral ingestion of the organism, colonization and bacterial adhesion to mucosal surfaces followed either by toxin production or mucosal invasion[25]. This review will focus on adhesion and internalization as potential virulence properties of *H. pylori*.

ADHESION

In vivo adherence

During infection *in vivo H. pylori* colonizes the surface of the gastric epithelium especially in the antrum. *H. pylori* does not reside within the acidic climate present in the lumen of the stomach. Rather, the organism colonizes a microenvironment with a more neutral pH that is formed by the mucus–bicarbonate layer immediately adjacent to the gastric epithelial surface[26]. Electron microscopy shows direct adhesion of the bacterium to the apical plasma membrane of gastric epithelial cells[27–29]. Initial reports suggested a predilection of *H. pylori* colonization in the region of intercellular junctions[30,31]. Subsequent studies, however, have not confirmed this observation[32]. During adhesion of *H. pylori* to gastric surfaces there is disruption of the normal apical microvillus membrane and intimate contact formed between the surface of the organism and the plasma membrane of the epithelial cell[28,29]. Comparable histopathology is evident following *H. pylori* infection of gnotobiotic piglets[33]. These findings are morphologically similar to the intimate adhesion of certain types of diarrhoeagenic *E. coli* to enterocytes and colonocytes during infection of both humans and domesticated animals *in vivo*, and following incubation with cultured epithelial cells *in vitro*[34].

Polymerization of actin in the cytosol subjacent to foci of bacterial adhesion is characteristic of *E. coli* 'attachment–effacement'. There is controversy regarding the induction of cytoskeletal rearrangements in eukaryotic cells infected with *H. pylori*. One group has reported F-actin accumulation following *H. pylori* infection of gastric cells grown in organ culture explants[35]. Two other groups, however, have shown no evidence of cytoskeletal rearrangements using tissue culture cell lines as model systems for bacterial infection of eukaryotic cells[29,36].

In vitro adhesion

In vitro binding of *H. pylori* to a variety of epithelial cell lines has been described including HEp-2 cells[36,37], Intestine 407[36], Y1 adrenal cells[38] and HeLa cells[39]. Adhesion of the bacterium to tissue culture cell lines derived from gastric carcinoma (e.g. KATO-III cells)[40,41] and gastric explants[42,43] have also been demonstrated. During infection of KATO-III cells, as shown in Fig. 1, there is initial binding of the organism to intact microvilli and evidence of disruption of the microvillus membrane with close adhesion of the infecting organism to the underlying plasma membrane[40]. A recent report indicates that *in vitro* binding of *H. pylori* to both KATO-III cells and differentiated epithelial cells isolated from gastric mucosal biopsies is greater than the degree of bacterial adhesion to isolated duodenal enterocytes and colonocytes[44].

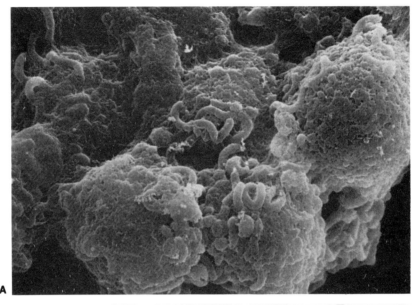

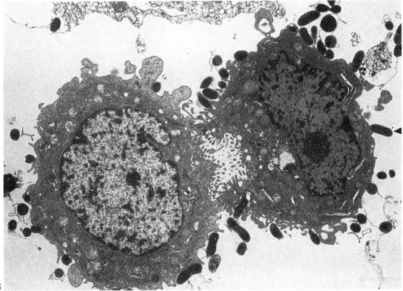

Fig. 1 Panel **A**: scanning electron micrograph of *H. pylori* (strain LC-3) adherent to KATO-III cells after infection for 3.5 h at 37°C. Panel **B**: transmission electron micrograph of *H. pylori* adherent to KATO-III cells. Arrowhead points to intimate bacterial adhesion to the plasma membrane of the infected eukaryotic cell. Taken from ref. 40, with permission

Mucus binding

H. pylori also adheres to isolated gastric mucus glycoproteins in vitro[45]. Sodium metaperiodate-induced oxidation of mucin carbohydrate side-chains reduces binding of H. pylori to mucin. This indicates that the carbohydrate side-chains on the mucus glycoprotein are involved in mediating attachment of the organism. Other investigators have shown that gastric mucus is degraded by urease[46,47], a preformed enzyme that is present and exposed on the bacterial cell surface[48].

Surface hydrophobicity in the stomach is conferred by the overlying gastric mucus layer[49-51]. Measurements of the contact angle of water droplets formed on the surfaces of gastrointestinal mucosa serve as a quantitative marker of surface hydrophobicity[52]. Contact angles formed on gastric mucosa obtained from the endoscopic biopsy of patients with H. pylori infection (59°) are significantly lower than the contact angle of water droplets formed on mucosal biopsies obtained from subjects without H. pylori infection (70°)[53]. The contact angles return towards normal values following eradication of the H. pylori infection[54]. Disruption of the integrity of gastric mucus by H. pylori and its products likely accounts for the observed changes in surface hydrophobicity. The urease enzyme could reduce the surface hydrophobicity of the infected antral mucosa by degrading mucus[46,47]. One group has reported that H. pylori also elaborates a protease that is capable of degrading native gastric mucus glycoproteins[55]. However, evidence of proteolytic activity in H. pylori strains has not been confirmed by other investigators[56].

ADHESINS

The bacterial product mediating adhesion of H. pylori to gastric mucus and to gastric epithelial surfaces is not yet known. It is likely, however, that multiple adhesion determinants are involved in binding of the organism to surface receptors[57]. Knockout mutations of candidate adhesin genes are required to definitively establish whether a single virulence determinant or multiple genes encode the adhesins which promote binding of H. pylori to mucosal surfaces (Table 1).

Flagellin

Motility conferred by flagella is an important virulence factor for this bacterium. H. pylori are flagellated organisms characterized by rapid darting movements when visualized under phase-contrast microscopy[58]. Flagella have been described as adhesins for enteric campylobacters[59]. The role of flagella in mediating adhesion of H. pylori, therefore, required investigation. Eaton et al.[60] tested non-motile variants of H. pylori in a gnotobiotic piglet model of H. pylori-induced chronic gastritis. Only two of eight piglets infected with the non-motile strain developed colonization of the stomach compared to nine of 10 piglets challenged with a motile H. pylori isolate. Although

Table 1 Factors reported to mediate *H. pylori* adhesion to eukaryotic cell surface receptors

Non-specific binding
Hydrophobicity
Charge
Specific adhesins
Flagellin
Urease
Haemagglutinins
63 kDa exoenzyme H
31 kDa OMP
20 kDa NANA-binding protein
19.6 kDa OMP (really an iron-binding cytosolic protein)

isogenic mutants were not employed in this study, these initial findings suggest that the motility properties of this organism increase access to both the gastric epithelium and the overlying mucus layer. Genes encoding the flagellin structural subunit proteins have now been cloned and sequenced[61,62]. Use of isogenic knockout strains deficient only in the production of *Fla*A or *Fla*B should now be employed to establish whether flagellin proteins are involved in adhesion of *H. pylori* to mucosal surfaces.

Urease

Urease has also been proposed as a virulence determinant mediating both bacterial adhesion and cytopathic effects on tissue culture epithelial cells[63]. The genes encoding for production of the structural subunits of the urease enzyme, as well as regulatory and accessory proteins, have been cloned and sequenced[64,65]. A recent study indicates that isogenic urease-negative *H. pylori* strains still adhere to porcine gastric explants *in vitro*[66]. Thus urease may not serve as a specific *H. pylori* attachment factor.

Haemagglutinins

H. pylori strains agglutinate erythrocytes in the presence of D-mannose[67–70]. Some *H. pylori* strains may also elaborate a soluble haemagglutinin that is suggested to be an adhesive factor[71,72]. Whether mannose-resistant haemagglutinin correlates directly with binding of *H. pylori* to gastric epithelial cells and gastric mucus is not clearly defined. One *H. pylori* haemagglutinin described by Evans *et al.*[73] binds to a specific neuraminyl lactose-containing membrane receptor[74]. This haemagglutinin is expressed by *H. pylori in vivo* as evidenced by a specific humoral response in infected individuals[75].

Outer membrane proteins

H. pylori and the ferret gastric pathogen *Helicobacter mustelae* also express a 63 kDa protein, referred to as exoenzyme H, which acts as a ligand

Table 2   Receptors reported to mediate *H. pylori* binding to gastric epithelial surfaces

---

Hydrophobic domains
Mucin
Extracellular matrix
  Laminin
  Collagen type IV
  Heparin sulphate
  Vitronectin
Membrane constituents
  Carbohydrates: fucose, sialic acid
  Glycerolipids: phosphatidylethanolamine, lyso-phosphatidylethanolamine
  Gangliosides: asialo GM-1 (Gg4), asialo GM-2 (Gg3), GM-3
  Cholesterol

---

mediating attachment of the organisms to lipid receptors *in vitro*[76,77].

Another report described the identification, cloning and sequencing of a gene coding for a surface-exposed 19.6 kDa outer membrane protein on *H. pylori*. This fibrillar protein was reported to function as a bacterial adhesin[78]. However, subsequent publications indicate that the cloned gene product is in fact a cytosolic iron-binding protein rather than a surface exposed adhesin candidate[79,80].

Hydrophobic domains

For many bacterial pathogens surface hydrophobicity properties are involved in the initial establishment of contact between the organism and mucosal surfaces[81,82]. The surface hydrophobicity properties of *H. pylori* have shown varying results[83,84]. These differences might well be explained by the use of varying bacterial strains and differing growth conditions. The roles of surface charge and hydrophobicity in the *in vivo* adhesion of *H. pylori* have yet to be defined.

RECEPTORS (Table 2)

Carbohydrates

Sugars present on proteins and lipids frequently serve as cell surface receptor to which bacterial ligands adhere[85]. Pretreatment of erythrocytes with neuraminidase abolishes *H. pylori*-mediated haemagglutination[72]. Sialic acid-rich glycoproteins such as fetuin and orosomucoid also completely inhibit *H. pylori* binding to erythrocytes[71,86]. These findings suggest that terminal sialic acid residues on glycoproteins and glycolipids could serve as receptors for bacterial ligand-mediated adhesion[67,87].

A subsequent study using differentiated gastric epithelium has shown, however, that L-fucose is more likely to function as a receptor for *H. pylori*-mediated adhesion[88]. Binding of *H. pylori* to human gastric mucosa sections that were fixed and placed onto microscope slides was inhibited by fucose, the fucose-binding lectin *Ulex europaeus*, and pretreatment of mucosal sections with either α-ʟ-fucosidase or a monoclonal antibody specific for fucosylated blood group antigens. Proteinase K pretreatment of tissue sections also abolished binding of the gastric pathogen. These findings suggest that there is a fucose-containing glycoprotein receptor that is present on gastric epithelial cells (and not a glycolipid receptor). In contrast, sialoproteins and selective cleavage of sialic acid residues with metaperiodate did not inhibit *H. pylori* adhesion. Moreover, plant lectins specific for sialic acid receptors did not bind to the prefixed gastric epithelial cells[88]. Characterization of the functional role of this fucosylated receptor for bacterial adhesion *in vivo* is now required to establish the biological relevance of this glycoprotein in *H. pylori* adhesion in human infection.

Extracellular matrix

H. pylori binds *in vitro* to selected extracellular matrix constituents. These include laminin[89], type IV collagen[89], vitronectin[90], and heparin sulphate[91]. Trust *et al.*[89] showed that a protein adhesin and surface hydrophobicity both promoted *H. pylori* binding to laminin. Whether these extracellular matrix proteins serve as receptors for *H. pylori* adhesion *in vivo* must now be demonstrated in order to confirm the biological relevance of these *in vitro* findings.

Lipids

Overlay binding assays following lipid separation using thin-layer chromatography demonstrate *H. pylori* adhesion to glycerolipids and gangliosides extracted from both erythrocytes and tissue culture cells[92] (Fig. 2). The lipid receptor is also present in the antrum and, to a lesser extent, in the fundus of humans[92]. The glycerolipid receptor for *H. pylori* binding *in vitro* has been characterized subsequently as a form of phosphatidylethanolamine[93]. Human embryonic lung (HEL) fibroblasts contain little of the lipid compared to both HEp-2 and KATO-III (gastric-derived) tissue culture cell lines of epithelial origin[29]. Adhesion of *H. pylori* to intact cells is least for the HEL cell line. Thus, as shown in Table 3, *H. pylori* adhesion to tissue culture cells correlates with the amount of the phosphatidylethanolamine receptor[29]. *H. pylori* also binds to a deacylated form of phosphatidylethanolamine[77], gangliotetraosylceramide (Gg4, asialo-GM-1) and gangliotriosylceramide (Gg3, asialo-GM-2)[94,95]. Others have reported *H. pylori* binding to the ganglioside GM3[95] and cholesterol[96]. Whether these membrane structures are surface exposed and mediate binding of *H. pylori* during infection *in vivo* requires further investigation.

INTERNALIZATION

Most histopathological studies of biopsy material obtained from *H. pylori*-infected humans have not provided evidence demonstrating bacterial invasion

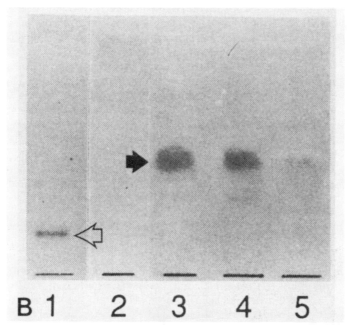

Fig. 2 *H. pylori* (strain LC-11) binding to lipids extracted from HEp-2 cells and separated by polarity using thin-layer chromatography (arrow, lanes 3–5). Lane 1 shows *H. pylori* binding to Gg4 (open arrow). Taken from ref. 77, with permission

Table 3 Adhesion of *H. pylori* (strain LC-11) to eukaryotic tissue culture cell lines (adapted from ref. 29, with permission)

		Bacterial adhesion	
Cell line	PE receptor[a]	Percentage of cells with adherent bacteria	Mean no. adherent bacteria/cell
HEp-2	+	72	8
KATO-III	+	71	7
CHO	+	79	10
HEL	−	43	2

[a] + and − denote presence and absence of receptor, respectively

into either the cytoplasm of surface gastric epithelial cells or through the basement membrane into the underlying interstitium. There are isolated reports, however, identifying the organism within the lamina propria of gastric epithelium[97,98]. Three groups have reported that there is internalization of intact, viable organisms into the cytoplasm of the eukaryotic cell following *H. pylori* infection of cultured epithelial cells[99–101]. In contrast, Megraud *et al.*[102] were not able to culture viable intracellular organisms from infected HEp-2 cells using the same gentamicin-invasion assay. In addition, Smoot *et al.*[35] observed occasional intracellular bacteria following *H. pylori* infection of gastric explants using transmission electron microscopy. However, evidence of morphological changes in the infected eukaryotic cells were present, and the viability of the intracellular organisms was not confirmed. Transmission electron microscopy did not detect intracellular organisms in KATO-III cells infected with *H. pylori*[40]. Whether *H. pylori* is internalized by differentiated gastric epithelial cells therefore requires further investigation.

Concerns have been raised about potential artifacts arising from employing the gentamicin assay as a measure of bacterial invasion[103]. Recent work indicates, for example, that there is internalization of pathogenic organisms such as enterotoxigenic *E. coli*[104] and enterohaemorrhagic *E. coli*[105] that are classically considered as non-invasive bacterial pathogens. The relevance of these *in vitro* findings to infection *in vivo* also must be defined. Genes encoding the ability of this organism to internalize into susceptible epithelial cells should be identified in order to confirm these laboratory observations, as well as to support their biological relevance.

Recent studies indicate that *H. pylori* infection induces production of interleukin-8 by infected gastric epithelial cells[106,107]. This cytokine is a potent neutrophil chemoattractant, which might explain the presence of a polymorphonuclear leukocyte infiltrate in the chronic–active gastritis that is evident in many *H. pylori*-infected individuals. Interleukin-8 responses by epithelial cells following infection with well-established invasive enteric pathogens have been described recently[108]. Whether *H. pylori* must be internalized to induce an IL-8 response in infected epithelial cells therefore requires further clarification.

CONCLUSION

Following the initial identification and culture of *H. pylori* by Drs Marshall and Warren some 10 years ago there has been a great deal written about the virulence properties of this gastric pathogen. There remain, however, a number of unanswered questions. To more clearly understand the virulence properties of *H. pylori* it is essential to define the biological relevance of bacterial adhesion and internalization. The relative importance of the adhesins and receptors identified to date in *in vitro* experiments requires additional evaluation using appropriate animal models of human gastroduodenal disease. The relative importance of *H. pylori* adhesion determinants and invasion should be undertaken by focusing on defining the genetic basis of these virulence factors. New methods of *in vivo* expression technology[109] should greatly facilitate such an approach.

Defining the adhesin, or adhesins, which mediate *H. pylori* binding *in vivo* and thereby promote bacterial colonization of gastric surfaces could then result in the development of effective vaccine candidates. Both active and passive vaccines are currently available for preventing enteric infections in domesticated animals[110] and they are in the rapid phase of development for use in the prevention of enteric bacterial infections in humans[111].

The development of vaccines to prevent primary infection in high-risk uninfected populations and possibly to prevent recurrence of *H. pylori* infection among successfully treated individuals should become possible with an improved understanding of the pathogenesis of disease. Recent findings indicate that indeed it should be possible to develop vaccines for the prevention of *H. pylori* infection[112]. Using a murine model, studies have shown that when *H. felis* is given in conjunction with small amounts of cholera toxin as an oral mucosal adjuvant[113], an immune response develops that effectively prevents bacterial colonization during subsequent challenge[114,115]. These preliminary studies indicate that safe and effective oral vaccines should now be developed to assess their application for future use in the prevention of gastroduodenal diseases in humans.

SUMMARY

Adhesion of pathogenic bacteria to mucosal surfaces promotes disease by increasing colonization of the infected host, by enhancing delivery of bacterial toxins and by facilitating entry of invasive pathogens into the eukaryotic cell cytoplasm. During *H. pylori* infection of humans there is intimate binding of the organism to the apical plasma membrane of surface epithelial cells in regions where the microvillus membrane is disrupted. *H. pylori* also adheres to a variety of tissue culture cell lines and to organ culture explants *in vitro*. Receptors for *H. pylori* adhesion *in vitro* include extracellular matrix proteins, mucus glycoproteins, glycerolipids, and gangliosides. Non-specific adhesion properties of the organism, including surface charge and hydrophobicity, may mediate initial interactions with host epithelia. Specific bacterial ligands that promote subsequent *H. pylori* adhesion *in vitro* include fibrillar proteins, outer membrane proteins, haemagglutinins and an exoenzyme S-like surface protein. As with other Gram-negative pathogens, multiple adhesins probably promote *H. pylori* binding to mucosal surfaces. Internalization of viable *H. pylori* into the cytosol of infected cell lines has been reported. The bacterial factors and host responses promoting internalization of this gastric pathogen require clarification, as does the biological relevance of this *in vitro* response. Characterization of both the bacterial and host factors which mediate *H. pylori* adhesion and internalization should result in the development of novel strategies for the prevention and treatment of *H. pylori* infection in humans.

Acknowledgements

P.S. is the recipient of a Career Scientist Award from the Ontario Ministry of Health. The author thanks Dr Benjamin Gold, Emory University, Atlanta, GA for his critical review of this manuscript.

References

1. Goodwin CS, Armstrong JA, Chilvers T *et al.* Transfer of *Campylobacter pylori* and *Campylobacter mustelae* to Helicobacter gen. nov. as *Helicobacter pylori* comb. nov. and *Helicobacter mustelae* comb. nov., respectively. Int J Syst Bacteriol. 1989;39:397–405.

2. Marshall BJ, Warren JR. Unidentified curved bacilli in the stomach of patients with gastritis and peptic ulceration. Lancet. 1984;1:1311–15.
3. Blaser MJ. *Helicobacter pylori* and the pathogenesis of gastroduodenal inflammation. J Infect Dis. 1990;161:626–33.
4. Marshall BJ, Armstrong JA, McGechie DB, Glancy RJ. Attempt to fulfill Koch's postulates for *pyloric Campylobacter*. Med J Aust. 1984;142:436–9.
5. Morris A, Nicholson G. Ingestion of *Campylobacter pyloridis* causes gastritis and raised fasting gastric pH. Am J Gastroenterol. 1987;82:192–9.
6. Fox JG, Lee A. Gastric Campylobacter-like organisms: their role in gastric diseases in laboratory animals. Lab Anim Sci. 1989;39:1543–53.
7. Drumm B, Sherman P, Chiasson D, Karmali M, Cutz E. Treatment of *Campylobacter pylori*-associated antral gastritis in children with bismuth subsalicylate and ampicillin. J Pediatr. 1988;113:908–12.
8. Drumm B, Sherman P, Cutz E, Karmali M. Association of *Campylobacter pylori* on the gastric mucosa with antral gastritis in children. N Engl J Med. 1987;316:1557–61.
9. Drumm B, O'Brien A, Cutz E, Sherman P. *Campylobacter pyloridis*-associated primary gastritis in children. Pediatrics. 1987;80:192–5.
10. Ormand JE, Talley NJ, Shorter RG *et al.* Prevalence of *Helicobacter pylori* in specific forms of gastritis. Dig Dis Sci. 1991;36:142–5.
11. Rauws EAJ, Tytgat GNJ. Cure of duodenal ulcer associated with eradication of *Helicobacter pylori*. Lancet. 1990;335:1233–5.
12. Graham DY, Lew GM, Klein PD *et al.* Effect of treatment of *Helicobacter pylori* infection on the long-term recurrence of gastric or duodenal ulcer. A randomized, controlled study. Ann Intern Med. 1992;116:705–8.
13. Hentschel E, Brandstatter G, Dragosics B *et al.* Effect of ranitidine and amoxicillin plus metronidazole on the eradication of *Helicobacter pylori* and the recurrence of duodenal ulcer. N Engl J Med. 1993;328:308–12.
14. Taylor DN, Blaser MJ. The epidemiology of *Helicobacter pylori* infection. Epidemiol Rev. 1991;13:42–59.
15. Moss S, Calam J. *Helicobacter pylori* and peptic ulcers: the present position. Gut. 1992;33:289–92 (Editorial).
16. Forman D, Newell DG, Fullerton F *et al.* Association between infection with *Helicobacter pylori* and risk of gastric cancer: evidence from a prospective investigation. BMJ. 1991;302:1302–5.
17. Wotherspoon AC, Ortiz-Hidalgo C, Falzon MR, Isaacson PG. *Helicobacter pylori*-associated gastritis and primary B-cell gastric lymphoma. Lancet. 1991;338:1175–6.
18. Doglioni C, Wotherspoon AC, Moschini A, De Boni M, Isaacson PG. High incidence of primary gastric lymphoma in northeastern Italy. Lancet. 1992;339:834–5.
19. Eurogast Study Group. An international association between *Helicobacter pylori* infection and gastric cancer. Lancet. 1993;341:1359–62.
20. Newell DG. Virulence factors of *Helicobacter pylori*. Scand J Gastroenterol. 1991;26(Suppl. 187):31–8.
21. Marshall BJ III. Virulence and pathogenicity of *Helicobacter pylori*. J Gastroenterol Hepatol. 1991;6:121–4.
22. Sinclair P. Virulence factors of *Helicobacter pylori*. Can J Gastroenterol. 1991;5:214–18.
23. Lee A, Fox J, Hazell S. Pathogenicity of *Helicobacter pylori*: a perspective. Infect Immun. 1993;61:1601–10.
24. Dunn BE. Pathogenic mechanisms of *Helicobacter pylori*. Gastroenterol Clin N Am. 1993;22:43–57.
25. Finlay BB, Falkow S. Common themes in microbial pathogenicity. Microbiol Rev. 1989;53:210–30.
26. Marshall BJ, Barrett LJ, Prakash C, MacCallum RW, Guerrant RL. Urea protects *Helicobacter pylori* from the bactericidal effect of acid. Gastroenterology. 1990;99:697–702.
27. Tricottet V, Bruneval P, Vire O *et al.* *Campylobacter*-like organisms and surface epithelium abnormalities in active, chronic gastritis in humans: an ultrastructural study. Ultrastruct Pathol. 1986;10:113–22.
28. Hessey SJ, Spencer J, Wyatt JI *et al.* Bacterial adhesion and disease activity in *Helicobacter* associated chronic gastritis. Gut. 1990;31:134–8.

29. Dytoc M, Gold B, Louie M *et al.* Comparison of *Helicobacter pylori* and attaching-effacing *Escherichia coli* adhesion to eukaryotic cells. Infect Immun. 1993;61:448–56.
30. Hazell SL, Lee A, Brady L, Hennessy W. *Campylobacter pyloridis* and gastritis: association with intercellular spaces and adaptation to an environment of mucus as important factors in colonization of the gastric epithelium. J Infect Dis. 1986;153:658–63.
31. Kazi JL, Sinniah R, Zaman V *et al.* Ultrastructural study of *Helicobacter pylori*-associated gastritis. J Pathol. 1990;161:65–70.
32. Thomsen LL, Gavin JB, Tasman-Jones C. Relation of *Helicobacter pylori* to the human gastric mucosa in chronic gastritis of the antrum. Gut. 1990;31:1230–6.
33. Rudmann DG, Eaton KA, Krakowka S. Ultrastructural study of *Helicobacter pylori* adherence properties in gnotobiotic piglets. Infect Immun. 1992;60:2121–4.
34. Tesh VL, O'Brien AD. Adherence and colonization mechanisms of enteropathogenic and enterohemorrhagic *Escherichia coli*. Microb Pathogen. 1992;12:245–54.
35. Smoot DT, Resau JH, Naab T *et al.* Adherence of *Helicobacter pylori* to cultured human gastric epithelial cells. Infect Immun. 1993;61:350–5.
36. Neman-Simha V, Megraud F. *In vitro* model for *Campylobacter pylori* adherence properties. Infect Immun. 1988;56:3329–33.
37. Figueroa G, Portell DP, Soto V, Troncoso M. Adherence of *Helicobacter pylori* to HEp-2 cells. J Infect. 1992;24:263–7.
38. Evans DG, Evans Jr DJ, Graham DY. Receptor-mediated adherence of *Campylobacter pylori* to mouse Y-1 adrenal cell monolayers. Infect Immun. 1989;57:2272–8.
39. Fauchere J-L, Blaser MJ. Adherence of *Helicobacter pylori* cells and their surface components to HeLa cell membranes. Microb Pathogen. 1990;9:427–39.
40. Hemalatha S, Drumm B, Sherman P. Adherence of *Helicobacter pylori* to human gastric epithelial cells in vitro. J Med Microbiol. 1991;35:197–202.
41. Dunn BE, Altmann M, Campbell GP. Adherence of *Helicobacter pylori* to gastric carcinoma cells: analysis by flow cytometry. Rev Infect Dis. 1991;13(Suppl. 8):S57–S64.
42. Smoot DT, Rosenthal LE, Mobley HLT, Iseri O, Zhu S, Resau JH. Development of a human stomach explant organ culture system to study the pathogenesis of *Helicobacter pylori*. Digestion. 1990;46:46–54.
43. Rosberg K, Berglindh T, Gustavsson S, Hubinette R, Rolfsen W. Adhesion of *Helicobacter pylori* to human gastric mucosal biopsy specimens cultivated *in vitro*. Scand J Gastroenterol. 1991;26:1179–87.
44. Clyne M, Drumm B. Adherence of *Helicobacter pylori* to primary human gastrointestinal cells. Infect Immun. 1993;61:4051–7.
45. Tzouvelekis LS, Mentis AF, Makris AM, Spiliadis C, Blackwell C, Weir DM. *In vitro* binding of *Helicobacter pylori* to human gastric mucin. Infect Immun. 1991;59:4252–4.
46. Sidebothom RL, Batten JJ, Karim QN, Spencer J, Baron JH. Breakdown of gastric mucus in the presence of *Helicobacter pylori*. J Clin Pathol. 1991;44:52–7.
47. Sidebothom RL, Baron JH. Hypothesis: *Helicobacter pylori*, urease, mucus, and gastric ulcer. Lancet. 1990;335:193–5.
48. Hawtin PR, Stacey AR, Newell DG. Investigation of the structure and localization of the urease of *Helicobacter pylori* using monoclonal antibodies. J Gen Microbiol. 1990;136:1995–2000.
49. Hills BR, Kirwood CA. Gastric mucosal barrier: barrier to hydrogen ions imparted by gastric surfactant in vitro. Gut. 1992;33:1039–41.
50. Kao Y-CJ, Lichtenberger LM. Phospholipid- and neutral lipid-containing organelles of rat gastroduodenal mucous cells. Possible origin of the hydrophobic mucosal lining. Gastroenterology. 1991;101:7–21.
51. Goddard PJ, Kao Y-CJ, Lichtenberger LM. Luminal surface hydrophobicity of canine gastric mucosa is dependent on a surface mucous gel. Gastroenterology. 1990;98:361–70.
52. Mack D, Neumann AW, Policova Z, Sherman P. Surface hydrophobicity of the intestinal tract. Am J Physiol. 1992;262:G171–7.
53. Spychal RT, Goggin PM, Marrero JM *et al.* Surface hydrophobicity of gastric mucosa in peptic ulcer disease. Relationship to gastritis and *Campylobacter pylori* infection. Gastroenterology. 1990;98:1250–4.
54. Goggin PM, Marrero JM, Spychal RT, Jackson PA, Corbishley CM, Northfield TC. Surface hydrophobicity of gastric mucosa in *Helicobacter pylori* infection: effect of clearance and

eradication. Gastroenterology. 1992;103:1486–90.

55. Slomiany BL, Bilski J, Sarosiek J et al. Campyolobacter pyloridis degrades mucin and undermines gastric mucosal integrity. Biochem Biophys Res Commun. 1987;144:307–14.

56. Baxter A, Campbell CJ, Cox DM, Grinham CJ, Pendlebury JE. Proteolytic activities of human Campylobacter pylori and ferret gastric Campylobacter-like organism. Biochem Biophys Res Commun. 1989;163:1–7.

57. Wadstrom T, Ascencio F, Ljungh A, et al. Helicobacter pylori adhesins. Eur J Gastroenterol Hepatol. 1993;5(suppl.2):S12–S15.

58. Drumm B, Sherman P. Long-term storage of Campylobacter pylori. J Clin Microbiol. 1989;27:1655–6.

59. Newell DG, McBride H, Dolby JM. Investigations on the role of flagella in the colonization of infant mice with Campylobacter jejuni and attachment of Campylobacter jejuni to human epithelial cell lines. J Hyg (Cambridge). 1985;95:217–27.

60. Eaton KA, Morgan DR, Krakowka S. Motility as a factor in the colonisation of gnotobiotic piglets by Helicobacter pylori. J Med Microbiol. 1992;37:123–7.

61. Leying H, Suerbaum S, Geis G, Haas R. Cloning and the genetic characterization of a Helicobacter pylori flagellin gene. Mol Microbiol. 1992;6:2863–74.

62. Suerbaum S, Josenhans C, Labigne A. Cloning and genetic characterization of the Helicobacter pylori and Helicobacter mustelae flaB flagellin genes and construction of H. pylori flaA- and fla-B negative mutants by electroporation-mediated allelic exchange. J Bacteriol. 1993;175:3278–88.

63. Eaton KA, Brooks CL, Morgan DR, Krakowka S. Essential role of urease in pathogenesis of gastritis induced by Helicobacter pylori in gnotobiotic piglets. Infect Immun. 1991;59:2470–5.

64. Cussac V, Ferraro RL, Labigne A. Expression of Helicobacter pylori urease genes in Escherichia coli grown under nitrogen-limiting conditions. J Bacteriol. 1992;174:2466–73.

65. Ferraro RL, Cussac V, Courcaux P, Labigne A. Construction of isogenic urease-negative mutants of Helicobacter pylori by allelic exchange. J Bacteriol. 1992;174:4212–17.

66. Eaton KA, Labigne AF, Krakowka S. An isogenic urease-deficient mutant of Helicobacter pylori colonizes gastric epithelia but not germ-free piglets. Gastroenterology. 1993;104:A694(abstract).

67. Emody L, Carlsson A, Ljungh A, Wadstrom T. Mannose-resistant haemagglutination by Campylobacter pylori. Scand J Infect Dis. 1988;20:353–4.

68. Huang J, Smyth CJ, Kennedy NP, Arbuthnott JP, Keeling PWN. Haemagglutinating activity of Campylobacter pylori. FEMS Microbiol Lett. 1988;56:109–12.

69. Nakazawa T, Ishibashi M, Konishi H, Takemoto T, Shigeeda M, Kochiyama T. Hemagglutination activity of Campylobacter pylori. Infect Immun. 1989;57:989–91.

70. Taylor NS, Hasubski AT, Fox JG, Lee A. Haemagglutination profiles of Helicobacter species that cause gastritis in man and animals. J Med Microbiol. 1992;37:299–303.

71. Armstrong JA, Cooper M, Goodwin CS et al. Influence of soluble haemagglutinins on adherence of Helicobacter pylori to HEp-2 cells. J Med Microbiol. 1991;34:181–7.

72. Lelwala-Guruge J, Ascencio F, Kreger AS, Ljungh A, Wadstrom T. Isolation of a sialic acid-specific surface haemagglutinin of Helicobacter pylori strain NCTC 11637. Zbl Bakt. 1993;280:93–106.

73. Evans DG, Karjalainen TK, Evans DJ, Graham DY, Lee C-H. Cloning, nucleotide sequence, and expression of a gene encoding an adhesin subunit protein of Helicobacter pylori. J Bacteriol. 1993;175:674–83.

74. Evans DG, Evans Jr DJ, Moulds JJ, Graham DY. N-acetylneuraminyllactose-binding fibrillar hemagglutinin of Campylobacter pylori: a putative colonization factor antigen. Infect Immun. 1988;56:2896–906.

75. Evans DG, Evans Jr DJ, Smith KE, Graham DY. Serum antibody responses to N-acetylneuraminyllactose-binding hemagglutinin of Campylobacter pylori. Infect Immun. 1989;57:664–7.

76. Lingwood CA, Wasfy G, Han H, Huesca M. Receptor affinity purification of a lipid-binding adhesin from Helicobacter pylori. Infect Immun. 1993;61:2474–8.

77. Gold B, Huesca M, Sherman PM, Lingwood CA. Helicobacter mustelae and Helicobacter pylori bind to common lipid receptors in vitro. Infect Immun. 1993;61:2632–8.

78. Doig P, Austin JW, Kostrzynska M, Trust TJ. Production of a conserved adhesin by the

human gastroduodenal pathogen *Helicobacter pylori*. J Bacteriol. 1992;174:2539–47.

79. Doig P, Austin JW, Trust TJ. The *Helicobacter pylori* 19.6-kilodalton protein is an iron-containing protein resembling ferritin. J Bacteriol. 1993;175:557–60.

80. Frazier BA, Pfeifer JD, Russell DG *et al*. Paracrystalline inclusions of a novel ferritin containing nonheme iron, produced by the human gastric pathogen *Helicobacter pylori*: evidence for a third class of ferritins. J Bacteriol. 1993;175:966–72.

81. Doyle RJ, Rosenberg M. Microbial cell surface hydrophobicity. Washington, DC: ASM Press; 1990.

82. Drumm B, Neumann AW, Policova Z, Sherman P. Bacterial cell surface hydrophobicity properties in the mediation of in vitro adhesion by the rabbit enteric pathogen *Escherichia coli* strain RDEC-1. J Clin Invest. 1989;84:1588–94.

83. Pruul H, Goodwin CS, McDonald PJ, Lewis G, Pankhurst D. Hydrophobic characterisation of *Helicobacter* (Campylobacter) *pylori*. J Med Microbiol. 1990;32:93–100.

84. Smith JI, Drumm B, Neumann AW, Policova Z, Sherman PM. *In vitro* surface properties of the newly recognized gastric pathogen *Helicobacter pylori*. Infect Immun. 1990;58:3056–60.

85. Karlsson K-A, Angstrom J, Bergstrom J, Lanne B. Microbial interaction with animal cell surface carbohydrates. APMIS 1991;100(Suppl 27):71–83.

86. Lelwalwa-Guruge J, Ascencio F, Ljungh A, Wadstrom T. Characterization of sialic acid-specific surface lectins of *Helicobacter pylori*. Abstr Annu Mtg Am Soc Microbiol. 1993;35(abstract B-53).

87. Evans DG, Karjalainen TK, Evans Jr DJ, Graham DY, Lee C-H. Cloning, nucleotide sequence, and expression of a gene encoding an adhesin subunit protein of *Helicobacter pylori*. J Bacteriol. 1993;175:674–83.

88. Falk P, Roth KA, Boren T, Westblom TU, Gordon JI, Normark S. An *in vitro* adherence assay reveals that *Helicobacter pylori* exhibits cell lineage-specific tropism in the human gastric epithelium. Proc Natl Acad Sci USA. 1993;90:2035–9.

89. Trust TJ, Doig P, Emody L, Kienle Z, Wadstrom T, O'Toole P. High-affinity binding of the basement membrane proteins collagen type IV and laminin to the gastric pathogen *Helicobacter pylori*. Infect Immun. 1991;59:4398–404.

90. Ringner M, Paulsson M, Wadstrom T. Vitronectin binding by *Helicobacter pylori*. FEMS Microbiol Immunol. 1992;105:219–24.

91. Ascencio F, Fransson LA, Wadstrom T. Affinity of the gastric pathogen *Helicobacter pylori* for the *N*-sulphated glycosaminoglycan heparin sulphate. J Med Microbiol. 1993;38:240–4.

92. Lingwood C, Law H, Pellizzari A, Sherman P, Drumm B. A gastric glycerolipid as receptor for *Campylobacter pylori*. Lancet. 1989;2:238–41.

93. Lingwood CA, Huesca M, Kuksis A. The glycerolipid receptor for *Helicobacter pylori* (and exoenzyme S) is phosphatidylethanolamine. Infect Immun. 1992;60:2470–4.

94. Saitoh T, Natomi H, Zhao W *et al*. Identification of glycolipid receptors for *Helicobacter pylori* by TLC-immunostaining. FEBS Lett. 1991;282:385–7.

95. Slomiany BL, Piotrowski J, Samanta A, Van Horn K, Murty VLN, Slomiany A. *Campylobacter pylori* colonization factor shows specificity for lactosylceramide sulfate and GM3 ganglioside. Biochem Int. 1989;19:929–36.

96. Ansorg R, Muller K-D, Von Recklinghausen G, Nalik HP. Cholesterol binding of *Helicobacter pylori*. Zbl Bakt. 1992;276:323–9.

97. Andersen LP, Holck S. Possible evidence of invasiveness of *Helicobacter* (Campylobacter) *pylori*. Eur J Clin Microbiol Infect Dis. 1990;9:135–8.

98. Wyle FA, Tarnawski A, Schulman D, Dabros W. Evidence for gastric mucosal cell invasion by *C. pylori*: an ultrastructural study. J Clin Gastroenterol. 1990;12(Suppl 1):S92–8.

99. Evans DG, Evans Jr DJ, Graham DY. Adherence and internalization of *Helicobacter pylori* by HEp-2 cells. Gastroenterology. 1992;102:1557–67.

100. Michetti P, Porta N, Racine L, Krachenbuhl JP, Blum AL. Polarized Madin Darby Canine Kidney epithelial cell monolayers as a model to study *Helicobacter pylori* adherence and invasion. Ir J Med Sci. 1992;161(Suppl. 10):46(abstract).

101. Wilkinson SM, Uhl JR, Cockerill III FR. Evaluation of adherence and invasion of HEp-2 cells by *Helicobacter pylori* strains. Abstr Annu Mtg Am Soc Microbiol. 1993;p.29(abstract D-31).

102. Megraud F, Trimoulet P, Lamouliatte H, Boyanova L. Bactericidal effect of amoxicillin on *Helicobacter pylori* in an in vitro model using epithelial cells. Antimicrob Agents Chemother. 1991;35:869–72.

103. Konkel MB, Hayes SF, Joens LA, Cieplak Jr W. Characteristics of the internalization and intracellular survival of *Campylobacter jejuni* in human epithelial cell cultures. Microb Pathogen. 1992;13:357–70.

104. Ibarra A, Rico G, Gonzalez G, Zepeda H. Invasion to HEp-2 cells by enterotoxigenic *Escherichia coli*. Abstr Annu Mtg Am Soc Microbiol. 1993;82(abstract B-318).

105. Oeleschalaeger TA, Barrett TJ, Kopecko DJ. Characterization of EHEC internalization into human epithelial cell lines. Abstr Annu Mtg Am Soc Microbiol. 1993;81(abstract B-309).

106. Crabtree JE, Peichl P, Wyatt JI, Lindley IJD. Gastric interleukin-8 and IgA IL-8 autoantibodies in *Helicobacter pylori* infection. Scand J Immunol. 1993;37:65–70.

107. Crowe S, Hunt RH, Jordana M *et al*. Interleukin-8 secretion by gastric epithelium following *Helicobacter pylori* infection in vitro. Gastroenterology. 1993;104:A687.

108. Eckmann L, Fierer J, Kagnoff MF. Bacterial invasion of epithelial cells induces secretion of the chemoattractant interleukin-8. Gastroenterology. 1993;104:500(abstract).

109. Mahan MJ, Slauch JM, Mekalanos JJ. Selection of bacterial virulence genes that are specifically induced in host tissues. Science. 1993;259:686–8.

110. Greenwood PE, Clark SJ, Cahill AD, Trevallyn-Jones J, Tsipori S. Development and protective efficacy of a recombinant-DNA derived fimbrial vaccine against enterotoxic collibacillosis in neonatal piglets. Vaccine. 1988;6:389–92.

111. Tackett CO, Losonsky G, Link H *et al*. Protection by milk immunoglobulin concentrate against oral challenge with enterotoxigenic *Escherichia coli*. N Engl J Med. 1988;318:1240–3.

112. Czinn SJ, Nedrud JG. Oral immunization against *Helicobacter pylori*. Infect Immun. 1991;59:2359–63.

113. Elson CO. Cholera toxin as a mucosal adjuvant: effects of H-2 major histocompatibility complex and *lps* genes. Infect Immun. 1992;60:2874–9.

114. Chen M, Lee A, Hazell S. Immunisation against gastric *Helicobacter* infection in a mouse/*Helicobacter felis* model. Lancet. 1992;339:1120–1 (Letter).

115. Czinn S, Cai A, Nedrud J. Oral immunization protects germ-free mice against infection from *Helicobacter felis*. Gastroenterology. 1992;102:A611(abstract).

12
Mechanisms of ammonia-induced gastric mucosal injury: role of glutathione and cysteine proteases

S. SZABO, S. KUSSTATSCHER, L. NAGY and Zs. SANDOR

The pathogenesis of cell and tissue injury produced by micro-organisms such as *Helicobacter pylori* is a complex process. Unlike lesions induced by a single chemical or physical agent, tissue damage caused by ischaemia and infectious agents are increasingly complex and multifactorial[1,2]. After the identification of *H. pylori* as a major cause of chronic gastritis[3] and duodenal and gastric ulcer[4,5], special attention was paid to elucidating the mechanism of tissue injury and mucosal inflammation[6,7].

Among the many products and properties of *H. pylori* that might be implicated in the pathogenesis of gastritis, the role of exotoxins has been extensively investigated. The *H. pylori* exotoxins include urease, which catalyses the production of ammonia, cytotoxins, proteases, phospholipase A_2 and platelet-activating factor[7]. We focused our research efforts on the role of ammonia and proteases in gastric mucosal injury. Our previous studies revealed that ammonia was about three times more damaging to the gastric mucosa than HCl on a molar basis, and about 75 times more toxic than ethanol (on %v/v basis) in the rat[8]. We also detected a rapidly developing vascular injury preceding the occurrence of haemorrhagic mucosal lesions after exposure to ammonia. We recently tested the hypothesis that this potent toxicity of ammonia might be multifactorial, and involve the depletion of protective non-protein sulphydryls such as glutathione (GSH) and release of damaging cysteine proteases such as cathepsins B, L and H. We review our recent results on the new endogenous mediators of ammonia-induced gastric mucosal injury.

SULPHYDRYLS

Sulphydryls are endogenous protective substances which, unlike prostaglandins, *directly* participate in mucosal defensive reactions (e.g., scavenge free

Table 1 GSH/GSSG ratios in the rat gastric mucosa after ammonia
or ethanol administration

	Controls	*1 min*	*3 min*	*6 min*	*12 min*
1% ammonia	104	58	35	45	—
75% ethanol	104	117	63	45	31

Groups of fasted rats were given 1 ml of 1% ammonia water or 75%
ethanol by gavage, and killed at times indicated. Mucosa of glandular
stomach was scraped, homogenized and processed for measurement of
GSH, GSSG and protein sulphydryls fractions by a spectrophotometric
and enzyme-coupled technique

radicals, and modulate membrane permeability and integrity, as well as
enzyme activities). Prostaglandins, on the other hand, stimulate the release
of protective substances such as mucus and bicarbonate, and hence indirectly
offer protection in the gastrointestinal tract. After the demonstration of a
protective role of sulphydryls, especially GSH[9], in the pathogenesis of
chemically induced gastric mucosal injury[10,11], we tested the hypothesis that
endogenous protective compounds which are present in large concentration
in the gastric mucosa might have a role in the mechanisms of defence
reactions against products of infectious agents such as the ammonia of *H.
pylori*. We thus performed biochemical and pharmacological experiments in
fasted Sprague–Dawley rats (150–200 g).

Ammonia was administered by gavage (1 ml) as 0.1, 0.5, 1 or 2% aqueous
solution (Sigma) to fasted rats which were killed 1 h later. The area of
haemorrhagic mucosal lesions as evaluated by stereo-microscopic planimetry
involved 0, 0.5 ± 0.1, $12.5 \pm 2\%$ or $28.7 \pm 4.1\%$ of the glandular stomach,
respectively. Comparable lesions can be produced in rats by 1 ml of 25, 50,
75 or 100% ethanol.

Following these preliminary experiments to choose the appropriate doses of
ammonia and ethanol which produce roughly equivalent acute haemorrhagic
lesions, additional groups of rats were fasted and killed 1, 3, 6 and 12 min
following administration of 1 ml of 1% ammonia or 75% ethanol. In
these biochemical studies we wanted to measure the changes in mucosal
concentration *before* and during the *early* stages of ammonia-induced tissue
injury, in comparison with the deleterious effect of alcohol. Thus, after
autopsy, the mucosa of the glandular stomach was rapidly scraped, homogenized and processed for the determination of sulphydryl derivatives by a
spectrophotometric and enzyme-coupled method recently adopted in our
laboratory[12]. GSH/GSSH ratios changed from 104 in controls to 58, 35, 45
or 117, 63, 45 and 31 after 1, 3, 6 and 12 min following ammonia or ethanol,
respectively (Table 1). Protein sulphydryl levels did not markedly change,
while protein disulphides and mixed disulphides were slightly increased by
ammonia.

Pharmacological experiments also implicated sulphydryls in the pathogenesis of ammonia-induced injury: the haemorrhagic mucosal lesions induced
by 1 ml of 1% ammonia intragastrically (i.g.) were decreased ($p < 0.0005$)
from $13.2 \pm 2.5\%$ of the glandular stomach in controls to 1.1 ± 0.7 or
$2.4 \pm 1.1\%$ after 30 min i.g. pre-treatment with the sulphydryl-containing

cysteamine (30 mg/100 g) or egualen (Kotobuki KT$_1$-32) (5 mg/100 g), respectively.

We conclude from these experiments that ammonia, just like ethanol in much larger concentration, rapidly depletes the levels of most prominent and multi-functional protective agents, such as glutathione. This reductionist approach indicates that although the pathogenesis of tissue injury produced by microbial agents such as *H. pylori* might be very complex, similar mechanistic changes may be detected in the pathogenesis of both chemically induced and infectious mucosal lesions. This can be detected only if a single chemical agent, a product of micro-organisms (e.g. ammonia produced by *H. pylori*), is tested in comparison with well-known damaging compounds such as alcohol.

CYSTEINE PROTEASES

These proteolytic enzymes are also common mediators of cell and tissue injury[13,14]. In comparison, aspartic (e.g. pepsin), and serine (e.g. trypsin) proteases, and metallo-proteases are mainly involved in luminal digestion and metabolism. Cysteine or thiol proteases (e.g., cathepsins B, H and L), on the other hand, are especially involved in intracellular catabolic processes and often related to extracellular damage and adaptation such as the spread of malignant tumour cells, and migration of endothelial cells during angiogenesis. Our previous results indicated that protein sulphydryls, especially cysteine proteases, might also play a role in gastric mucosal injury and protection[11-14]. We tested the hypothesis that these potent proteinases might mediate, in part, the early gastric mucosal damage produced by ammonia, again in comparison with ethanol.

The release of activated cysteine proteases by ammonia was tested in fasted anaesthetized rats using continuous gastric perfusion (1.5 ml saline/min): 1 ml of 1% ammonia solution or 50% ethanol was administered intragastrically (i.g.) and left in the stomach for 1 min after 5 min of stabilization. Gastric samples were collected at 1 min intervals during 5 min before and 15 min after the damaging agents. Specific substrates (5 nmol) were used for direct fluorimetric assays of cathepsins B, L and H in Barrett's buffer (0.1 mol/l, pH 6.0 or 6.8) containing 2 μmol cysteine and 1 μmol Na$_2$EDTA (37°C, 10 min). The haemorrhagic mucosal lesions were quantified with stereomicroscopic planimetry.

The activity (μmol/ml) of cathepsin B increased from 2.7 $\pm$ 1.1 during 5 min before ammonia to 70.7 $\pm$ 19.0, 43.4 $\pm$ 15.0 and 27.0 $\pm$ 12.0 at 1, 2 and 3 min after ammonia, respectively: cathepsin B + L from 4.2 $\pm$ 1.8 to 131.0 $\pm$ 33.0, 91.0 $\pm$ 34.0 and 47.0 $\pm$ 17.0; and cathepsin H from 7.6 $\pm$ 1.3 to 117 $\pm$ 16.0, 74.0 $\pm$ 14.0 and 43.0 $\pm$ 4 (Fig. 1). The activity of cathepsin B increased from 5.1 $\pm$ 2.5 during 5 min before ethanol to 57.0 $\pm$ 19.0, 36.0 $\pm$ 10.0 and 21.0 $\pm$ 7.0 at 1, 2 and 3 min after ethanol, respectively: cathepsin H from 14.6 $\pm$ 1.1 to 25.0 $\pm$ 11.0, 21.0 $\pm$ 9.0 and 9.1 $\pm$ 5.0.

Haemorrhagic mucosal lesions produced by ammonia or 50 times more concentrated ethanol developed after release of proteases and involved

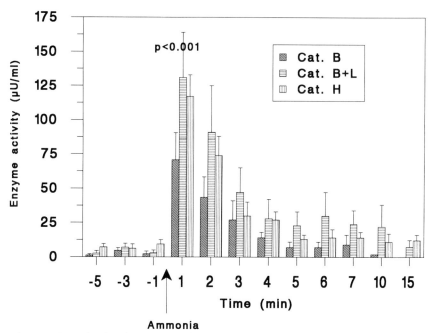

Fig. 1 Release of cathepsins B, L and H into the gastric lumen after intragastric administration of 1 ml of 1% ammonia in anaesthetized rats which were prepared for gastric perfusion as described in the text

$2.9 \pm 0.2\%$ or $5.1 \pm 1.1\%$ of the glandular stomach, respectively. Pre-treatment of rats with the thiol protease inhibitor N-ethylmaleimide (NEM) (1 mg/100 g i.g., 30 min before 1% of ammonia) diminished the release of mucosal cysteine proteases, and prevented the development of acute haemorrhagic lesions. In additional preliminary experiments we pretreated groups of fasted rats with lower than previously used dose of NEM, i.e. 0.1 mg/100 g i.g., 30 min before 1 ml of 50% ethanol (Fig. 2). This low dose of cysteine protease inhibitor also significantly ($p < 0.001$) diminished the ethanol-induced gastric haemorrhagic lesions (Fig. 2). Similar studies with the low dose of NEM need to be performed in the ammonia-induced mucosal injury as well.

These biochemical and pharmacological experiments again indicate common mediators, i.e. release of cysteine proteases (e.g. cathepsins B, H and L) in the mechanism of early tissue injury caused by low (0.5–1%) concentrations of ammonia and more concentrated (50–75%) ethanol. Ammonia seems to be more potent in releasing these damaging proteases than alcohol, and pre-treatment of rats with the cysteine protease inhibitor NEM diminished the acute haemorrhagic mucosal lesions induced by either ammonia or alcohol.

SUMMARY

Our toxicological and pharmacological experiments indicate that ammonia was more damaging to the rat gastric mucosa than ethanol or HCl. Depletion

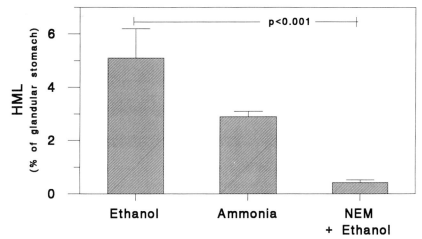

Fig. 2 Acute haemorrhagic mucosal lesions (HML) induced by 1 ml of 50% ethanol or 1% ammonia in fasted rats. An additional group of animals was pretreated with the cysteine protease inhibitor N-ethylmaleimide (NEM) (0.1 mg/100 g by gavage) 30 min before the administration of alcohol

of mucosal GSH levels preceded the occurrence of haemorrhagic mucosal lesions after administration of either ammonia or alcohol, and pretreatment with sulphydryl drugs offered gastroprotection. Rapid activation and release of the cysteine protease cathepsins B, L and H were also detected following ammonia or ethanol exposure of the rat stomach preceding the development of acute mucosal damage. Thus, depletion of mucosal sulphydryls, release of cysteine proteases and early vascular injury may play a role in the pathogenesis of ammonia and *H. pylori*-induced gastric injury.

References

1. Cotran RS, Kumar V, Robbins SI. Robbins pathologic basis of disease, 4th edn. Philadelphia: WB Saunders; 1989.
2. Szabo S, Kovacs K. Causes and mechanisms of cell and tissue injury in endocrine glands. In: Kovacs K, Asa A, eds. Endocrine pathology. Boston: Blackwell Scientific Publications; 1990:914–33.
3. Warren JR, Marshall B. Unidentified curved bacilli on gastric epithelium in active chronic gastritis. Lancet. 1983;2:1273–5.
4. Goodwin CS, Armstrong JA, Marshall BJ. *Campylobacter pyloridis*, gastritis and peptic ulceration. J Clin Pathol. 1986;39:353–65.
5. Tytgat GNJ, Rauws EA, De Koster E. *Campylobacter pylori*. Scand J Gastroenterol. 1988;155(suppl):68–81.
6. Blaser MJ. *H. pylori* and the pathogenesis of gastroduodenal inflammation. J Infect Dis. 1990;161:626–33.
7. Wyle FA, Chang KJ, Tarnawski A. *Helicobacter pylori*: pathogenetic mechanisms. In: Domschke W, Konturek SJ, eds. The stomach: physiology, pathophysiology and treatment. Berlin, Heidelberg, New York, London, Paris, Tokyo, Hong Kong, Barcelona, Budapest: Springer-Verlag; 1993:198–211.
8. Szabo S, Nagy L, Morales RE, Sandor Z. Ammonia is more damaging to the gastric mucosa than ethanol: Role of sulfhydryls and vascular injury. Gastroenterology. 1992;102:A703.

 9. Meister A. On the antioxidant effects of ascorbic acid and glutathione. Biochem Pharmacol. 1992;44(suppl. 10):1905–15.
10. Szabo S, Trier JS, Franke PW. Sulfhydryl compounds may mediate gastric cytoprotection. Science. 1981;214:200–2.
11. Dupuy D, Szabo S. Protection by metals against ethanol-induced gastric mucosal injury in the rat. Comparative biochemical and pharmacologic studies implicate protein sulfhydryls. Gastroenterology. 1986;91:966–74.
12. Nagy L, Jenkins JM, Morales RE, Nagy G, Szabo S. Protein and nonprotein sulfhydryls and disulfides in the early phase of gastric mucosal injury caused by ammonia, ethanol, HCL, NaOH and NaCl in rats. Gastroenterology. 1993;104:A154.
13. Szabo S, Nagy L, Plebani M. Glutathione, protein sulfhydryls and cysteine proteases in gastric mucosal injury and protection. Clin Chim Acta. 1992;206:95–105.
14. Nagy L, Johnson BR, Saha B, LeQuesne P, Neumeyer JL, Plebani, Szabo S. Correlation between gastroprotection and inhibition of cysteine proteases by new maleimide derivatives. Dig Dis Sci. 1990;35:1037.

13
Lipopolysaccharide (LPS)-related damage by *H. pylori*

A. LEE and A. P. MORAN

LIPOPOLYSACCHARIDE (LPS): WHAT IS IT AND WHAT IS ITS FUNCTION IN BACTERIA?

The outer membrane of the cell wall of Gram-negative bacteria is a protective layer that controls the entry of many large molecules and protects the cell from potentially damaging agents. For those bacteria that come in contact with animals an important component of the Gram-negative outer membrane is lipopolysaccharide (LPS), a complex molecule not found elsewhere in nature. LPS, also termed endotoxin, represents the main surface antigen (O-antigen) for Gram-negative bacteria. The term endotoxin was coined by Pfeiffer in 1982, when he noted that certain toxic material was not excreted from living bacteria, as an exotoxin, but rather was released when the bacteria underwent lysis[1]. LPS is firmly bound to the bacterial cell and is composed of three main domains[2] (Fig. 1). An outer polysaccharide chain, called the O-specific chain, contributes to the antigenicity and serospecificity of the molecule and is composed of repeating units that may contain up to seven different sugars. This O-specific chain is thus a polymer of identical repeating units, and is of large size since it can be up to 50 repeating units in length. The second component of the molecule is a short series of core sugars (approximately 10–15) while the innermost lipid component, termed lipid A, anchors LPS in the outer leaflet of the membrane. The fatty acids in lipid A vary with the microbial species, and endow hydrophobicity to the molecules. Thus LPS is an essential structure of all Gram-negative bacteria whether their natural habitat is salt lakes, ocean sediments, root nodules or the human gut. LPS is not a specific component to bacterial pathogens, rather it is a universal component of these organisms, be they friend or foe.

LPS AS TRIGGER FOR NATURAL IMMUNITY

For survival in a competitive world, humans have needed to develop a sophisticated defence system to protect them from various potentially noxious

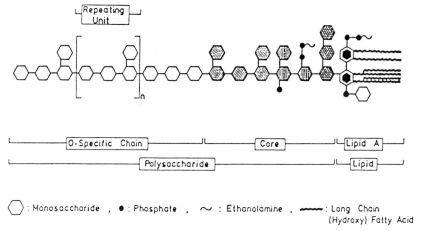

Fig. 1   Basic structure of lipopolysaccharide (LPS)

environmental agents. One such group of agents were the bacteria who evolved equally rapidly and acquired the ability to survive in every available niche. We, as human hosts, have a highly adapted system that can sense the presence of bacteria once they come in contact with the host, and as a result induce a series of protective defence mechanisms. Not surprisingly, the molecules that trigger this response are those that are most exposed, e.g. the LPS of the outer envelope of Gram-negative bacteria. These alarm responses are designed to be helpful to the host, i.e.

1. LPS activates complement directly by the alternate pathway, thus allowing bacterial cell lysis, opsonization and phagocyte recruitment.
2. LPS stimulates B lymphocytes. This immunopotentiation is aimed at the development of a more rapid protective antibody response.
3. LPS activates macrophages. The phagocytes are more able to scavenge invading bacteria.
4. LPS acts as a pyrogen and induces fever.

The main mediators of the latter two responses appear to be the cytokines, interleukin-1 (IL-1) and tumour necrosis factor (TNF), released from mononuclear phagocytes.

Humans harbour a mass of approximately 1 kg of bacteria in the gut lumen, of which many are Gram-negative. The integrity of the large bowel mucosa ensures that not many of these bacteria enter the tissues. However, the small amount of LPS that does pass the mucosal surface is believed to play a positive role in priming our immune defences. Indeed, the bacterial microbiota (flora) of the bowel, mainly through LPS, is considered to play a crucial immunostimulatory role[3].

LPS AS A VIRULENCE FACTOR IN HUMAN DISEASE

Whereas contact with low-dose LPS is immunostimulatory, exposure to high doses poses real problems for the host. Injection of LPS into animals will induce various pathologies, i.e. intravenous administration results in hypotension, disseminated intravascular coagulation and death, so-called endotoxic shock[1]. If an LPS injection given intradermally is followed by an intravenous injection 24 h later there is haemorrhagic necrosis at the site of intradermal injection. Both these effects of LPS can be mimicked by the cytokine TNF, suggesting an indirect effect. In human sepsis or endotoxic shock it is suggested that there are ordered cascades of cytokine production, i.e. LPS induces TNF which induces IL-1 which induces IL-6. In excess these cytokines are detrimental to the host. This, therefore, is the key to the role of LPS in any disease process: a situation occurs whereby the body tissues come in contact with excess LPS such that the beneficial immunoregulatory threshold is exceeded, the host defences fail and the excess cytokine produced induces immunopathological sequelae.

Entry of excess LPS may be due to mechanical action such as when a cytoscope breaks the integrity of an infected bladder and millions of *E. coli* are released into the tissue. Of more relevance here is the situation where an evolved pathogen has acquired traits which permit it to evade the host defences, enter the tissues and multiply in large numbers. Examples would be *Salmonella typhi* and *Neisseria meningitidis*.

Except in the case of *S. typhimurium*, where structures in the O-specific chain contribute to virulence[2], LPS is generally not a virulence factor of a pathogen. Rather, LPS may contribute to pathology if an evolved characteristic of an organism allows it to invade and survive in tissue, e.g. the antiphagocytic capsule of *N. meningitidis*. For non-invasive bacteria that survive on mucosal surfaces increased biological activity of LPS is no advantage; indeed it may be a disadvantage. This is an important concept that needs to be considered as we review the literature on a role for LPS in *H. pylori*-associated disease, especially when we bear in mind that *H. pylori* is a successful mucosal colonizer that can inhabit the gastric surface for most of the life of the host.

THE STRUCTURE OF *H. PYLORI* LPS

Preliminary studies on the general architecture of LPS of *H. pylori* indicated that some strains produce LPS with O-specific chains (smooth-form LPS), whereas other lacked such chains (rough-form LPS)[4]. From these results it was hypothesized that the LPS type might correlate with the pathogenicity of *H. pylori* strains. This was of interest since *E. coli* smooth-form LPS binds to mucus glycoproteins[5] potentially impeding colonization of the underlying intestinal epithelium[6], and thus strains with rough-form LPS would be relatively unimpeded in their movement through the mucus to the epithelium. However, a subsequent study by one of us found that all fresh clinical isolates of *H. pylori* produce smooth-form LPS, whereas strains which have been

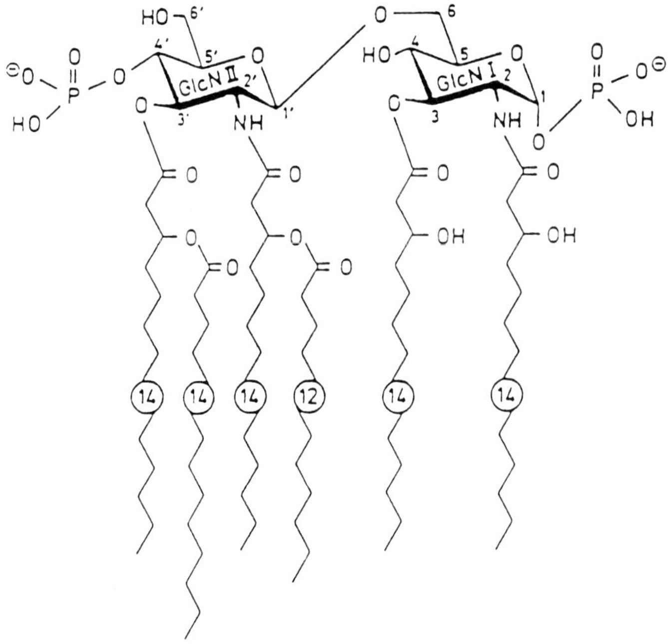

Fig. 2 Lipid A of *Escherichia coli*

grown *in vitro* for extended periods all produce rough-form LPS[7]. Furthermore, it was demonstrated that *in vitro* bacterial cultivation on conventional solid media can result in the loss of the O-specific chain and production of rough-form LPS by *H. pylori* strains[7,8], thus explaining the observations in preliminary studies[4]. Nevertheless, the phase shift from smooth- to rough-form LPS can be reversed when strains are grown in liquid media[8], possibly because *in vitro* conditions mimic the fluid environment where *H. pylori* is found *in vivo*.

Compared with the structure of lipid A normally encountered in Gram-negative bacteria, e.g. *E. coli* (Fig. 2), preliminary structural evidence[7,9] indicates that *H. pylori* lipid A possesses unique features (Fig. 3). *E. coli* lipid A (Fig. 2) is composed of a glucosamine (GlcN) disaccharide which carries two phosphate groups (one at carbon-1 of GlcN I, the other at carbon-4' of GlcN II), and six fatty acids at carbons-2, 3, 2', and 3' (two fatty acids on GlcN I and four on GlcN II). In contrast, *H. pylori* lipid carries only one phosphate group (at carbon-1 of GlcN). Aslo *H. pylori* lipid A contains longer saturated fatty acids (16 and 18 carbon atoms in length) that are present in *E. coli* lipid A (12 and 14 carbon atoms in length). This is also true when the 3-hydroxy fatty acids are compared; 16 and 18 carbon atoms in length in *H. pylori*, but only 14 carbon atoms in length in *E. coli*. Thus, the deduced structure of *H. pylori* lipid A bears a striking resemblance to the lipid A of *Bacteroides fragilis*, a member of the normal gut microbiota, which lacks 4'-phosphate and contains unusual fatty acids[10].

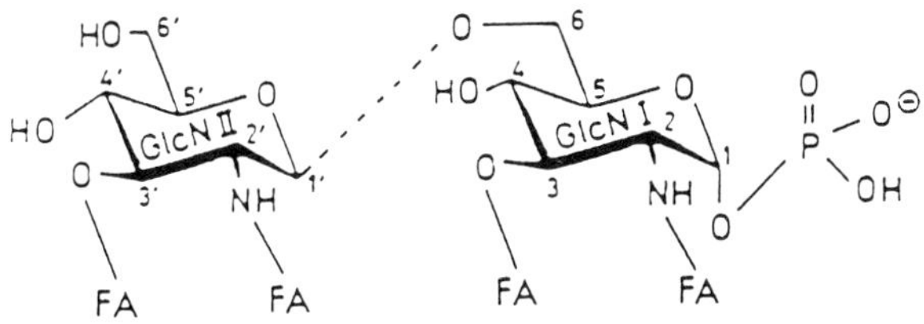

FA = Fatty acids

14:0	18:0
16:0	3-OH-16:0
	3-OH-18:0

Fig. 3 Lipid A of *Helicobacter pylori*

POSTULATED CONTRIBUTION OF *H. PYLORI* LPS TO HUMAN GASTRODUODENAL DISEASE

Interaction of *H. pylori* LPS with laminin

In early studies on *H. pylori* in human gastric epithelium, the bacterium was seen to congregate close to intercellular junctions[11,12]. It was initially considered that this might be a fixation artefact[13], yet many microscopic studies showed that there often appeared to be significant penetration between cells and a weakening of adhesion between the gastric epithelial cells. The integrity of the gastric epithelium is normally very tight. This is the barrier that has to be protected from the myriad of potentially noxious agents we ingest from time to time. As *H. pylori* antigens such as urease have been shown deep in the gastric mucosa[14] and have been implicated in the immunopathology that is *H. pylori*-associated gastritis[15] the gastric barrier must have been weakened. The disruption of tight junctions seen in *H. pylori*-infected tissue may be the origin of gastric leakiness. Two independent research groups, those of Trust *et al.* and Slomiany *et al.*[16,17], showed a high affinity of binding of the basement membrane protein laminin to *H. pylori*, and postulated that this binding might be responsible for a weakening of tissue cell integrity, particularly at intercellular junctions. Slomiany and colleagues showed that adhesion of a specific laminin receptor on epithelial cells to laminin was prevented by LPS from *H. pylori*[17]. Slomiany's group isolated the laminin receptor from rat gastric epithelial cell membrane by affinity chromatography on laminin coupled Sepharose of membrane solubilized with octyl glucoside. The 67 kDa receptor protein was eluted, iodinated and incorporated into liposomes which subsequently showed specific affinity towards laminin-coated surfaces. The binding of the labelled liposomes to wells of a polystyrene microtitre plate coated with laminin was 96% inhibited by a concentration of 50 μg/ml of *H. pylori* LPS. As a result of these studies these authors proposed the interesting hypothesis that LPS on the surface of *H. pylori* close to the gastric epithelium is responsible for disrupting gastric mucosal integrity, particularly cells at intercellular junctions. They also showed that a number of cytoprotective anti-ulcer drugs counteract the *in vitro* anti-adhesive effects of *H. pylori* LPS, i.e. nitecapone[18], sucralfate[19], ebrotidine[20] and sulglycotide[21]. Further studies by one of us have shown that laminin binding by different *H. pylori* strains varies from 0% to 30%[22], and that some strains can also bind extracellular matrix proteins other than laminin[23], suggesting potential pathogenic or virulence differences between strains. As to the mechanisms involved in the interaction between *H. pylori* LPS and laminin, the situation appears complex. A phosphorylated structure in the core of LPS of some strains of *H. pylori* is involved[22].

INTERFERENCE OF *H. PYLORI* LPS WITH THE SYNTHESIS OF SULPHATED GASTRIC MUCIN

Changes in gastric mucin structure, including decreased sulphation, have long been associated with the onset of gastric disease[24-27]. In a series of *in vitro* studies Slomiany and colleagues showed that inclusion of *H. pylori* LPS in small segments of rat stomach led to a decrease in mucin synthesis with a maximum 3-fold inhibition occurring as early as 15 min, with 20% inhibition being present after 120 min[28]. This inhibitory effect was maximal at an LPS concentration of 100 μg/ml, and the mucus glycoprotein that was secreted initially in response to *H. pylori* LPS was different from that elaborated following prolonged exposure. Furthermore the extent of sulphation of mucus glycoprotein was decreased. These authors inferred that these mucin changes *in vitro* are relevant to *H. pylori* infection *in vivo*. This important hypothesis is in urgent need of assessment *in vivo*.

Stimulation of pepsinogen secretion by *H. pylori* LPS

Pepsin is a proteolytic enzyme with powerful mucolytic and barrier-breaking properties, and is potentially an aggressive factor in the development of duodenal ulcer disease[29,30]. Furthermore, stimulated gastric pepsin secretion has been shown to correlate with serum pepsinogen I[31], the endocrine component of pepsinogen secreted by chief cells, and elevated levels are considered a major risk factor for the development and recurrence of duodenal ulcers[32,33].

Young and colleagues[34], using mucosa from guinea pigs mounted in Ussing chambers, demonstrated a 50-fold stimulation of pepsinogen secretion by *H. pylori* LPS compared with only a 12-fold stimulation with *E. coli* LPS 20 min post-treatment. Acid secretion was similar in control and LPS-treated tissues. These workers also noted, in electron microscopic studies, that the histology of chief cells appeared normal with prominent zymogen granules, although there was evidence of degranulation in LPS-treated tissue, particularly that treated with *H. pylori* LPS. From their *in vitro* studies these investigators concluded that *in vivo* elevated pepsinogen levels in patients with duodenal ulcers reflect the consequences of *H. pylori* infection, specifically the action of the bacterium's LPS. Although Cave and Cave[35], using isolated rabbit gastric glands, did obtain stimulation of pepsinogen with preparations of *H. pylori* strains, not all the strains tested induced stimulation. Therefore, further investigations are required to establish the pathogenic importance of stimulation by pepsinogen by *H. pylori* LPS *in vivo*, and to determine whether variations between strains in their stimulatory ability could be related to virulence differences.

The biological activity of *H. pylori* LPS

The biological activity of *H. pylori* LPS has been assessed in both experimental animals and humans. In both cases, comparisons were made with LPS from typical human pathogens known to induce significant toxic effects. In mice, *H. pylori* LPS exhibited mitogenic activity, as measured by tritiated thymidine uptake in mouse spleen cells, that was 1000 times lower than the LPS of *S. typhimurium*[36]. In a lethal toxicity test with D-galactosamine-sensitized mice *H. pylori* LPS also showed greatly reduced toxicity compared to that of *Salmonella*[36], e.g. LD_{50} 2 µg compared to 4 ng. The pyrogenicity of *H. pylori* LPS was likewise 500-fold less than that of *Salmonella* LPS. When the immunological activity of *H. pylori* LPS was tested on human peripheral mononuclear blood cells and compared with LPS from other intestinal bacteria, lowered activity was also observed[37]. Mitogenicity was similar to that of *Campylobacter jejuni* LPS, but much reduced compared to *E. coli* LPS. Nevertheless, *H. pylori* LPS was able to induce the cytokines TNF, IL-1 and IL-6 but to a lesser extent than the LPS of the other bacteria tested.

Whole *H. pylori* and extracted LPS have been shown to induce expression of the monocyte surface antigen HLA-DR and IL-2 receptors in purified human monocytes[14]. However, in this study an LPS-independent activation of human monocytes was demonstrated by soluble *H. pylori* surface proteins, and was considered by the authors to be more important, given that *H. pylori* does not invade mucosal tissue. Nevertheless, the kinetics of the responses induced by *H. pylori* LPS were unusual and require further investigation.

Antigenicity of *H. pylori* LPS

The somatic (O) antigens, namely LPS, are highly immunogenic and stable molecules. As these antigens, in particular their O-specific chains, vary from strain to strain, specific antisera raised in animals such as rabbits may be used to separate strains into antigenic groups, and so form the basis of a typing scheme that may be useful in epidemiological studies. This has proved successful with the Salmonellae[38] and the Campylobacters[39]. With respect to *H. pylori* LPS, structural studies have indicated that variations exist in the composition and structure of the O-specific chain of LPS of different strains[7,8]. In investigations of the antigenicity of *H. pylori* LPS, a diversity of *H. pylori* LPS structures was demonstrated, and it was suggested that this may form the basis of an O-antigen serotyping system[40]. Although the growing sophistication of genetic fingerprinting schemes may make LPS-based typing systems appear less practical, the equipment required for the performance of genetic tests may not be available in a clinical reference laboratory. In contrast, equipment and materials required for LPS-based tests are generally available in clinical laboratories, but even if these are limited, boiled preparations from bacteria, which are enriched for LPS, can be sent through the mail to a central reference laboratory for typing, as LPS preparations are highly stable.

Low biological activity of *H. pylori* LPS as a consequence of a highly evolved host–parasite relationship

The low biological activity of *H. pylori* LPS is no coincidence, but a consequence of a long and continually evolving host–parasite relationship. *H. pylori* has adapted to a niche external to human tissue. In its location on the gastric surface it is to the organism's advantage to stimulate the immune system as little as possible, and thus it has acquired an LPS with a structure that stimulates less biological activity than more aggressive and short-lived pathogens. There is precedent for this concept. *Bacteroides fragilis*, another organism that survives for the life of the human host, in the intestinal tract as part of the normal gut microbiota (flora), also has an LPS with low biological activity[10].

Thus it may be that LPS does not play a direct role via the immune system in *H. pylori*-associated tissue damage. However, *H. pylori* is not as benign as the lower intestinal organism *B. fragilis*. *H. pylori* colonization of the human antral mucosa is always associated with inflammation. Crabtree and colleagues have shown the severity of this inflammation via induction of the cytokine IL-8 to be linked with the production of cytotoxin and cytotoxin-associated proteins[41,42]. The latter is also consistent with the idea that LPS plays a minimal role in *H. pylori* gastritis via stimulation of the immune system. However, the hypotheses that *H. pylori* LPS contributes to the epithelium-disrupting effect of the organism via its effect on laminin–laminin receptor interaction, interference of synthesis of sulphated gastric mucin and stimulation of pepsinogen secretion are in urgent need of confirmation *in vivo*. Thus, the situation could be that, although *H. pylori* LPS has evolved to induce a low level of immunological response – hence allowing the organism to remain in human mucosa for long periods without clearance, other properties of the LPS can contribute to tissue damage and *H. pylori*-associated pathology.

CONCLUSION

As stated earlier, the *in vitro* observations that *H. pylori* LPS interferes with laminin–laminin receptor interaction and synthesis of sulphated gastric mucin, and stimulates pepsinogen secretion, need to be confirmed *in vivo*. Nevertheless, these observations raise important questions regarding the pathogenesis and virulence of *H. pylori* strains.

First, however, before the postulate becomes dogma that the LPS–laminin interaction is primarily responsible for disrupting gastric mucosal integrity, it will be necessary to test this hypothesis by electron microscopic examination of the gastric mucosa of *H. pylori*-infected persons on monotherapy with the various anti-ulcer agents which have been shown to inhibit the LPS–laminin interaction *in vitro*. Also why does LPS of some *H. pylori* strains bind to laminin and others not? Is this related to the virulence of strains? The *in vitro* observation that *H. pylori* strains bind to extracellular matrix proteins, other than laminin, requires further investigation, particularly regarding pathogenesis *in vivo* and virulence of strains.

Second, the observations on inhibition of sulphated mucin synthesis were performed only with isolated LPS. Do whole living bacteria have the same effect? The optimal concentration to induce these effects was $100\,\mu g/ml$, which is a very high concentration of LPS. What concentration of LPS is likely to come in contact with mucin-secreting cells in an *H. pylori*-colonized stomach? Would such levels of LPS be capable of inducing a similar effect on mucin *in vivo*? In addition, if this effect on mucin results in a weakened barrier, why is ulcer disease not more common in *H. pylori*-infected persons?

Finally, what is the extent of the role played by pepsinogen secretion stimulated by *H. pylori* LPS in the loss of mucosal integrity *in vivo*? Is there damage to the mucosa by *H. pylori* because of the concerted action of LPS-induced changes to the composition of mucin and increased pepsinogen secretion? Is the LPS of only certain strains of *H. pylori* capable of stimulating pepsinogen secretion, and are these strains specifically associated with the development of duodenal ulcer disease?

The questions posed above are intriguing questions, the answers to which, we believe, will give new insight into the pathogenesis and virulence of *H. pylori* and the role of the bacterium in gastric mucosal damage.

Acknowledgements

The support of the National Health and Medical Research Council of Australia to Professor Adrian Lee, and the support of the Irish Health Research Board to Dr Anthony P. Moran for research on *H. pylori* LPS, is gratefully acknowledged.

References

1. Rietschel ET, Brade H. Bacterial endotoxins. Sci Am. 1992;267:54–61.
2. Rietschel ET, Brade L, Holst O *et al.* Molecular structure of bacterial endotoxin in relation to bioactivity. In: Nowotny A, Spitzer JJ, Ziegler EJ, editors. Cellular and molecular aspects of endotoxin reactions. Amsterdam: Elsevier; 1990:15–32.
3. Bocci V. The neglected organ: bacterial flora has a crucial immunostimulatory role. Prospect Biol Med. 1992;35:249–58.

4. Perez Perez GI, Blaser MJ. Conservation and diversity of *Campylobacter pyloridis* major antigens. Infect Immun. 1987;55:1256–63.
5. Cohen PS, Arruda JC, Williams TJ, Laux DC. Adhesion of a human faecal *Escherichia coli* strain to mouse colonic mucus. Infect Immun. 1985;48:139–45.
6. Myhal ML, Cohen PS, Laux DC. Altered colonising ability for mouse large intestine of a surface mutant of a human faecal isolate of *Escherichia coli*. J Gen Microbiol. 1993;129: 1549–58.
7. Moran AP, Helander IM, Kosunen TU. Compositional analysis of *Helicobacter pylori* rough-form lipopolysaccharides. J Bacteriol. 1992;174:1370–7.
8. Moran AP, Walsh EJ. Expression and electrophoretic characterisation of smooth-form lipopolysaccharides of *Helicobacter pylori*. Acta Gastroenterol Belg. 1993;56(S):97.
9. Mattsby-Baltzer I, Mielniczuk Z, Larsson L, Lindgren K, Goodwin S. Lipid-A in *Helicobacter pylori*. Infect Immun. 1992;60:4383–7.
10. Weintraub A, Zahringer U, Wollenweber HW, Seydel U, Rietschel ET. Structural characterisation of the lipid A component of *Bacteroides fragilis* strain NCTC 9343 lipopolysaccharide. Eur J Biochem. 1989;183:425–31.
11. Hazell SL, Lee A, Brady L, Hennessy W. *Campylobacter pyloridis* and gastritis: association with intercellular spaces and adaptation to an environment of mucus as important factors in colonization of the gastric epithelium. J Infect Dis. 1986;153:658–63.
12. Steer HW. The gastro-duodenal epithelium in peptic ulceration. J Pathol. 1985;146: 355–62.
13. Thomsen LL, Gavin JB, Tasman Jones C. Relation of *Helicobacter pylori* to the human gastric mucosa in chronic gastritis of the antrum. Gut. 1990;31:1230–6.
14. Mai UE, Perez Perez GI, Wahl LM, Wahl SM, Blaser MJ, Smith PD. Soluble surface proteins from *Helicobacter pylori* activate monocytes/macrophages by lipopolysaccharide-independent mechanism. J Clin Invest. 1991;87:894–900.
15. Blaser MJ. Hypothesis on the pathogenesis and natural history of *Helicobacter pylori*-induced inflammation. Gastroenterology. 1992;102:720–7.
16. Trust TJ, Doig P, Emody L, Kienle Z, Wadstrom T, O'Toole P. High affinity binding of the basement membrane proteins collagen type IV and laminin to the gastric pathogen *Helicobacter pylori*. Infect Immun. 1991;59:4398–404.
17. Slomiany BL, Piotrowski J, Sengupta S, Slomiany A. Inhibition of gastric mucosal laminin receptor by *Helicobacter pylori* lipopolysaccharide. Biochem Biophys Res Commun. 1991;175:963–70.
18. Slomiany BL, Piotrowski J, Rajiah G, Slomiany A. Inhibition of gastric mucosa laminin receptor by *Helicobacter pylori* lipopolysaccharide: effect of nitecapone. Gen Pharmacol. 1991;22:1063–9.
19. Piotrowski J, Yamaki K, Slomiany A, Slomiany BL. Inhibition of gastric mucosal laminin receptor by *Helicobacter pylori*: effect of sucralfate. Am J Gastroenterol. 1991;86:1756–60.
20. Piotrowski J, Morita M, Slomiany A, Slomiany BL. Inhibition of gastric mucosal laminin receptor by *Helicobacter pylori* lipopolysaccharide – effect of ebrotidine. Biochem Int. 1992;27:131–8.
21. Slomiany A, Piotrowski J, Yotsumoto F, Czajkowski A, Slomiany BL. *H. pylori* lipopolysaccharide inhibition of gastric mucosal laminin receptor: effect of sulglycotide. Acta Gastroenterol Belg. 1993;65(suppl.):120.
22. Valkonen KH, Ringner M, Ljungh A, Wadstrom T. High-affinity binding of laminin by *Helicobacter pylori* – evidence for a lectin-like interaction. FEMS Immunol Med Microbiol. 1993;7:29–37.
23. Moran AP, Kuusela P, Kosunen TU. Interaction of *Helicobacter pylori* with extracellular matrix proteins. J Appl Bacteriol. 1993;75:184–9.
24. Glass GBJ, Slomiany BL. Derangements of biosynthesis, production and secretion of mucus in gastrointestinal injury and disease. In: Elstein M, Parke DV, editors. Mucus in health and disease. New York: Plenum Press; 1977:311–47.
25. Murakami S, Mori Y. Changes in the incorporating activity of ^{35}S-sulphate into gastric sulfated glycoproteins in the rat with erosions by restraint and water immersion stress. Jpn J Pharmacol. 1984;35:279–86.
26. Azumi Y, Ohara S, Ishihara K, Okabe H, Hotta K. Correlation of quantitative changes of gastric mucosal glycoproteins with aspirin-induced gastric damage in rats. Gut. 1980;21:

533–6.

27. Younan F, Pearson J, Allen A, Venables C. Changes in the structure of the mucous gel on the mucosal surface of the stomach in association with peptic ulcer disease. Gastroenterology. 1982;82:827–31.

28. Slomiany BL, Liau YH, Lopez RA, Piotrowski J, Czajkowski A, Slomiany A. Effect of *Helicobacter pylori* lipopolysaccharide on the synthesis of sulfated gastric mucin. Biochem Int. 1992;27:687–97.

29. Pearson JP, Ward R, Allen A, Roberts NB, Taylor WH. Mucus degradation by pepsin: comparison of mucolytic activity of human pepsin 1 and pepsin 3: implications in peptic ulceration. Gut. 1986;27:243–8.

30. Venables CW. Mucus, pepsin, and peptic ulcer. Gut. 1986;27:233–8.

31. Waldrum HL, Burhol PG, Straume BK. Serum group I pepsinogens and gastrin in relation to gastric H^+ and pepsin outputs before and after subcutaneous injection of pentagastrin. Scand J Gastroenterol. 1978;13:943–6.

32. Sumii K, Inbe A, Uemura N *et al.* Increased serum pepsinogen 1 and recurrence of duodenal ulcer. Scand J Gastroenterol. 1989;24:1200–4.

33. Samloff IM, Stemmermann GN, Heilbrun LK, Nomura A. Elevated serum pepsinogen I and II levels differ as risk factors for duodenal ulcer and gastric ulcer. Gastroenterology. 1986;90:570–6.

34. Young GO, Stemmet N, Lastovica A *et al. Helicobacter pylori* lipopolysaccharide stimulates mucosal pepsinogen secretion. Aliment Pharmacol Ther. 1992;6:169–77.

35. Cave TR, Cave DR. *Helicobacter pylori* stimulates pepsin secretion from isolated rabbit gastric glands. Scand J Gastroenterol. 1991;26:9–14.

36. Muotiala A, Helander IM. Low biological activity of *Helicobacter pylori* lipopolysaccharide. Infect Immun. 1992;60:1714–16.

37. Birkholz S, Knipp U, Nietzki C, Adamek RJ, Opferkuch W. Immunological activity of lipopolysaccharide of *Helicobacter pylori* on human peripheral mononuclear blood cells in comparison to lipopolysaccharides of other intestinal bacteria. FEMS Immunol Med Microbiol. 1993;6:317–24.

38. Kauffman F. The bacteriology of the Enterobacteriaeceae. Copenhagen: Munksgaard; 1966:55–309.

39. Penner JL, Hennessy JN. Possible haemagglutination technique for serotyping *Campylobacter fetus* subs. *jejuni* on the basis of heat-stable antigens. J Clin Microbiol. 1983;12:732–7.

40. Mills SD, Kurjanczyk LA, Penner JL. Antigenicity of *Helicobacter pylori* lipopolysaccharides. J Clin Microbiol. 1992;30:3175–80.

41. Crabtree JE, Plusa S, Farmery S, Peichl P, Lindley IJD. Cytokine regulation of interleukin-8 secretion by gastric epithelial cell lines. Acta Gastroenterol Belg. 1993;56(S):52.

42. Crabtree JE, Farmery S, Lindley IJD, Peichl P. Cytotoxic strains of *Helicobacter pylori* induce IL-8 production by gastric epithelial cells. Acta Gastroenterol Belg. 1993;56(S):48.

14
The cpn60 heat shock protein homologue of *H. pylori*

B. E. DUNN

INTRODUCTION

Infection by *Helicobacter pylori* is the causative agent of chronic active gastritis in humans[1–3]; chronic infection with this bacterium appears to play an important role in gastric and duodenal ulcers, and in at least some forms of gastric carcinoma and gastric lymphoma[4,5]. Essentially all strains of *H. pylori* are associated with gastric inflammation, although not all isolates produce identifiable toxins[6–8]. The mechanisms whereby *H. pylori* induces gastric inflammation and mucosal injury *in vivo* are not known.

IDENTIFICATION OF Hp54K as a cpn60 HEAT SHOCK PROTEIN HOMOLOGUE

We have identified and purified a major surface-exposed protein of 54 000 kDa in *H. pylori* which is homologous with members of the chaperonin cpn60 family of heat shock proteins (HSP)[9]. Purification of this protein, which we refer to as Hp54K, was facilitated by its recovery in water extracts of whole cells of *H. pylori* and co-purification with urease by size exclusion chromatography[10,11]. Hp54K was then separated from urease by anion exchange chromatography[9,11].

Hp54K was identified as a cpn60 homologue on the basis of its N-terminal amino acid sequence and its cross-reactivity with monospecific antibodies against a variety of known cpn60 homologues[9]. Evans *et al.* purified a 62 kDa protein (HSP62) from *H. pylori* which was recognized by a monoclonal antibody against the 65 kDa HSP common antigen of *Mycobacterium leprae*[12]. Independently, Austin *et al.* purified a protein they termed Hp60K from *H. pylori*[13]. Based on identical N-terminal amino acid sequences and immune cross-reactivity with antibodies against cpn60 homologues, Hp54K, HSP62 and Hp60K all appear to represent the same protein.

It is now clear that Hp54K is Protein 3, identified previously by two-dimensional gel electrophoresis (2DGE[9,14]). Based on 2DGE analyses, Hp54K is a major antigen of all strains of *H. pylori*, grown on sheep blood agar plates, which have been studied to date. Native molecular mass of Hp54K is 740–750 kDa[9,13], thus Hp54K apparently comprises a 14-mer, similar to other cpn60 homologues[9]. The isoelectric point (pI)[14] of Hp54K is 5.2–5.5, which is in good agreement with the pI based on the amino acid composition of the protein predicted from the DNA sequence (see below). On the basis of immunoblot analysis, Hp54K induces a strong antibody response in humans infected with *H. pylori*[9,14].

GENERAL CHARACTERISTICS OF cpn60 HOMOLOGUES

The HSP are highly conserved proteins found in all prokaryotic and eukaryotic cells that have been examined for their presence[15-18]. HSP can be induced by a variety of environmental stresses including elevated temperature, inflammation, irradiation, viral infection, malignant transformation, reactive oxygen metabolites, heavy metals, ethanol and anoxia[15,16]. A subset of HSP, known as the cpn60 family of chaperonins, which includes GroEL of *Escherichia coli* and the 65 kDa immunodominant antigen of *Mycobacterium* sp., is thought to facilitate the folding, unfolding and translocation of polypeptides as well as the assembly and disassembly of oligomeric protein complexes[19,20]. The cpn60 homologues are important antigens of a variety of infectious agents[21,22]. In addition, there is increasing evidence that some cpn60 homologues can induce tissue injury in infected hosts via autoimmune responses[17,18,21,22].

ULTRASTRUCTURE OF Hp54K

Austin *et al.* have recently described the ultrastructural appearance of purified Hp54K[13]. Hp54K forms rings or discs 13 mm diameter with seven-fold symmetry, when viewed on end. When viewed from the side, Hp54K appears as a stack of four linear structures each 13 nm in length and 2–3 nm in width. Thus, Hp54K appears to be formed from discs stacked side by side in a manner analogous to that observed for other cpn60 homologues[23,24]. In contrast, purified urease appears as a 13 nm diameter doughnut-like structure with a 3–5 nm darkly staining 'hole' in the centre[13].

CELLULAR LOCALIZATION OF Hp54K

Based on surface radioiodination and protein analysis by 2DGE, Hp54K and the 62-kDa subunit of urease are the two major surface-exposed proteins identified in *H. pylori* grown on blood agar for 72 h[9]. Supporting this observation, Eschweiler *et al.* demonstrated surface localization of Hp54K by immunostaining ultrathin sections of *H. pylori* using an antibody directed against the 65 kDa HSP of *M. tuberculosis*[25]. In addition, *H. pylori* expresses three major Sarkosyl-insoluble membrane proteins of approximately 61, 54 and 30 kDa[26-28], which presumably represent Hp54K (54 kDa peptide) and urease (61 and 30 kDa peptides). In general, Sarkosyl-insoluble membrane proteins are thought to represent a subset of integral membrane proteins of Gram-negative bacteria[29]. However, based on analogy with other cpn60 homologues and the known characteristics of Hp54K, it seems unlikely that the latter protein is a true integral membrane protein. In broth culture, large amounts of Hp54K are found in the supernatant[9], suggesting either that the protein is secreted selectively or that it may be a normal cell surface component which is shed during the course of incubation[9]. *H. pylori* cultures older than 48 h typically express increased amounts of Hp54K[13].

In our laboratory, preliminary experiments attempting to localize Hp54K ultrastructurally using a two-stage technique with colloidal gold-labelled antibodies demonstrated a significant amount of Hp54K within the cytoplasmic compartment of intact *H. pylori* (Dunn BE, Ilver D, Phadnis S, unpublished observations). Colloidal gold particles were also observed in juxtaposition with the outer bacterial membrane. Taken together, these results seem to suggest that Hp54K is synthesized within the cytoplasm prior to becoming associated with the outer cell membrane.

Since both Hp54K and urease lack a leader sequence (see below), the mechanism by which these proteins become associated with the outer membrane of *H. pylori* is not known. There is a precedent for this type of protein behaviour, however. Blaser and colleagues have characterized a surface array protein of *Campylobacter fetus* which is apparently secreted onto the surface of the bacterium, despite the fact that the protein lacks a leader sequence[30,31].

It has been suggested previously that surface localization of Hp54K and urease in *H. pylori* grown on agar plates may be an artifact resulting from rupture of senescent bacteria and subsequent adsorption of these abundant proteins onto the surface of remaining viable bacteria[9]. Unfortunately our ultrastructural and surface-labelling experiments performed to date are not sufficient to determine whether Hp54K is actively secreted onto the surface of the bacterium, or whether passive adsorption of protein released from senescent bacteria is involved. Of interest, most bacterial cpn60 homologues, which typically evoke a strong immune response, are thought to be cytoplasmic in nature[15,16]. Thus, surface localization is not necessary for cpn60 molecules to be recognized by the immune system. Molecular studies are needed to determine the mechanisms whereby Hp54K and urease become associated with cell membranes of *H. pylori*.

CLONING AND SEQUENCING OF Hp54K

Hp54K has recently been cloned and sequenced[32,33] (Dunn BE, Ilver D, Phadnis S, unpublished data). The open reading frame encodes a protein of 542[32] or 546[33] amino acids with a predicted molecular mass of 58.2 kDa[32] or 58.3 kDa[33] and a predicted pI of 5.37[33]. The predicted protein sequence is hydrophilic in nature[33] and lacks a predicted leader peptide or other transmembrane domains[33]. Extensive homology with other cpn60 homologues was noted by all groups. In addition, Macchia and colleagues reported that Hp54K was expressed in all *H. pylori* strains tested, including a urease-negative strain and several cytotoxin-negative strains[33]. Suerbaum and Labigne identified a second open reading frame (which they designated *hspA*, in contrast to *hspB*, which encodes the gene for Hp54K), encoding a protein of 118 amino acids corresponding to a calculated molecular weight of 13 kDa. HspA exhibited 35.6% and 20.3% identity to the HspA and GroES proteins of *Legionella pneumophila* and *E. coli*, respectively[32]. A consensus heat shock promoter region was identified upstream of the *hspA* gene, whereas no obvious promoter sequences were detected upstream of *hspB*[32].

Suerbaum and Labigne were unable to construct an isogenic mutant of *H. pylori* in the *hspB* gene, suggesting that this gene is essential for bacterial survival[32]. The cpn60 homologues appear to be essential proteins in other bacteria as well[15,17].

Hp54K, similar to almost all other members of the cpn60 family, exhibits a striking motif consisting of glycine and methionine residues at the carboxy-terminus of the protein[32–34]. This glycine- and methionine-rich motif may be essential to ATP hydrolysis, since mutant *E. coli* strains containing GroEL lacking the final 16 residues (including nine glycine and five methionine residues) hydrolyse ATP at a slower rate than do wild-type bacteria[34].

POSSIBLE PATHOGENIC ROLE OF Hp54K

Two recent studies have indirectly implicated Hp54K in the pathogenesis of *H. pylori*-associated gastric inflammation[35,36]. Engstrand and co-workers have demonstrated that human gastric mucosa infected with *H. pylori*, but not uninfected mucosa, is recognized by monoclonal antibodies against the 65 kDa mycobacterial cpn60 homologue[35]. The latter antibody also recognizes intact *H. pylori*. *H. pylori* infection also appears to be associated with an increased number of $\gamma\delta$ T cells in the adjacent gastric mucosa[35]. The $\gamma\delta$ cells represent a primitive set of T cells which may have evolved to recognize antigens such as the cpn60 homologue in pathogens exposed to a stressful environment[17]. In addition, seropositivity in humans naturally infected with *H. pylori* is strongly correlated with the presence of autoantibodies against gastric mucosal cells[36]. Several monoclonal antibodies made against *H. pylori* also cross-react with human gastric mucosa[36]. The induction of antibodies cross-reacting with antigens of the gastric mucosa in mice immunized with *H. pylori* extracts, could be explained by the presence of anti-HSP antibodies[33]. Taken together, these data suggest that *H. pylori* and human gastric mucosal cells share common epitopes. This immunological cross-reactivity may represent an important pathogenic link between *H. pylori* and gastritis.

By analogy with mycobacterial and chlamydial HSP[37–39], Hp54K may contribute to gastric injury by stimulating $\gamma\delta$ T cells which cross-react with similar determinants on the endogenous 'self' HSP from stressed host cells[9]. This hypothesis might explain why *H. pylori* is essentially always associated with inflammation *in vivo*, although only a subset of *H. pylori* isolates produces cytotoxins[1-3,6-8]. Thus, *H. pylori* cytotoxins may not be responsible for evoking inflammation *per se*, but may contribute to more extensive gastric injury, possibly leading to ulcer formation[7,8]. *H. pylori*-induced activation of macrophages may also contribute to gastric injury[9]. Several cpn60 homologues, including the 65 kDa mycobacterial HSP, are thought to promote tissue injury through cell-mediated immune cross-reactivity[17,21,22].

However, the significance of Hp54K as a mediator of gastric inflammation is not clear. Macchia *et al.*[33] tested the immune response of individuals infected with *H. pylori* by immunoblotting for the presence of antibodies against Hp54K. They reported that 50% of the sera of infected individuals recognized Hp54K. The degree of recognition varied greatly between individuals, and did not show any obvious correlation with the type of gastroduodenal disease. Sera of uninfected people did not recognize Hp54K[33]. These data seem to suggest that immunological recognition of Hp54K is not essential for induction of *H. pylori*-associated gastritis. In addition, the rapid and essentially complete reversal of inflammation known to be associated with eradication of *H. pylori* suggests that a continuing autoimmune reaction is unlikely[1,40]. It is possible that inflammation *per se* is sufficient to induce increased expression of HSP within gastric mucosal cells and the resultant immunological cross-reactivity is merely an epiphenomenon. Further, Trejdosiewicz *et al.* did not observe an increase in $\gamma\delta$ T cells in *H. pylori*-associated gastritis[41]. Finally, Burroni and colleagues reported a significantly higher prevalence of specific antibodies directed against Hp54K in *H. pylori*-infected individuals with mild chronic gastritis compared with those with peptic ulcer, active moderate gastritis or normal histology[42]. The latter authors have proposed that antibodies against Hp54K may, in fact, protect against development of more serious gastroduodenal disease[42]. Experimental studies to assess the role of Hp54K as a mediator of gastric inflammation are needed.

CHAPERONE FUNCTIONS OF cpn60 HOMOLOGUES

Molecular chaperones are defined as a family of unrelated classes of protein which mediate the correct assembly of other polypeptides, but are not themselves components of the final functional structures (reviewed in ref. 15). In general, chaperone proteins are thought to bind to specific structural components that may be exposed only in the early stages of polypeptide assembly, and inhibit unproductive assembly pathways that would produce incorrect tertiary structure, hence act as 'kinetic dead-end traps'[15]. The best-studied example of a cpn60 chaperonin is GroEL of *E. coli*, whose function was first identified by its requirement in the assembly of bacteriophages (reviewed in ref. 15). A second chaperonin, known as cpn10 or GroES, is required for correct phage head formation, since it is involved in the release of the phage protein from GroEL[15]. These two chaperonins have been implicated in a number of processes in uninfected bacterial cells including DNA replication, cell division and protein secretion[15-18].

Evans *et al.* have speculated that Hp54K functions in the transmembrane export of the urease subunit molecules, assembly of the urease complex after

Table 1 Possible roles of *H. pylori* cpn60 homologue (Hp54K)

Immune mimicry
  Immunologically cross-reactive with gastric mucosal cells
Chaperone function
  Urease
  Outer membrane proteins
Essential protein for bacterial survival
Activation of cellular immune system
Immune evasion
  Surface layer protein which masks outer membrane proteins

---

export, or both[12]. They also suggest that Hp54K may serve to stabilize the urease complex thought to be secreted onto the surface of intact *H. pylori*, in the presence of gastric acidity local pH changes and protease activity[12]. In this regard, Suerbaum and Labigne recently reported that when the operon encoding both HspA and HspB was introduced together with the urease gene cluster into an *E. coli* host strain, activity of the expressed urease protein was increased significantly[43]. This observation is consistent with a chaperone function for Hp54K in processing or stabilizing the urease molecule. Further investigations are necessary to define the mechanisms of interaction between Hp54K and urease.

SUMMARY

In summary, Hp54K shares many characteristics with the cpn60 family of heat shock proteins including molecular sequence, size of native molecule and subunits, immunological cross-reactivity and ability to stimulate a strong immune response within infected hosts. Possible roles of the protein are summarized in Table 1. As a cpn60 homologue which appears to be surface-exposed, is highly immunogenic and is expressed in relatively large amounts (at least *in vitro*), Hp54K is a likely candidate protein to promote immune mimicry between *H. pylori* and gastric mucosal cells *in vivo*. In addition, Hp54K may serve as a chaperonin which promotes subunit association or stabilization of urease, outer membrane proteins and/or other proteins. Analogous to other cpn60 homologues, Hp54K appears to be essential to bacterial survival.

Hp54K, known to be present in soluble preparations of surface proteins from *H. pylori*[9,11], may, along with urease, play a role in activation of the cellular immune system[44,45]. In contrast, it seems possible, based on its apparent association with the surface of intact bacteria, that Hp54K and/or urease may facilitate immune evasion by *H. pylori* by masking integral outer membrane proteins from immune surveillance. In conclusion, Hp54K is likely to play an important role in the physiology and pathogenesis of *H. pylori*. Currently the functions of this interesting protein are not known.

Acknowledgements

This work was supported in part by the Medical Research Service of the Veterans Administration.

References

1. Graham DY, Go MF. *Helicobacter pylori*: current status. Gastroenterology. 1993;105: 279–82.
2. Marshall BJ. *Campylobacter pylori*: its link to gastritis and peptic ulcer disease. Rev Infect Dis. 1990;12:S87–93.
3. Blaser MJ. Hypotheses on the pathogenesis and natural history of *Helicobacter pylori*-induced inflammation. Gastroenterology. 1992;102:720–7.
4. Genta RM, Hamner HW, Graham DY. Gastric lymphoid follicles in *Helicobacter pylori* infection: frequency, distribution, and response to triple therapy. Human Pathol. 1993;24:577–83.
5. Parsonnet J, Friedman GD, Vandersteen DP et al. *Helicobacter pylori* infection and risk for gastric cancer. N Engl J Med. 1991;325:1127.
6. Leunk RD, Johnson PT, David BC, Kraft WG, Morgan DR. Cytotoxic activity in broth-culture filtrates of *Campylobacter pylori*. J Med Microbiol. 1988;26:93–9.
7. Cover TL, Dooley CP, Blaser MJ. Characterization of and human serologic response to proteins in *Helicobacter pylori* broth culture supernatants with vacuolizing cytotoxin activity. Infect Immun. 1990;58:603–10.
8. Figura N, Gugliemetti P, Rossolini A et al. Cytotoxin production by *Campylobacter pylori* strains isolated from patients with peptic ulcers and from patients with chronic gastritis only. J Clin Microbiol. 1990;28:1181–4.
9. Dunn BE, Roop RM II, Sung CC, Sharma SA, Perez-Perez GI, Blaser MJ. Identification and purification of a cpn60 heat shock protein homolog from *Helicobacter pylori*. Infect Immun. 1992;60:1946–51.
10. Stacey AR, Hawtin PR, Newell DG. Antigenicity of fractions of *Helicobacter pylori* prepared by fast protein liquid chromatography and urease captured by monoclonal antibodies. Eur J Clin Microbiol Inf Dis. 1990;9:732–7.
11. Dunn BE, Campbell GP, Perez-Perez GI, Blaser MJ. Purification and characterization of urease from *Helicobacter pylori*. J Biol Chem. 1990;265:9464–9.
12. Evans DJ, Evans DG, Engstrand L, Graham DY. Urease-associated heat shock protein of *Helicobacter pylori*. Infect Immun. 1992;60:2125–7.
13. Austin JW, Doig P, Stewart M, Trust TJ. Structural comparison of urease and a GroEL analog from *Helicobacter pylori*. J Bacteriol. 1992;174:7470–3.
14. Dunn BE, Perez-Perez GI, Blaser MJ. Characterization of *Campylobacter pylori* proteins by two-dimensional gel electrophoresis and immunoblotting. Infect Immun. 1989;57: 1825–33.
15. Ellis RJ. Molecular chaperones. Annu Rev Biochem. 1991;60:321–47.
16. Young DB. Chaperonins and the immune response. Semin Cell Biol. 1990;1:27–35.
17. Murray PJ, Young RA. Stress and immunological recognition in host-pathogen interactions. J Bacteriol. 1992;174:4193–6.
18. Hill Gaston JS. Heat shock proteins and autoimmunity. Immunology. 1991;3:35–42.
19. Creighton TE. Unfolding protein folding. Nature. 1991;352:17–18.
20. Hemmingsen SM, Woolford C, van der Vies SM et al. Homologous plant and bacterial proteins chaperone protein assembly. Nature (London). 1988;333:330–4.
21. Born W, Happ MP, Dallas A et al. Recognition of heat shock proteins and $\gamma\delta$ cell function. Immunol Today. 1990;11:40–3.
22. Kaufman SHE, Schoel B, Wand-Wurttenburger A, Steinhoff U, Munk ME, Koga T. T-cells, stress proteins, and pathogenesis of mycobacterial infections. Curr Top Microbiol Immunol. 1990;155:125–41.
23. Hendrix RW. Purification and properties of groE, a host protein involved in bacteriophage assembly. J Mol Biol. 1979;129:375–92.

24. Hohn T, Hohn B, Engel A, Wurtz M, Smith PR. Isolation and characterization of the host protein groE involved in bacteriophage lambda assembly. J Mol Biol. 1979;129:359–73.
25. Eshweiler B, Bohrmann B, Gerstenecker B, Schlitz E, Kist M. *In situ* localization of the 60 K protein of *Helicobacter pylori*, which belongs to the family of heat shock proteins, by immune electron microscopy. Acta Gastroenterol Belg. 1993;56:110.
26. Newell DG. Identification of the outer membrane proteins of *Campylobacter pyloridis* and antigenic cross-reactivity between *C. pyloridis* and *C. jejuni*. J Gen Microbiol. 1987;133:163–70.
27. Czinn S, Carr H, Sheffler L, Aranoff S. Serum IgG antibody to the outer membrane proteins of *Campylobacter pylori* in children with gastroduodenal disease. J Infect Dis. 1989;159:586–9.
28. Drouet EB, Dnoyel GA, Boude M, Wallano E, Andujar M, De Montclos HP. Characterization of an immunoreactive species-specific 19-kilodalton outer membrane protein from *Helicobacter pylori* by using a monoclonal antibody. J Clin Microbiol. 1991;29:1620–5.
29. Schnaitman CA. Outer membrane proteins of *Escherichia coli*. II. Heterogeneity of major outer membrane polypeptides. Arch Biochem Biophys. 1973;157:553–60.
30. Blaser MJ, Gotschlich EC. Surface array protein of *Campylobacter fetus*. Cloning and gene structure. J Biol Chem. 1990;265:19372–4.
31. Blaser MJ, Pei Z. Pathogenesis of *Campylobacter fetus* infections: critical role of high-molecular-weight S-layer proteins in virulence. J Infect Dis. 1993;167:372–7.
32. Suerbaum S, Labigne A. Cloning and sequencing of the HspA and HspB heat shock protein genes of *Helicobacter pylori*. Programs and Abstracts of the 93rd Annual Meeting of the American Society for Microbiology. 1993;127.
33. Macchia G, Massone A, Burroni D, Covacci A, Censini S, Rappuoli R. The Hsp60 protein of *Helicobacter pylori*: structure and immune response in patients with gastroduodenal disease. Mol Microbiol. 1993;9:645–52.
34. McLennan NF, Girshovich AS, Lissin NM, Charters Y, Masters M. The strongly conserved carboxyl-terminus glycine-methionine motif of the *Escherichia coli* GroEL chaperonin is dispensable. Mol Microbiol. 1993;7:49–58.
35. Engstrand L, Scheynius A, Pahlson C. An increased number of $\gamma\delta$ T-cells and gastric epithelial cell expression of the groEL stress-protein homologue in *Helicobacter pylori*-associated chronic gastritis of the antrum. Am J Gastroenterol. 1991;86:976–80.
36. Negrini R, Lisato L, Zanella I et al. *Helicobacter pylori* infection induces antibodies cross-reacting with human gastric mucosa. Gastroenterology. 1991;101:437–5.
37. Fu YX, Cranfill R, Vollmer M, Van Der Zee R, O'Brien RL, Born W. *In vivo* response of murine gamma delta T cells to a heat shock protein-derived peptide. Proc Natl Acad Sci. 1993;90:322–6.
38. Nomoto K, Yoshikai Y. Heat-shock proteins and immunopathology: regulatory role of heat-shock protein-specific T cells. Springer Semin Immunopathol. 1991;13:63–80.
39. Winfield J, Jarjour W, Minota S. Stress protein autoantibodies and the expression of stress proteins on the surface of human gamma–delta cells and other cells of the immune system. Chem Immunol. 1992;53:47–60.
40. Lee A, Fox J, Hazell S. Pathogenicity of *Helicobacter pylori*: a perspective. Infect Immun. 1993;61:1601–10.
41. Trejdosiewicz LK, Calabrese A, Smart CJ et al. $\gamma\delta$ T cell receptor-positive cells of the human gastrointestinal mucosa: occurrence and V region gene expression in *Helicobacter pylori*-associated gastritis, coeliac disease and inflammatory bowel disease. Clin Exp Immunol. 1991;84:440–4.
42. Burroni D, Figura N, Bugnoli M et al. Are antibodies to *Helicobacter pylori* heat-shock proteins protective? Acta Gastroenterol Belg. 1993;56:64.
43. Suerbaum S, Labigne A. *Helicobacter pylori* HspA-B heat shock protein operon: nucleotide sequence, expression, and putative role. Acta Gastroenterol Belg. 1993;56:51.
44. Mai UEH, Perez-Perez GI, Wahl LM, Blaser MJ, Smith PD. Soluble surface proteins from *Helicobacter pylori* activate monocytes/macrophages by lipopolysaccharide-independent mechanism. J Clin Invest. 1991;87:894–900.
45. Mai UE, Perez-Perez GI, Allen JB, Wahl SM, Blaser MJ, Smith PD. Surface proteins from *Helicobacter pylori* exhibit chemotactic activity for human leukocytes and are present in gastric mucosa. J Exp Med. 1992;15:517–25.

15
Gastric mucosal injury: interactions of mast cells, cytokines and nitric oxide

K. P. RIOUX, C. M. HOGABOAM and J. L. WALLACE

INTRODUCTION

The discovery of an association between gastric colonization by *Helicobacter pylori* and peptic ulcer disease has stimulated a re-evaluation of the role of the mucosal immune system in the pathogenesis of ulceration. One of the key mucosal immunocytes that might contribute to the modulation of mucosal integrity is the mast cell. Recent studies have suggested that the mast cell, through the release of a variety of mediators, can profoundly affect mucosal resistance to injury. There is also recent evidence that cytokines (e.g. IL-1) and prostaglandins can modulate mast cell reactivity and gastric acid secretion. Some of the actions of these cytokines, including modulation of mast cell reactivity, appear to be mediated through the generation of nitric oxide. In this chapter we review the interactions between cytokines, mast cells and nitric oxide, with reference in particular to the impact of such interactions on gastric mucosal integrity.

MAST CELLS AND GASTRIC MUCOSAL INTEGRITY

There is considerable evidence to suggest that mast cells contribute to the development of gastric mucosal injury. Foremost is the fact that mast cells are a source of a variety of potent, pro-ulcerogenic and pro-inflammatory mediators. Mast cell mediators shown to be important in the development of gastrointestinal injury include leukotriene C_4 (LTC_4)[1-3], platelet-activating factor (PAF)[3,4], histamine[5,6], endothelin[7], and tumour necrosis factor-α[8-10]. Furthermore, agents which cause activation of mast cells leading to mediator release have been shown to produce mucosal injury[11-13]; whereas mast cell 'stabilizers' have been reported to reduce gastric mucosal injury caused by ethanol[14-17]. Such evidence, however, is largely circumstantial since mast cells are not the exclusive source of inflammatory mediators in the stomach, and mast cell activators and stabilizers almost certainly have effects on other cell types. The situation is further complicated by the fact that mast cells are capable of producing IL-1[18], prostaglandins[19], and nitric oxide[20], each of which can protect the stomach from injury[21-23].

More convincing evidence of the contribution of mast cells to the development of mucosal injury comes from studies of ethanol-induced gastric damage in genetically mast cell-deficient mice[24]. These mice have significantly increased resistance to acute gastric damage induced by ethanol compared to normal littermates. Moreover, when mast cell populations were reconstituted by bone marrow transplantation, susceptibility of the stomach to injury was restored.

Another useful approach for examining the role of mast cells in gastric mucosal injury is to study animals in which mast cell numbers have been elevated. In rats, infection with the nematode *Nippostrongylus brasiliensis* increases the number of mucosal mast cells in the gastrointestinal tract and provides a means of mast cell activation, through re-exposure to *N. brasiliensis* antigen[25]. It has been shown that despite a two- to three-fold increase in the number of gastric mucosal mast cells after *N. brasiliensis* infection, ethanol-induced gastric damage was not significantly increased[26,27]. However, when mast cells were activated by antigen challenge prior to ethanol exposure, a significant increase in gastric injury was observed in sensitized rats compared to sham-sensitized controls. Depletion of mucosal mast cells by dexamethasone did not significantly reduce ethanol-induced gastric damage in control rats, but abolished the increased damage in sensitized rats challenged with antigen[27]. Rather than the number of mast cells *per se*, the state of mast cell activation seems to be the important determinant of the stomach's susceptibility to injury. Subsequent studies in our laboratory have identified LTC_4 as the principal mediator released in response to antigen administration which accounts for increasing the susceptibility of the gastric mucosa to injury (unpublished observations).

If mast cells do, in fact, play a role in gastric injury, there can be little doubt that it relates to their ability to release potent inflammatory mediators. It is possible, then, that susceptibility of the stomach to ulceration relates to the sensitivity of mast cells to stimuli which cause activation. The remainder of this chapter will describe factors which regulate mast cell reactivity, and how these factors might contribute to the pathogenesis of ulcer disease.

HELICOBACTER PYLORI AND MAST CELLS

H. pylori is a curved, Gram-negative, microaerophilic bacterium which was cultured for the first time in 1983 from the stomach of a patient with chronic gastritis[28]. The importance of this discovery is highlighted by the fact that *H. pylori* has since been linked to gastrointestinal disease in humans. For example, it is now recognized that *H. pylori* is the cause of chronic–active gastritis, and is closely associated with gastric and duodenal ulceration[29]. There is also a growing body of evidence that links *H. pylori* infection to gastric carcinoma[30].

Since its discovery there has been intense interest in the mechanisms by which *H. pylori* causes inflammation and ulceration of the stomach. Whereas much effort has gone into identifying the factors responsible for the pathogenicity of *H. pylori*[31], an emerging concept is that the host's immune response to persistent infection leads to mucosal injury[32]. This concept has stimulated renewed interest in the immunology of the stomach which had previously been neglected due to the firmly established belief that the human stomach is inhospitable to micro-organisms.

A strong antibody response is a consistent feature of infection with *H. pylori*, and has been exploited in the development of serological methods for its detection. Several studies have examined the presence of *H. pylori*-specific IgG in serum and IgA in gastric juice of colonized patients[33–35]. Despite the production of specific immunoglobulin the organism is not eliminated, and in most patients infection persists indefinitely, leading to chronic inflammatory changes in the gastric mucosa.

Of particular interest in the context of this review is a study of the IgE response in 26 patients infected with *H. pylori*[36]. *H. pylori*-specific serum IgE was found in 69% of colonized subjects compared to 5% in uninfected controls. Furthermore, 84% of colonized subjects had specific IgE bound to basophils, and histamine could be released upon stimulation with antigen. Although not examined in this study, mast cells in the stomachs of *H. pylori*-infected patients may be sensitized for release of damaging mediators upon encounter with antigen from adjacent sites of infection.

H. pylori infection manifests histologically as chronic–active gastritis, diagnosed when intra-epithelial and interstitial neutrophil polymorphs are present in addition to lymphocytes and plasma cells[37]. Eosinophil infiltration and degranulation has also been observed in gastric biopsy specimens of *H. pylori*-colonized patients[38]. Thus, the histological features of *H. pylori* infection are similar to allergic disease in humans[39,40].

There is considerable evidence that mast cells in the stomach may initiate IgE-mediated hypersensitivity reactions[41,42], and that these reactions may even result in gastric mucosal damage[43,44]. For example, gastric mucosal swelling and haemorrhage can be endoscopically observed after antigen challenge in patients with food allergy[45]. Furthermore, in humans it is noted that activated mast cells and IgE-producing plasma cells are abundant in the gastric mucosa surrounding ulcer lesions[42]. In humans, mast cells are the major source of histamine in the gastric mucosa[46]. It has been reported that children with *H. pylori*-associated gastritis have lower gastric mucosal histamine levels[47]. This suggests that histamine and possibly other mast cell mediators are released as a result of *H. pylori* infection. Whether this is primary to the development of gastritis or consequent to it remains to be established. It is also not known if mediator release is the result of IgE-dependent or IgE-independent mechanisms. Nevertheless, it is conceivable that mast cells may play a role in the pathogenesis of mucosal ulceration associated with *H. pylori* infection (Fig. 1).

Clearly it is possible that IgE-mediated type I hypersensitivity reactions play a role in the production of gastric mucosal damage in *H. pylori* infection. Although the pathological features of *H. pylori* infection may point to local

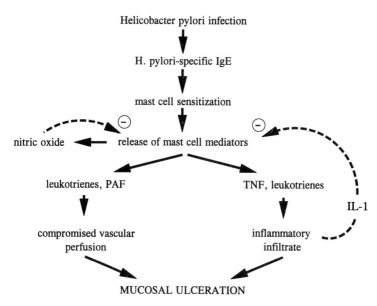

Fig. 1 Proposed scheme for the role of mast cells in the pathogenesis of *H. pylori*-associated ulceration. Mast cells sensitized to *H. pylori* would become activated when exposed to the antigen. A number of mediators released from mast cells could affect mucosal susceptibility to injury through their vasoactive effects and through the recruitment of inflammatory cells. Other mediators released from mast cells, such as IL-1 and nitric oxide, would exert down-regulatory effects on this cascade

allergic disease, no systemic allergic manifestations have yet been noted. However, in a large number of patients with chronic gastritis and peptic ulceration, features of an atopic condition have been reported[49].

As final evidence of a role for the mast cell in *H. pylori*-associated gastritis, one group has shown that *H. pylori* potentiates compound 48/80- and calcium ionophore-induced release of histamine from rat serosal mast cells *in vitro*[50]. Interestingly, this effect was observed when various preparations of both live and killed *H. pylori* were used. This implies that *H. pylori* has effects on mast cells that may contribute to the injury associated with colonization by this organism. Indeed, it has been shown that histamine can be released from human basophils by bacterial lectins, and this effect may contribute to the pathological features of bacterial infection[51,52]. It is conceivable that *H. pylori* profoundly influences mast cell function through combined immunological and non-immunological effects.

Mast cell mediators have known effects on vascular, secretory, and neural function in the stomach. But how might mast cell activation contribute to the production of the active gastric mucosal inflammation which characterizes *H. pylori* infection? Local infiltration of inflammatory cells following IgE-dependent mast cell degranulation is the result of late-phase reactions which are mediated by cytokines. TNF-α is known to mediate the late-phase reactions associated with immediate hypersensitivity[53]. Human and mouse mast cells have been shown to be a source of TNF-α[54,55]. It is reasonable to suggest that release of TNF-α from mast cells may contribute to the histological features of *H. pylori*-associated gastritis. Of course, mast cells are also capable of releasing a number of other chemotaxins, including PAF and LTB$_4$, which could contribute to the recruitment of lymphocytes and granulocytes in gastritis.

PROSTAGLANDINS AND MAST CELL REACTIVITY

Injury to the gastric mucosa is the most common and serious adverse effect associated with the use of non-steroidal anti-inflammatory drugs (NSAID)[56]. The mechanism by which NSAID produce injury to the stomach probably relates to their ability to block the enzyme cyclo-oxygenase and thereby inhibit production of prostaglandins. However, it remains unclear exactly how inhibition of prostaglandin synthesis in the stomach promotes mucosal ulceration. In a variety of models of experimental gastrointestinal mucosal injury, exogenous prostaglandins have been shown to lessen the severity of damage[22,57]. Furthermore, misoprostol, a PGE$_1$ analogue, has proven clinically effective in reducing the incidence of gastric and duodenal ulceration in patients taking NSAID[58,59].

The protective effects of prostaglandins have been linked to their ability to stimulate mucus and bicarbonate secretion and to maintain mucosal blood flow[60]. It has also been suggested that their effects may be attributable to stabilization of mast cells[61]. Raud *et al.*, using the hamster cheek pouch model of allergic inflammation, showed that exogenous PGE$_2$ reduced histamine release and plasma leakage evoked by antigen challenge, whereas NSAID enhanced histamine release, plasma leakage, and leukocyte accumulation following both antigen- and compound 48/80-induced mast cell activation[62,63]. Hogaboam *et al.* recently tested the hypothesis that prostaglandins can stabilize mast cells, by assessing their effects *in vitro* using both connective tissue (i.e. peritoneal) and intestinal mucosal mast cells[64]. They reported that PGE$_2$, 16,16-dimethyl PGE$_2$ and misoprostol significantly inhibited the release of PAF, TNF-α, and histamine. These inhibitory effects of the prostaglandins were observed at concentrations in the picomolar to nanomolar range. Thus, prostaglandins are potent modulators of mast cell reactivity, possibly contributing to their cytoprotective actions. Suppression of prostaglandin synthesis by NSAID probably increases the reactivity of mast cells, and it is possible that this contributes to the pathogenesis of mucosal injury caused by these drugs.

IL-1 AND GASTRIC MUCOSAL FUNCTION

There has been a great deal of interest in IL-1 as a potential modulator of gastric mucosal integrity and function since this cytokine was reported to be a very potent gastroprotective agent in experimental ulcer models. For example, nanogram to microgram doses of IL-1 were shown to prevent gastric damage induced by ethanol, aspirin and indomethacin[65-69] and duodenal ulceration induced by cysteamine[67]. At least part of the action of IL-1 is mediated centrally through prostaglandin-dependent pathways[65,66]. These studies suggest that this central action of IL-1 results in suppression of acid secretion. In other studies, gastroprotective effects of IL-1 against NSAID-induced gastric injury were shown to be at least in part independent of its actions on acid secretion[66]. We demonstrated that IL-1, at gastroprotective doses, markedly suppressed neutrophil functions such as migration in response to chemotaxins. Such actions of IL-1 might contribute to its gastroprotective effects, since NSAID-induced gastric damage in experimental models has been shown to be neutrophil-dependent[70-72].

The antisecretory effects of IL-1 appear to be secretagogue-specific, at least in the rat[73]. We demonstrated that IL-1 could dose-dependently inhibit gastric acid secretion stimulated by pentagastrin, but not that stimulated by histamine or bethanechol. We suggested that IL-1 might be acting at the level of a histamine-releasing cell, such as the enterochromaffin-like cell and/or the mast cell. Subsequent studies in our laboratory and others have supported this hypothesis, and implicated nitric oxide as a secondary mediator of the effects of IL-1[74,75]. For example, Barrachina *et al.* recently reported that inhibition of pentagastrin-stimulated acid secretion by IL-1 is mediated by nitric oxide[75].

NITRIC OXIDE, IL-1 AND MAST CELL REACTIVITY

Nitric oxide is a highly reactive substance which exerts effects on many cells, and can be released by many cells[76]. Mast cells have been shown to release nitric oxide constitutively[20,77], and it has been suggested that this acts as an autoregulator of mast cell activation[78], since addition of exogenous sources of nitric oxide to isolated mast cells results in inhibition of histamine release[79]. The nitric oxide released from mast cells also contributes to the ability of these cells to kill other cells[77]. We recently examined the effects of IL-1 on mast cell release of nitric oxide, and the impact this might have on the release of a pro-ulcerogenic mediator, PAF[74]. IL-1 was found to rapidly stimulate nitric oxide release from peritoneal mast cells at doses in the picogram to nanogram per millilitre range. This effect is consistent with the ability of IL-1 to stimulate nitric oxide release from a number of other cell types[80-84]. When PAF release from mast cells was stimulated with calcium ionophore, those cells pretreated with IL-1 were found to release markedly less[74]. The inhibition of PAF release by IL-1 was dose-dependent and could be reversed by pre-exposure of the mast cells to a nitric oxide synthase inhibitor. While we did not examine the effects of IL-1 on histamine release, it is conceivable that IL-1, through generation of nitric oxide, would inhibit histamine release. Such a mechanism could contribute to the inhibition of pentagastrin-stimulated acid secretion by IL-1, which has been previously shown to be nitric oxide-dependent.[75]

SUMMARY

The mast cell plays a key role as an 'alarm cell', initiating defensive responses when it encounters antigen. This cell also appears to play an important role in modulating gastric mucosal defence. In recent years a great deal has been learned about the many inflammatory mediators released from mast cells and their effects on gastric mucosal integrity and function (e.g. acid secretion). There is now emerging evidence for autoregulatory feedback by some of these mediators (e.g. IL-1, nitric oxide) on mast cell reactivity. While a role for the mast cell in the gastric injury associated with *H. pylori* infection has not been established, there is considerable evidence to suggest that this may be the case.

Acknowledgements

This work was supported by grants from the Medical Research Council of Canada (MRC). K.P.R. and C.M.H. are supported by studentships from the Alberta Heritage Foundation for Medical Research (AHFMR). J.L.W. is an MRC Scientist and AHFMR Scholar.

References

1. Wallace JL, McKnight GW, Keenan CM, Byles NIA, MacNaughton WK. Effects of leukotrienes on susceptibility of the rat stomach to damage and investigation of the mechanism of action. Gastroenterology. 1990;98:1178–86.
2. Peskar BM. Role of leukotriene C_4 in mucosal damage caused by necrotizing agents and indomethacin in the rat stomach. Gastroenterology. 1991;100:619–26.
3. Konturek SJ, Brzozowki T, Drozdowicz D, Garlicki J, Beck G. Role of leukotrienes and platelet-activating factor in acute gastric mucosal lesions in rats. Eur J Pharmacol. 1989;164:285–92.
4. Wallace JL, Steel G, Whittle BJR, Lagente V, Vargaftig B. Evidence for platelet-activating factor as a mediator of endotoxin-induced gastrointestinal damage in the rat. Gastroenterology. 1987;93:765–73.
5. Franco-Brown S, Masson GMC, Corcoran AC. Induction of acute gastric lesions by histamine liberators in rats: effects thereon of pharmacologic blocking agents. J Allergy. 1959;30:1–10.
6. Bommelaer G, Guth PH. Protection by histamine receptor antagonists and prostaglandin against gastric mucosal barrier disruption in the rat. Gastroenterology. 1979;77:303–8.
7. Wallace JL, Cirino G, Denucci G, McKnight GW, MacNaughton WK. Endothelin has potent ulcerogenic and vasoconstrictor actions in the stomach. Am J Physiol. 1989;256:G661–6.
8. Tracey KJ, Beutler B, Lowry SF et al. Shock and tissue injury induced by recombinant human cachectin. Science. 1986;234:470–4.
9. Sun X, Hsueh W. Bowel necrosis induced by tumour necrosis factor in rats is mediated by platelet-activating factor. J Clin Invest. 1988;81:1328–31.
10. Mahatma M, Agawal N, Dajane EZ, Nelson S, Nakamura C, Sitton J. Misoprostol but not antacid prevents endotoxin-induced gastric mucosal injury: role of tumour necrosis factor-alpha. Dig Dis Sci. 1991;36:1562–8.
11. Takeuchi K, Ohtsuki H, Okabe S. Pathogenesis of compound 48/80-induced gastric lesions in rats. Dig Dis Sci. 1986;31:392–400.
12. Cho CH, Ogle CW. Cholinergic-mediated gastric mast cell degranulation with subsequent histamine H_1- and H_2-receptor activation in stress ulceration in rats. Eur J Pharmacol. 1979;55:23–33.

13. Guth PH, Hall P. Microcirculatory and mast cell changes in restraint-induced gastric ulcer. Gastroenterology. 1966;50:562–70.
14. Beck PL, Morris GP, Wallace JL. Reduction of ethanol-induced gastric damage by sodium cromoglycate and FPL-52694. Role of leukotrienes, prostaglandins, and mast cells in the protective mechanism. Can J Physiol Pharmacol. 1989;67:287–93.
15. Takeuchi K, Nishiwaki H, Okabe S. Cytoprotective action of mast cell stabilizers against ethanol-induced gastric lesions in rats. Jpn J Pharmacol. 1986;42:297–307.
16. Goosens J, Van Reempts J, Van Wauwe JP. Cytoprotective effects of disodium cromoglycate on rat stomach mucosa. Br J Pharmacol. 1987;91:165–9.
17. Karmeli F, Eliakim R, Okon E, Rachmilewitz D. Gastric mucosal damage by ethanol is mediated by substance P and prevented by ketotifen, a mast cell stabilizer. Gastroenterology. 1991;100:1206–16.
18. Gordon JR, Burd PR, Galli SJ. Mast cells as a source of multifunctional cytokines. Immunol Today. 1990;11:458–64.
19. Heavey DJ, Ernst PB, Stevens RL, Befus AD, Bienenstock J, Austen KF. Generation of leukotriene C_4, leukotriene B_4, and prostaglandin D_2 by immunologically activated rat intestinal mucosal mast cells. J Immunol. 1988;140:1953–7.
20. Salvemini D, Masini E, Anggard E, Mannaioni PF, Vane J. Synthesis of a nitric oxide-like factor from L-arginine by rat serosal mast cells: stimulation of guanylate cyclase and inhibition of platelet aggregation. Biochem Biophys Res Commun. 1990;169:596–601.
21. MacNaughton WK, Cirino G, Wallace JL. Endothelium-derived relaxing factor (nitric oxide) has protective actions in the stomach. Life Sci. 1989;45:1869–76.
22. Robert A. Cytoprotection by prostaglandins in rats. Prevention of gastric necrosis produced by alcohol, HCl, NaOH, hypertonic NaCl, and thermal injury. Gastroenterology. 1979;77:433–43.
23. Wallace JL, Keenan CM, Mugridge KG, Parente L. Reduction of the severity of experimental gastric and duodenal ulceration by interleukin-1β. Eur J Pharmacol. 1990;186:279–84.
24. Galli SJ, Wershil BK, Bose R, Walker PA, Szabo S. Ethanol-induced acute gastric injury in mast cell-deficient and congenic normal mice. Evidence that mast cells can augment the area of damage. Am J Pathol. 1988;128:131–40.
25. Miller HRP, Woodbury RG, Huntley JF, Newlands GFJ. Systemic release of mucosal mast cell protease in primed rats challenged with *Nippostrongylus brasiliensis*. Immunology. 1983;49:471–9.
26. Chiverton SG, Perdue MH, Hunt RH. Do mast cells have a role in gastric injury? Gastroenterology. 1989;96:A87.
27. Rioux KP, Wallace JL. Activation of mucosal mast cells augments gastric mucosal injury. Gastroenterology. 1993;104:A1059.
28. Warren JR. Unidentified curved bacilli on gastric epithelium in active chronic gastritis. Lancet. 1983;1:1273.
29. Buck GE. *Campylobacter pylori* and associated gastroduodenal disease. Clin Microbiol Rev. 1990;3:1–12.
30. Loffeld RJ, Willems I, Flendrig JA, Arends JW. *Helicobacter pylori* and gastric carcinoma. Histopathology. 1990;17:537–41.
31. Blaser MJ. *Helicobacter pylori* and the pathogenesis of gastroduodenal inflammation. J Infect Dis. 1990;161:626–33.
32. Lee A, Fox J, Hazell S. Pathogenicity of *Helicobacter pylori*: a perspective. Infect Immunol. 1993;61:1601–10.
33. Rathbone BJ, Wyatt JI, Worsley BW et al. Systemic and local antibody responses to gastric *Campylobacter pyloridis* in non-ulcer dyspepsia. Gut. 1986;27:642–7.
34. Kazi JI, Sinniah R, Jaffrey NA et al. Cellular and humoral immune responses in *Campylobacter pylori*-associated chronic gastritis. J Pathol. 1989;159:231–7.
35. Ireland A, Bamforth J, DuBoulay CE, Lloyd RS, Pearson AD. Clinical importance of *Campylobacter pyloridis* and association of serum IgG and IgA antibody responses in patients undergoing upper gastrointestinal endoscopy. J Clin Pathol. 1986;39:215–19.
36. Aceti A, Celestino D, Caferro M et al. Basophil-bound and serum immunoglobulin E directed against *Helicobacter pylori* in patients with chronic gastritis. Gastroenterology. 1991;101:131–7.
37. Andersen LP, Holck S, Povlsen CO, Elseborg L, Justesen T. *Campylobacter pyloridis* in

peptic ulcer disease. I. Gastric and duodenal infection caused by *C. pyloridis*: histopathologic and microbiologic findings. Scand J Gastroenterol. 1987;22:219–24.

38. McGovern TW, Talley NJ, Kephart GM, Carpenter HA, Gleich GJ. Eosinophil infiltration and degranulation in *Helicobacter pylori*-associated gastritis. Dig Dis Sci. 1989;36:435–40.
39. Gleich GJ. The late phase of the immunoglobulin E-mediated reaction: a link between anaphylaxis and common allergic disease? J Allergy Clin Immunol. 1982;70:160–9.
40. Lemanske RF, Kaliner MA. Mast cell-dependent late phase reactions. Clin Immunol Rev. 1982;1:547–80.
41. Catto-Smith AG, Patrick MK, Scott RB, Davison JS, Gall DG. Gastric response to mucosal IgE-mediated reactions. Am J Physiol. 1989;257:G704–8.
42. Brown WR, Borthistle KB, Chen ST. Immunoglobulin E (IgE) and IgE-containing cells in human gastrointestinal fluids. Clin Exp Immunol. 1975;20:227–37.
43. Shapiro PF, Ivy AC. Gastric ulcer: IV. Experimental production of gastric ulcer by local anaphylaxis. Arch Intern Med. 1926;38:237–58.
44. Andre F, Andre C. Gastric ulcer disease: gastric ulcer induced by mucosal anaphylaxis in ovalbumin-sensitized *Praomys* (*Mastomys*) *matalensis*. Am J Pathol. 1981;102:133–5.
45. Reimann H-J, Lewin J. Gastric mucosal reactions in patients with food allergy. Am J Gastroenterol. 1988;83:1212–19.
46. Wershil BK, Galli SJ. Gastrointestinal mast cells: new approaches for analyzing their function *in vivo*. Gastroenterol Clin N Am. 1991;20:613–27.
47. Quieroz DMM, Mendes EN, Rocha GA, Barbosa AJA, Carvalho AST, Cunha-Melo JR. Histamine concentration of gastric mucosa in *Helicobacter pylori* positive and negative children. Gut. 1991;32:464–6.
49. Romamski B, Bartuzi Z, Zbikowska-Gotz M, Korenkiewicz J. Allergy to cockroach antigens in patients with peptic ulcers and chronic gastritis. Allergol Immunopathol. 1988;16:219–24.
50. Bechi P, Dei R, DiBello MG, Masini E. *Helicobacter pylori* potentiates histamine release from serosal rat mast cells *in vitro*. Dig Dis Sci. 1993;38:944–9.
51. Norn S, Stahl Skov P, Jensen C *et al.* Intrinsic asthma and bacterial histamine release via lectin effect. Agents Actions. 1983;13:210–12.
52. Jensen C, Norn S, Stahl Skov P, Espersen F, Koch C, Permin H. Bacterial histamine release by immunological and non-immunological lectin mediated reactions. Allergy. 1984;39:371–7.
53. Galli SJ, Gordon JR, Wershil BK. Cytokine production by mast cells and basophils. Curr Opin Immunol. 1991;3:865–73.
54. Gordon JR, Galli JS. Mast cells as a source of both preformed and immunologically inducible TNF-α/cachectin. Nature. 1990;346:274–6.
55. Steffen M, Abboud M, Potter GK, Yung YP, Moore MAS. Presence of tumour necrosis factor or a related factor in human basophils/mast cells. Immunology. 1989;66:445–50.
56. Fries JF, Miller SR, Spitz BW, Williams CA, Hubert HB, Bloch DA. Toward an epidemiology of gastropathy associated with nonsteroidal anti-inflammatory drug use. Gastroenterology. 1989;96:647–55.
57. Hawkey CJ, Rampton DS. Prostaglandins and the gastrointestinal mucosa: are they important in its function, disease, or treatment? Gastroenterology. 1985;89:1162–8.
58. Graham DY, Agrawal NM, Roth SH. Prevention of NSAID-induced gastric ulcer with misoprostol: multicentre, double-blind, placebo-controlled trial. Lancet. 1988;2:1277–80.
59. Graham DY, Lidsky MD, Cox AM, Evans DJ, Evans DG, Albert L. Long term nonsteroidal anti-inflammatory drug use and *Helicobacter pylori* infection. Gastroenterology. 1991;100:1653–7.
60. Whittle BJR, Vane JR. Prostanoids as regulators of gastrointestinal function. In: Johnson LR, editor. Physiology of the gastrointestinal tract, vol. 1, 2nd edn. New York: Raven Press; 1987:143–80.
61. Reimann HJ, Lewin J, Schmidt U, Wendt P, Bluemi G, Dajani EZ. Misoprostol prevents damage to the gastric mucosa by stabilizing the mast cells. Prostaglandins. 1987;33(Suppl):105–16.
62. Raud J, Dahlen S.-E, Smedegard G, Hedqvist P. Enhancement of acute allergic inflammation by indomethacin is reversed by prostaglandin E_2: apparent correlation with *in vivo* modulation of mediator release. Proc Natl Acad Sci USA. 1989;85:2315–19.

63. Raud J, Sydbom A, Dahlen SE, Heqvist P. Prostaglandin E_2 prevents diclofenac-induced enhancement of histamine release and inflammation evoked by in vivo challenge with compound 48/80 in the hamster cheek pouch. Agents Actions. 1989;28:108–14.

64. Hogaboam CM, Bissonnette EY, Chin BC, Befus AD, Wallace JL. Prostaglandins inhibit inflammatory mediator release from rat mast cells. Gastroenterology. 1993;104:122–9.

65. Saperas ES, Yang H, Rivier C, Taché Y. Central action of recombinant interleukin-1 to inhibit acid secretion in rats. Gastroenterology. 1990;99:1599–606.

66. Robert A, Saperas E, Zhang W et al. Gastric cytoprotection by intracisternal interleukin-1β in the rat. Biochem Biophys Res Commun. 1991;174:1117–24.

67. Wallace JL, Keenan CM, Mugridge KG, Parente L. Reduction of the severity of experimental gastric and duodenal ulceration by interleukin-1β. Eur J Pharmacol. 1990;186:279–84.

68. Wallace JL, Keenan CM, Cucala M, Mugridge KG, Parente L. Mechanisms underlying the protective effects of interleukin-1 in experimental NSAID-gastropathy. Gastroenterology. 1992;102:1176–85.

69. Robert A, Olafsson AS, Lancaster C, Zhang W. Interleukin-1 is cytoprotective, antisecretory, stimulates PGE_2 synthesis by the stomach, and retards gastric emptying. Life Sci. 1991;48:123–34.

70. Wallace JL, Keenan CM, Granger DN. Gastric ulceration induced by nonsteroidal anti-inflammatory drugs is a neutrophil-dependent process. Am J Physiol. 1990;259:G462–7.

71. Wallace JL, Arfors KE, McKnight GW. A monoclonal antibody against the CD18 leukocyte adhesion molecule prevents indomethacin-induced gastric damage in the rabbit. Gastroenterology. 1991;100:878–83.

72. Wallace JL, Granger DN. Pathogenesis of NSAID gastropathy: are neutrophils the culprits? Trends Pharmacol Sci. 1992;13:129–31.

73. Wallace JL, Cucala M, Mugridge K, Parente L. Secretagogue-specific effects of interleukin-1 on gastric acid secretion. Am J Physiol. 1991;261:G559–64.

74. Hogaboam CM, Befus AD, Wallace JL. Modulation of mast cell reactivity by interleukin-1β: divergent effects on nitric oxide and platelet-activating factor release. J Immunol. 1993: in press.

75. Barrachina MD, Calatayud S, Moreno L, Pique JM, Whittle BJR, Esplugues JV. Nitric oxide generation modulates the inhibition by interleukin-1β of pentagastrin-stimulated gastric acid secretion in the rat. Gut. 1993;34:S11.

76. Moncada S, Palmer RMJ, Higgs EA. Nitric oxide: physiology, pathophysiology, and pharmacology. Pharmacol Rev. 1991;43:109–42.

77. Bissonnette EY, Hogaboam CM, Wallace JL, Befus AD. Potentiation of tumor necrosis factor-α-mediated cytotoxicity of mast cells by their production of nitric oxide. J Immunol. 1991;147:3060–5.

78. Salvemini D, Masini E, Pistelli A, Mannaioni PF, Vane JR. Nitric oxide: a regulatory mediator of mast cell reactivity. J Cardiovasc Pharmacol. 1991;17:S258–64.

79. Van Overveld FJ, Bult H, Vermeire PA, Herman AG. Nitroprusside, a nitrogen oxide generating drug, inhibits release of histamine and tryptase from human skin mast cells. Agents Actions. 1993;38(Suppl):C237–8.

80. Beasley D, Schwartz JH, Brenner BM. Interleukin 1 induces prolonged L-arginine-dependent cyclic guanosine monophosphate and nitrite production in rat vascular smooth muscle cells. J Clin Invest. 1991;87:602–8.

81. Pfeilschifter J, Vosbeck J. Transforming growth factor β inhibits interleukin 1β- and tumour necrosis factor α-induction of nitric oxide synthase in rat renal mesangial cells. Biochem Biophys Res Commun. 1991;175:372–9.

82. Schini VB, Junquero DC, Scott-Burden T, Vanhoutte PM. Interleukin-1β induces the production of an L-arginine-derived relaxing factor from cultured smooth muscle cells from rat aorta. Biochem Biophys Res Commun. 1991;176:114–21.

83. Corbett JA, Wang JL, Sweetland MA, Lancaster JR, McDaniel ML. Interleukin 1β induces the formation of nitric oxide by β-cells purified from rodent islets of Langerhans. Evidence for the β-cell as a source and site of action of nitric oxide. J Clin Invest. 1992;90:2384–91.

84. Xenos ES, Stevens RB, Gores PF et al. IL-1β-induced inhibition of β-cell function is mediated through nitric oxide. Transplant Proc. 1993;25:994.

16
H. pylori supernatant contains a novel chemotactic factor for monocytes different from FMLP

P. A. ANTON, J. R. REEVE JR, D. QUISMORIO, K. SMELA,
M. C. TERRITO and J. H. WALSH

INTRODUCTION

Significant evidence exists that *Helicobacter pylori* causes superficial antral gastritis, duodenitis as well as ulcer disease[1], even though the bacterium rarely invades the tissue[2]. Inflammatory infiltrates are observed just below regions of *H. pylori* that are on the gastric luminal side and gastric mucosa remains intact[3]. The bacteria are rarely observed in non-inflamed tissue[4]. There is a strong correlation between the number of bacteria seen and the amount of inflammation[1], and gastritis ceases after the bacteria are eradicated[3].

Nevertheless, mechanisms to explain the immunoinflammatory recruitment are lacking. One hypothesis for the association between *H. pylori* and gastritis is that the bacterium secretes a factor which attacks leukocytes. Evidence for this hypothesis is a recent demonstration that *H. pylori* grown in culture secretes a factor which is chemotactic for monocytes and neutrophils[5].

Many bacteria have been shown to secrete chemotactic peptides[6]. Most of these peptides have an amino terminus that has been modified after translation by an amino terminal formyl group. The first chemotactic factor was purified from *E. coli* in 1984. Structural analysis of this factor showed that it was a tripeptide with a formylated amino terminus, f-Met-Leu-Phe[7]. This factor, and other *N*-formylated peptides, are normally present throughout much of the gastrointestinal tract without inducing inflammation[8-11].

The report on a chemotactic factor of *H. pylori* by Craig *et al.*[5] did not permit its differentiation from FMLP. It is known that *H. pylori* contains significant amounts of FMLP (V. Chadwick, personal communication) emphasizing the importance of distinguishing the factors stimulating chemotaxis.

The studies reported here were performed to evaluate whether the chemotactic factor was related to FMLP. A low molecular weight, hydrophobic factor derived from *H. pylori* culture medium that is chemotactic for monocytes has been purified. This factor is different from FMLP and may contribute to the inflammation in *H. pylori* infection after absorption through the gastric mucosa.

MATERIALS AND METHODS

Chemicals and supplies

Brucella broth (Difco Laboratories, Detroit, MI); vancomycin, polymixin B, *N*-formyl-methionyl-leucyl-phenylalanine (Sigma, St Louis, MO); fetal bovine serum (Gemini, Calabasas, CA); phosphate buffered saline (Irvine Sci., Irvine, CA); 48-well chemotaxis chambers (Neuroprobe, Cabin John, MD); 5 μm chemotaxis filters (Costar, Livermore, CA); C-18 Sep-pak columns (Millipore, Milford, MA).

Bacterial strains and culture conditions

The *H. pylori* isolates examined were obtained from (1) American Tissue Cell Culture (ATCC) strain no. 43579 and (2) consenting patients undergoing routine upper gastrointestinal endoscopy. Isolated *H. pylori* was identified by urease, catalase, oxidase activity and microscopy (Gram-negative spiral bacilli). Strains were grown under microaerophilic conditions at 37°C in brucella broth with 1% heat-inactivated PBS, vancomycin (10 μg/ml) and poly-B (2.5 units/ml) for 48–72 h.

Supernatant collection

Bacteria were harvested during log phase growth. Cultures were centrifuged (3000 rpm) and washed twice with phosphate buffered saline (PBS without Ca^{2+} and Mg^{2+}). The pellet was resuspended with PBS (prescreened for chemotactic activity) to give an absorbance at 620 nm of 0.9 (approximately 10^7 colony-forming units (c.f.u.) per millilitre). Resuspended bacteria were incubated in PBS for 4 h at 37°C and harvested again by centrifugation (3000 rpm, 30 min at 25°C). The resultant supernatant was filtered through a 0.22 μm filter unit. If necessary, supernatant was stored at −80°C for up to 2 months without loss of activity.

Solid-phase extraction concentration (Sep-pak)

Supernatant (100 ml) was processed through a Waters C-18 Sep-pak cartridge, prepared with 100% ETOH, equilibrated with distilled H_2O, and eluted with 50% acetonitrile containing 0.1% TFA (24-fold concentrate). A control of cultured medium that had f-Met-Leu-Phe added in amounts sufficient for optical detection was also treated in the same manner.

Gel permeation chromatography

Neighbouring fractions (1 ml each) of *H. pylori* supernatant demonstrating chemotactic activity after Sep-pak purification were pooled together and vacuum centrifuged to a final volume of 2 ml. This sample was then loaded onto a G-50 Sephadex column (1×80 cm). Buffer used was non-chemotactic PBS; 1 ml fractions were collected at $4°C$.

Chemotaxis assay

Chemotactic response was determined in 48-well chemotactic chambers (Neuro-Probe, Inc., Cabin John, MD). Monocytic chemotaxis was performed in triplicate by placing $50\,\mu l$ of the cell suspension (10^6/ml) in the upper compartment of the chamber, separated from the lower compartment by a PVP-free nitrocellulose filter with a pore size of $5\,\mu m$ (Costar, Pleasanton, CA). The lower compartment was filled with $27\,\mu l$ of the appropriate dilutions of sample to be tested. FMLP (10^{-8} mol/l) and PBS were run simultaneously as controls. The chambers were incubated for 90 min at $37°C$; monocytes that migrated completely through the filter were counted in 20 random fields in each well. Results are expressed as the number of monocytes per high-powered field. Chemokinesis activity was distinguished from chemokinetic activity by checkerboard analysis. Most movement of leukocytes has been shown to be chemotactic[4]. Serial dilutions of the test sample were placed in the lower compartment of the chamber and similar concentrations of the factor were used to dilute the monocytes in the upper compartment. Directional movement of the cells in response to a concentration gradient indicates chemotaxis, whereas increased movement of the cells induced by the factor unrelated to the concentration gradient indicates chemokinesis.

Isolation of monocytes

Peripheral venous blood of healthy donors was separated on Ficoll-Hypaque density gradient separation (Histopaque, Sigma, MO) to obtain mononuclear cells. The cells were washed and resuspended in DME Low Glucose containing 0.1% heat-inactivated PBS. Determination of monocyte concentration was achieved using Wright stain for microscopic characterization; mononuclear cell population was resuspended to give a corrected monocyte concentration of 10^6 monocytes/ml.

HPLC purification

Reverse-phase HPLC chromatography was done directly on Sep-pak concentrated chemotactic factor or on chemotactic factor previously purified by gel permeation chromatography. For Sep-pak concentrated factor, the 50% acetonitrile eluant was diluted 5-fold with 0.1% trifluoroacetate (TFA) before loading onto the HPLC. The factor first purified by gel permeation chromatography was brought to pH 4.0 with acetic acid before loading onto HPLC. These mixtures were loaded in 5 ml aliquots onto an analytical Vydac C-4 reverse-phase HPLC column (Vydac 214TP54, 4.6 mm × 25 cm, 5 micron; Separations Group, Hesperia, CA) and equilibrated in 0.1% TFA. After loading, the column was rinsed in 0.1% TFA for 5 min, then brought to 35% buffer B (50% acetonitrile in 0.1% TFA) over 5 min, and eluted with a gradient from 35% to 65% of buffer B over 60 min. For bioactivity, from each 2 ml HPLC fraction, 100 μl was diluted with 2 ml of distilled H_2O, loaded on to a Sep-pak column, eluted with 100% ETOH and rotary evaporated. Each fraction was reconstituted with non-chemotactic PBS to the appropriate dilution before bioassay.

Statistical analysis

All values are expressed as means $\pm$ SE. Data were analysed using Student's *t*-test.

RESULTS

Characterization of chemotactic assay

Phosphate buffered saline (PBS) used to dilute all samples had very low chemotactic activity (5.1 $\pm$ 0.8 monocytes per high-power field). FMLP at concentrations from 10^{-10} to 10^{-8} mol/l demonstrated a dose-related increase in monocyte chemotaxis. Higher concentrations show characteristic inhibition by supermaximal concentration of FMLP. Therefore, FMLP at a concentration of 10^{-8} mol/l was selected as a control in all studies.

Initial purification of non-FMLP *H. pylori*-chemotactic factor

Bacterial supernatant from *H. pylori* was prepared as described in Methods and concentrated from 2000 ml to 1 ml using solid-phase extraction concentration (Sep-pak) techniques. Chemotactically active material was eluted with 50% acetonitrile.

In order to contrast elution profiles of our *H. pylori*-chemotactic peptide with that of FMLP, equal volumes of bacterial supernatant, concentrated by Sep-pak, were evaluated by reverse-phase HPLC and bioassay; FMLP (10^{-6} mol/l) was added to one of the two samples prior to initial purification. Chemotactic assay of all HPLC-eluted fractions from the cultured medium with added FMLP demonstrated two chemotactic fractions, one associated with an absorbance peak which was absent when FMLP was not added. The other absorbance peak associated with chemotactic activity was the same as the chemotactic factor observed during runs of cultured media

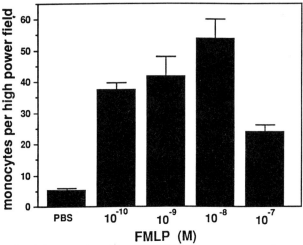

Fig. 1 Dose-related chemotactic activity of FMLP for human monocytes. Increasing concentrations of FMLP are shown to variably stimulate monocyte chemotaxis. Baseline chemotactic activity of PBS is demonstrated. Figures represent the mean of three wells ± SE

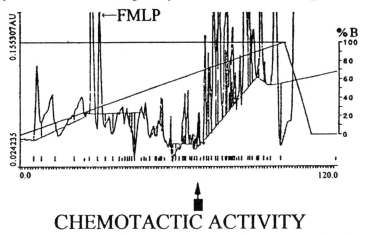

CHEMOTACTIC ACTIVITY

Fig. 2 HPLC elution profile of *H. pylori* supernatant after Sep-pak concentration. Tubes demonstrating chemotactic activity after Sep-pak concentration were diluted and loaded onto reverse-phase HPLC column, then eluted with increasing concentrations of acetonitrile. FMLP eluted at 15% acetonitrile; *H. pylori* chemotactic factor eluted at 32.5% acetonitrile

without added FMLP. These absorbance peaks are identified in Fig. 2. Chemotactic activity for monocytes of the non-FMLP absorbance peak identified in Fig. 2 is shown in Fig. 3. Although many absorbance peaks are present in *H. pylori* supernatant initially purified by C-18 Sep-pak, one absorbance peak (separate from FMLP) associated with chemotactic activity is identified, eluting at 32.5% acetonitrile (Fig. 2).

Purification of bacterial supernatant obtained from an ATCC strain of *H. pylori* was processed as above. Chemotactic activity was associated with the

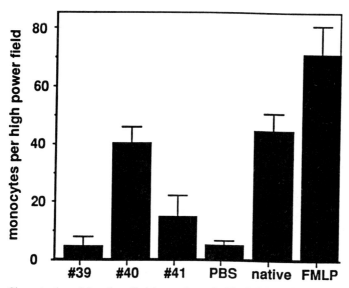

Fig. 3 Chemotactic activity of purified factor shown in Fig. 2. HPLC fractions (100 ml) were all tested for chemotactic activity as described in Methods to remove acetonitrile. This figure shows the main chemotactic activity seen in tube 40 as well as the activity from flanking elution tubes (39, 41). FMLP (10^{-8} mol/l) and PBS are controls. 'Native' refers to the chemotactic activity of unprocessed bacterial cultured supernatant from *H. pylori*. Figures are the mean of three wells ± SE

absorbance peak eluting at 32.5% acetonitrile from reverse-phase HPLC purification. This is the same elution point detected from the patient isolate (Fig. 2). This demonstrates that the identified chemotactic factor in a patient strain of *H. pylori* and ATCC strain no. 43579 co-elute; it is not unique to an individual patient sample.

Gel permeation purification of Sep-pak concentrated supernatant

Although reverse-phase HPLC purification of Sep-pak concentrated material identified only one absorbance peak associated with chemotactic activity, it was unclear whether several factors co-eluted in this region. Additional separation techniques were utilized to address this question. The peak of chemotactic activity (tubes 56–63) eluted later than the salt peak during gel permeation chromatography, suggesting the chemotactic factor is a small, hydrophobic compound (Fig. 4).

Reverse-phase HPLC of G-50 purified chemotactic factor

Figure 5 shows two absorbance peaks on reverse-phase HPLC elution obtained from G-50 purified chemotactic factor. The chemotactic activity co-eluted with the major absorbance peak. The elution profile is consistent with the chemotactic factor being a single compound. In this gradient system, FMLP would elute much earlier.

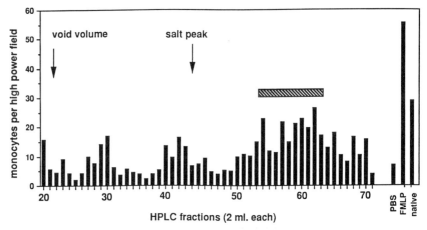

Fig. 4 Chemotactic profile of G-50 eluant. Fractions from Sep-pak concentration demonstrating chemotactic activity were pooled and loaded (2 ml volume) onto G-50 column, eluted with PBS. Figure shows chemotactic activity associated with each collected fraction. Areas of void volume, salt peak, and chemotactic factor are identified. The bar shows the tubes pooled for further purification

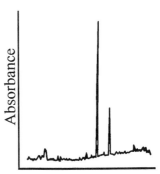

Fig. 5 HPLC purification of G-50 purified chemotactic factor. Two-millilitre fractions from the gel permeation column which demonstrated associated chemotactic activity were pooled and loaded onto reverse-phase HPLC. Two separate absorbance peaks at 220 nm are shown; chemotactic activity was associated with the earlier and larger absorbance peak only

DISCUSSION

H. pylori supernatants contain a factor chemotactic for monocytes that is different from FMLP. This novel factor is of low molecular weight, hydrophobic and is present in multiple strains of *H. pylori*. A three-step purification procedure has been designed allowing recovery of $> 50\%$ non-FMLP-related chemotactic activity detected in culture supernatants.

Although *H. pylori* appears to play an integral role in the pathogenesis of gastroduodenal inflammation and ulceration, the mechanism initiating the inflammatory response remains enigmatic. The bacteria rarely invade yet are nonetheless essential for inflammation[1–4]. One explanation suggests that *H.*

pylori secretes a factor which is able to cross the gastric mucosal lining and subsequently stimulate an inflammatory response, directly or indirectly. This paradigm is consistent with a non-invasive bacterium; the secreted factor may be absorbed through the gastric barrier via a receptor-dependent or receptor-independent mechanism. The demonstrated hydrophobic nature of the chemotactic factor may allow it to diffuse through membranes via a receptor-independent pathway.

An important contribution of this work is that there is a novel bacterial factor, different from FMLP, that is capable of stimulating an immune response. Even though the factor is not FMLP, it may exert its actions through the FMLP receptor. Another example of a naturally occurring non-peptide working through an endogenous peptide receptor is asperlicin[12]. This fungally derived factor binds to the CCK-A receptor with high affinity; this shows non-mammalian species can produce factors capable of binding to mammalian peptide receptors. Chemical characterization of the *H. pylori* chemotactic factor is being addressed presently for future synthetic and labelling studies.

SUMMARY

H. pylori is strongly associated with antral gastritis in which gastric luminal or non-invasive bacteria cause a submucosal inflammatory infiltrate. The mechanism explaining the interaction between the bacterial infection and the immune response remains unclear. It was previously demonstrated that conditioned medium from cultured *H. pylori* contained a factor chemotactic for human monocytes and neutrophils. We report purification of a hydrophobic factor of low molecular weight that is chemotactic for monocytes. This factor could be purified to a single absorbance peak by Sep-pak concentration, gel permeation chromatography and reverse-phase HPLC. The chemotactic factor elutes during reverse-phase HPLC in a position clearly different from *N*-formyl-methionyl-leucyl-phenylalanine (FMLP). This factor elutes in the same position during reverse-phase HPLC when purified from supernatants of *H. pylori* obtained from a patient biopsy as well as from the American Tissue Cell Culture (ATCC). These results suggest *H. pylori* secretes a factor chemotactic for monocytes that is present in multiple strains. This factor is different from FMLP, with features that may contribute to the immunopathogenesis characteristic of *H. pylori* gastritis.

Acknowledgements

This work was supported by the Veterans Administration and by NIH Center Grant DK 41301. Funds were received to do these studies as a Pilot and Feasibility Research Project from this Center Grant. Support by the Peptide Biochemistry Core of the CURE: Gastroenteric Biology Center is gratefully acknowledged. In addition, the authors are supported by the following NIH grants: DK 01879 (P.A.). The support of Linda Doornbos Fellowship and Fund for Stress-Immune Research is acknowledged and appreciated.

References

1. Graham DY, Klein PD. *Campylobacter pyloridis* gastritis: the past, the present, and speculations about the future. Am J Gastroenterol. 1987;82:282–6.
2. Anderson LP, Holck S. Possible evidence of invasiveness of *Helicobacter (Campylobacter) pylori*. Eur J Clin Microbiol Infect Dis. 1990;9:135–8.
3. Rauws EAJ, Langenberg W, Houthoff HJ, Zanen HC, Tytgat GNJ. *Campylobacter pyloridis*-associated chronic active antral gastritis: a prospective study of its prevalence and the effects of antibacterial and antiulcer treatment. Gastroenterology. 1988;94:44–50.
4. Dooley CP, Cohen H. The clinical significance of *Campylobacter pylori*. Ann Intern Med. 1988;108:70–9.
5. Craig PM, Territo MC, Karnes WE, Walsh JH. *Helicobacter pylori* secretes a chemotactic factor for monocytes and neutrophils. Gut. 1992;33:1020–3.
6. Chadwick VS, Mellor DM, Meyers DB *et al.* Production of peptides inducing chemotaxis and lysozomal enzyme release in human neutrophils by intestinal bacteria *in vitro* and *in vivo*. Scand J Gastroenterol. 1988;23:121–8.
7. Marasco WA, Phan SH, Krutzsch H *et al.* Purification and identification of formyl-methionyl-leucyl-phenylalanine as the major peptide neutrophil chemotactic factor produced by *Escherichia coli*. J Biol Chem. 1984;259:5430–9.
8. Ferry DM, Butt TJ, Broom MF, Hunter J, Chadwick VS. Bacterial chemotactic oligopeptides and the intestinal mucosal barrier. Gastroenterology. 1989;97:61–7.
9. Magnusson KE, Dahlgren C, Sjolander A. Effect of *N*-formylated-methionyl-leucyl-phenylalanine on gut permeability. Inflammation. 1985;9:365–73.
10. Nash SJ, Stafford J, Madera JL. Effects of polymorphonuclear leukocyte transmigration on the barrier function of cultured intestinal epithelial monolayers. J Clin Invest. 1987;80:1104–12.
11. Schiffman E, Corcoran BA, Wahl SM. *N*-formylated peptides as chemoattractants for leukocytes. Proc Natl Acad Sci USA. 1975;72:1059–62.
12. Chang RS, Lotti VJ, Monaghan RL *et al.* A potent non-peptide cholecystokinin antagonist selective for peripheral tissues isolated from *Aspergillus alliaceus*. Science. 1985;230:177–9.

17
H. pylori-induced neutrophil activation and production of toxic oxygen radicals

V. S. CHADWICK

INTRODUCTION

Helicobacter pylori infection of the gastric mucosa is a chronic infection, but unlike many chronic bacterial infections where lymphocytes and plasma cells predominate, the cellular infiltrate in *H. pylori* infection is, in addition, composed of large numbers of polymorphonuclear leukocytes (PMNs)[1]. A second unusual feature of this infection is that the bacterium is rarely found within the mucosa itself[2,3], apparently able to produce a profound host inflammatory response from a distance. This has naturally led to studies of leukocyte chemotactic factor production by *H. pylori*, the idea being that factors secreted by the bacterium, within the juxtamucosal mucus layer, may permeate the mucosal barrier, recruit and subsequently activate inflammatory leukocytes[4]. Not all the bacteria are free within the mucus layer, however; some are closely associated with the epithelium via 'adhesion pedestals'[5,6] providing a possible route of direct transfer of bacterial products across the mucosal barrier.

Little is known about the permeability of the gastric epithelium. The healthy canine stomach is less permeable to low molecular weight polyethylene glycols than the small intestine or colon[7], so that only very small polar molecules would be expected to traverse gastric tight junctions. Lipid chemotactic factors may traverse the epithelium more easily. Once inflamed or damaged, epithelial permeability would increase, permitting more bacterial products across in a similar way to that described for back-diffusion of hydrogen ions[8]. Another possibility is that cytotoxins produced by the bacterium damage the gastric epithelial cells, impairing the mucosal barrier function. Several toxins have been described[9]. These provide the basis for destruction of the mucus coat, alteration of epithelial phospholipids and direct cytotoxic damage or indirect damage caused by ammonia generation by bacterial urease. Direct tissue damage would initiate generation of host chemotactic

207

factors such as leukotrienes, and may permit permeation of bacterial lipopolysaccharide (LPS, or endotoxin) with activation of macrophages leading to TNF production and of complement leading to C_{5a} production. Factors responsible for leukocyte recruitment and activation in *H. pylori* infection may arise from either the bacterium or the host, and these will now be considered in turn.

N-FORMYL-PEPTIDES AND *H. PYLORI*

Two groups have reported secretion of low molecular weight factors by *H. pylori*, which induce chemotaxis, oxidative burst and degranulation in neutrophil leukocytes. Craig and co-workers[10] identified chemotactic activity for both neutrophils and monocytes in *H. pylori* culture supernatants. All strains tested, both those from patients with active ulcer disease and those from patients without ulcers, produced chemotactic activity. This activity was resistant to freezing, boiling, pH 2 or pH 10 for 30 min and passed through a M_r 3000 filter. Mooney and co-workers[11], in collaboration with our own laboratory, showed that *H. pylori* secreted substances which induced the oxidative burst in neutrophils. This material was subjected to reverse-phase HPLC and fractions tested for ability to stimulate release of vitamin B_{12} binding protein from neutrophils[12]. Fraction 25 contained the majority of the bioactivity. The same fraction contained substantial immunoreactivity using an antiserum raised against fMet-Leu Phe. Authentic fMet-Leu-Phe eluted in the same fraction 25. Thus, the secreted neutrophil-activating substance co-chromatographed and was antigenically cross-reactive with the known bacterial chemotactic factor fMet-Leu-Phe. Subsequently, using reverse-phase and affinity chromatography, the substance was purified and its structure confirmed by amino-acid sequencing[13].

The confirmation that *H. pylori* is a producer of fMet-Leu-Phe supports the contention that accumulation, retention and activation of PMNs in chronic gastritis may result from permeation of this pro-inflammatory peptide across the gastric mucosal epithelium. Recently, the source of fMet-Leu-Phe in *E. coli* has been identified as the amino-terminal of the 15 kDa UmuD protein of the SOS operon[14]. When the bacterium is exposed to oxidative stress and DNA damage, UmuD protein production increases markedly, and so does fMet-Leu-Phe production as a consequence. If this peptide arises by a similar mechanism in *H. pylori*, then the oxygen tensions of its juxtamucosal environment may subject the bacterium to oxidative stress, and result in enhanced fMet-Leu-Phe production *in vivo*.

In vitro and probably *in vivo* neutrophil activation may be enhanced by the presence of other bacterial products[12]. Mooney *et al.*[11] showed that opsonized *H. pylori* prolonged the oxidative burst induced by fMet-Leu-Phe, suggesting that the presence of bacterial antigens and opsonizing host antibody may potentiate inflammatory responses. Priming of responses to fMet-Leu-Phe by other bacterial products such as endotoxin is also a well-established phenomenon[12,15].

However, evidence for fMet-Leu-Phe production *in vivo* by *H. pylori* is lacking, and the gastric barrier to peptides has not been characterized. In the small and large intestine there are both enzymic[16] and anatomical barriers, but fMet peptides can traverse the intact intestine, especially when mucosal permeability is increased[17]. *In vitro* fMet-Leu-Phe can induce neutrophil chemotaxis across epithelial cell monolayers[18] and *in vivo* increase permeability and blood flow in rat small intestine[19].

SURFACE PROTEINS FROM *H. PYLORI* AS CHEMOTACTIC FACTORS

Mai *et al.*[20] showed that *H. pylori* released products into culture supernatants with chemotactic activity for monocytes and neutrophils by a mechanism not involving fMet-peptides. The chemotactic activity was inhibited by antisera to whole bacteria or *H. pylori*-derived urease enzyme. Purified urease showed dose-dependent antibody-inhibitable chemotactic activity which was localized into the amino-terminal portion of the 61 kDa subunit of urease. A synthetic 20 amino acid peptide based on the known sequence of the amino-terminus was also chemotactic. Immunohistochemistry was used to show that *H. pylori* urease antigens were present in the lamina propria, even though no bacteria were identified inside the epithelial barrier. The authors point out that *H. pylori* is the first Gram-negative organism shown to release chemotactic factors other than fMet peptides.

NEUTROPHIL CHEMOTACTIC FACTORS IN *H. PYLORI* BUT NOT *H. MUSTELAE*

Kozol *et al.*[21] compared neutrophil chemotactic activity (NCA) in culture supernatants from *H. pylori* and *H. mustelae*. These organisms produce antral gastritis in humans and in the ferret respectively, but histologically, only *H. pylori* gastritis is associated with neutrophil accumulation. A 10.5 kDa chemotactic factor was isolated by sequential gel permeation and electrophoresis. This factor was only found in *H. pylori* supernatants, not in *H. mustelae*. The precise nature of the NCA was not defined.

CHEMOTACTIC ACTIVITY AND STIMULATION OF PHAGOCYTE OXIDATIVE BURST BY FACTORS IN *H. PYLORI* SONICATES

Nielsen and Andersen[22,23] prepared sonicates of *H. pylori* and showed that both chemotactic and chemiluminescence-inducing activity for neutrophils and monocytes resided predominantly in a 25–35 kDa fraction. The material was susceptible to protease digestion and prolonged boiling, the latter generating smaller fragments which were still biologically active. Preincubation with crude sonicate primed phagocytes for increased chemiluminescence responses to fMet-Leu-Phe and phorbol-myristate-acetate. The putative protein factor was present in high activity in water-extracted surface proteins. However, the sonicate also contained priming activity which was in a

12–14 kDa fraction, totally resistant to heating, and was not directly chemotactic. This latter activity was probably LPS, which is known to prime phagocytes for increased responses to fMet-Leu-Phe and to increase fMet-Leu-Phe receptor numbers on PMNs. Whether the 25–30 kDa protein is related to the urease-derived chemotactic factor described by Mai *et al.*[20], and referred to above, is not clear. Furthermore, whether the antibody-dependent immune complex-mediated stimulant for neutrophil oxidative burst described by Mooney *et al.*[11] is relevant to this study is also unclear.

PLATELET ACTIVATING FACTOR

Platelet activating factor (PAF) is a potent inflammatory mediator synthesized by macrophages, neutrophils, endothelial cells and platelets. Denizot *et al.*[24] presented evidence that *H. pylori* synthesized PAF when grown on blood agar, but not when grown in liquid broth culture, unless lyso-PAF and acetyl-CoA were added. This suggested that *H. pylori* has the enzymic apparatus to complete the synthesis if supplied with precursors. Lyso-PAF is abundant in inflamed mucosa, so PAF could be synthesized in the vicinity of *H. pylori*. PAF induces leukocyte chemotaxis and marked changes in vascular permeability. Not all clinical isolates of *H. pylori* could produce PAF from precursors, however, and significant PAF levels in inflamed mucosa were difficult to demonstrate.

LEUKOTRIENES IN *H. PYLORI*-ASSOCIATED GASTRITIS

Fukuda *et al.*[25] showed that leukotriene (LTB_4) concentrations in gastric mucosal biopsies correlated with the severity of gastritis evaluated histologically, and in particular the density of neutrophil infiltration. Neutrophils are the major source of LTB_4 and the finding of high concentrations of LTB_4 may result from neutrophil infiltration and activation rather than arising endogenously. In any event LTB_4 is a very potent chemotactic factor. Other endogenously generated leukotrienes such as LTC_4 and LTD_4 were not measured in this study, but are recognized as important in gastric mucosal injury caused by other agents.

TUMOUR NECROSIS FACTOR α AND INTERLEUKIN-6 IN *H. PYLORI*-ASSOCIATED GASTRITIS

Crabtree *et al.*[26] measured the production of TNF-α and IL-6 in antral mucosa in short-term organ culture. TNF-α and IL-6 concentrations were greater in supernatants of tissue from patients with *H. pylori* infection. TNF-α concentrations were highest in those with active gastritis and neutrophil infiltration, whereas IL-6 levels were raised in both active and inactive gastritis. This difference may be explained by the different effects of these cytokines. TNF-α is produced mainly by macrophages when stimulated with bacterial products, particularly lipopolysaccharide (LPS or endotoxin). It up-regulates endothelial adhesion molecules, stimulates production of IL-8[27], a potent neutrophil chemotactic factor from endothelium and fibroblasts, activates neutrophils and promotes T and B cell proliferation. IL-6, on the other hand, is not chemotactic for neutrophils, though it amplifies neutrophil oxidative burst and degranulation responses. Its other major effects are to stimulate maturation of B cells.

OVERVIEW OF MECHANISMS FOR NEUTROPHIL RECRUITMENT AND ACTIVATION

It is impossible at this point in time to discern the exact sequence of events leading to leukocyte recruitment and activation, in *H. pylori*-associated gastritis. In established inflammation, multiple inflammatory mediators are generated and *H. pylori* gastritis is no exception. The mediators identified so far, including the bacterial products and host-derived lipid and cytokine chemotactic factors, probably represent an incomplete list. Nevertheless there are some unusual features in *H. pylori*-associated inflammation, suggesting that factors elaborated by the bacterium itself may stimulate mucosal inflammation, and yet do not appear to result in its own elimination.

In experimental[28] and spontaneous inflammation[29] elsewhere in the gastrointestinal tract recruited PMNs traverse the epithelium and can be seen to ingest and kill bacteria[30]. While *in vitro*, PMNs can phagocytose and kill opsonized *H. pylori*[31-34], *in vivo*, in spite of strong secretory and systemic antibody response the infection persists. It is not known why recruited neutrophils do not migrate across the gastric mucosa and engulf and destroy *H. pylori* in its juxtamucosal ecological niche. It is possible that neutrophils are subjected to activation by chemotactic factors at such a high level in the gastric mucosa that motility is arrested, and oxidative burst and degranulation occur prematurely. Neutrophil activation is a hierarchical event and preactivation, for example in the circulation by bacterial chemotactic factors, has been shown to inhibit appropriate migratory responses to the pleural cavity in response to carrageenan-induced pleurisy[24]. If *H. pylori* has adapted so that is can arrest neutrophil migration from a distance, this could explain the inability of host responses to eliminate the infection, once established.

It appears that, while the host immune and inflammatory response is not effective in eradication of *H. pylori*, once this infection is eradicated using antibiotics or other agents, early reinfection is rare[35]. Eradication of bacteria from porcine small intestine loops is much more rapid and efficient on second or third challenge with the same bacterial serotype, and involves neutrophil emigration and immune phagocytosis[30]. It remains possible, therefore, that neutrophils may play a more effective role in prevention of reinfection than in eradication of the initial infection. Much more work is required before we will have the answers to these intriguing questions.

References

1. Robert ME, Weinstein WM. *Helicobacter pylori*-associated gastric pathology. Gastroenterol Clin N Am. 1993;22:59–72.
2. Hazell SL, Lee A, Brady L, Hennessy W. *Campylobacter pyloridis* and gastritis: association with intracellular spaces and adaptation to an environment of mucus as important factors in colonization of the gastric epithelium. J Infect Dis. 1986;153:658–63.
3. Buck GE, Gourley WK, Lee WK, Subramanyam K, Latnier JM, Dinuzzo AR. Relation of *Campylobacter pyloridis* to gastritis and peptic ulcer. J Infect Dis. 1986;163:644–9.
4. Wallace JL. Possible mechanisms and mediators of gastritis associated with *Helicobacter pylori* infection. Scand J Gastroenterol. 1991;26(Suppl. 187):65–70.
5. Dazi JL, Sinniah R, Zaman V *et al.* Ultrastructural study of *Helicobacter pylori*-associated gastritis. J Pathol. 1990;161:65–70.
6. Hessey SJ, Spencer J, Wyatt JI *et al.* Bacterial adhesion and disease activity in *Helicobacter*-associated chronic gastritis. Gut. 1990;31:134–8.
7. Chadwick VS, Phillips SF, Hofmann AF. Measurements of intestinal permeability using low molecular weight polyethylene glycols (PEG 400). II. Application to normal and abnormal permeability states in man and animals. Gastroenterology. 1977;73:247–51.
8. Davenport HW. Destruction of the gastric mucosal barrier by detergents and urea. Gastroenterology. 1968;54:175–81.
9. Dunn BE. Pathogenic mechanisms of *Helicobacter pylori*. Gastroenterol Clin N Am. 1993;22:43–57.
10. Graig PM, Territo MC, Karnes WE, Walsh JH. *Helicobacter pylori* secretes a chemotactic factor for monocytes and neutrophils. Gut. 1992;33:1020–3.
11. Mooney C, Keenan J, Munster D *et al.* Neutrophil activation by *Helicobacter pylori*. Gut. 1991;32:853–7.
12. Chadwick VS, Ferry DM, Butt TJ. Assessment of neutrophil leukocyte secretory response to fMLP in whole blood *in vitro*. J Leuk Biol. 1992;42:143–50.
13. Broom MF, Sherriff RM, Munster D, Chadwick VS. Identification of formyl Met-Leu-Phe in culture filtrates of *Helicobacter pylori*. Microbios. 1992;72:239–45.
14. Broom MF, Sherriff RM, Ferry DM, Chadwick VS. Formylmethionyl-leucylphenylalanine and the SOS operon in *Escherichia coli*: a model of host-bacterial interactions. Biochem J. 1993;291:895–900.
15. Allen CA, Broom MF, Chadwick VS. Flow cytometry analysis of the expression of neutrophil FMLP receptors. J Immunol Methods. 1992;149:159–64.
16. Chadwick VS, Schlup MMT, Cooper BT, Broom MF. Enzymes degrading bacterial chemotactic F-met peptides in human ileal and colonic mucosa. J Gastroenterol Hepatol. 1990;5:375–81.
17. Ferry DM, Butt TJ, Broom MF, Hunter J, Chadwick VS. Bacterial chemotactic oligopeptides and the intestinal mucosal barrier. Gastroenterology. 1989;97:61–7.
18. Nash S, Stafford J, Madara JL. Effects of polymorphonuclear leukocyte transmigration on the barrier function of cultured intestinal epithelial monolayers. J Clin Invest. 1987;80:1104–13.
19. Von Ritter C, Sekizuka E, Grisham MB, Granger DN. The chemotactic peptide N-formyl-methionyl-leucyl-phenylalanine increases permeability in the distal ileum of the rat. Gastroenterology. 1988;95:651–6.
20. Mai UEH, Perez-Perez GI, Allen JB, Wahl SM, Blaser MJ, Smith PD. Surface proteins from *Helicobacter pylori* exhibit chemotactic activity for human leukocytes and are present in gastric mucosa. J Exp Med. 1992;175:517–25.
21. Kozol R, McCurdy B, Czanko R. A neutrophil chemotactic factor present in *H. pylori* but absent in *H. mustelae*. Dig Dis Sci. 1993;38:137–41.
22. Nielsen H, Andersen LP. Chemotactic activity of *Helicobacter pylori* sonicate for human polymorphonuclear leucocytes and monocytes. Gut. 1992;33:738–42.
23. Nielsen H, Andersen LP. Activation of human phagocyte oxidative metabolism by *Helicobacter pylori*. Gastroenterology. 1992;103:1747–53.
24. Denizot Y, Sobhani I, Rambaud J-C, Lewin M, Thomas Y, Benveniste J. Paf-acether synthesis by *Helicobacter pylori*. Gut. 1990;31:1242–5.
25. Fukuda T, Kimura S, Arakawa T, Kobayashi K. Possible role of leukotrienes in gastritis

associated with *Campylobacter pylori*. J Clin Gastroenterol. 1990;12(Suppl. 1):S131–4.

26. Crabtree JE, Shallcross TM, Heatley RV, Wyatt JI. Mucosal tumour necrosis factor a and interleukin-6 in patients with *Helicobacter pylori* associated gastritis. Gut. 1991;32:1473–7.

27. Strieter RM, Kunkel SL, Showell HJ, Marks RM. Monokine-induced gene expression of a human endothelial cell-derived neutrophil chemotactic factor. Biochem Biophys Res Commun. 1988;156:1340–5.

28. Bellamy JEC, Nielsen NO. Immune-mediated emigration of neutrophils into the lumen of the small intestine. Infect Immun. 1974;9:615–19.

29. Saverymuttu SH, Peters AM, Lavender JP, Pepys MB, Hodgson HJF, Chadwick VS. Quantitative fecal indium 111-labeled leukocyte excretion in the assessment of disease in Crohn's disease. Gastroenterology. 1983;85:1333–9.

30. Walker PD. Interactions between microorganisms and the host. In: Chadwick VS, Phillips S, editors. Gastroenterology 2. The small intestine. London: Butterworths International Medical Reviews; 1982:131–50.

31. Pruul H, Lee PC, Goodwin CS, McDonald PJ. Interaction of *Campylobacter pyloridis* with human immune defence mechanisms. J Med Microbiol. 1987;23:233–8.

32. Das SS, Karim QN, Easmon CSF. Opsonophagocytosis of *Campylobacter pylori*. J Med Microbiol. 1988;27:125–30.

33. Bernatowska E, Jose P, Davies H, Stephenson M, Webster D. Interaction of *Campylobacter* species with antibody, complement and phagocytes. Gut. 1989;30:906–11.

34. Allen CA, Ferry DM, Chadwick VS. Anti-inflammatory effects of LPS, MDP and FMLP on carrageenan pleurisy in the rat. Agents Actions. 1994: in press.

35. George LL, Borody TJ, Andrews P *et al.* Cure of duodenal ulcer after eradication of *Helicobacter pylori*. Med J Aust. 1990;153:145–9.

18
Polymorphonuclear leukocytes traffic into the gastric mucosa and through the gastric mucosal barrier in *H. pylori* infection: is that bad?

D. Y. GRAHAM

INTRODUCTION

One of the characteristic histological features of *Helicobacter pylori* infection is neutrophil infiltration of the gastric mucosa. Neutrophils (PMN) are important and active participants in the normal inflammatory response. PMN are able to traverse essentially every epithelium in the body regardless of the mucosa's permeability[1,2]. Inflammatory cells are sparse in normal gastric mucosa, with neutrophils being rare to absent[3]. Neutrophilic infiltration of the mucosa is thought to be a direct response to the presence of *H. pylori*. The initial steps in infection are probably ingestion followed by penetration of the mucus layer, 'swimming' through the mucus layer to the mucosa, attachment, and multiplication[4]. The first reaction of the host is neutrophilic. This is an important phase of the infection and one in which the bacterium and any bacterial toxins are unfettered by a local humoral immune response. The mediators of the neutrophilic reaction at this stage are unknown, but local or systemic antibody is unlikely to be involved. Recent studies have been directed towards examination of cytokine production by epithelial cells in contact with *H. pylori*[5–8].

In acute *H. pylori* infections polymorphonuclear cells are evident wherever *H. pylori* are present. High magnification of thin sections of gastric mucosa of recently infected patients shows numerous PMN moving into the areas where *H. pylori* are present (Fig. 1). At this early stage there is tissue damage and the whole host of reactions to bacterial damage to tissue and the presence of bacterial products in and on the tissue (e.g. endotoxin, peptidoglycans, and formyl-peptides) may occur, including complement activation. This process results in a vigorous local and systemic immune response. There is little information as to the proportion of *H. pylori* infections that start as a

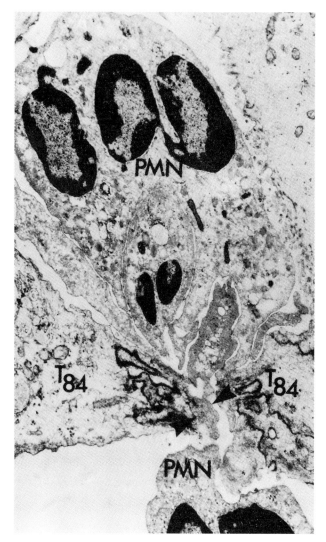

Fig. 1 Electron micrograph of PMN indenting a monolayer of T84 cells and passing single file through a tight junction. Arrowheads show extension of pseudopodia through the site of epithelial discontinuity. Kindly provided by Dr James L. Madara. From ref. 16

vigorous acute neutrophilic reaction and what proportion start insidiously.

The second phase of the infection includes continuation of acute inflammation, but with the addition of infiltration with chronic inflammatory cells. Later, the acute inflammatory response seems to fade but never to resolve completely. Thus, the PMN response is not only the initial gastric mucosal response to *H. pylori* infection, but it continues throughout the life of the infection.

There is considerable interest in what the neutrophils are doing in the tissue, what brought them there, and whether their transit through tight junctions leads to measurable untoward effects. There are a number of well-studied examples of microbial/mucosal interactions. *H. pylori* infection does not represent an entirely new form of bacteria/mucosal interaction, and lessons learned from other mucosal infections are not only applicable to the *H. pylori* story but can, in many instances, help in the planning and interpretation of experiments. The two models of mucosal bacterial interactions that seem to hold the promise are urinary tract epithelial/*E. coli* interactions and the interactions of *Pseudomonas* sp. with the bronchial epithelium in patients with cystic fibrosis[9–15]. For example, recent *in vitro* experiments have demonstrated that the association of *H. pylori* with gastric epithelial cells resulted in a brisk release of the major chemotactic cytokine IL-8 from epithelial cells[5–8]. These results are reminiscent of experiments done with *E. coli* urinary tract infections in both animals and humans[9,12–14].

One question that might be asked from the perspective of both the host and the bacterium is whether the PMN response is helpful, harmful, or both. For example, is there evidence for PMN damage to the gastric mucosa? Are the PMN effective in reducing the bacterial load and, if not, what strategies do the bacteria use to avoid being cleared by them?

EFFECTS OF MIGRATION OF PMN THROUGH EPITHELIAL TIGHT JUNCTIONS

There are considerable *in vitro* data regarding neutrophil migration through epithelium and the effect of migration on epithelial permeability and viability. Such data should serve as a guide for studies of *H. pylori*/mucosal/PMN interactions. Events in a neutrophil's response to chemotactic stimuli include adherence to vascular epithelium followed by migration to the extravascular space via the intercellular junctions[2]. Once in the tissue, PMN migrate to the epithelial surface through the intercellular junctions. Examination of histological material in *H. pylori* gastritis shows PMN both in the lumen and in the process of traversing the mucosal cells. One might ask whether migration of PMN through the mucosa damages the barrier function of the gastric epithelium. Although *in vitro* one can measure changes in mucosal resistance and permeability associated with PMN migration, migration through intercellular junctions does not affect the viability of the epithelial cell. PMN apparently cross the tight junctions by extending pseudopods into them to force them open[16]. Focal alterations in the cytoskeleton are seen (condensation of intermediate and microfilaments) adjacent to the sites of contact between PMN and the plasma cell membrane of the epithelial cell as if the PMN must get a good grip to force the tight junction open (Fig. 1)[16]. Any effects on resistance and permeability are consequences of the physical opening of the tight junctions, and not the result of damage caused by release of PMN secretory products[17]. Opening and resealing of the epithelial tight junctions does not require new protein synthesis; nor is it a function of a protein synthesis-dependent mechanism that has been demonstrated experimentally[17]. For example, neither PMN transmigration nor tight junction resealing is influenced by the presence of catalase or cycloheximide.

EFFECT OF PMN MIGRATION ON EPITHELIAL PERMEABILITY

Typically, transmigration of PMN is associated with minimal or no increase in transjunctional flux of paracellular tracers[1,16–18]. The number of PMN transmigrating is a function of the number of 'invasion sites'[1]. When the number of transmigration PMN is low, the tight junctions have sufficient time to reseal, and there is minimal or no change in conductance or passage of paracellular tracers. Whatever changes in mucosal resistance or permeability occur are a reflection of the number and density of transmigrating PMN[1,16]. One might consider these changes to be a function of the overall duration and number of tight junctions open during any period. Because there is no differential enhancement of permeability of paracellular tracers of different molecular dimension, it is thought that the defects in the junctional barrier are confined to the foci of the transmigrating PMN, which is further evidence that results are mechanical[16]. After the transmigration of PMN, the tight junctions rapidly reseal and regain their barrier function. Transmigration has an effect on the PMN. This effect of transmigration has been studied in the lung and in skin blisters, where transmigration has been shown to result in loss of secondary granules and an increase in C3bi and FMLP receptors[18]. Importantly, transmigration is not associated with a loss of PMN function[18].

The ability of PMN to transmigrate is limited by the tightness of the tight junction. It is not known whether this limitation is secondary to the inability of the chemoattractant to diffuse across the epithelium, the inability of the PMN to penetrate the tight junction, or both[1,19].

If transmigration of PMN across the gastric mucosa had a deleterious effect, one might see this to be reflected in a reduction in gastric transmembrane potential difference. None has been described.

CAN TRANSMIGRATION GO BOTH WAYS?

Although we generally think of transmucosal migration of PMN to be a one-way phenomenon, it may be bidirectional. For example, a series of elegant experiments using microspheres of different colour have shown that, at least in the lung, PMN can migrate to the surface and then return to the mucosa, carrying with them the engulfed antigen[20]. This provides still another mechanism for the systemic immune system to access *H. pylori* antigens.

DOES THE PRESENCE OF PMN (OR REACTIVE OXYGEN METABOLITES) EQUATE WITH DAMAGE?

PMN are a source of reactive oxygen metabolites (ROM). There has been a tendency to equate the presence of ROM in tissue with injury or damage. The three prerequisites necessary to ascribe free radicals a role in tissue injury include: (1) a source of free radical species, (2) evidence that the free-radical scavenging systems are either deficient or have not dynamically altered to adjust to the altered rates of radical generation, and (3) biomolecular evidence that free-radical injury has occurred[21]. Studies with cardiac muscle have shown that the concept that one can equate the presence of ROM with damage is probably too simplistic[22-24]. Oxidative injury may be highly compartmented[22]. For example, in ROM injury associated with cardiac ischaemia, the critical step required is adherence of PMN to myocytes. Once an activated PMN adhered to a myocyte, neither the extracellular oxygen radical scavengers superoxidase, dismutase and catalase, nor the presence of an extracellular iron chelator was able to reduce ROM damage to the myocyte[22]. In contrast, administration of anti-ROM agents which are active intracellularly was effective in reducing or preventing ROM damage. Without PMN adherence myocytes were not damaged. Thus, ROM damage should be thought of as localized damage acting only over very short distances.

Increased mucosal ROM has been demonstrated in patients with duodenal ulcer, with the majority of evidence suggesting that they were derived from myeloperoxidase from activated PMN[25]. This finding may simply be a reflection of the increased number of PMN in the tissue, as well as the presence of activated PMN on the surface of the mucosa. Previous studies in humans have suggested that the antibacterial compounds hypochlorous acid and monochloramine are not damaging to mucosal surfaces[26]. Whether PMN-associated proteases are present and active in gastric tissue is unknown. There is a tendency to associate focal microscopic abnormalities with functional changes, but there is little or any evidence to justify such a belief. Finally, there is one published study reporting reduced ulcer recurrence with administration of allopurinol or DMSO compared to placebo[27]. This report suggests a role for ROM in peptic ulcer. Unfortunately, that report is probably an example of scientific misconduct (the experiments were never actually performed) and cannot be taken at face value, or as evidence one way or the other.

WHAT DO PMN DO WHEN THEY ARE ON THE SURFACE?

Very little is known about *H. pylori*/PMN interactions *in vivo*. The outcome of the phagocyte/micro-organism interaction is influenced by a large number of factors including the microenvironment, the microbicidal mechanisms available to the phagocyte, and the organism's repertoire of defensive factors[4]. Examination of histological sections of *H. pylori*-infected gastric mucosa often reveals *H. pylori* within PMN. Generally, *H. pylori* within PMN appear injured or dying. Both granulocytes and eosinophils are microbicidal, and the majority of killing is intracellular within phagosomes. Phagocytosis of bacteria is followed by a series of events including a process called the respiratory burst[28]. Killing is associated with fusion of cytoplasmic granules with the plasma membrane and degranulation, which delivers their contents into the phagosomes, and the generation of toxic products of the reduction of oxygen[29]. The respiratory burst is accompanied by an increase in oxygen consumption of granulocytes, and microbial killing is impaired under anaerobic conditions. Bacterial killing is impaired by the presence of endogenous catalase[29]. Effective degranulation and production of the respiratory burst is accompanied by acidification of the phagosome. Ammonium chloride inhibits acidification of lysosomal compartments, thus impairing microbicidal activity of PMN[30]. Tosi and Czinn[15] suggested that generation of ammonium chloride as a product of *H. pylori* urease may be a protective strategy of *H. pylori*; this has not been tested directly. Tosi and Czinn[15] also drew the parallel between *H. pylori* gastritis and the chronic lung infection with *Pseudomonas* seen in patients with cystic fibrosis. In both instances the host responds with high titre specific antibody, but is unable to clear the infection[31].

Immunohistochemical staining of *H. pylori* in tissue sections has demonstrated that *H. pylori* organisms are coated with immunoglobulin[32]. IgA-coated bacteria were most common, but IgG- and IgM-positive bacteria were also present. Whether the immunoglobulin coating *H. pylori* is intact or Fab fragments is unknown. In chronic *Pseudomonas* infection in patients with cystic fibrosis IgG is fragmented, lacking the Fc portion required to bind to surface receptors and initiate internalization and killing, and is thus ineffective as an opsonin[15].

SUMMARY

Neutrophil infiltration of the mucosa is one of the characteristic histological features of *H. pylori* infection and is thought to be a direct response to the presence of the bacteria. Although in model systems *in vitro*, one can measure changes in mucosal resistance and permeability associated with neutrophil migration, migration through intercellular junctions does not affect the viability of the epithelial cell or polymorphonuclear function. In the lung neutrophils have been demonstrated to migrate to the surface and then return, delivering antigens to the mononuclear cells. Whether this occurs in the stomach is unknown. The presence of neutrophils in the mucosa is associated with an increase in tissue levels of reactive oxygen metabolites, but there is no convincing evidence that this can be equated with injury. Neutrophils on the surface are unable to cure the infection. Neutrophil function may be reduced by bacterial catalase, production of ammonium, coating of the bacteria with the Fab portion of secreted antibodies, or the local environment may be unfavourable (pH, oxygen tension, etc.) for neutrophils to kill *H. pylori*.

Acknowledgements

This work was supported by the Department of Veterans Affairs and by the generous support of Hilda Schwartz.

References

1. Milks LC, Brontoli MJ, Cramer EB. Epithelial permeability and the transepithelial migration of human neutrophils. J Cell Biol. 1983;96:1241–7.
2. Jutila MA. Leukocyte traffic to sites of inflammation. APMIS. 1992;100:191–201.
3. Genta RM, Lew GM, Graham DY. Changes in gastric mucosa following eradication of *Helicobacter pylori*. Mod Pathol. 1993;6:281–9.
4. Graham DY. Pathologic mechanism leading to *Helicobacter pylori*-induced inflammation. Eur J Gastroenterol Hepatol. 1993;4(Suppl.2):S9–16.
5. Crabtree JE, Farmery S, Lindley IJD, Peichl P. Cytotoxic strains of *Helicobacter pylori* induce IL-8 production by gastric epithelial cells. Acta Gastroenterol Belg. 1993;56:48.
6. Crabtree JE, Plusa S, Farmery S, Peichl P, Lindley IJD. Cytokine regulation of interleukin-8 secretion by gastric epithelial cells. Acta Gastroenterol Belg. 1993;56:52.
7. Crabtree JE, Peichl P, Wyatt JI, Stachl U, Lindley IJ. Gastric interleukin-8 and IgA IL-8 autoantibodies in *Helicobacter pylori* infection. Scand J Immunol. 1993;37:65–70.
8. Crowe SE, Hunt RH, Jordana M *et al*. Interleukin-8 secretion by gastric epithelium following *Helicobacter pylori* infection *in vitro*. Gastroenterology. 1993;104:A687.
9. Agace WW, Hedges SR, Ceska M, Svanborg C. Interleukin-8 and the neutrophil response to mucosal gram-negative infection. J Clin Invest. 1993;92:780–5.
10. Hedges S, Stenqvist K, Lidin-Janson G, Martinell J, Sandberg T, Svanborg C. Comparison of urine and serum concentrations of interleukin-6 in women with acute pyelonephritis or asymptomatic bacteriuria. J Infect Dis. 1992;166:653–6.
11. Agace W, Hedges S, Svanborg C. Lps genotype in the C57 black mouse background and its influence on the interleukin-6 response to *E. coli* urinary tract infection. Scand J Immunol. 1992;35:531–8.
12. Hedges S, Svensson M, Svanborg C. Interleukin-6 response of epithelial cell lines to bacterial stimulation *in vitro*. Infect Immun. 1992;60:1295–301.
13. Linder H, Engberg I, Hoschutzky H, Mattsby-Baltzer I, Svanborg C. Adhesion-dependent activation of mucosal interleukin-6 production. Infect Immun. 1991;59:4357–62.
14. Hedges S, Anderson P, Lidin-Janson G, de Man P, Svanborg C. Interleukin-6 response to deliberate colonization of the human urinary tract with gram-negative bacteria. Infect Immun. 1991;59:421–7.
15. Tosi MF, Czinn SJ. Opsonic activity of specific human IgG against *Helicobacter pylori*. J Infect Dis. 1990;162:156–62.
16. Nash S, Stafford J, Madara JL. Effects of polymorphonuclear leukocyte transmigration on the barrier function of cultured intestinal epithelial monolayers. J Clin Invest. 1987;80:1104–13.
17. Parsons PE, Sugahara K, Cott GR, Mason RJ, Henson PM. The effect of neutrophil migration and prolonged neutrophil contact on epithelial permeability. Am J Pathol. 1987;129:302–12.
18. Martin TR, Pistorese BP, Chi EY, Goodman RB, Matthay MA. Effects of leukotriene B4 in the human lung. Recruitment of neutrophils into the alveolar spaces without a change in protein permeability. J Clin Invest. 1989;84:1609–19.
19. Casale TB, Abbas MK. Comparison of leukotriene B4-induced neutrophil migration through different cellular barriers. Am J Physiol. 1990;258:C639–47.
20. Harmsen AG, Mason MG, Muggenburg BA, Gillett NA, Jarpe MA, Bice DE. Migration of neutrophils from lung to tracheobronchial lymph node. J Leukoc Biol. 1987;41:95–103.
21. Del Mestro R. Free radicals as mediators of tissue injury. In: Dreosti IE, editor. Trace elements, micronutrients, and free radicals. New York: Humana Press; 1991:25–51.
22. Entman ML, Youker K, Shoji T *et al*. Neutrophil induced oxidative injury of cardiac myocytes. A compartmented system requiring CD11b/CD18-ICAM-1 adherence. J Clin

Invest. 1992;90:1335–45.
23. Youker K, Smith CW, Anderson DC *et al.* Neutrophil adherence to isolated adult cardiac myocytes. Induction by cardiac lymph collected during ischemia and reperfusion. J Clin Invest. 1992;89:602–9.
24. Gasic AC, McGuire G, Krater S *et al.* Hydrogen peroxide pretreatment of perfused canine vessels induces ICAM-1 and CD18-dependent neutrophil adherence. Circulation. 1991;84:2154–66.
25. Davies GR, Simmonds NJ, Stevens TR, Grandison A, Blake DR, Rampton DS. Mucosal reactive oxygen metabolite production in duodenal ulcer disease. Gut. 1992;33:1467–72.
26. Weiss SJ. Tissue destruction by neutrophils. N Engl J Med. 1989;320:365–76.
27. Salim AS. Oxygen-derived free radicals and the prevention of duodenal ulcer relapse: a new approach. Am J Med Sci. 1990;300:1–6.
28. Clark RA. The human neutrophil respiratory burst oxidase. J Infect Dis. 1990;161:140–7.
29. Root RK, Cohen MS. The microbicidal mechanisms of human neutrophils and eosinophils. Rev Infect Dis. 1981;3:565–98.
30. Klempner MS, Styrt B. Alkalinizing the intralysosomal pH inhibits degranulation of human neutrophils. J Clin Invest. 1983;72:1793–1800.
31. Fick RB, Naegel GP, Squier SU, Wood RE, Gee JBL, Reynolds HY. Proteins of the cystic fibrosis respiratory tract. Fragmented immunoglobulin G opsonic antibody causing defective opsonophagocytosis. J Clin Invest. 1984;74:236–48.
32. Wyatt JI, Rathbone BJ. Immune response of the gastric mucosa to *Campylobacter pylori.* Scand J Gastroenterol. Suppl 1988;142:44–9.

19
H. pylori vacuolating toxin

N. FIGURA and J. E. CRABTREE

INTRODUCTION

Helicobacter pylori is the agent of chronic gastritis, the most widespread infection in the world after dental caries; it is also the *condicio sine qua non* for the development of duodenal ulcer[1], and a concomitant cause of gastric cancer[2]. Despite the world-wide occurrence of these illnesses, the natural history of *H. pylori* infection is still far from understood. The study of the pathogenicity characteristics of these micro-organisms is required to understand the pathway between infection and the development of mucosal lesions. It is currently unclear why only a small percentage of *H. pylori*-infected patients develop serious gastroduodenal lesions, and why most infected individuals can carry this organism in their stomach throughout their life, seemingly without problems.

Recent studies suggest strains of *H. pylori* may vary in pathogenicity. Strains producing a toxin which induces vacuolation of eukaryotic cells in culture are more frequently isolated from patients with ulcers than from those with only chronic gastritis[3], suggesting that cytotoxigenicity could be involved in the development of peptic ulcers, and that cytotoxic strains could be more ulcerogenic than non-cytotoxic ones. This observation also raised the question of whether *H. pylori* strains differ from each other in other virulence and pathogenicity characteristics.

The study of genomic and phenotypic characteristics of *H. pylori* in relation to gastroduodenal disease is an important current area of research. *H. pylori* is extremely genomically diverse and almost every patient is infected with a unique strain[4]. In the field of bacteriology there are numerous examples of species, *Escherichia coli* for example, which can behave as perfect saprophytes or as perfect pathogens depending on whether they possess genomic material which enhances their pathogenicity potential or which confers them selective advantage. It is not unreasonable, therefore, to think that there exist strains of *H. pylori* potentially more pathogenic than others.

WHY SHOULD WE LOOK FOR A CYTOTOXIN IN *H. PYLORI*-ASSOCIATED DISEASES?

Production of substances which cause morphological changes or toxic effects on epithelial cells *in vitro* is a characteristic common to bacteria associated with enteric infections. Therefore, when 'new' enteric organisms are discovered, in order to study their virulence characteristics, microbiologists test broth cultures for cytopathic effect on cells in tissue culture. Johnson and Lior[5] and Leunk *et al.*[6] initially demonstrated cytotoxigenicity in *H. pylori*. The fact that the first study observed cytotoxic and cytotonic effects[5], and the second study[6] a different cytopathic effect characterized by intracytoplasmic vacuolation, was attributed to differences in cultivation of the organisms.

In reality, cytopathic effects, different from cytovacuolation, can sometimes be observed when testing supernatants of cultures carried out in conditions that are considered to be optimum for the growth, i.e. *Brucella* broth with fetal bovine serum incubated in a shaker. Cytotonic-like and cytotoxic effects, however, are rare (less than 1% of strains tested) and therefore have no relevance from a pathogenic point of view[7]. World-wide studies have demonstrated that the incidence of cytotoxicity in *H. pylori* strains is about 55%[6].

The importance of cytotoxigenicity was appreciated following the observations that the isolation of strains which induce vacuolation of cells *in vitro* is significantly more frequent from patients with ulcers (and histological gastritis) or with atrophic gastric pathology than from patients with chronic superficial gastritis[3,8,9]. In addition, Eaton *et al.*[10] observed in gnotobiotic piglets experimentally infected with *H. pylori* that a cytotoxic, weakly motile strain was more virulent than a non-cytotoxic non-motile one (infection rate = 40% versus 17%). A fully motile cytotoxic strain infected 100% of animals. These latter studies provided the first experimental evidence that there can possibly be variability in *H. pylori* virulence.

In vivo vacuolation in gastric mucosa samples has also been described by different groups[11,12]. Fiocca *et al.*[12] observed that the degree of histological gastritis and the presence of vacuoles in epithelial cells did not correlate with the number of bacteria which colonized the epithelium, and suspected that a cytotoxin could be involved in the determination of epithelial lesions. These observations suggest that vacuolating activity of *H. pylori* identifies a group of organisms which could possibly contribute to the development of serious gastroduodenal pathologies.

ACTIVITIES OF CYTOTOXIC *H. PYLORI* CULTURES AND ASSOCIATION OF CYTOTOXICITY WITH OTHER BACTERIAL CHARACTERISTICS

H. pylori cytotoxin causes consistent vacuolation in several mammalian cell lines[3,6]. Although vacuolated cells exposed to toxic filtrates are still vital, since they exclude Trypan blue[6], after a long exposure they lose their morphology and die far sooner than do cells exposed to non-cytotoxic supernatants[7]. This is in agreement with the observation that cytotoxic broth cultures reduce the replication index of EBV-transformed B lymphocytes[7]. It is not yet clear whether the target of the growth inhibition and of vacuolation activity is the same. However, the possibility that the toxin can interfere with the function of non-epithelial cells is suggested by the observation that phagocytosis of polymorphonuclear cells, after contact with cytotoxic *H. pylori* broth cultures for 45 min, was reduced by about 20%[7]. The phagocyte oxygen metabolism, examined by the nitro blue tetrazolium reduction assay, seemingly was not influenced. Non-cytotoxic supernatants had no effect on phagocytosis. The fact that the intracellular oxidative metabolism was maintained, indicates that the toxin most probably damaged cell membrane structures of PMN cells[7].

Some toxins produced by enteric pathogens, *Vibrio cholerae* and enterotoxigenic *E. coli* for instance, also stimulate the production of cyclic AMP *in vitro*. Cytotoxic and non-cytotoxic *H. pylori* supernatants have been tested. Even though some strains possessed an adenylate cyclase activity, this activity was not associated with cytotoxin production[7].

Cytotoxin production is also not associated with biotypes, ribopatterns, and plasmid DNA content of *H. pylori* strains[13]. However, it was found to be associated with motility in 64% of strains from patients with peptic ulcers; 75% of strains from patients without ulcer were non-cytotoxic and non-motile[13]. Motility and cytotoxicity should also give a selective advantage to the strains which possess them. Strains which lack one or both characteristics are in fact a minority[13,14]. Recently it has been demonstrated that the cytotoxin may facilitate colonization. The cytotoxin was found to be surface-located and to enable strains to adhere to mammalian cells *in vitro*[15]. Both cytotoxin and motility could therefore favour successful colonization of the gastric epithelium.

MECHANISM OF VACUOLE FORMATION

Papini *et al.*[16] found that the *in vitro* vacuolation of cells could be blocked and even reversed by inhibitors of vacuolar-type ATPases such as bafilomycin A1. Thus the cytotoxin may possibly work by interfering with the endocellular ion-transporting protein mechanisms. This alteration creates a transmembrane pH gradient and favours the accumulation of basic substances inside the endocytic compartments where they are protonated. Since protonated substances are not membrane permeable, if the alteration of the proton pump is not reversed, they remain inside the organelles and attract water osmotically, which induces vacuole formation[16,17]. *In vitro*, vacuoles originate around nuclei (Fig. 1a), increase in number and become bigger and confluent. Finally, the cells break up and degenerate (Fig. 1b) in a couple of days.

Numerous stimuli and substances can cause intracytoplasmic vacuolation *in vitro*. Ammonia, for instance, and other bases can induce vacuolation (Fig. 1c), and can potentiate the vacuolating activity of cytotoxic supernatants (Fig. 1d)[17-19]. Non-cytotoxic *H. pylori* strains can also induce vacuolation if they are grown in the presence of appropriate amounts of urea (≥ 10 mmol/l,

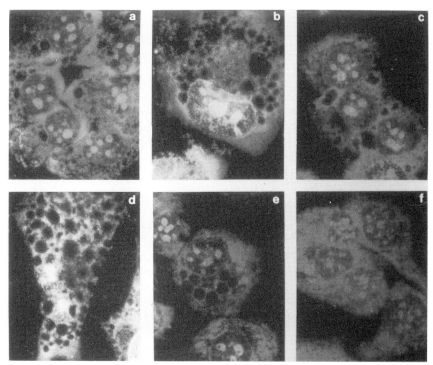

Fig. 1 Vacuolization of HeLa cells *in vitro*. Cells under the effect of a cytotoxic broth culture filtrate show few perinuclear vacuoles after a few hours of incubation (**a**); after 48 h of incubation the vacuoles become bigger and confluent (**b**). Ammonia alone at ≥ 10 mmol/l can cause vacuole formation (**c**) and can potentiate vacuolation induced by the toxin (**d**). Filtrates of non-cytotoxic strains can cause vacuolation if grown in presence of 10 mmol/l urea (**e**). (**f**) HeLa cells exposed to a non-cytotoxic supernatant in the absence of urea (fetal bovine serum was previously dialysed). No vacuolation is evident

in our experience) (Fig. 1e). These *in vitro* experiments indicate that the toxin-induced cytovacuolation, should it also occur *in vivo*, could be potentiated by high concentrations of urea (which can be attained in uraemic patients, for instance), and associated production of ammonia. The observation that omeprazole, a proton pump inhibitor, competitively inhibits *H. pylori* urease[20] could help to explain the amelioration of gastroduodenal lesions observed after treatment with this drug[21] even when the bacteria are not eradicated.

Whilst vacuoles can be observed histologically in gastroduodenal biopsy samples they are not a frequent occurrence. In part this could be a consequence of paraffin processing or perhaps haematoxylin–eosin staining does not allow a good definition of vacuoles. The inclusion of biopsies in methacrylate and Giemsa or toluidine blue staining improves the histological detection of vacuoles (Fig. 2; personal observation). Sometimes it is also possible to observe, in smeared biopsy samples stained with acridine orange, epithelial vacuolar formations which resemble vacuoles induced by the toxin

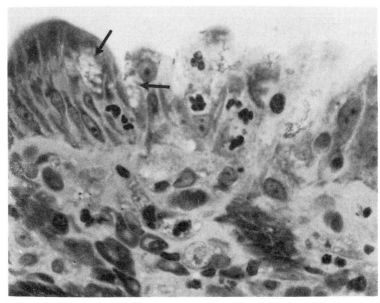

Fig. 2 *In vivo* vacuolation. Section of methacrylate-processed gastric antral biopsy. Giemsa stained. Vacuoles (arrows), *H. pylori* organisms, mononuclear and polymorphonuclear cells, and mucosal erosions are visible (original magnification × 400)

in tissue culture cells (Fig. 3). Ultrastructurally there is also evidence of vacuolation *in vivo* (Fig. 4). However, it is difficult to say if those features result from the *in vivo* activity of the toxin. Eaton *et al.*[10] did not find any vacuolar activity in the gastric juice of pigs infected with cytotoxic strains. Others observed vacuolating effects on cells *in vitro* directly exerted by biopsy specimens in only one out of 15 cases in which *in vitro* cytotoxic HP strains were isolated[7]. An explanation could be that the toxin *in vivo* is released when strains are strictly adherent to gastric cells.

NATURE OF *H. PYLORI* CYTOTOXIN

Since the first report[6], it was suggested that the vacuolating toxin was proteinaceous in nature (but what else can an exotoxin be if not a protein?). It took 4 years to definitively demonstrate that the toxin is a molecular complex made up by proteic subunits of about 87 kDa mass[22]. At the beginning it seemed that two proteins accounted for the vacuolating activity of cytotoxic strains. Silver staining of broth culture filtrates demonstrated the presence of a protein of 82 kDa mass (later assigned to a weight of 87 kDa) in 19% of supernatants inducing vacuolation, and in none of 14 broth cultures which did not exert vacuolating activity[23]. This protein was also recognized by serum from rabbits immunized with cytotoxic *H. pylori* strains. However, human serum samples reacted by the Western blotting

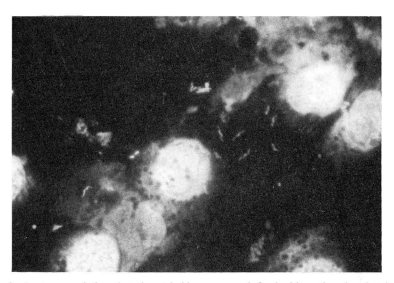

Fig. 3 *In vivo* vacuolation. Antral gastric biopsy smeared, fixed with methanol and stained with 0.01% acridine orange in 0.5 mol/l acetate buffer pH 4.0 for 2 min. Numerous *H. pylori* organisms and vacuolated cells are visible (original magnification × 1250)

technique with a protein of 128 kDa which was present in all 16 vacuolating supernatants, and also in 64% of non-vacuolating ones[23]. Silver staining did not reveal any 128-kDa polypeptide in vacuolating supernatants, suggesting that it was produced in very small amounts[23]. Serum samples from patients infected with cytotoxic strains immunoreacted with this protein significantly more often than did samples from patients infected by non-cytotoxic *H. pylori* (80% versus 45%, in one study[23], and 100% versus 70% in another study[7]). To complicate things even more, out of 18 serum samples which recognized 128 kDa protein in the supernatant of a cytotoxic strain, only four also immunoreacted with 82 kDa protein[23].

More recent studies have clarified the biochemical molecular nature of the toxin. Cover and Blaser[22] showed that the toxin, in its native form, is a proteic aggregate of ≥970 kDa mass, composed by subunits of 87 kDa molecular weight, and that the 128 kDa protein does not induce any vacuolation. The N-terminal sequence of the toxin was found to have some homology with internal segments of cellular ATPases deputed to the cellular ion trafficking[22]. This similarity could account for the formation of a pH gradient in the intracellular compartments which in the end leads to vacuolation[16,22].

The gene which codifies for the cytotoxin has been cloned recently[15,24]. Starting from the published 23 amino acid terminal sequence of the purified toxin[22], Telford *et al.*[24] created oligonucleotides codifying for the first six and the last six vacuolating toxin amino acids, and amplified a 69 bp *H. pylori* genomic fragment by PCR. The products of the amplification were used to screen a *H. pylori* DNA library. Two regions of the DNA containing

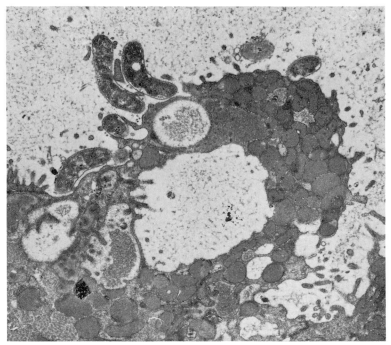

Fig. 4 *In vivo* vacuolation. Transmission electron micrograph of gastric mucosa. Some *H. pylori* organisms and vacuoles are visible. Courtesy of Dr M. Caselli. Reproduced with the permission of *Current Therapeutic Research*

the entire gene were isolated. Fusion proteins, obtained by cloning different segments of the gene in a plasmid expression vector, were used to immunize rabbits. Polyclonal serum immunoreacted with polypeptides of 94 kDa which were present in supernatants of cytotoxic *H. pylori* strains, and absent in those of cytotoxin negative organisms[24]. (This protein is the same 87 kDa protein described by Cover and Blaser[22]. Technical differences in performing electrophoretic runs account for the difference in their molecular masses.) Interestingly, it was also found that the toxin gene was present in non-cytotoxic strains, since fragments of the cytotoxin gene hybridized with the genome of cytotoxic negative organisms[24].

Why should this organism bother to replicate the gene for the toxin if it is not expressed? In the field of bacteriology no character is carried for long enough if it is not expressed. Most probably the gene that codifies for the toxin is inducible. If so, what is the substance(s) which induces it? We have seen that the presence of cytotoxin-producing strains is strongly associated with peptic ulceration[3,8]. We also know that the toxin is also produced *in vivo*, because serum samples from patients mostly infected by cytotoxic strains neutralize *in vitro* the vacuolating activity of cytotoxic supernatants[7,23]. Telford *et al.*[24] confirmed a potential role of the toxin in the development of gastroduodenal lesions, since sera from patients with histological epithelial damage of any type immunoreacted with the purified toxin significantly more often than did sera from *H. pylori*-colonized subjects, seropositive for other *H. pylori* antigens, but with reduced epithelial lesions. In addition, they also demonstrated extensive, destructive effects exerted on the epithelium of the stomach by the purified cytotoxin administered intragastrically to mice[15]. Thus the cytotoxin is likely to have a role in determining human gastroduodenal epithelial lesions.

The observation that non-cytotoxic *H. pylori* strains also possess the toxin gene is of particular interest[15]. Gastric ulcerations are characterized by long periods of remission. Could phases of remission correspond to periods in which the toxin gene is switched off? Is the expression of the gene regulated by other cistrons? Cytotoxic strains also express a protein of 128 kDa which is not present in cytotoxic negative supernatants and whole cell extracts[7,23,25,26]. The gene which codifies for this protein has been cloned recently by two different groups, and called *cagA* (cytotoxin-associated gene A)[27,28]. Studies to date show *cagA* is nearly always absent in non-cytotoxic strains. The CagA antigen seems to be an important phenotypic characteristic of virulence, because it more often immunoreacts with mucosal and systemic antibodies of adults and children with the most serious gastroduodenal diseases, cancer included[7,23,29,33]. In addition, supernatants of gastric biopsy cultures which neutralize the vacuolation *in vitro* induced by water extracts of cytotoxic strains contain IgA which react by Western blotting with CagA antigen (Fig. 5). These observations, together with that on the absence of *cagA* in cytotoxic-negative strains[15,24] could indicate that the expression of the toxin is under the control of the gene that codes for 128 kDa protein.

CONCLUSIONS

In conclusion, despite the high genomic variability of *H. pylori*, recent molecular and immunological studies have divided *H. pylori* into two major groups based on the presence of the CagA antigen and the vacuolating cytotoxin. Insertion of the genes for CagA and the cytotoxin and expression of these virulence associated *H. pylori* proteins in other *Helicobacter* species such as *H. mustelae* and *H. felis* would allow *in vivo* analysis of their functional importance in animal models.

Acknowledgements

We are grateful to Massimo Bugnoli (IRIS, Siena) for his skilful technical assistance, and to Rino Rappuoli (IRIS, Siena) for critical reading of the manuscript.

References

1. Desforges JF. *Helicobacter pylori* and peptic ulcer disease. N Engl J Med. 1991;324: 1043–8.

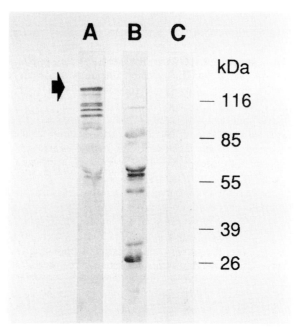

Fig. 5 Immunoblot of a 6 mol/l guanidine extract of *H. pylori* CCUG 17874 (cytotoxic strain) and immunoglobulin A antibodies contained in the supernatants of *in vitro* cultured antral biopsies. Supernatant which neutralized vacuolation *in vitro* also reacted with CagA protein (arrow, line A); line B, supernatant which did not neutralize vacuolation; line C, supernatant from a non-infected patient

2. Eurogast Study Group. An international association between *Helicobacter pylori* infection and gastric cancer. Lancet. 1993;341:1359–62.

3. Figura N, Guglielmetti P, Rossolini A *et al.* Cytotoxin production by *Campylobacter pylori* strains isolated from patients with peptic ulcers and from patients with chronic gastritis only. J Clin Microbiol. 1989;27:225–6.

4. Owen RJ, Bickley J, Costas M, Morgan DR. Genomic variation of *Helicobacter pylori*: application to identification of strains. Scand J Gastroenterol. 1991;26(Suppl. 181):43–50.

5. Johnson WM, Lior H. Production of heat-labile cytotoxin by *Campylobacter pyloridis*. Abstr. 86th Gen Meet Am Soc Microbiol, Washington, 1986. Washington, DC: American Society for Microbiology, abstract B234, p. 63.

6. Leunk RD, Johnson PT, David BC, Kraft WG, Morgan DR. Cytotoxic activity in broth-culture filtrates of *Campylobacter pylori*. J Med Microbiol. 1988;26:93–9.

7. Figura N, Bugnoli M, Cusi MG *et al.* Pathogenic mechanisms of *Helicobacter pylori*: production of cytotoxin. In: Malfertheiner P, Ditschneit H, editors. *Helicobacter pylori*, gastritis and peptic ulcer. Berlin, Heidelberg: Springer-Verlag; 1990:86–95.

8. Goossens H, Glupczynski Y, Burette A, Lambert J-P, Vlaes L, Butzler J-P. Role of the vacuolating toxin from *Helicobacter pylori* in the pathogenesis of duodenal and gastric ulcer. Med Microbiol. 1992;1:153–9.

9. Fox JG, Correa P, Taylor NS *et al.* High prevalence and persistence of cytotoxin-positive *Helicobacter pylori* strains in a population with high prevalence of atrophic gastritis. Am J Gastroenterol. 1992;87:1554–60.

10. Eaton KA, Morgan DR, Krakowka S. *Campylobacter pylori* virulence factors in gnotobiotic piglets. Infect Immun. 1989;57:1119–25.

11. Tricottet V, Bruneval P, Vire O. *Campylobacter*-like organisms and surface epithelium abnormalities in active chronic gastritis in humans: an ultrastructural study. Ultrastruct

Pathol. 1986;10:113–22.

12. Fiocca R, Villani L, De GC, Perego M, Trespi E, Solcia E. Morphological evidence of *Campylobacter pylori* pathogenicity in chronic gastritis and peptic ulcer. Acta Gastroenterol Belg. 1989;52:324–31.

13. Owen RJ, Figura N, Moreno M. Biotypes and DNA fingerprints of cytotoxigenic *Helicobacter pylori* from patients with gastritis and peptic ulceration in Italy. Eur J Epidemiol. 1992;8:15–21.

14. Owen RJ, Desai M, Figura N *et al*. Comparison between degree of histological gastritis and DNA fingerprints, cytotoxicity and adhesivity of *Helicobacter pylori* from different gastric sites. Eur J Epidemiol. 1993;9:315–21.

15. Telford JL, Dell'Orco M, Comanducci M *et al*. Gene structure of *Helicobacter pylori* cytotoxin and evidence of its key role in gastric disease. (submitted).

16. Papini E, Bugnoli M, De Bernard M, Figura N, Rappuoli R, Montecucco C. Bafilomycin A1 inhibits *Helicobacter pylori*-induced vacuolization of HeLa cells. Mol Microbiol. 1993;7:323–7.

17. Catrenich CE, Chestnut MH. Character and origin of vacuoles induced in mammalian cells by the cytotoxin of *Helicobacter pylori*. J Med Microbiol. 1992;37:389–95.

18. Cover TL, Puryear W, Perez-Perez GI, Blaser MJ. Effect of urease on HeLa cell vacuolation induced by *Helicobacter pylori* cytotoxin. Infect Immun. 1991;59:1264–70.

19. Cover TL, Vaughn SG, Cao P, Blaser MJ. Potentiation of *Helicobacter pylori* vacuolating toxin activity by nicotine and other weak bases. J Infect Dis. 1992;166:1073–8.

20. Bugnoli M, Bayeli PF, Rappuoli R, Pennatini C, Figura N, Crabtree JE. Inhibition of *Helicobacter pylori* urease by omeprazole. Eur J Gastroenterol Hepatol. 1993;5:683–5.

21. Daw MA, Deegan P, Leen E, O'Morain C. The effect of omeprazole on *Helicobacter pylori* and associated gastritis. Aliment Pharmacol Ther. 1991;5:435–9.

22. Cover TL, Blaser MJ. Purification and characterization of the vacuolating toxin from *Helicobacter pylori*. J Biol Chem. 1992;267:10570–5.

23. Cover TL, Dooley CP, Blaser MJ. Characterization of and human serologic response to proteins in *Helicobacter pylori* broth culture supernatants with vacuolizing cytotoxin activity. Infect Immun. 1990;58:603–10.

24. Telford JL, Dell'Orco M, Burroni D *et al*. Molecular analysis of the *H. pylori* cytotoxin gene. Eur J Gastroenterol Hepatol. 1993;5(Suppl. 2):522–4.

25. Crabtree JE, Figura N, Taylor JD, Bugnoli M, Armellini D, Tompkins DS. Expression of 120 kilodalton protein and cytotoxicity in *Helicobacter pylori*. J Clin Pathol. 1992;45:733–4.

26. Bugnoli M, Armellini D, Rappuoli R, Rossolini A, Xiang Y, Figura N. The 130 kDa vacuolating cytotoxin-associated protein is a component of cytotoxic *Helicobacter pylori* organisms. In: Gasbarrini G, Pretolani S, editors. Basic and clinical aspects of *H. pylori* infection. Berlin, Heidelberg: Springer-Verlag; 1993:225–8.

27. Covacci A, Censini S, Bugnoli M *et al*. Molecular characterization of the 128 kDa immunodominant antigen of *Helicobacter pylori* associated with cytotoxicity and duodenal ulcer. Proc Natl Acad Sci USA. 1993;90:5791–5.

28. Tummuru MKR, Cover TL, Blaser MJ. Cloning and expression of a high-molecular-mass major antigen of *Helicobacter pylori*: evidence of linkage to cytotoxin production. Infect Immun. 1993;61:1799–809.

29. Figura N, Bugnoli M, Guglielmetti P, Musmanno RA, Russi M, Quaranta S. Antibodies to vacuolating toxin of *Helicobacter pylori* in dyspeptic patients. In: Pajares JM, editor. *Helicobacter pylori* and gastroduodenal pathology. Berlin, Heidelberg: Springer-Verlag; 1992:181–6.

30. Crabtree JE, Taylor JD, Wyatt JI *et al*. Mucosal IgA recognition of *Helicobacter pylori* 120 kDa protein, peptic ulceration, and gastric pathology. Lancet. 1991;338:332–5.

31. Crabtree JE, Wyatt JI, Sobala GM *et al*. Systemic and mucosal humoral responses to *Helicobacter pylori* in gastric cancer. Gut. 1993;34:1339–43.

32. Oderda G, Figura N, Bayeli PF *et al*. Serologic IgG recognition of *Helicobacter pylori* cytotoxin-associated protein, peptic ulcer and gastroduodenal pathology in childhood. Eur J Gastroenterol Hepatol. 1993;5:695–9.

33. Xiang Z, Bugnoli M, Rappuoli R, Covacci A, Ponzetto A, Crabtree JE. *Helicobacter pylori*: host responses in peptic ulceration. Lancet. 1993;341:900.

20
H. pylori alcohol dehydrogenase

M. SALASPURO

INTRODUCTION

The pathogenetic mechanisms behind *Helicobacter pylori*-associated morbidity have so far not been fully elucidated[1]. It has been proposed that *H. pylori* contributes to gastroduodenal injury either by impairing local mucosal defence[2] or by increasing antral gastrin release, which leads to increased gastric acidity[3]. The 'leaking roof' theory – impaired mucosal defence – has been related to many inflammatory and toxic factors[1]. One of these could be acetaldehyde produced by *H. pylori* alcohol dehydrogenase (HPADH).

Alcohol dehydrogenase (ADH)-catalysed fermentation of sugars to ethanol provides a source of anaerobic energy for ethanologenic bacteria. Such bacterial ethanol production has been shown to occur in the intestine of both humans[4] and experimental animals[5]. In bacteria the ADH-catalysed fermentation reaction runs from acetaldehyde to ethanol. On the other hand in somatic cells (e.g. in the liver) ADH catalyses the oxidation of ethanol to acetaldehyde that is effectively oxidized to acetate by mitochondrial aldehyde dehydrogenase[6]. The oxidation and fermentation reactions catalysed by ADH run according to the following schemes:

Ethanol oxidation in somatic cells

$$\text{Ethanol} \xrightarrow{\text{ADH}} \text{Acetaldehyde} \xrightarrow{\text{ALDH}} \text{Acetate}$$

Alcoholic fermentation in bacteria

$$\text{Glucose} \longrightarrow \text{Acetaldehyde} \xrightarrow{\text{ADH}} \text{Ethanol}$$

(in excess of ethanol)

However, as will be indicated subsequently, ADH-mediated fermentation reaction in bacteria may in the presence of excess ethanol be reversed, and under these conditions ethanol is oxidized to acetaldehyde, which is a highly reactive and toxic substance.

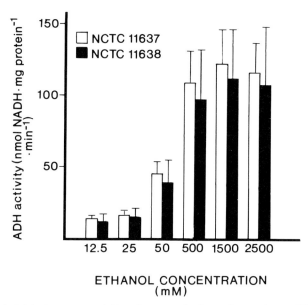

Fig. 1 Alcohol dehydrogenase activities of two standard *H. pylori* strains at different ethanol concentrations (with permission of *Gastroenterology*)[8]

H. PYLORI ALCOHOL DEHYDROGENASE AND ACETALDEHYDE PRODUCTION

We have recently demonstrated that two standard *H. pylori* strains (NCTC 11637 and 11638) exhibit significant ADH activity both at low and high ethanol concentrations[7,8] (Fig. 1). The mean ADH activity of these strains was more than 10-fold higher than that found in *Escherichia coli* and *Campylobacter jejuni*, and it was more than 20 times higher than that we have found in histologically normal human gastric mucosal biopsy samples[7]. In subsequent studies we have been able to show that 34 different *H. pylori* strains of human, and three of animal, origin contain alcohol dehydrogenase[9]. In line with the observed ADH activity the cytosols of both *Helicobacter* strains produced in the presence of excess ethanol larger amounts of acetaldehyde (Fig. 2) than that produced by the cytosols prepared from two other ADH-containing bacteria *Escherichia coli* and *Campylobacter jejuni*[7].

  H. pylori alcohol dehydrogenase (HPADH) is active already at an ethanol concentration comparable to the low endogenous ethanol level known to prevail in the stomach, for instance during the use of H_2-blockers[4]. The relatively high K_m (65–104 mmol/l)[7,8,10] of the bacterial enzyme for ethanol oxidation, however, indicates that maximal ethanol-oxidizing activity and acetaldehyde production could be observed after drinking of alcoholic beverages. The high optimal pH (9.6)[8] of HPADH is similar to that found for the majority of ADHs from different origins. Significant bacterial ADH activity and acetaldehyde production was, however, detected even at pH 7.2. Accordingly, ADH-mediated reactions could, at least theoretically, also be

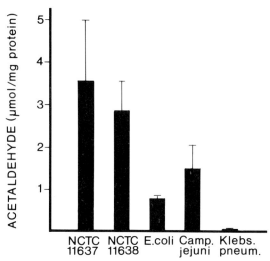

Fig. 2 Acetaldehyde production in the excess of ethanol by two standard *H. pylori* strains and by three other bacteria (with permission of *Life Sciences*)[7]

possible *in vivo* in the neutral mucin layer covering gastric mucosa. By virtue of its high urease activity[11], *H. pylori* is known to be able to break down urea to ammonia. Thereby the organism may even be able to create an alkaline environment favouring ADH-associated acetaldehyde production. Optimal conditions for *H. pylori*-associated acetaldehyde formation from ethanol – and possible consequent mucosal injury – can also be assumed to prevail in the duodenal bulb where gastric acid is neutralized by pancreatic bicarbonate secretion.

As already mentioned in somatic cells acetaldehyde is effectively removed by aldehyde dehydrogenase[6] and consequently only very low levels of acetaldehyde can be detected outside the liver[6,12,13]. In sharp contrast to gastric mucosal and liver cells neither *H. pylori* strain studied showed any NAD-linked aldehyde dehydrogenase activity[8]. The lack of ALDH in *H. pylori* may favour the accumulation of the very active and toxic acetaldehyde, at least in the close vicinity of bacterial clusters.

PURIFICATION AND CHARACTERIZATION OF HPADH

Alcohol dehydrogenase of *H. pylori* was purified from cytosol of cultured bacteria (strain NCTC 11637) by anion exchange and affinity chromatography[10]. On sodium dodecyl sulphate polyacrylamide-gel electrophoresis the 160-fold purified enzyme displayed one protein band[10] with a mobility that corresponded to a M_r of 38 000. Accordingly the subunit size of the enzyme is in the range of typical values for the medium-chain alcohol dehydrogenases. Purified HPADH represents approximately 0.5% of the cytosolic protein which supports its metabolic function.

HPADH shows distinct kinetic characteristics when compared to human gastric alcohol dehydrogenases. Contrary to human ADH isoenzymes HPADH has a strong preference for NADP ($K_m = 80\,\mu$mol/l) over NAD ($K_m = 4.4$ mmol/l) as a cofactor in alcohol oxidation[10]. Although HPADH has a relatively high K_m for ethanol, at the same time it has several-fold higher specific activity for ethanol (32 U/mg) than human gastric isoenzymes[14]. 4-Methylpyrazole inhibits HPADH in a competitive manner, but in contrast to class I gastric alcohol dehydrogenases HPADH is inhibited first at millimolar concentrations of 4-methylpyrazole[8,10]. Isoelectric focusing of the bacterial enzyme shows activity bands[8] with pI at 7.1–7.3, a pattern different from that described previously for gastric mucosal alcohol dehydrogenases. The kinetic differences mentioned above could form the basis for the separation and determination of bacterial and human gastric ADH activities in order to evaluate the possible role of HPADH in gastric 'first-pass' metabolism of ethanol[15]. Differences in *H. pylori* infection status could therefore explain some of the conflicting results concerning the significance of gastric ethanol metabolism and its inhibition by H_2-receptor antagonists[16–19].

ETHANOL AND ACETALDEHYDE PRODUCTION BY INTACT *H. PYLORI*

Several observations suggest that HPADH is a metabolic enzyme taking part in the production of anaerobic energy. As already mentioned it is a rather abundant enzyme comprising approximately 0.5% of cytosolic proteins[10]. Therefore, it presumably has a basic role in the functions and maintenance of *H. pylori*. Its K_m for acetaldehyde is approximately 100 times lower than the K_m for ethanol[10]. These kinetic results indicate that the main function of HPADH is to reduce acetaldehyde to ethanol and concomitantly oxidize NADPH/NADH to NADP/NAD, and by that means produce energy in anaerobic conditions. On the other hand, the microaerophilic bacteria may also be capable of producing energy aerobically. The use of nuclear magnetic resonance (NMR) spectroscopy in metabolic studies of *H. pylori* has revealed Krebs cycle activities in the bacteria[20]. Therefore the inhibition of HPADH by citrate – the main metabolite of citric acid cycle – may reflect possible regulation between aerobic and anaerobic energy production by *H. pylori*[10].

In line with our kinetic observations we have recently been able to demonstrate[21] that *H. pylori* strains (NCTC 11637 and NCTC 11638) are capable of producing ethanol when incubated in sealed vials for 2 h at 37°C. In similar incubations, but in the presence of ethanol, intact *H. pylori* cultures formed significant amounts of acetaldehyde already at a low (0.1%) ethanol concentration, and at a higher (2.5%) ethanol concentration acetaldehyde production was even more pronounced[21].

INHIBITION OF *H. PYLORI* ADH

Although the value of colloidal bismuth subcitrate (CBS) in the treatment of *H. pylori*-induced gastric and duodenal diseases is well established, less is known about the mechanism by which the drug exerts its effect[22]. Similarly, omeprazole is known to suppress *H. pylori*[23], but the mechanism remains speculative. In our hands CBS at a drug concentration of 0.01 mmol/l inhibited the activity of the cytosolic ADH of the organism by 93%[24]. This was associated with almost as effective inhibition of acetaldehyde production in the presence of 22 mmol/l ethanol[24]. In our most recent studies CBS also suppressed acetaldehyde production by intact *H. pylori*[25]. However, rather high drug concentrations were required for this to occur[25]. The reason for the sensitivity difference between cytosol and intact bacteria remains obscure, as CBS has been shown to penetrate fairly rapidly into *H. pylori*[26]. *In vivo*, however, the degree of inhibition may also depend on the prevailing amount of bacteria in the gastric mucosa, as shown to be case for omeprazole, which inhibited *H. pylori* urease only when low bacterial inocula were incubated at high drug concentrations[27].

Omeprazole inhibited HPADH and suppressed bacterial acetaldehyde formation mediated by the bacterial cytosol to 69% of control[24] at a drug concentration of 0.1 mmol/l. By contrast, the H_2-receptor antagonists ranitidine and famotidine showed only modest effect on HPADH and acetaldehyde production[24].

We have recently also tested the inhibitory effect on acetaldehyde formation of nitecapone, 3-(3,4-dihydroxy-5-nitrobenzylidine)-2,4-pentanedione, a novel gastroprotective drug presently undergoing clinical trials[28]. Nitecapone has been shown to interfere with the mechanisms that may be important in the pathogenesis of *H. pylori*-associated diseases[29] and, furthermore, it has a direct bactericidal effect on *H. pylori* (MIC 128 mg/l)[30]. In our hands, nitecapone turned out to be a potent inhibitor of acetaldehyde production by the cytosol of *H. pylori* at concentrations that can be achieved in gastric mucosa after a therapeutic dose of the drug (300 mg BID). Nitecapone has previously been shown to be able to inhibit *H. pylori* protease and lipase at similar concentrations to those used in the present study[31]. A potential mechanism for enzyme inhibition by nitecapone is its ability to react with sulphydryl groups[32]. A similar mechanism may also play a role in bismuth-mediated enzyme inhibition[33], a concept of interest since ADH also possesses sulphydryl groups.

As mentioned above, 4-methylpyrazole, a well-known ADH inhibitor[34], inhibited HPADH and *in vitro* formation of acetaldehyde from ethanol by the organism[8,10]. Both phenomena, however, occurred only at relatively high concentrations of the compound[8]. Supporting the hypothesis about the role of ADH for the energy metabolism of *H. pylori*, 4-methylpyrazole also inhibited growth of the bacterium under microaerophilic culture conditions[8]. Again, however, as for ADH inhibition, high concentrations of the compound were required for this to occur.

HPADH is an abundant enzyme which prefers NADP(H) as a cofactor contrary to human alcohol dehydrogenase[10]. Consequently, the difference

SCHIFF BASE

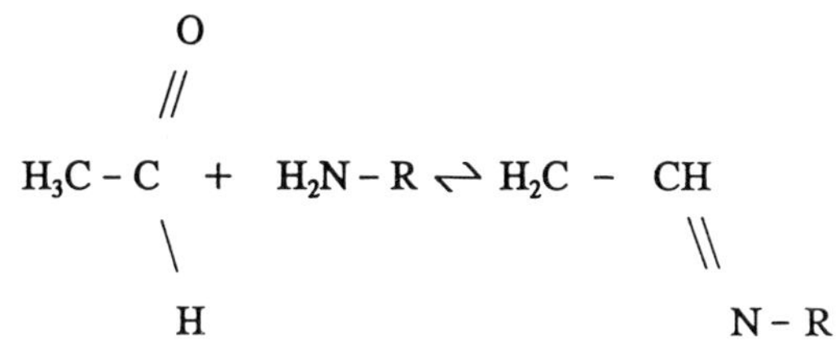

$$\underset{H}{\overset{\overset{\displaystyle O}{\parallel}}{H_3C - C}} \quad + \quad H_2N - R \; \rightleftharpoons \; \underset{N - R}{\overset{\overset{\displaystyle }{}}{H_2C - \overset{\displaystyle \backslash\backslash}{CH}}}$$

Fig. 3 The formation of Schiff base, i.e. the binding of acetaldehyde with the free amino groups of proteins

in the active site of bacterial ADH could form the basis for the development and use of a specific inhibitory drug against the enzyme and the energy-producing metabolic activities of *H. pylori*. The inhibition of energy-producing metabolic activities of the bacteria could for its part facilitate the eradication of *H. pylori* from human stomach.

TOXICITY OF ACETALDEHYDE

Acetaldehyde is both pharmacologically and chemically a very potent and reactive compound, and has been suggested as a major initiating factor in the pathogenesis of alcoholic liver damage[6,13,35,36]. Local bacterial acetaldehyde production has been incriminated as a possible pathogenic factor behind upper respiratory tract cancer in alcoholics[37], and in alcohol-related rectal carcinogenesis in rats[38]. The toxicity of acetaldehyde has been related to several important metabolic and cellular factors.

Covalent binding of acetaldehyde–acetaldehyde adducts

In vitro acetaldehyde has been shown to form adducts with phospholipids[39]. However, most probable target macromolecules are proteins, for instance erythrocyte membrane proteins[40], haemoglobin[41], hepatic microsomal proteins[42] and liver tubulin[43]. The formation of protein–acetaldehyde adducts may occur through at least three mechanisms[44]. A Schiff base can be formed between the electrophilic carbonyl carbon of acetaldehyde and nucleophilic sites on proteins such as the free epsilon-amino group of lysine residues (Fig. 3). Alternative possibilities are the formation of cyclic imidazolidinone at the N-terminal ends of proteins, or the reaction of acetaldehyde with cysteine yielding 2-methyl-1-thiazolidine-4-carboxylic acid[44].

The biochemical background of the possible toxicity associated with the covalent binding of acetaldehyde with tissue proteins is not yet fully understood. Acetaldehyde–protein adducts could inhibit protein secretion[45], displace pyridoxal phosphate from its binding sites in proteins[46] or impair some biological functions of enzyme proteins. According to our preliminary studies similar acetaldehyde–protein adduct formation may also occur in gastric mucosa[47]. Since acetaldehyde–adduct formation has been shown to occur even at rather low acetaldehyde concentrations, even low endogenous ethanol levels demonstrated in gastric juice[4] might initiate the reaction.

Accordingly, conversion of endogenous or exogenous ethanol to acetaldehyde by *H. pylori*, if it also occurs *in vivo*, could lead to the formation of acetaldehyde adducts with gastric mucin or proteins of the gastric epithelial cells in analogy to the adducts formed with hepatic proteins in the liver. This potential acetaldehyde-mediated interference with the mucosal defence factors may contribute to *H. pylori*-linked gastrointestinal morbidity.

Antibodies against acetaldehyde adducts

It has been shown that mice immunized by acetaldehyde–protein adduct produce specific antibodies against binding epitopes[48]. Humoral immune response to acetaldehyde–protein adducts is also produced in acute alcoholic liver disease[49] and even in alcoholics without liver injury. The immune response has been suggested to contribute to the aggravation or perpetuation of alcoholic liver injury. It remains to be established whether similar immune reactions could also occur in gastric mucosa infected by *H. pylori*.

Acetaldehyde and lipid peroxidation

Under certain *in vitro* conditions the metabolism of acetaldehyde may produce free radicals and mediate lipid peroxidation[50]. In addition to the mitochondrial aldehyde dehydrogenase of gastric mucosal cells, acetaldehyde may also be oxidized to acetate via xanthine oxidase[51]. In this reaction oxygen may be metabolized to free radical, superoxide, which is a well-known lipid peroxidative agent. Normally free radicals are inactivated by glutathione. Acetaldehyde, however, may bind with glutathione or with cysteine, which is needed in the synthesis of glutathione. As in the liver this might depress gastric glutathione with a secondary increase in lipid peroxidation[52].

Acetaldehyde and *N*-nitroso compounds

N-nitroso compounds within gastric juice have been implicated in the aetiology of gastric cancer[53]. One of the main precarcinogenic lesions induced by *N*-nitroso compounds in DNA is alkylation of guanine[53] at position O^6. On the other hand, gastric mucosal cells have been shown to contain DNA repair protein, O^6-alkylguanine-DNA-alkyltransferase (AGT), which can eliminate modifications at this premutagenic site[54]. Human O^6-methylguanine-transferase – as well as other methyltransferases[55,56] – have, however, been shown to be inhibited by acetaldehyde even at nanomolar concentrations[57]. Accordingly, acetaldehyde produced by *H. pylori* ADH may severely hamper the AGT-mediated repair mechanism by inactivating the gastric enzyme. In rapidly proliferating gastric mucosal cells this effective inactivation of AGT and concomitant inhibition of DNA repair may give rise to a transition mutation – adenine replacing guanine – during cell replication[58] and ultimately result in the development of gastric cancer. Another possible mechanism could be the intragastric nitrate $\rightarrow$ nitrite $\rightarrow$ nitrosocarcinogen conversion that has been shown to be enhanced by aldehydes[59].

CONCLUSIONS

We have recently shown that 34 different *H. pylori* strains of human, and three of animal, origin contain alcohol dehydrogenase (ADH) and produce acetaldehyde (Ach) even from low (0.1%) ethanol concentrations. The primary function of *H. pylori* alcohol dehydrogenase (HPADH), however, appears to be the production of energy under anaerobic conditions. The K_m value of HPADH for ethanol oxidation ranges from 64 to 104 mmol/l. Based on isoelectric focusing and coenzyme requirements HPADH differs clearly from gastric mucosal alcohol dehydrogenases. 4-Methylpyrazole (an ADH-inhibitor) also inhibits HPADH, and suppresses the growth of *H. pylori* during culture. Commonly used bismuth compounds are potent inhibitors of HPADH and inhibit also Ach production from excess ethanol by intact bacteria. On the other hand *H. pylori* has no aldehyde dehydrogenase activity, which may lead to high Ach concentrations in the vicinity of bacterial accumulations. Acetaldehyde is a highly reactive substance and readily forms adducts with cellular proteins. Ach-modified proteins may be immunogenic and induce the formation of antibodies. Furthermore Ach may lead to tissue injury by producing free radicals and by inducing lipid peroxidation. Our most recent results indicate that Ach forms stable adducts with rat gastric and duodenal mucosa both *in vitro* and *in vivo*. Consequently HPADH-mediated acetaldehyde formation may be of importance in the pathogenesis of gastric injury associated with the organism.

References

1. Dunn BE. Pathogenic mechanisms of *Helicobacter pylori*. Gastroenterol Clin N Am. 1993;22:1–43.
2. Goodwin CS. Duodenal ulcer, *Campylobacter pylori*, and the 'leaking roof' concept. Lancet. 1988;2:1467–9.
3. Levi S, Beardshall K, Haddad G, Playford R, Ghosh P, Calam J. *Campylobacter pylori* and duodenal ulcers: the gastrin link (see comments). Lancet. 1989;1:1167–8.
4. Bode JC, Rust S, Bode C. The effect of cimetidine treatment on ethanol formation in the human stomach. Scand J Gastroenterol. 1984;19:853–6.
5. Baraona E, Julkunen R, Tannenbaum L, Lieber CS. Role of intestinal bacterial overgrowth in ethanol production and metabolism in rats. Gastroenterology. 1986;90:103–10.
6. Salaspuro M. Epidemiological aspects of alcohol and alcoholic liver disease, ethanol metabolism, and pathogenesis of alcoholic liver injury. In: McIntyre N, Benhanmou J-P, Bircher J, Rizzetto M, Rodes J, editors. Oxford textbook of clinical hepatology, vol. 2. Oxford, New York, Tokyo: Oxford University Press; 1991:791–810.
7. Roine RP, Salmela KS, Höök-Nikanne J, Kosunen TU, Salaspuro MP. Alcohol dehydrogen-

ase mediated acetaldehyde production by *Helicobacter pylori* – a possible mechanism behind gastric injury. Life Sci. 1992;51:1333–7.

8. Salmela KS, Roine RP, Koivisto T, Höök-Nikanne J, Kosunen TU, Salaspuro M. Characteristics of *Helicobacter pylori* alcohol dehydrogenase. Gastroenterology. 1993;105:325–30.

9. Höök-Nikanne J, Roine RP, Salmela KS, Kosunen TU, Salaspuro M. Alcohol dehydrogenase activities of different *Helicobacter* strains. Gastroenterology. 1993;104:A103 (abstract).

10. Kaihovaara P, Salmela KS, Roine R, Kosunen TU, Salaspuro M. Purification and characterization of *Helicobacter pylori* alcohol dehydrogenase. Alcohol Clin Exp Res. 1994;in press.

11. Mobley HL, Cortesia MJ, Rosenthal LE, Jones BD. Characterization of urease from *Campylobacter pylori*. J Clin Microbiol. 1988;26:831–6.

12. Nuutinen HU, Salaspuro MP, Valle M, Lindros KO. Blood acetaldehyde concentration gradient between hepatic and antecubital venous blood in ethanol-intoxicated alcoholics and controls. Eur J Clin Invest. 1984;14:306–11.

13. Salaspuro M, Lindros K. Metabolism and toxicity of acetaldehyde. In: Seitz HK, Kommerell B, editors. Alcohol related diseases in gastroenterology. Berlin: Springer-Verlag; 1985: 106–23.

14. Moreno A, Pares X. Purification and characterization of a new alcohol dehydrogenase from human stomach. J Biol Chem. 1991;266:1128–33.

15. Julkunen RJ, Di-Padova C, Lieber CS. First pass metabolism of ethanol – a gastrointestinal barrier against the systemic toxicity of ethanol. Life Sci. 1985;37:567–73.

16. DiPadova C, Roine R, Frezza M, Gentry RT, Baraona E, Lieber CS. Effects of ranitidine on blood alcohol levels after ethanol ingestion. Comparison with other H_2-receptor antagonists (see comments). JAMA. 1992;267:83–6.

17. Fraser AG, Prewett EJ, Hudson M, Sawyerr AM, Rosalki SB, Pounder RE. The effect of ranitidine, cimetidine or famotidine on low-dose post-prandial alcohol absorption (see comments). Aliment Pharmacol Ther. 1991;5:263–72.

18. Palmer RH, Frank WO, Nambi P, Wetherington JD, Fox MJ. Effects of various concomitant medications on gastric alcohol dehydrogenase and the first-pass metabolism of ethanol. Am J Gastroenterol. 1991;86(12):1749–55.

19. Guram M, Howden CW, Holt S. Further evidence for an interaction between alcohol and certain H_2-receptor antagonists. Alcohol Clin Exp Res. 1991;15:1084–5.

20. Dick JD. *Helicobacter* (*Campylobacter*) *pylori*: a new twist to an old disease. Annu Rev Microbiol. 1990;44:249–69.

21. Salmela KS, Roine RP, Höök-Nikanne J, Kosunen TU, Salaspuro M. Acetaldehyde and ethanol production by *Helicobacter pylori* Scand J Gastroenterol. 1994;29:in press.

22. Gorbach SL. Bismuth therapy in gastrointestinal diseases. Gastroenterology. 1990;99: 863–75.

23. Mainguet P, Delmee M, Debongnie JC. Omeprazole, *Campylobacter pylori*, and duodenal ulcer (letter; comment) (see comments). Lancet. 1989;2:389–90.

24. Roine RP, Salmela KS, Hook-Nikanne J, Kosunen TU, Salaspuro M. Colloidal bismuth subcitrate and omeprazole inhibit alcohol dehydrogenase mediated acetaldehyde production by *Helicobacter pylori*. Life Sci. 1992;5-1:PL195–200.

25. Salmela KS, Roine RP, Höök-Nikanne J, Kosunen TU, Salaspuro M. Effect of bismuth and nitecapone on acetaldehyde production by *Helicobacter pylori*. Scand J Gastroenterol. 1994;29:in press.

26. Marshall BJ, Armstrong JA, Francis FJ, Nokes NT, Wee SH. Antibacterial action of bismuth in relation to *Campylobacer pyloridis* colonization and gastritis. Digestion. 1987;37(Suppl. 2):16–30.

27. Vogt K, Hahn H. Influence of omeprazole on urease activity of Helicobacter pylori *in vitro*. Ir J Med. 1992;161(Suppl. 10):89(abstract).

28. Aho PA, Linden IB. Role of gastric mucosal eicosanoid production in the cytoprotection induced by nitecapone. Scand J Gastroenterol. 1992;27(2):134–8.

29. Slomiany BL, Piotrowski J, Rajiah G, Slomiany A. Inhibition of gastric mucosal laminin receptor by *Helicobacter pylori* lipopolysaccharide: effect of nitecapone. Gen Pharmacol. 1991;22:1063–9.

30. Rautelin H, Renkonen OV, Kosunen TV. *In vitro* susceptibility of *Helicobacter pylori* to

nitecapone (letter). Eur J Clin Microbiol Infect Dis. 1992;11:274–5.

31. Piotrowski J, Slomiany A, Liu J, Fekete Z, Slomiany BL. Effect of nitecapone on the proteolytic and lipolytic activities of *Helicobacter pylori*. Biochem (Life Sci Adv.) 1991;10: 79–83.

32. Korkolainen T, Nissinen E, Aho P, Lotta T, Lindén I-B. Gastroprotective agent nitecapone reacts with sulfhydryl groups (abstract). Eur J Pharmacol. 1990;183:315–16.

33. Lambert JR, Way DJ, King RG, Eaves ER, Lianeas K, Wan A. DeNol vs Pepto-Bismol-Bismuth pharmacokinetics in the human gastric mucosa. Gastroenterology. 1989;96:A284(abstract).

34. Salaspuro M. Inhibitors of alcohol metabolism. Acta Med Scand. Suppl. 1985;703:219–24.

35. Lieber CS. Biochemical and molecular basis of alcohol-induced injury to liver and other tissues (see comments). N Engl J Med. 1988;319:1639–50.

36. Sorrell MF, Tuma DJ. Hypothesis: alcoholic liver injury and the covalent binding of acetaldehyde. Alcohol Clin Exp Res. 1985;9:306–9.

37. Miyakawa H, Baraona E, Chang JC, Lesser MD, Lieber CS. Oxidation of ethanol to acetaldehyde by bronchopulmonary washings: role of bacteria. Alcohol Clin Exp Res. 1986;10:517–20.

38. Seitz HK, Simanowski UA, Garzon FT et al. Possible role of acetaldehyde in ethanol-related rectal cocarcinogenesis in the rat. Gastroenterology. 1990;98:406–13.

39. Kenney WC. Acetaldehyde adducts of phospholipids. Alcohol Clin Exp Res. 1982;6: 412–16.

40. Gaines KC, Salhany JM, Tuma DJ, Sorrell MF. Reaction of acetaldehyde with human erythrocyte membrane proteins. FEBS Lett. 1977;75:115–19.

41. Stevens VJ, Fantl WJ, Newman CB, Rims RV, Cerami A, Peterson CM. Acetaldehyde adducts with hemoglobin. J Clin Invest. 1981;67:361–9.

42. Nomura F, Lieber CS. Binding of acetaldehyde to rat liver microsomes: enhancement after chronic alcohol consumption. Biochem Biophys Res Commun. 1981;100:131–7.

43. Tuma DJ, Jennett RB, Sorrell MF. The interaction of acetaldehyde with tubulin. Ann NY Acad Sci. 1987;492:277–86.

44. Lauterburg BH, Bilzer M. Mechanisms of acetaldehyde hepatotoxicity. J Hepatol. 1988;7:384–90.

45. Matsuda Y, Baraona E, Salaspuro M, Lieber CS. Effects of ethanol on liver microtubules and Golgi apparatus. Possible role in altered hepatic secretion of plasma proteins. Lab Invest. 1979;41:455–63.

46. Lumeng L. The role of acetaldehyde in mediating the deleterious effect of ethanol on pyridoxal 5'-phosphate metabolism. J Clin Invest. 1978;62:286–93.

47. Roine RP, Sillanaukee P, Itälä L et al. Binding of acetaldehyde to rat gastric mucosa. Scand J Gastroenterol. 1993;28(Suppl. 197):72(abstract).

48. Israel Y, Hurwitz E, Niemela O, Arnon R. Monoclonal and polyclonal antibodies against acetaldehyde-containing epitopes in acetaldehyde-protein adducts. Proc Natl Acad Sci USA. 1986;83:7923–7.

49. Hoerner M, Behrens UJ, Worner TM et al. The role of alcoholism and liver disease in the appearance of serum antibodies against acetaldehyde adducts. Hepatology. 1988;8:569–74.

50. Shaw S, Jayatilleke E, Ross WA, Gordon ER, Leiber CS. Ethanol-induced lipid peroxidation: potentiation by long-term alcohol feeding and attenuation by methionine. J Lab Clin Med. 1981;98:417–24.

51. Lewis KO, Paton A. Could superoxide cause cirrhosis? Lancet. 1982;2:188–9.

52. Shaw S, Rubin KP, Lieber CS. Depressed hepatic glutathione and increased diene conjugates in alcoholic liver disease. Evidence of lipid peroxidation. Dig Dis Sci. 1983;28:585–9.

53. Pegg AE. Methylation of the O_6 position of guanine in DNA is the most likely initiating event in carcinogenesis by methylating agents. Cancer Invest. 1984;2:223–31.

54. Kyrtopoulos SA, Ampatzi P, Davaris P, Haritopoulos N, Golematis B. Studies in gastric carcinogenesis. IV. O^6-methylguanine and its repair in normal and atrophic biopsy specimens of human gastric mucosa. Correlation of O^6-alkylguanine–DNA alkyltransferase activities in gastric mucosa and circulating lymphocytes. Carcinogenesis. 1990;11:431–6.

55. Garro AJ, McBeth DL, Lima V, Lieber CS. Ethanol consumption inhibits fetal DNA methylation in mice: implications for the fetal alcohol syndrome. Alcohol Clin Exp Res. 1991;15:395–8.

56. Barak AJ, Beckenhauer HC. The influence of ethanol on hepatic transmethylation. Alcohol Alcoholism. 1988;23:73–7.
57. Espina N, Lima V, Lieber CS, Garro AJ. *In vitro* and *in vivo* inhibitory effect of ethanol and acetaldehyde on O^6-methylguanine transferase. Carcinogenesis. 1988;9:761–6.
58. Loveless A. Possible relevance of O^6 alkylation of deoxyguanosine to the mutagenicity and carcinogenicity of nitrosamines and nitrosamides. Nature. 1969;223:206–7.
59. Hartman PE. Nitrates and nitrites: ingestion, pharmacodynamics and toxicology. Chem Mutagen. 1982;7:211–94.

Section IV
Hormonal disturbances in
H. pylori infection

21
Effect of *H. pylori* infection on gastrin and gastric acid secretion

K. E. L. McCOLL and E. EL-OMAR

INTRODUCTION

It is now well established that *Helicobacter pylori* is the major acquired factor in the pathogenesis of duodenal ulcer (DU) disease. The infection is found in > 95% of DU patients and numerous studies have demonstrated that eradicating the infection markedly lowers the ulcer relapse rate[1-5]. The mechanism by which the infection predisposes to ulceration of the duodenum has been the subject of much speculation. The fact that the infection is most pronounced in the stomach, whereas the associated ulceration occurs in the duodenum, suggests that the ulceration is not merely due to local damage of the mucosa by the organism. The antrum plays an important role in the regulation of gastric acid secretion via the release of the hormone gastrin. One hypothesis linking *H. pylori* infection and duodenal ulceration is that the infection stimulates an increased release of gastrin, which in turn produces increased acid secretion, and that the excessive duodenal acid load causes the ulceration[6].

Numerous studies have confirmed that *H. pylori* infection is associated with increased basal, meal-stimulated and gastrin releasing peptide-stimulated gastrin concentrations which rapidly return to normal following eradication of the infection[7-13]. The degree of hypergastrinaemia caused by *H. pylori* is the same in DU patients and healthy volunteers[8]. The elevated gastrin level associated with *H. pylori* infection is due to an increase in the biologically active G17 form of the hormone[14] (Fig. 1). Gastrin-17 is mainly produced in the gastric antrum whereas G34 is mainly produced in the duodenum. The increase in the G17 form is consistent with *H. pylori* predominantly affecting the antral mucosa. In addition G17 is the main gastrin which increases in response to eating[14], and this is consistent with *H. pylori*-associated hypergastrinaemia being most marked postprandially.

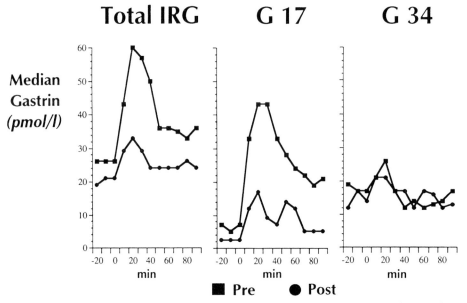

Fig. 1 Median serum concentrations of total immunoreactive gastrin (IRG), gastrin 17 and gastrin 34 basally and in response to a meal, before (■) and 1 month following (●) eradication of *H. pylori* in 13 DU patients. The meal was commenced at time 0. (Reproduced by kind permission of *Gut*)

MECHANISM OF *H. PYLORI*-ASSOCIATED HYPERGASTRINAEMIA

The mechanism by which *H. pylori* infection causes increased antral gastrin release is unclear. Levi *et al.* postulated that the ammonia produced by the high bacterial urease activity might raise antral surface pH and thereby prevent the physiological inhibition of gastrin release by intragastric acid[6]. We have performed a number of studies in order to test this very plausible hypothesis. In the first study we increased *H. pylori* ammonia production *in vivo* by the intragastric infusion of urea to infected subjects, but found no change in the serum gastrin[15]. Graham *et al.* performed a similar study with the same result[12]. We also assessed the effect of inhibiting *H. pylori* urease activity *in vivo* by the oral administration of acetohydroxamic acid to infected subjects[16]. Despite inhibiting bacterial urease activity by more than 80% we could not detect any change in serum gastrin. In a further study we completely suppressed *H. pylori* urease activity by 36 h of triple therapy, but again could not demonstrate any fall in either basal or meal-stimulated gastrin concentrations[17].

If *H. pylori* were raising gastrin by its ammonia production blocking the inhibitory effect of intragastric acid, then *H. pylori*-associated hypergastrinaemia should be most marked at low intragastric pH, and least in the absence of acid. However, we found that *H. pylori* infection raised gastrin by a similar percentage in the presence and absence of gastric acid[18]. Likewise, Moss *et* al.[19] and Karnes et al.[20] found that *H. pylori* infection was associated with a similar percentage increase in gastrin at pH 5.5 and pH 2.5.

The studies to date, therefore, do not support the hypergastrinaemia being secondary to bacterial ammonia interfering with the acid-inhibitory control of gastrin release.

Another possible cause of *H. pylori*-induced hypergastrinaemia is that it is a compensatory response to the infection reducing gastric acid secretion. There is some evidence that acute *H. pylori* infection may cause hypochlorhydria, and in some subjects this could persist and thus produce reflex hypergastrinaemia. Both our own group and Dr Calam's have studied the acid response to increasing doses of gastrin in DU patients before and following eradication of *H. pylori* and have found no change in parietal cell sensitivity[21,22]. This excludes the increased gastrin being secondary to the infection impairing parietal cell function in patients with DU. However, there are no data on the effect of chronic infection on parietal cell function in non-DU subjects.

The release of gastrin by the antral mucosa is under inhibitory control by somatostatin release from the antral D cells. The hypergastrinaemia could therefore be secondary to a relative deficiency of somatostatin. As somatostatin mainly exerts its effects locally in a paracrine fashion, it is necessary to look at the concentrations of the hormone in the mucosa rather than in the serum. Kaneko et al. reported reduced immunoreactive-somatostatin concentrations in gastric mucosal biopsies of patients with *H. pylori* infection[23]. However, a wide variety of upper gastrointestinal disorders were included in the study, and it is difficult to be sure whether the changes in somatostatin were related to the infection, to specific gastrointestinal disorders or to drug therapy. However, a significant correlation was noted between the severity of chronic inflammation and degree of depletion of somatostatin. In a study of 18 DU patients Moss et al. reported a rise in antral mucosal somatostatin-immunoreactive cell density at 4 weeks following eradication of *H. pylori* infection[24]. In a similar study in 10 such patients they noted a rise in antral mucosal somatostatin mRNA at 4 weeks following eradication of the infection[24]. Recently Graham et al. studied D cell numbers in volunteers with and without *H. pylori* and in DU patients before and following eradication of the infection[25]. There was a trend towards reduced D cell numbers in the infected healthy volunteers, but this did not reach statistical significance. In addition, there was no difference in D cell numbers between patients and volunteers, or between DU patients before and following *H. pylori* eradication. At present, therefore, the mechanism of *H. pylori*-induced hypergastrinaemia remains unclear.

EFFECT OF *H. PYLORI*-ASSOCIATED HYPERGASTRINAEMIA ON ACID SECRETION

Gastrin is generally accepted to be the major mediator of the gastric phase of acid secretion[26]. The fact that *H. pylori* increases biologically active gastrin, together with the finding in DU patients that this is not accompanied by any reduction in parietal cell responsiveness to gastrin, suggests that the infection should be causing significantly increased acid secretion. A number of studies have examined acid secretion by a variety of methods and these are discussed below.

Basal acid output

There are only a few adequately controlled prospective studies examining the effect of *H. pylori* on basal acid output. Montbriand *et al.* studied basal acid output in 10 patients with functional dyspepsia before and following suppression of *H. pylori*[27]. There was no statistically significant change, but eight of the 10 did show a fall, suggesting that larger numbers might have produced a significant result. Levi *et al.* did not observe any fall in basal acid output in 10 DU patients examined after 4 weeks of triple therapy[28]. However, in a more recent study the same group did observe a significant fall in a group of nine DU patients examined at 4 weeks following completion of eradication therapy[21].

These studies indicated that *H. pylori* might be increasing basal acid output, but that larger studies were required to clarify the question. Recently we have examined basal acid output in 25 *H. pylori*-negative healthy volunteers, 25 *H. pylori*-positive healthy volunteers and 25 *H. pylori*-positive DU patients, with all groups closely matched for age, sex and body weight[29–31]. The healthy volunteers were re-examined at 1 month following *H. pylori* eradication and the DU patients at 1 month and 1 year. Reproducibility studies of basal acid output measurement were performed and showed a coefficient of variation of 32%[32].

Median basal acid output (mmol/h) was slightly higher in the *H. pylori*-positive (2.9) compared to negative (1.8) healthy volunteers ($p < 0.05$). It was more markedly increased in the *H. pylori*-positive DU patients at 6.6 mmol/h. At 1 month following eradication of *H. pylori* the basal acid output in the healthy volunteers fell to 1.8 mmol/h. In the DU patients eradication of *H. pylori* lowered basal acid output to 4.5 mmol/h at 1 month and to 2.5 mmol/h at 1 year ($p < 0.01$ for each versus pretreatment).

The above studies indicate that *H. pylori* infection produces a small increase in basal acid output in healthy volunteers and a greater increase in DU patients.

Maximal acid output

There are few adequately controlled studies examining the effect of *H. pylori* infection on maximal acid output. The only clear message is that eradication of *H. pylori* infection does not cause any early reduction in maximal acid output in DU patients[27,28]. There is a need for well-controlled studies with adequate numbers of patients comparing DU patients and healthy volunteers with and without *H. pylori*. In addition, studies are required of the longer-term effects of eradicating *H. pylori* on maximal acid output.

Intragastric acidity and 24 h pH

In 1988 we examined intragastric pH by means of *in situ* electrodes in 12 DU patients before and 1 month following eradication of the infection[33]. There was no overall change in the median intragastric pH. However, we noted that there was a significantly greater rise in pH in response to the buffering effect of the meals following eradication of the infection. This was consistent with reduced acid secretion in response to the meals. However, when we re-examined a smaller number of the subjects 7 months later, the changes were no longer significant[7]. Smith *et al.* found no difference in median 24 h intragastric acidity in a retrospective analysis comparing eight *H. pylori*-seropositive and 87 seronegative young healthy volunteers[34]. Eradication of the infection in the eight subjects did not produce any change in intragastric acidity when re-examined 1 month or 6 months later[35].

At present, therefore, the effect of *H. pylori* on intragastric acidity remains unclear. One problem with intragastric pH is that it is a relatively insensitive method of assessing changes in gastric acid secretion. This is partly due to its poor reproducibility. Fimmel *et al.* found that the day-to-day variation in median 24 h pH using *in situ* electrodes was in the region of 1 pH unit[36]. This variability can be explained by the fact that *in situ* electrodes can move within the gastric lumen and daytime pH varies by approximately 1 pH unit between the antrum and body[37]. In addition, alkaline reflux of duodenal contents or close contact between the electrode and mucosa can cause intermittent and marked rises in pH through the night[37]. Day-to-day variations in the order of 1 pH unit are a major problem, as this represents a 10-fold variation in hydrogen ion concentration. Another weakness of intragastric pH or acidity studies is that they only assess hydrogen ion concentration and not the volume of gastric juice secreted, which is a major determinant of acid output. These problems associated with intragastric acidity measurements are exemplified by the fact that ranitidine 300 mg, which markedly inhibits gastric acid secretion, may only increase median 24 h intragastric pH in DU subjects from 1.1 to 1.4, i.e. an increase of only 0.3 pH unit[38].

In view of the insensitivity of intragastric pH studies, the lack of consistent change following eradication of *H. pylori* in the small number of subjects examined to date in no way excludes a significant change in acid secretion.

ACID SECRETION IN RESPONSE TO GASTRIN-RELEASING PEPTIDE

Gastrin is the major mediator of meal-stimulated acid secretion[26] and therefore changes in acid secretion due to increased gastrin release should be most marked following a meal. Unfortunately, there is no simple means of measuring acid secretion in response to a meal under physiological conditions. Meal-stimulated acid secretion has been measured by means of constantly titrating the acid in the stomach to a predetermined value, but this blocks the physiological acid-inhibitory control mehanisms which could

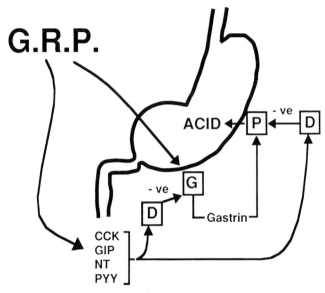

Fig. 2 Diagrammatic representation of the mechanism by which gastrin-releasing peptide (GRP) stimulates acid secretion. It stimulates the release of gastrin from antral G cells which then stimulates acid secretion by the parietal cells. GRP also stimulates the release of various hormones which exert inhibitory control on both the G cell and parietal cell. Many of these hormones exert their inhibitory effect by stimulating the release of somatostatin from D cells within the mucosa

be particularly important in *H. pylori*-associated disturbances of acid secretion.

In order to overcome some of the problems associated with the conventional methods available for assessing gastric acid secretion, and in an attempt partly to simulate the response to eating, we studied acid secretion in response to stimulation with gastrin-releasing peptide (GRP).

GRP is a neuropeptide present in nerves in the gastrointestinal tract and in particularly high concentrations in the gastric antrum. It is one of the major mediators by which food entering the stomach stimulates acid secretion[39]. The neuropeptide does this by stimulating the release of gastrin from G cells in the antral mucosa, and this hormone then circulates and in turn stimulates the parietal cells to secrete acid (Fig. 2). GRP thus stimulates acid secretion indirectly via stimulating gastrin release, and simulates the effect of food in the stomach. GRP also stimulates the release of other hormones which exert an inhibitory control on acid secretion, including somatostatin, cholecystokinin and gastric inhibitory peptide[40]. In this way GRP-stimulated acid secretion simulates acid secretion in response to an ingested meal.

We have recently examined the effect of *H. pylori* infection on gastrin release and acid secretion in response to stimulation with GRP administered intravenously at a rate of 40 pmol/kg per hour. Twenty-five *H. pylori*-negative

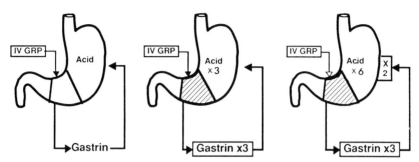

Fig. 3 Diagrammatic representation of the defects in GRP-stimulated acid secretion in *H. pylori*-positive healthy volunteers and DU patients. The increased acid responses fully resolve following eradication of the infection, though in the DU patients it takes up to 1 year to do so

healthy volunteers, 25 *H. pylori*-positive healthy volunteers and 25 *H. pylori*-positive DU patients were examined[29–31]. The *H. pylori*-positive healthy volunteers and DU patients were re-examined at 1 month following eradication of the infection and the DU patients again 1 year later.

Both the *H. pylori*-positive healthy volunteers and DU patients had a three-fold increased gastrin response to GRP compared to the *H. pylori*-negative healthy volunteers. This exaggerated gastrin response fully resolved in both groups within 1 month of eradication of the organism.

The acid output in the *H. pylori*-positive healthy volunteers was three times higher than that of the *H. pylori*-negative healthy volunteers, consistent with their three-fold increased gastrin response (Fig. 3). This increased acid response resolved within 1 month of eradication of the infection, again concomitant with resolution of the hypergastrinaemia.

The acid output in the *H. pylori*-positive DU patients was six times that of the *H. pylori*-negative healthy volunteers and twice that of the *H. pylori*-positive healthy volunteers (Fig. 3). The DU patients with *H. pylori* were therefore producing twice as much acid as the *H. pylori*-positive healthy volunteers despite both having a similar degree of hypergastrinaemia. At 1 month following eradication of *H. pylori* the acid output in the DU patients had fallen by 66%, but was still twice that of the *H. pylori*-negative healthy volunteers. By this time the gastrin levels in the DU patients were similar to those of the *H. pylori*-negative healthy volunteers and thus the DU patients were again producing twice the acid for the same level of gastrin. When the DU patients were re-examined at 1 year following eradication of *H. pylori* their acid response to GRP had completely normalized, representing a fall of 85%.

These studies indicate that DU patients with *H. pylori* have two disturbances in response to stimulation with GRP. The first is a three-fold increase in the gastrin response by the antral mucosa, which can be explained by the *H. pylori* infection, and which is similar to that seen in infected healthy volunteers. The second disturbance is an exaggerated acid response of the body of the stomach to gastrin stimulation, and which is not present in infected healthy volunteers. It is the combination of these two defects which causes six-fold increased acid response in the DU patients.

The cause of the second defect in the DU patients, i.e. the increased acid response to gastrin stimulation, is unclear. It could represent the increased parietal cell mass which is characteristic of DU patients[41]. This could be caused by the long-term trophic effects of *H. pylori*-associated hypergastrin-aemia on the oxyntic mucosa[42,43]. The fact that resolution of the second defect was slow would be consistent with it being due to resolution of an increased parietal cell mass, which would take considerable time due to the long half-life of these cells[44]. If this second defect is due to an increased parietal cell mass then it should be possible to see a corresponding fall in maximal acid output to pentagastrin. To date there are no published studies of the effect of eradication of the infection on maximal acid output in DU patients over the time period.

An alternative explanation for the increased acid response to gastrin stimulation seen in the DU patients during GRP stimulation is that it is due to impairment of the inhibitory pathways controlling the acid response to gastrin stimulation. In addition to stimulating gastrin release, GRP also stimulates the release of other peptides such as cholecystokinin and somato-statin which are known to inhibit the acid response to gastrin[40]. Failure of the inhibitory control would therefore produce an exaggerated response to gastrin. Somatostatin is an important mediator in the inhibitory control of parietal cell function and *H. pylori* infection has been reported to reduce somatostatin concentration in the antrum and thereby possibly explain the increased antral gastrin response[22,23]. It is possible that *H. pylori* infection might similarly be depleting somatostatin in the body of the stomach and thereby increasing the acid response to gastrin during GRP stimulation.

It is interesting to compare our recent findings using GRP with those of Hirschowitz *et al.* using the closely related peptide bombesin which exerts a similar biological effect[45]. They studied the gastrin and acid response in DU patients and healthy controls prior to the recognition of *H. pylori*. Acid output to bombesin was increased approximately three-fold in the DU patients. The exaggerated acid response was due to the combination of two defects: (1) increased antral gastrin release and (2) an increased acid response by the oxyntic mucosa to gastrin stimulation, which was most apparent at higher bombesin infusion rates. They concluded that the second defect was due to failure of an inhibitory control mechanism controlling the acid response to gastrin release. The findings by Hirschowitz *et al.* are thus very similar to our own. The fact that we have found a six-fold exaggerated acid response compared to their three-fold exaggerated response may be explained by the fact that we had a group of *H. pylori*-negative volunteers to define true normal, whereas a proportion of the 'normals' in the earlier study would have had an exaggerated response due to unrecognized *H. pylori* infection. Our own studies extend the work of Hirschowitz *et al.* by showing that the defects in acid regulation are secondary to *H. pylori* in that they fully resolve following eradication.

As already discussed, GRP-stimulated acid secretion simulates a meal in that it assesses the combined functional response of the antrum and body of the stomach, and also by the fact that it activates both stimulatory and inhibitory control pathways. However, it is clearly inappropriate to assume that a six-fold exaggerated response to GRP indicates a similarly exaggerated acid response to eating a meal. Other factors contribute to the acid response to a meal, including stimulation via the vagal nerve. In addition, food will initially predominantly activate the stimulatory pathways of acid secretion and only later, when it enters the small intestine, activate the inhibitory pathway. In contrast, the intravenous administration of GRP will *simultaneously* activate both the stimulatory and inhibitory pathways. The main message from the GRP findings is probably that there is a failure of an important inhibitory pathway regulating gastric acid secretion, and which probably normally exerts an effect on both gastrin release and acid response to gastrin. This inhibitory control is likely to be of particular importance in protecting the duodenum from excessive acid exposure.

Irrespective of its explanation, the fact that GRP-stimulated acid secretion is increased six-fold in DU patients, and completely differentiates DU patients from true normals, indicates that the defective control which it detects is likely to be an important factor in the pathogenesis of DU disease.

CONCLUSION

There is now consistent evidence that *H. pylori* infection causes increased gastrin release by the antral mucosa, and that this is due to biologically active G17. Initial studies of changes in acid secretion produced confusing results, largely due to the small size and inappropriate design of the studies and variations in selection of patients. More recent studies demonstrate a modest increase in basal acid output and GRP-stimulated acid response in infected healthy volunteers and marked increase in both basal and GRP-stimulated acid secretion in infected DU patients. More importantly, the increased acid secretion fully resolves following eradication of the infection, though it may take up to 1 year to do so. These findings suggest that disturbed regulation of gastric secretion may be an important mechanism by which *H. pylori* infection predisposes to DU disease.

SUMMARY

H. pylori infection causes a modest increase in basal serum gastrin concentrations and a more marked increase in gastrin stimulated by either a meal or by gastrin-releasing peptide (GRP). The degree of hypergastrinaemia is similar in DU patients and infected healthy volunteers. The increased circulating gastrin is due to an increase in the biologically active gastrin G17. Recent studies also indicate that the chronic infection is altering gastric acid secretion. In infected healthy volunteers it is associated with a small increase in basal and GRP-stimulated acid output, which can be explained by the increased gastrin, and which resolves within 1 month of eradication therapy. DU patients with *H. pylori* have a 6-fold increase in both basal and GRP-stimulated acid output, which is due to the combination of increased gastrin release and an increased acid response by the oxyntic mucosa to stimulation by gastrin. This increased acid secretion in the DU patients fully resolves following eradication of the infection, but takes up to 1 year to do so. This disturbed regulation of gastric secretion is likely to be an important mechanism by which *H. pylori* infection predisposes to duodenal ulceration.

References

1. Marshall BJ, Goodwin CS, Warren JR *et al.* Prospective double-blind trial of duodenal ulcer relapse after eradication of *Campylobacter pylori.* Lancet. 1988;2:1437–41.
2. Coghlan JG, Gilligan D, Humphries H *et al. Campylobacter pylori* and recurrence of duodenal ulcers – a 12 month follow-up study. Lancet. 1987;2:1109–11.
3. Rauws EAJ, Tytgat GNJ. Cure of duodenal ulcer associated with eradication of *Helicobacter pylori.* Lancet. 1990;335:1233–5.
4. Fiocca R, Solcia E, Santoro B. Duodenal ulcer relapse after eradication of *Helicobacter pylori.* Lancet. 1991;337:1614.
5. Hentschel E, Brandstatter G, Dragosics B *et al.* Effect of ranitidine and amoxycillin plus metronidazole on the eradication of *Helicobacter pylori* and the recurrence of duodenal ulcer. N Engl J Med. 1993;1:308–12.
6. Levi S, Beardshall K, Haddad G, Playford R, Ghosh P, Calam J. *Campylobacter pylori* and duodenal ulcers: the gastrin link. Lancet. 1989;1:1167–8.
7. McColl KEL, Fullarton GM, Chittajallu R *et al.* Plasma gastrin, daytime intragastric pH, and nocturnal acid output before and at 1 and 7 months after eradication of *Helicobacter pylori* in duodenal ulcer subjects. Scand J Gastroenterol. 1991;26(3):339–46.
8. Chittajallu RS, Ardill JES, McColl KEL. The degree of hypergastrinaemia induced by *Helicobacter pylori* is the same in duodenal ulcer patients and asymptomatic volunteers. Eur J Gastroenterol Hepatol. 1992;4:49–53.
9. Levi S, Beardshall K, Swift I *et al.* Antral *Helicobacter pylori*, hypergastrinaemia and duodenal ulcers: effect of eradicating the organism. BMJ. 1989;299:1504–5.
10. Graham DY, Opekum A, Lew GM, Evans DJ, Klein PD, Evans DG. Ablation of exaggerated meal-stimulated gastrin release in duodenal ulcer patients after clearance of *Helicobacter (Campylobacter) pylori* infection. Am J Gastroenterol. 1990;85(4):394–8.
11. Prewett EJ, Smith JTL, Nwokolo CU, Hudson M, Sawyerr AM, Pounder RE. Eradication of *Helicobacter pylori* abolishes 24-hour hypergastrinaemia: a prospective study in healthy subjects. Aliment Pharmacol Ther. 1991;5:283–90.
12. Graham DY, Opekun A, Lew GM, Klein PD, Walsh JH. *Helicobacter pylori*-associated exaggerated gastrin release in duodenal ulcer patients. Gastroenterology. 1991;100:1571–5.
13. Beardshall K, Moss S, Gill J, Levi S, Ghosh P, Playford RJ, Calam J. Suppression of *Helicobacter pylori* reduces gastrin releasing peptide stimulated gastrin release in duodenal ulcer patients. Gut. 1992;33:601–3.
14. Mulholland G, Ardill JES, Fillmore D, Chittajallu RS, Fullarton GM, McColl KEL. *Helicobacter pylori*-related hypergastrinaemia is due to a selective increase in gastrin 17. Gut. 1993;34:757–61.
15. Chittajallu RS, Neithercut WD, Madonald AMI, McColl KEL. Effect of increasing *Helicobacter pylori* ammonia production by urea infusion on plasma gastrin concentrations. Gut. 1991;32:21–4.
16. Nujumi AM El, Dorrian CA, Chittajallu RS, Neithercut WD, McColl KEL. Effect of inhibition of *Helicobacter pylori* urease activity by acetohydroxamic acid on serum gastrin in duodenal ulcer subjects. Gut. 1991;32:866–70.
17. Chittajallu RS, Dorrian CA, Neithercut WD, Dahill S, McColl KEL. Is *Helicobacter pylori*

associated hypergastrinaemia due to the bacterium's urease activity or the antral gastritis? Gut. 1991;32:1286–90.

18. Chittajallu RS, Neithercut WD, Ardill JES, McColl KEL. *Helicobacter pylori*-related hypergastrinaemia is not due to elevated antral surface pH. Studies with antral alkalinisation. Scand J Gastroenterol. 1992;27:218–22.

19. Moss SF, Ayesu K, Li SK, Calam J. pH dependent secretion of gastrin, acid and pepsin in duodenal ulcer disease: effect of suppressing *Helicobacter pylori*. Digestion. 1992;52:173–8.

20. Karnes WE Jr, Ohning GV, Sytnik B, Kim SWR, Walsh JH. Elevation of meal-stimulated gastrin release in subjects with *Helicobacter pylori* infection: reversal by low intragastric pH. Rev Infect Dis. 1991;13(Suppl. 8):S665–70.

21. Chittajallu RS, Howie A, McColl KEL. Effect of *Helicobacter pylori* on parietal cell sensitivity to pentagastrin in duodenal ulcer subjects. Scand J Gastroenterol. 1992;10: 857–63.

22. Moss SF, Calam J. Acid secretion and sensitivity to gastrin in patients with duodenal ulcer: effect of eradication of *Helicobacter pylori*. Gut. 1993;34:888–92.

23. Kaneko H, Nakada K, Mitsuma T *et al*. *Helicobacter pylori* infection induces a decrease in immunoreactive-somatostatin concentrations of human stomach. Dig Dis Sci. 1992;37(3):409–16.

24. Moss SF, Legon S, Bishop AE, Polak JM, Calam J. Effect of *Helicobacter pylori* on gastric somatostatin in duodenal ulcer disease. Lancet. 1992;340:930–2.

25. Graham DY, Lew GM, Lechago J. Antral G-cell and D-cell numbers in *Helicobacter pylori* infection: effect of *H. pylori* eradication. Gastroenterology. 1993;104:1655–60.

26. Kovacs TOG, Walsh JH, Maxwell V, Wong HC, Azuma T, Katt E. Gastrin is a major mediator of the gastric phase of acid secretion in dogs: proof by monoclonal antibody neutralization. Gastroenterology. 1989;97:1406–13.

27. Montbriand JR, Appelman HD, Cotner EK, Nostrant TT, Elta GH. Treatment of *Campylobacter pylori* does not alter gastric acid secretion. Am J Gastroenterol. 1989;84(12):1513–16.

28. Levi S, Beardshall K, Desa LA, Calam J. *Campylobacter pylori*, gastrin, acid secretion and duodenal ulcers. Lancet. 1989;2:613.

29. El-Omar E, Penman I, Dorrian CA, Ardill JES, McColl KEL. Eradicating *H. pylori* lowers gastrin-mediated acid secretion by 70% in DU patients and by 50% in healthy volunteers. Gastroenterology. 1993;104(Suppl.4):A75.

30. El-Omar E, Penman I, Ardill JES, McColl KEL. The exaggerated acid response to GRP in DU patients completely resolves following eradication of *H. pylori*. Gut. 1993;34(Suppl.4):S49.

31. El-Omar EM, Penman ID, Ardill JES, McColl KEL. The effect of *Helicobacter pylori* on acid secretion in healthy volunteers or duodenal ulcer patients (Submitted).

32. El-Omar E, Penman I, Ardill JES, McColl KEL. The GRP test – a new clinical test of acid secretion – reproducibility data. Gut. 1993;34(Suppl.1):G13.

33. McColl KEL, Fullarton GM, Nujumi AM, Macdonald AM, Brown IL, Hilditch TE. Lowered gastrin and gastric acidity after eradication of *Campylobacter pylori* in duodenal ulcer. Lancet. 1989;2:499–500.

34. Smith JTL, Pounder RE, Nwokolo CU *et al*. Inappropriate hypergastrinaemia in asymptomatic healthy subjects infected with *Helicobacter pylori*. Gut. 1990;31:522–5.

35. Prewett EJ, Smith JTL, Nwokolo CU, Hudson M, Sawyerr AM, Pounder RE. Eradication of *Helicobacter pylori* abolished 24-hour hypergastrinaemia: a prospective study in healthy subjects. Aliment Pharmacol Ther. 1991;5:283–90.

36. Fimmel CJ, Etienne A, Ciluffo T *et al*. Long-term ambulatory gastric pH monitoring: validation of a new method and effect of H_2-antagonists. Gastroenterology. 1985;88: 1842–51.

37. McLauchlan G, Fullarton GM, Crean GP, McColl KEL. Comparison of gastric body and antral pH: a 24 hour ambulatory study in healthy volunteers. Gut. 1989;30:573–8.

38. Merki HS, Witzel L, Walt RP *et al*. Comparison of ranitidine 300 mg twice daily, 300 mg at night and placebo on 24-hour intragastric acidity of duodenal ulcer patients. Aliment Pharmacol Ther. 1987;1:217–23.

39. Schubert ML, Coy DH, Makhloaf GM. Peptone stimulates gastrin secretion from the stomach by activating bombesin/GRP and cholinergic neurones. Am J Physiol.

1992;262:G685–9.

40. Ghatei MA, Jung RT, Stevenson JC *et al.* Bombesin: action on gut hormones and calcium in man. J Clin Endocrinol Metab. 1982;54:980–5.
41. Cox AJ. Stomach size and its relation to chronic peptic ulcer. Arch Pathol. 1952;54:407.
42. Willems G, Lehy T. Radioautographic and quantitative studies on parietal and peptic cell kinetics in the mouse. A selective effect of gastrin on parietal cell proliferation. Gastroenterology. 1975;69:416–26.
43. Crean GP, Marshall MW, Ramsey RDE. Parietal cell hyperplasia induced by the administration of pentagastrin (ICI 50, 123) to rats. Gastroenterology. 1969;57:147–55.
44. Ragins H, Wincze F, Liu SM, Dittbrenner M. The origin and survival of gastric parietal cells in the mouse. Anat Rec. 1968;162:99–110.
45. Hirschowitz BI, Tim LO, Helman CA, Molina E. Bombesin and G-17 dose responses in duodenal ulcer and controls. Dig Dis Sci. 1985;30(11):1092–103.

22
H. pylori, gastrin and somatostatin

J. CALAM, S. MOSS, N. TOKER and S. LEGON

INTRODUCTION

Helicobacter pylori causes duodenal ulcers (DU), and various lines of research are examining the roles of bacterial and host factors in this effect. We and others have examined whether the abnormalities of gastroduodenal physiology that were previously described in DU disease are actually due to *H. pylori* infection.

PATHOPHYSIOLOGY OF PEPTIC ULCER DISEASE

'Before' *H. pylori*, studies of the aetiology and treatment of DU concentrated on the associated abnormalities of acid secretion. Compared with controls, DU patients showed a trend to a greater maximal acid output (MAO), in response to histamine or pentagastrin. This was because they have more parietal cells[1,2]. In addition, DU patients were found to have abnormalities in the physiological control of acid secretion: basal acid was increased more than MAO[2], so the increase was not due solely to the greater parietal cell mass. Meal-stimulated acid output increased in line with MAO[2], but meal-stimulated acid secretion was inhibited less by a low intragastric pH than in controls[3] and, perhaps because of this, acid secretion persisted for longer after meals in DU patients[4]. Acid secretion was also inhibited less by gastric distension[5] and by intraduodenal fat[6] in DU patients. It is interesting to note that all of these abnormalities point to a defect in the inhibition of acid secretion.

Studies of the hormonal control of acid secretion focused on the antral acid-stimulating hormone gastrin. Inhibition of gastrin release by intragastric acid was also found to be decreased in DU patients[3]. Some studies showed increased peak postprandial plasma gastrin concentrations in DU patients v. controls[7]. Others did not, and in retrospect this probably depended on the prevalence of *H. pylori* in the control group. Somatostatin was discovered to be an important mediator of gastric inhibition, and studies showed that both the number of immunoreactive somatostatin cells and the amount of somatostatin peptide in gastric antral mucosa were diminished in DU disease[8].

GASTRIN AND SOMATOSTATIN: THE EFFECT OF *H. PYLORI*

Gastrin

Gastrin peptides are released from mucosal endocrine cells located in the gastric antrum, and to a lesser extent in the duodenum. Gastrin acts via the circulation to stimulate secretion of acid and pepsin from the gastric body and corpus. The two main forms in plasma are gastrin-17 and gastrin-34. Initial studies suggested that gastrin-17 is more potent than gastrin-34, but studies with high-quality synthetic peptides showed them to be equipotent on a molar basis[9]. Gastrin-34 has a longer plasma half-life, however. About 95% of gastrin in the antrum is gastrin-17, but about 60% of duodenal gastrin is gastrin-34[10].

In 1989 we showed that postprandial plasma gastrin concentrations were significantly higher in DU patients with a positive biopsy urease test for *H. pylori*, than in the few patients in whom the test was negative[11]. We and others confirmed the gastrin-releasing effect of *H. pylori* by demonstrating a decrease in gastrin release after eradication therapy[12]. It is now apparent that this infection increases gastrin release during fasting, after meals, and during stimulation with gastrin-releasing peptide[13] or its amphibian equivalent bombesin[14]. The increase in gastrin is predominantly due to a rise in gastrin-17, with no significant rise in gastrin-34[12,15], suggesting that excessive release is from gastric antrum, rather than the duodenum. This is consistent with the predominant location of bacteria in the antrum. We recently examined the inhibition of peptone-stimulated gastrin release by luminal acid in infected non-ulcer patients, and found that this reflex, which is known to be mediated via release of somatostatin, is significantly diminished[16].

Somatostatin

Somatostatin peptides are released from D cells in many organs of the body and all regions of the gastrointestinal tract, including the stomach. Somatostatin acts in a paracrine manner, inhibiting the activity of adjacent cells within each organ[17]. In the stomach, somatostatin acts as the final common pathway for several reflexes which inhibit gastrin release from G cells in the antrum[18], and acid secretion from parietal cells in the corpus[19]. D cells of the gastric antrum have apical microvilli and release somatostatin in response to luminal acid[20,21]. Antral D cells are also activated during fasting[22]. This is probably because the lumen is most acidic when the stomach is empty, with no food to buffer the acid. D cells of the gastric fundus are not in contact with the gastric lumen, but release somatostatin in response to neural reflexes, and hormones released by the small and large intestines. These include secretin which is released from the upper small intestine by

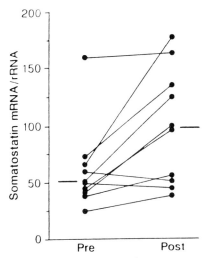

Fig. 1 The rise in the expression of somatostatin RNA in gastric antral mucosa on eradication of *H. pylori* from patients with duodenal ulcers. From ref. 25, with permission

luminal acid[23]. The various neural, hormonal and luminal factors which affect D-cell function have been reviewed by Yamada and Chiba[17].

We asked whether *H. pylori* infection attenuates the normal inhibition of gastric function by somatostatin. The rate of somatostatin release cannot be assessed by measuring circulating concentrations, because somatostatin is released in many organs and is destroyed locally[17]. However, studies in experimental animals showed that the rate of peptide release is reflected by the tissue concentration of the mRNA encoding it[24]. Therefore we measured somatostatin mRNA in extracts of endoscopic biopsies taken from DU patients before and 4 weeks after 'World Congress' triple therapy, which successfully eradicated *H. pylori*. Biopsies were taken from the gastric corpus on the midpoint of the greater curve, the gastric antrum 2 cm proximal from the pylorus on the greater curve, and the duodenal bulb avoiding any areas of ulceration or obvious inflammation. RNA was extracted and analysed by Northern blotting as described previously[25]. Control experiments have demonstrated that there is considerable variation in somatostatin mRNA levels between individual biopsies from the same region of a single patient. We find that it is necessary to take at least three biopsies per region to avoid unacceptable scatter in the results. Despite this, when small differences are being measured, some patients will inevitably show changes which appear to contradict the trend, and it is likely that much of this is due to variation in sampling. In the antrum, somatostatin mRNA levels rose significantly (median 1.9) on eradication of *H. pylori*[25] (Fig. 1). A similar increase of 2.1-fold was seen in the duodenal bulb (Fig. 2) but no significant change in somatostatin mRNA levels was seen after eradication in the gastric corpus (Fig. 3). Thus it appears that *H. pylori* inhibits expression of somatostatin similarly in the gastric antrum and duodenal bulb, but not at all in the

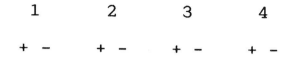

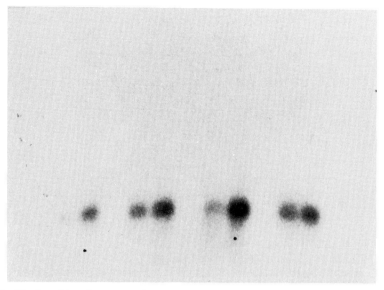

Fig. 2 Northern blot of somatostatin RNA in the duodenum of four patients with duodenal ulcers, before (+) and after (−) eradication of *H. pylori*. Somatostatin RNA/16S rRNA rose an average of 2.1-fold

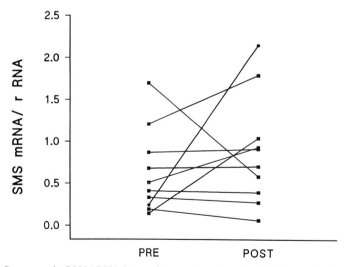

Fig. 3 Somatostatin RNA/rRNA in gastric corpus mucosa of patients with duodenal ulcers, before and after eradication of *H. pylori*. There was no significant change

gastric corpus of duodenal ulcer patients. This pattern of change reflects the typical distribution of H. pylori bacteria in these patients, with sparing of the gastric corpus[26]. Kaneko et al. have shown a decrease in mucosal somatostatin-like immunoreactivity in H. pylori-infected versus non-infected antral mucosa[27].

We found no change in gastrin RNA in the duodenal bulb or gastric antrum of duodenal ulcer patients after eradication of H. pylori. Therefore we wanted to investigate the relationship between gastrin RNA and circulating gastrin peptide, and did so by studying hypergastrinaemia patients with pernicious anaemia. Their plasma gastrin levels were 130 times normal but their gastrin RNA/rRNA ratio was only 6 times normal ($p < 0.02$). Therefore it is not surprising that the rise of about 3 times in circulating gastrin produced by H. pylori is not associated with a detectable change in antral gastrin RNA. Antral somatostatin RNA was about 40% of normal in patients with pernicious anaemia ($p < 0.05$)[28].

H. PYLORI AND GASTRIC ACID SECRETION

Do the hormonal changes that H. pylori produces actually lead to a change in gastric acid secretion? It has become apparent that this infection can have (at least) three different effects on acid secretion:

Suppression of acid secretion on first infection

Before the discovery of H. pylori clinical physiologists noted 'epidemic achlorhydria'; a condition transmitted by gastric intubation which results in the disappearance of acid secretion for a period of months. Retrospective serology and further work has shown that this phenomenon is actually due to first infection with H. pylori[29]. The mechanism is not established, but H. pylori releases at least one factor which suppresses parietal cell function[30]. Alternatively a factor released during the immunological response to infection might be responsible. In support of this, patients with other infections such as pneumonia also often develop transient achlorhydria[31]. Certain cytokines released from inflammatory cells, such as interleukin-1, can inhibit acid secretion[32].

Loss of acid secretory capacity through atrophic gastritis

Longitudinal epidemiological studies in Finland and Estonia indicate that the active superficial gastritis produced by H. pylori often progresses to atrophic gastritis[26]. Parietal cells may be lost initially by atrophy, and later by replacement of the gastric epithelium with intestinal-type mucosa through the process of intestinal metaplasia. If this occurs, H. pylori infection may eventually disappear, either because no gastric-type mucosa remains for the bacteria to adhere to, or because the intragastric pH becomes too high for the bacteria to survive[33]. Acid secretion is diminished if gastritis affects the acid-secreting parts of the stomach. This typically occurs in patients with gastric ulcers or cancers. If this were reversible one would expect a rise in maximal acid output after eradication of H. pylori from populations with atrophy, including older 'normal' people, but not in patients with duodenal ulcer disease who lack atrophy in the acid-secreting part of the stomach[26]. It is distinctly possible that the lack of atrophy seen in DU patients explains their tendency to have a greater parietal cell mass and maximal acid output than controls[1,2].

Increased acid secretion through altered physiological control

H. pylori infection has recently been shown to be associated with increased gastric acid secretion, particularly in DU patients, and at times when acid secretion would normally be inhibited by somatostatin release. Recently in Los Angeles we re-examined whether the failure of luminal acid to suppress peptone-stimulated acid secretion and gastrin release in DU patients, first observed in the same laboratory 18 years earlier[3], was actually due to H. pylori infection. We studied non-ulcer patients and found that a low pH did indeed inhibit peptone-stimulated acid secretion and gastrin release less in those infected with H. pylori[16]. Dr McColl's group report in the preceding chapter their interesting finding that H. pylori infection increases acid secretion in response to gastrin-releasing peptide[34]. It should be noted that these studies involved the measurement of acid secretion by aspiration. Under these conditions the intragastric pH is low, so somatostatin release would normally be stimulated. Furthermore gastrin-releasing peptide itself is a potent stimulator of somatostatin release, both in the antrum and in the acid-secreting region of the stomach[35]. Therefore it is interesting to speculate that this finding also reflects defective somatostatin release in H. pylori infection. We noted a significant fall in basal acid secretion on eradication of H. pylori from patients who had active duodenal ulcers[36]. The median rate of acid secretion fell from 8.3 to 2.6 mmol/h. The idea that H. pylori increases acid secretion during fasting is particularly interesting in view of the clinical correlation between duodenal ulcer disease and pain at night, which is the longest period of fasting, and the marked ulcer-healing effect of suppressing nocturnal acid secretion[37]. According to gastrin-17 : acid dose–response curves in the same patients, the fall in basal acid was attributable to a fall in basal gastrin. The sensitivity of parietal cells to gastrin-17 did not change after eradication of H. pylori[36]. However, when interpreting these results it is necessary to consider the findings of Achord[38]. He noted significantly higher basal acid output in DU patients with active versus inactive DU in a study without eradication of H. pylori, although the finding was not significant when patients acted as their own controls. Thus it is possible that ulcer healing contributes to decreased basal acid output following eradication of H. pylori from DU patients. This might occur if ulceration diminishes normal inhibitory duodenogastric reflexes.

MECHANISMS OF INCREASED HORMONE RELEASE

Antral alkalinization

We initially proposed that *H. pylori* increases gastrin release because ammonia, produced by the bacteria's urease, alkalinizes the antral microenvironment[11]. This would be expected to decrease expression of somatostatin[20,21], and could produce all of the other abnormalities of gastric physiology that have since been attributed to *H. pylori* infection, as explained above. A variety of findings have put this theory out of favour, but it cannot be regarded as disproved. This is firstly because we know so little about the responses of human D cells to their microenvironment, particularly over longer periods of time. Secondly we are ignorant of the pH in the antral pits where the D cells are located at different times of the day with and without *H. pylori* infection. Direct measurements of the pH of the surface gastric mucus layer in *H. pylori* infection have shown that it is indeed more alkaline, but only slightly so[39-41]. Increasing intragastric urea in infected individuals did not elevate gastrin[42], but would not necessarily be expected to do so because urease's K_m of 0.3[43] is below the normal intragastric concentration of urea, 1–2.5 mmol/L[42]. Thus the main change in ammonia production and any ensuing effect on gastrin might be expected to occur at lower, rather than higher, concentrations of urea. Inhibition of urease either using acetohydroxamic acid[44] or bismuth plus antibiotics[45] did not decrease gastrin release in short-term experiments. However it is not clear that urease was completely inhibited in the gastric pits. Urease there might be missed by the urea breath test. Some ammonia production persisted during the study with acetohydroxamic acid[44]. Also it is not clear how long it takes for the results of long-term alkalinization on endocrine cells to fully reverse. Acidification of achlorhydric stomachs leads to a fall in plasma gastrin, but levels remain well above the normal range for as long as measurements have been made[46].

The possible role of inflammatory mediators

Currently the most popular view is that the inflammatory mediators (cytokines) released in *H. pylori* gastritis cause the changes in endocrine cell function. This infection increases the release of all of the cytokines that have been measured so far; interleukins 1, 6 and 8, tumour necrosis factor-alpha, interferon-gamma and platelet-activating factor (PAF)[47-54]. Several studies have shown that different cytokines release gastrin from various antral preparations *in vitro*. These include interleukins 1 and 2, interferon-gamma and leukotrienes C_4 and D_4[55-58]. Our work with Andrew Soll used his preparation of canine antral endocrine cells in primary culture. Gastrin was released by diffusible products of human peripheral blood mononuclear cells (lymphocytes plus monocytes)[59], and by pure tumour necrosis factor-alpha and interferon-gamma[60]. A number of questions remain. Do the mononuclear cells act via these, or other cytokines? Are the D cells in the preparation involved in the response? How do these findings relate to the situation *in vivo*?

CONCLUSIONS

In conclusion, *H. pylori* infection suppresses expression of the inhibitory peptide somatostatin in the gastric antrum and duodenum. This leads to increased gastrin release and defects in the inhibition of acid secretion during fasting, and when the gastric lumen is acidic. Increased acid secretion under these circumstances may contribute to the ulcerogenic effect of *H. pylori*. However *H. pylori* also decreases acid secretion at other times; on first infection and perhaps also eventually by initiating gastric atrophy. It is not really clear how *H. pylori* infection effects endocrine cells. Cytokines may be involved, but the evidence for their involvement is indirect.

References

1. Soll AH. Duodenal ulcer and drug therapy. In: Sleisenger MH, Fordtran JS, editors. Gastrointestinal disease, 4th edn. Philadelphia: Saunders; 1989:814–79.
2. Blair AJ, Feldman M, Barnett C, Walsh JH, Richardson CT. Detailed comparison of basal and food-stimulated gastric acid secretion rates and serum gastrin concentrations in duodenal ulcer patients and normal subjects. J Clin Invest. 1987;79:582–7.
3. Walsh JH, Richardson CT, Fordtran JS. pH dependence of acid secretion and gastrin release in normal and ulcer subjects. J Clin Invest. 1975;55:462–8.
4. Malagelada JR, Longstreth GF, Deering TB, Summerskill WHJ, Go VLW. Gastric secretion and emptying after ordinary meals in duodenal ulcer. Gastroenterology. 1977;73:989–96.
5. Sjovall M, Lindstedt G, Olbe L, Lundell L. Defective inhibition of gastrin release by antral distension in duodenal ulcer patients. Digestion. 1992;51:1–9.
6. Kihl B, Olbe L. Inhibition of pentagastrin-stimulated gastric acid secretion by graded intraduodenal administration of oleic acid in man. Scand J Gastroenterol. 1981;16:121–8.
7. Taylor IL, Dockray GJ, Calam J, Walker RJ. Big and little gastrin responses to food in normal and ulcer subjects. Gut. 1979;20:957–62.
8. McHenry L, Vuyyuru L, Schubert ML. *Helicobacter pylori* and duodenal ulcer disease; the somatostatin link? (Selected summaries). Gastroenterology. 1993;104:1573–5.
9. Eysselein VE, Maxwell V, Reedy T, Wunsch E, Walsh JH. Similar potencies of synthetic big and little gastrins in man. J Clin Invest. 1984;73:1284–90.
10. Calam J, Dockray GJ, Walker RJ, Tracey HJ, Owens D. Molecular forms of gastrin in peptic ulcer: a comparison of serum and tissue concentrations of G17 and G34 in gastric and duodenal ulcer subjects. Eur J Clin Invest. 1980;10:241–7.
11. Levi S, Beardshall K, Playford R, Ghosh P, Haddad G, Calam J. *Campylobacter pylori* and duodenal ulcers: the gastrin link. Lancet. 1989;1:1167–8.
12. Moss SF, Calam J. *Helicobacter pylori* and peptic ulcers: the present position. Gut. 1992;33:289–92.
13. Beardshall K, Moss S, Gill J, Levi S, Ghosh P, Playford RJ, Calam J. Suppression of *Helicobacter pylori* reduces gastrin releasing peptide stimulated gastrin release in duodenal ulcer patients. Gut. 1992;33:601–3.
14. Graham DY, Opekun A, Lew GM, Klein PD, Walsh JH. *Helicobacter pylori*-associated exaggerated gastrin release in duodenal ulcer patients. The effect of bombesin infusion and urea ingestion. Gastroenterology. 1991;100(6):1571–5.
15. Mulholland G, Ardill JES, Fillmore D, Chittajallu RS, Fullarton GM, McKoll KEL. *Helicobacter pylori* related hypergastrinaemia is the result of a selective increase in gastrin 17. Gut. 1993;34:757–61.
16. Kovaks TOG, Sytnik B, Calam J, Walsh JH. *Helicobacter pylori* infection impairs pH

inhibition in non-duodenal ulcer subjects. Gastroenterology. 1993;104:A123.

17. Yamada T, Chiba T. Somatostatin. In: Makhlouf GM, editor. Handbook of physiology – the gastrointestinal system, Section 6, vol 2. Bethesda: American Physiological Society; 1989:431–53.
18. Karnick PS, Monahan SJ, Wolfe MM. Inhibition of gastrin gene expression by somatostatin. J Clin Invest. 1989;83:367–72.
19. Park J, Chiba T, Yamada T. Mechanism for direct inhibition of canine gastric pareital cells by somastostatin. J Biol Chem. 1987;262:14190.
20. Holst JJ, Jensen SL, Knuhtsen S, Nielsen OV, Rehfeld JF. Effect of vagus, gastric inhibitory peptide and HCl on gastrin and somatostatin release from perfused pig antrum. Am J Physiol. 1983;244:G515.
21. Brand SJ, Stone D. Reciprocal regulation of antral gastrin and somatostatin gene expression by omeprazole-induced achlorhydria. J Clin Invest. 1988;82:1059–66.
22. Wu V, Sumii K, Tari A, Sumii M, Walsh JH. Regulation of rat antral gastrin and somatostatin gene expression during starvation and after refeeding. Gastroenterology. 1991;101:1552–8.
23. Chiba T, Taminato T, Kadawaki S et al. Effects of glucagon, secretin and vasoactive intestinal polypeptide on gastric somatostatin and gastrin release from isolated perfused rat stomach. Gastroenterology. 1980;79:67–71.
24. Dockray GJ, Hamer C, Evans C, Varro A, Dimaline R. The secretory kinetics of the G-cell in omeprazole-treated rats. Gastroenterology. 1991;100:1187–94.
25. Moss SF, Legon S, Bishop AE, Polak JM, Calam J. Effect of Helicobacter pylori on gastric somatostatin in duodenal ulcer disease. Lancet. 1992;340:930–3.
26. Kekki M, Sipponen P, Siurala M. Progression of antral and body gastritis in active and healed duodenal ulcer and duodenitis. Scand J Gastroenterol. 1984;19:382–8.
27. Kaneko H, Nakada K, Mitsuma T et al. H. pylori infection induces a decrease in immunoreactive-somatostatin concentrations of the human stomach. Dig Dis Sci. 1992;37:409–16.
28. Moss SF, Legon S, Calam J. Reciprocal changes in antral gastrin and somatostatin in pernicious anaemia. Dig Dis Sci. 1993 (in press).
29. Graham DY, Alpert LC, Lacey-Smith J, Yoshimura HH. Iatrogenic Campylobacter infection is a cause of epidemic achlorhydria. Am J Gastroenterol. 1988;83:971–80.
30. Cave DR, Vargas M. Effect of a Campylobacter pylori protein on acid secretion by parietal cells. Lancet. 1989;2:187–9.
31. Hunt RH. Campylobacter pylori and spontaneous hypochlorhydria. In: Rathbone BJ, Heatley RV, editors. Campylobacter pylori and gastroduodenal disease. London: Blackwell Scientific; 1989:175–84.
32. Saperas-ES, Yang-H, Rivier C, Tache Y. Central action of recombinant interleukin-1 to inhibit acid secretion in rats. Gastroenterology. 1990;99:1599–606.
33. Fong TL, Dooley CP, Dehesa M et al. Helicobacter pylori infection in pernicious anaemia: a prospective controlled study. Gastroenterology. 1991;100:328–32.
34. El-Omar E, Penman I, Dorrian CA, Ardill JES, McColl KEL. Eradicating Helicobacter pylori infection lowers gastrin-mediated acid secretion by two-thirds in duodenal ulcer patients. Gut. 1993;34:1060–5.
35. Schubert ML, Jong MJ, Maklouf GM. Bombesin/GRP-stimulated somatostatin secretion is mediated by gastrin in the antrum and intrinsic neurons in the fundus. Am J Physiol. 1991;261:G885–90.
36. Moss SF, Calam J. Acid secretion and sensitivity to gastrin in duodenal ulcer patients: effect of eradication of H. pylori. Gut. 1993;34:888–92.
37. Khasawneh-SM, Affarah-HB. Morning versus evening dose: a comparison of three H2-receptor blockers in duodenal ulcer healing. Am J Gastroenterol. 1992;87:1180–2.
38. Achord JL. Gastric pepsin and acid secretion in patients with acute and healed duodenal ulcer. Gastroenterology. 1981;81:15–20.
39. Beardshall K, Adamson D, Gill J, Unwin R, Calam J. Helicobacter pylori raises the pH of the juxta epithelial region of the mucus layer of the gastric antrum and body. Gut. 1991;32:A569.
40. Kelly SM, Crampton J, Hunter JO. Helicobater pylori increases the pH of the gastric mucosa in vivo. Gut. 1990;31:A1177–78(abstract).

41. Odera G, Kuvidi M, Garbo G et al. Antral and fundic surface mucosal pH in children with and without Helicobacter pylori. Gut. 1993;34:S36.
42. Chittajallu RS, Neitherdutt WD, Macdonald AMI, McColl KEL. Effect of increasing Helicobacter pylori ammonia production by urea infusion on plasma gastrin concentrations. Gut. 1991;32:21–4.
43. Dunn BE, Campbell GP, Perez Perez GI, Blaser MJ. Purification and characterization of urease from Helicobacter pylori. J Biol Chem. 1990;256(16):9464–9.
44. El Nujumi AM, Dorian CA, Chitajallu RS, Neithercut WD, McColl KEL. Effect of inhibition of H. pylori urease activity by acetohydroxamic acid on serum gastrin in duodenal ulcer subjects. Gut. 1991;32:866–70.
45. Chittajallu RS, Dorrian CA, Neithercut WD, Dahill S, McColl KEL. Is Helicobacter pylori-associated hypergastrinaemia due to the bacterium's urease activity or the antral gastritis? Gut. 1991;32:1286–90.
46. Fahrenkrug J, Schaffalitzky de Muckadell OB, Hornum I, Rehfeld JF. The mechanism of hypergastrinemia in achlorhydria. Effect of food, acid, and calcitonin on serum gastrin concentrations and component pattern in pernicious anemia, with correlation to endogenous secretin concentrations in plasma. Gastroenterology. 1976;71(1):33–7.
47. Blaser MJ. Hypothesis on the pathogenesis and natural history of Helicobacter pylori-induced inflammation. Gastroenterology. 1992;102:720–7.
48. Crabtree JE, Shallcross TM, Heatley RV, Wyatt JI. Mucosal tumour necrosis factor alpha and interleukin-6 in patients with Helicobacter pylori associated gastritis. Gut. 1991;32:1473–7.
49. Gupta R, Moss S, Thomas DM, Abbott F, Rees A, Calam J. Helicobacter pylori increases release of interleukin-8: a potent attractant of neutrophils. Gut. 1991;32:A1206.
50. Crabtree JE, Peichl P, Wyatt JI, Lindley IJ. Gastric interleukin-8 and anti-interleukin-8 IgA antibodies in Helicobacter pylori infection. Ir J Med Sci. 1992;161(Suppl. 10):20.
51. Atherton JC, Hudson N, Hale TL, Kirk GE, Spiller RC, Hawkey CJ. Interleukin-1B in gastric biopsy samples: relationship with inflammation and epithelial hyperplasia. Ir J Med Sci. 1992;161(Suppl. 10):57.
52. Nouch LA, Bosma NB, Jansen JE. Mucosal interleukin-1B and interleukin-8 production in patients with Helicobacter pylori infection. Ir J Med Sci. 1992;161(Suppl. 10):57.
53. Fan XJ, Chua CN, Shahi CN et al. Tumour necrosis factor-alpha and gamma-interferon production by patients with Helicobacter pylori. Ir J Med Sci. 1992;161(Suppl.10):58.
54. Denizot Y, Sobbani J, Rambaud JC, Lewin M, Thomas Y, Beneveniste J. Paf acether synthesis by Helicobacter pylori. Gut. 1990;31:1242–5.
55. Teichmann RK, Grab PJ, Hammer C, Brendel W. Gastrin release by interleukin-2 and gamma-interferon in vitro. Can J Phys Pharm. 1986;64(Suppl.):62.
56. Teichmann RK, Kramling HJ, Merle Y, Merkle R. Opposite effects of interleukin-1 on gastrin and bombesin release in cell suspensions of antral mucosa. Digestion. 1990;46(Suppl.1):114.
57. Teichmann RK, Utz E, Becker HD. Leukotrienes release gastrin and somatostatin from human antral mucosa in vitro. Digestion. 1990;46(Suppl.1):114.
58. Weigert N, Stolley S, Schusdziarra V, Calssen M, Schepp W. Interleukin-1B but not leukotriene-B4 stimulates gastrin release from rat antral G-cells in primary culture. Ir J Med Sci. 1992;161(Suppl.10):55.
59. Golodner EH, Territo MC, Walsh JH, Soll AH. Stimulation of gastrin release from cultured canine G cells by Helicobacter pylori and mononuclear cells. Gastroenterology. 1992;102:A630.
60. Golodner EH, Soll AH, Walsh JH, Calam J. Release of gastrin from cultured canine G-cells by interferon-gamma and tumour necrosis factor-alpha. Gastroenterology. 1993;104:A89.

23
Parietal cell responsiveness in *H. pylori* infections

D. R. CAVE

INTRODUCTION

Until 1983[1] the gastric mucosa was considered a sterile environment except for swallowed organisms. Since then *Helicobacter pylori* has been shown to colonize the gastric mucosa of a substantial proportion of the world's population, despite the hostile nature of the gastric environment. *H. pylori* is able to maintain long-term infection, and it has a predilection for the antral mucosa, where it is nearly always detectable. The body and fundic mucosa are also frequently colonized. The strategies that it employs to do this in the long term include production of NH_3 and chloramine[2] produced by the hydrolysis of readily available urea by its urease. The production of these alkaline substances helps to neutralize the local acidic environment. It has the ability to reside close to the epithelial cell surface sometimes adherent and sometimes free in the mucus at a pH that is believed to be near neutral. The organism has also been seen within the canalicular system of the parietal cell[3]. However, it also appears to be associated with the ability to profoundly alter parietal cell function for long periods. The data supporting this contention are still incomplete, but the voluntary ingestion of *H. pylori* by Morris and Nicholson[4] provided an insight into the early natural history of this organism. Spontaneous achlorhydria has often been reported in young people[5,6]. These reports are clearly not to be confused with reports of achlorhydria in pernicious anaemia, since the parietal cells are present and intact, in the presence of *H. pylori*.

The reasons why *H. pylori* should need to induce this state are speculative. The delay from onset of infection to achlorhydria in humans[4] and ferrets[7] suggests that the effect is unrelated to the early mechanisms of infection. The achlorhydria may provide an opportunity for the organism to be passed via the faeces without it being destroyed by acid degradation, thereby acting as a spreading mechanism. It is during this achlorhydric phase that Fox *et al.*[8] were able to recover *H. mustelae* from ferret faeces. There is one report of the recovery of viable *H. pylori* from the faeces, but in none of these individuals was any study done on acid secretion[9].

This chapter reviews the clinical and experimental data related to *Helicobacter* infection that suggest that it has developed a specific mechanism to reduce or eliminate acid secretion early in the natural history of infection.

CLINICAL OBSERVATIONS

In 1958 Spiro and Schwartz[5] reported on eight individuals with gastritis who produced little if any acid as judged by measurement of gastric pH. One of these was noted to have returned to normal acid secretion after 2 months and another, when tested 2 years later, had also returned to normal. One explanation offered for this was that necrotic cells blocked the gastric glands, thereby preventing egress of gastric acid. More recently, Barthels *et al.*[6] have looked at the prevalence of *H. pylori* in completely asymptomatic volunteers (in the 20–30-year age group). An unexpected finding in this age group was that 25% of the *H. pylori*-positive volunteers were also achlorhydric. They were otherwise completely healthy and on no medication. There have been several reports of epidemics of hypochlorhydria. The best-defined study was reported by Ramsey *et al.*[10]. In retrospect these cases appear to have been caused by *H. pylori*, possibly transmitted via a non-sterile pH probe. Fourteen out of 34 healthy volunteers developed achlorhydria that lasted from 50 to 250 days, and an additional three did not recover secretion within 1 year of follow-up. All of the volunteers developed a gastritis that contained a neutrophil infiltrate. The authors speculated that an infectious agent was involved, but were unable to find a viral or bacterial cause. Of particular note is that they performed studies of gastric permeability. The results of these were normal, implying that increased back-diffusion of hydrogen ion was not the cause of the reduced basal and peak acid secretion. Furthermore they noted that the parietal cell population was normal and intact without any evidence for loss of parietal cell mass. Despite the very low acid secretion, gastrin levels were only mildly increased. The volunteer study by Morris and Nicholson[4] provides additional clues as to the mechanism of the reduced acid secretion. Morris, after the ingestion of an isolate of *H. pylori* from a woman with chronic gastritis, developed a brief illness consisting of abdominal pain and vomiting for 2 days. By day 8 after ingestion he had developed a severe gastritis and had become achlorhydric. This state persisted for 25 days after ingestion. At that point he took an antibiotic to try to eradicate the infection. Doxycyline 100 mg **BID** did not eradicate *H. pylori* infection or heal the gastritis, but acid secretion returned to normal. This could be interpreted as the antibiotic somehow being able to turn off a factor produced by *H. pylori* that was inhibiting the parietal cells. The infection persisted despite the sequential use of four different antimicrobials. The organism was finally eradicated with triple therapy, and the gastritis resolved.

A serendipitous observation by Graham *et al.*[11] in a volunteer undergoing testing for the effects of aspirin on the gastric mucosa provides further clues. The volunteer had had several baseline studies performed, and then developed abdominal pain and nausea. Initially the individual showed increases in basal acid secretion, mucus output, pepsin secretion, DNA loss and bleeding. After 8 days acid secretion ceased, coincident with the development of gastritis spreading from the antrum to the body and fundus. Acid secretion slowly started to recover spontaneously at about 2 months after the acute event, and was normal 6 months later.

Wiersinga and Tytgat[12] reported a patient with Zollinger-Ellison syndrome who, in the middle of the evolution of his disease, suddenly lost his ability to secrete acid. They found that he had suddenly, during the course of an acute febrile gastroenteric illness, developed an acute gastritis with a polymorphonuclear cell infiltrate. Initially this was florid, but subsequently it diminished to a mild chronic gastritis. He remained profoundly hypo-chlorhydric despite well-documented evidence for the continued presence of the tumour, which in turn continued to secrete high levels of gastrin. At the time of this report *H. pylori* was unknown. However, the histology is consistent with a gastritis caused by this organism. A similar case is alluded to by Ramsey *et al.*[10].

These observations have led to a search for specific moieties produced by *H. pylori* and other *Helicobacter* species that could alter parietal cell function without overt parietal cell injury.

LABORATORY EVIDENCE FOR PARIETAL CELL INHIBITION

Cave and Vargas[13] reported that *H. pylori*, as a whole bacterium or as sonicates, was able to inhibit acid secretion in isolated gastric glands as measured by the retention of [^{14}C]aminopyrine in parietal cells. The effect took 2 h to reach a maximal level. Pretreatment of the sonicate with pronase abolished the effect, but treatment with trypsin, a more specific proteolytic enzyme, had no effect. This was interpreted as the inhibitor being protein-aceous in nature. The medium in which the bacteria were grown had no inhibitory effect until it was concentrated 10-fold, when near-complete acid inhibition occurred. There was no loss of activity of the inhibitor on dialysis, which suggested that the factor was too large to pass a 12 kDa cut-off membrane. Dilution experiments suggested that the inhibitor is present in low concentrations. Using $1 \times 10^{8.5}$ c.f.u./ml of *H. pylori*, they showed half the activity was gone at a 1:5 dilution and all activity had disappeared at a 1:10 dilution.

Defize *et al.*[14] reported inhibition of acid secretion by whole *H. pylori* with the [^{14}C]aminopyrine assay system, but using guinea pig gastric glands instead of rabbit glands. Subsequently, Jalanowski *et al.*[15] have shown that *H. pylori* will also inhibit acid secretion from isolated human gastric glands obtained from surgically resected specimens.

Fox *et al.*[7] have established the ferret (*Mustelae putorius furo*) infected with *H. mustelae* as a good comparative model of *H. pylori* infection in humans. A gastritis develops with some but not all the features of the condition in humans. They have recently reported that about 4 weeks after infection, four of four ferrets infected had impaired acid secretion for 2 weeks.

Their gastric pH was elevated to 4–5.2. The authors subsequently speculated that during this period *H. mustelae* could be cultured from the stool, but not at other times[8]. Similar observations were made in Beagle dogs using *H. felis* as the infecting organism. In this model two of five Beagles showed an elevation of pH to 6.4 at 5 weeks post-infection. Control animals had a pH in the 2–3.6 range[16].

Hoffman *et al.*[17] showed that the same isolates of *H. pylori* were able to inhibit acid secretion in both rabbit and ferret gastric glands. Furthermore the use of *H. felis* and *H. mustelae*, tested in the same way, showed that these too could cause inhibition of both systems. These data suggest that at least three species of *Helicobacter* are able to inhibit a variety of mammalian parietal cells *in vivo* or *in vitro*.

CHARACTERIZATION OF THE ACID INHIBITOR(S)

Initial characterization of the acid inhibitor produced by *H. pylori* suggested that it is a protein. Its mechanism of action has been investigated in a preliminary way. Cimetidine was used to inhibit acid secretion as measured by the $[^{14}C]$aminopyrine assay when rabbit gastric glands were stimulated by 8-bromo-cyclic AMP. It failed to do this, whereas *H. pylori* sonicates effectively did so. This was interpreted as *H. pylori* acting at a site other than the histamine-2 receptor. Review of individual data in the rabbit parietal cell assay shows that *H. pylori* is able to reduce acid secretion below basal levels. This in turn suggests the inhibition involves the final common pathway of secretion, as none of the current receptor blocking agents can do this. Protein synthesis was used to demonstrate that there was no toxic effect to the gastric glands during the incubation period, suggesting that the effect was physiological rather than toxic in nature[13].

Further characterization studies have shown that there are at least two inhibitory factors produced by *H. pylori*[18]. The second factor came to light when it became apparent that there was residual acid inhibitory activity after pronase treatment of the *H. pylori* sonicates. This activity was heat-stable, it withstood boiling, whereas the protein was inactivated by this treatment. Filtration experiments suggest that it is of small size, 1–2 kDa as compared with > 12 kDa for the inhibitory protein.

The second factor has been shown to be soluble in organic solvents such as benzene and toluene and insoluble in water. This has made progress very slow as the bioassay systems require the factor to be tested to be in aqueous solution. However, we have used gastric epithelial cell vesicles containing the H^+,K^+-ATPase as an additional assay for biological activity of crude sonicates[19]. The 'inside-out' vesicles have been used in three ways. Firstly we measured the effect of the sonicate on the rate of hydrolysis of ATP as an indicator of ATPase activity. Unexpectedly, the rate of hydrolysis, as measured by the release of phosphate, increased. This suggests that the H^+,K^+-ATPase is not inhibited, and that the explanation for the reduced acid secretion lies elsewhere. Secondly, the vesicles were incubated in a buffer containing acridine orange and placed in a fluorimeter. The addition of valinomycin allowed H^+ in the buffer to gain entry into the vesicles. This shift is associated with a reduction of fluorescence of the acridine orange. After a period of stabilization a sonicate of *H. pylori* was added. This allowed a dose-dependent release of H^+ back into the medium with a consequent increase in fluorescence. We interpreted this as either disruption of the vesicles or their permeabilization. In order to resolve this issue we treated the vesicles with albumin to remove any putative ionophore, and then retested the vesicles with valinomycin; they behaved in an identical fashion to the first experiment. These data taken together suggest that the second inhibitor is an ionophore, at least for H^+ and K^+. The factor is hydrophobic and has a solubility profile similar to, but different from, nigericin, a similar hydrophobic H^+/K^+ ionophore.

CONCLUSIONS

It is clear from clinical observations and from animal studies that *Helicobacter* species can inhibit secretion without destroying parietal cells. However, the effect is short-lived compared with the natural history of infection. In addition the inhibition often starts in humans at the time of a florid gastritis and persists at least until a chronic gastritis is established. A polymorphonuclear cell infiltrate is present during and after the recovery of acid secretion, making it unlikely that a neutrophil-associated cytokine is involved. A plausible explanation is as follows: *H. pylori* produces a water-soluble protein, soon after infection is initiated, that is able to completely inhibit acid secretion. This factor is produced until an environmental factor switches it off, e.g. doxycycline in the case reported by Morris and Nicholson. The isolate we have worked with in the laboratory eventually switched itself off on serial passage. The second factor, the ionophore, is constitutively expressed by the organism and acts only locally. Its insolubility in the aqueous phase necessitates direct delivery to the cell membrane for it to work. The local production of such a molecule could account for the survival of *H. pylori* within the canalicular system of a parietal cell, or deep in a gastric pit where there is little protective mucus. This local inhibition of secretion with relatively few organisms present on the fundic or body mucosa would have little impact on overall acid secretion and would be typical of most long-term chronic infections with *H. pylori*.

References

1. Marshall B. Unidentified curved bacilli on gastric epithelium in active chronic gastritis. Lancet. 1983;1:1273–5.
2. Hazell SL, Lee A. *Campylobacter pyloridis*, urease, hydrogen ion back diffusion and gastric ulcers. Lancet. 1986;1:15–17.
3. Chen XG, Correa P, Offerhaus J *et al.* Ultrastructure of the gastric mucosa harboring *Campylobacter*-like organisms. Am J Clin Pathol. 1986;86:575–82.
4. Morris A, Nicholson G. Ingestion of *Campylobacter pyloridis* causes gastritis and raises fasting gastric pH. Am J Gastroenterol. 1987;3:192–9.
5. Spiro H, Schwartz RD. Superficial gastritis. A cause of temporary achlorhydria and

hyperpepsinemia. N Engl J Med. 1958;259:682–4.

6. Barthel JS, Westblom AD, Havey F *et al.* Gastritis and *Campylobacter pylori* in healthy asymptomatic volunteers. Arch Intern Med. 1988;148:1149–51.

7. Fox JG, Otto H, Taylor NS *et al. Helicobacter mustelae* induced gastritis and elevated gastric pH in the ferret (*Mustela putorius furo*). Infect Immun. 1991;59:1875–80.

8. Fox JG, Paster BJ, Dewhirst FE *et al. Helicobacter mustelae* isolation from feces of ferrets: evidence to support fecal oral transmission of a gastric *Helicobacter*. Infect Immun. 1992;60:606–11.

9. Thomas JE, Gibson GR, Darboe MK *et al.* Isolation of *Helicobacter pylori* from human feces. Lancet. 1992;2:1194–5.

10. Ramsey EJ, Carey KV, Peterson WL *et al.* Epidemic gastritis with hypochlorhydria. Gastroenterology. 1979;76:1449–57.

11. Graham DY, Alpert LC, Smith JL *et al.* Iatrogenic *Campylobacter pylori* infection is a cause of epidemic achlorhydria. Am J Gastroenterol. 1988;83:974–80.

12. Wiersinga WM, Tytgat GN. Clinical recovery owing to target parietal cell failure in a patient with Zollinger-Ellison syndrome. Gastroenterology. 1977;73:1413–17.

13. Cave DR, Vargas M. Effect of *Campylobacter pylori* protein on acid secretion by parietal cells. Lancet. 1989;2:187–9.

14. Defize J, Goldie J, Hunt RH. Inhibition of acid production by *Campylobacter pylori* in isolated guinea pig parietal cells. Gastroenterology. 1989;96:A114.

15. Jablonowski H, Kramer N, Hengels KJ. Effect of *Helicobacter pylori* on acid secretion by isolated human gastric glands. Gastroenterology. 1991;100:A90.

16. Lee A, Krakowka S, Fox JG *et al.* Role of *Helicobacter felis* in chronic canine gastritis. Vet Pathol. 1992;29:487–94.

17. Hoffman JS, King WW, Taylor NS *et al.* Ferret and rabbit parietal cell inhibition is a property common to *Helicobacter* species. Gastroenterology. 1991;100:A84.

18. Cave DR, King WW, Hoffman J. Production of two chemically distinct acid inhibitory factors produced by *H. pylori*. Eur J Gastroenterol Hepatol. 1993;5(Suppl.):23–7.

19. King WW, Yu W, Hoffman J *et al.* Inhibition of parietal cell function by a pore forming factor produced by *Helicobacter pylori*. Gastroenterology. 1992;102:A646.

24
Role of bacterial amines in *H. pylori*-associated hypergastrinaemia

B. E. DUNN

INTRODUCTION

Increasing evidence suggests that *Helicobacter pylori* plays an important role in the pathogenesis of duodenal ulcer disease. The bacterium is present in the gastric antrum in over 90% of individuals with duodenal ulcer[1,2], and eradication of the organism decreases recurrence of duodenal ulcers significantly[3,4]. However, the pathogenic mechanisms whereby *H. pylori* infection predisposes to formation of duodenal ulcer disease are not known with certainty[5]. Possible mechanisms include: (1) disruption of the mucosal barrier by bacterial products such as ammonia, cytotoxin and phospholipase A_2[6-8]; (2) enhancement of aggressive factors such as acid, pepsin and platelet-activating factor[9,10]; (3) activation of monocytes and macrophages by release of cytokines such as tumour necrosis factor, interleukin 1 and reactive oxygen metabolites[11]; (4) immune crossreactivity between *H. pylori* and gastric tissue[12]; and (5) enhanced release of gastrin[13], possibly resulting in increased production of acid and/or pepsin.

Recent studies suggest that the hypergastrinaemia observed in patients with duodenal ulcer is probably due to infection with *H. pylori*. *H. pylori* infection is associated with increased basal as well as bombesin-, gastrin-releasing peptide- and meal-stimulated gastrin secretion, all of which are decreased after eradication of the bacterium[14-16].

The mechanisms whereby *H. pylori* might enhance secretion of gastrin include: (1) direct effect(s) of the bacterium or secreted products such as ammonia, amines or peptides directly on gastric G cells[17,18]; (2) elevation of antral surface pH with interference with the normal feedback inhibition of gastrin secretion by intragastric acid[13,19]; (3) compensatory response to reduced parietal cell sensitivity to gastrin[20,21]; (4) production of cytokines by the gastric inflammatory infiltrate[22,23]; and (5) inhibition of somatostatin secretion[24,25]. Somatostatin is produced by D cells present in the gastric mucosa. D cells are located in proximity to G cells (which produce gastrin) in the antrum and in proximity to parietal cells (which produce acid) in the

Classes of amines:

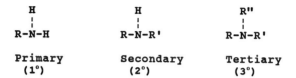

Examples of amines:

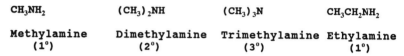

Fig. 1   Classes of amines and examples of each class

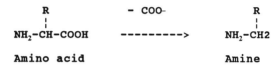

Fig. 2   Schematic diagram of amino acid decarboxylation to form primary amines

fundus. Somatostatin exerts an inhibitory paracrine effect on secretion of gastrin and gastric acid[26].

The focus of this discussion is on possible direct effects of bacterial amines on gastrin secretion by G cells. In this regard three questions come to mind: (1) Is there evidence that amines induce secretion of gastrin from G cells? (2) Does *H. pylori* produce amines *in vivo* or *in vitro*? (3) Does production of amines or ammonia by *H. pylori* account for the observed hypergastrinaemia observed in *H. pylori*-infected individuals?

PROPERTIES OF AMINES

An amine is an organic molecule which has the general formula RNH_2, R_2NH, or R_3N, where R is any alkyl or aryl group[27]. When a fourth substituent is bonded to the nitrogen the species is positively charged and called a quaternary ammonium ion[27]. Amines are classified as primary, secondary or tertiary according to the number of groups attached to the nitrogen atom. Figure 1 shows the structure of three classes of amines. Also shown are representative amines including methylamine in which R is a methyl group; dimethylamine and trimethylamine in which two and three methyl groups are present, respectively; and ethylamine, a primary amine in which R is an ethyl group. In many bacteria, decarboxylation of amino acids to form the corresponding primary amines is known to occur[28] (see Fig. 2).

Amines are basic molecules that will accept hydrogen ions (H^+) depending upon the pH of the environment[27]. At a pH below the pK_a of the particular amine the majority of the molecule is present in the protonated state. Above the pK_a the majority of the amine is present in the non-ionized form. Uncharged amines are highly lipid-soluble in nature and will freely diffuse across biological membranes. In contrast, protonated amines are insoluble in lipid and do not diffuse freely across biological membranes[29].

IS THERE EVIDENCE THAT AMINES INDUCE SECRETION OF GASTRIN BY G CELLS?

Lichtenberger *et al.* investigated the chemical constituents responsible for initiating the gastrin secretory response to a meal[29]. Specifically, these authors investigated the role of amino acid metabolites in the regulation of gastrin release. When standard rat chow was lyophilized under alkaline conditions, both ammonia and amines were volatilized and removed by condensation in a cold trap. The normal postprandial release of gastrin was found to be reduced by about 50% when rats consumed lyophilized chow with a reduced content of ammonia and amines. Addition of the crude condensate back to the chow restored meal-induced gastrin secretion to normal levels[29]. Analysis of the condensate by thin-layer chromatography revealed ammonia and four aliphatic amines: methylamine, ethylamine, dimethylamine and an unidentified amine. When lyophilized chow was supplemented, in separate experiments, to $100 \mu mol/g$ of diet with either ammonium chloride, methylamine, ethylamine or dimethylamine, serum gastrin levels increased significantly[29]. In addition, ammonia, methylamine, ethylamine and dimethylamine were shown significantly to stimulate release of gastrin from isolated rat G cells. These studies were among the first to demonstrate that dietary amines and ammonia play a key role in initiating the gastrin secretory response, and are capable of stimulating the release of gastrin from isolated G cells[29].

Subsequently, Lichtenberger and colleagues used three model systems to investigate the pH-dependence of meal-stimulated gastrin release and the permeability of the antral mucosa to dietary amines[30]. Ingestion by rats of standard chow resulted in elevated levels of gastrin and ammonia in plasma; pre-acidification of chow to pH 2.4 abolished the postprandial increases in plasma ammonia and gastrin. In separate experiments, uptake in rodent antral mucosa of quinacrine, a complex fluorescent cyclic amine, was inhibited in a stepwise fashion as pH was decreased. In addition, transport of [^{14}C]methylamine into canine antral mucosa isolated in Ussing chambers was pH-dependent, as was gastrin release. Based on these experiments it was suggested that meal-stimulated gastrin release is inhibited at low pH, in part due to protonation of dietary amines (rendering them less soluble in biological membranes), thus preventing their diffusion into G cells to stimulate gastrin secretion. Thus, amine trapping may help to explain the inhibitory effect of gastric acidity on the postprandial release of gastrin[30].

DelValle and Yamada[31] studied the effects of amino acids and amines on gastrin release from isolated G cells. In their experiments, canine gastric antral G cells were enriched by treatment with collagenase, filtration and elutriation. After 42–46 h of culture, $25 \pm 2\%$ of remaining viable cells were identified as G cells by immunohistochemistry. The remainder of the cells were identified as mucus cells and fibroblasts. These authors found that amino acids and, more potently, their corresponding amines, directly stimulated gastrin release. Amino acid-stimulated secretion of gastrin was unaffected by a variety of decarboxylase inhibitors, suggesting that the amino acids *per se* were capable of the stimulatory effect without being converted to amines. Amino acid-stimulated gastrin secretion was enhanced by bombesin; isobutylmethylxanthine, which is an inhibitor of phosphodiesterase; and dibutyryl cAMP. Somatostatin inhibited amino acid-stimulated gastrin release via a pertussis toxin-sensitive GTP-binding protein. In contrast, gastrin secretion induced by amines was unaffected by any of the latter agents. It was concluded that amino acids and amines, either as primary constituents of an ingested meal or as metabolites of dietary proteins, act directly via separate mechanisms to stimulate gastrin secretion from G cells[31].

Dial and colleagues studied the effects of amino acids and amines on gastrin release from isolated rat endocrine granules[32]. Granules were enriched by differential centrifugation of homogenized rat gastric antral tissue. The identity of endocrine granules was confirmed by electron microscopy and by release studies. Nine of 13 amino acids tested were ineffective at inducing gastrin release from isolated granules. In contrast, all 13 amine metabolites of the corresponding amino acids were potent stimulators of gastrin release and alkalinized the gastrin granule interior. Ammonium chloride, similarly to amines, induced gastrin release and reversed the pH gradient across the isolated endocrine granules. These studies suggest that amines may directly stimulate gastrin granules to release their contents by alkalinizing the gastrin granule interior[32].

DOES *H. PYLORI* PRODUCE AMINES *IN VIVO* OR *IN VITRO*?

It is well known that *H. pylori* produces large amounts of urease, an enzyme responsible for hydrolysis of intragastric urea to ammonia and CO_2[33]. The pK_a for ammonia/ammonium is 9.1[34], suggesting that in the stomach most of the ion would be present in the insoluble charged form, hence trapped within the lumen[30,33]. To my knowledge the only information in the literature regarding synthesis of amines other than ammonia by *H. pylori* is the statement '*H. pylori* produces amines *in vitro*...but the significance of this finding *in vivo* is unknown'[35]. A recently published list of enzymes produced by *H. pylori* does not include amino acid decarboxylases[36].

Golodner *et al.*[22] studied the effects of diffusible substances from *H. pylori* and/or monocytes on secretion of gastrin from isolated canine G cells. Transwell cell culture inserts were used to separate cultured G cells below from added monocytes and/or bacteria above. In these experiments, bombesin stimulated gastrin release 8-fold compared to basal levels. Monocytes stimulated gastrin release approximately 5-fold. *H. pylori* alone stimulated a 3-fold increase in the secretion of gastrin. Addition of *H. pylori* and monocytes together resulted in no increase in gastrin secretion over that observed in the presence of monocytes alone. These experiments demonstrate for the first time that diffusible factors from *H. pylori* are capable of directly stimulating gastrin release from G cells. However, they also demonstrate that recruited inflammatory cells in *H. pylori*-associated gastritis may function to stimulate gastrin secretion, possibly via the release of cytokines[22]. The identity of the soluble factor(s) produced by *H. pylori* responsible for inducing gastrin release is not yet known. However, based on the studies of Lichtenberger and colleagues[29,32], production of ammonia by *H. pylori* urease by hydrolysis of urea present in culture medium may be sufficient to induce gastrin release under the conditions used.

DOES PRODUCTION OF AMINES OR AMMONIA BY *H. PYLORI* ACCOUNT FOR THE OBSERVED HYPERGASTRINAEMIA OBSERVED IN *H. PYLORI*-INFECTED INDIVIDUALS?

It has been suggested that production of ammonia by *H. pylori* leads to elevation of gastric antral surface pH, resulting in interference with the normal feedback inhibition of gastrin secretion by intra-gastric acid[13,19]. However, while *H. pylori* does make the pH of the antral mucus layer more alkaline, the difference was only 0.5 and 0.2 pH units when measured *in vivo* and *in vitro*, respectively[19,37]. Manipulation of gastric pH, urea concentration and urease activity in individuals infected with *H. pylori* does not affect gastrin levels in short-term experiments. For example, Graham et al.[35] noted that serum gastrin levels were not increased by short-term feeding of urea (500 mg) to five *H. pylori*-affected individuals. McColl et al. demonstrated that inhibition of urease activity with acetohydroxamic acid[38] or bismuth[39] did not affect short-term plasma gastrin concentrations. Finally, Moss et al. reported that the ratio of peptone-stimulated gastrin at pH 2.5/pH 5.5 was similar before and after suppression of *H. pylori*[40]. Taken together, the results of a variety of experiments in *H. pylori*-infected humans suggest that access of hydrogen ion to the pH-sensitive sites governing gastrin release by mucosal ammonia produced by *H. pylori* urease is not a critical factor[35].

In contrast, Calam et al.[23] compared plasma gastrin levels during inhibition of acid secretion, induced with the histamine–H_2-receptor inhibitor loxtidine, between germ-free and conventional rats. Partial inhibition of acid secretion by administration of loxtidine at a dose of 10 mg/kg per day increased gastrin levels from 59 ± 11 pmol/l to 153 ± 30 pmol/l in germ-free rats and from 36 ± 8 to 181 ± 27 pmol/l in conventional rats. Complete inhibition of acid secretion by the administration of 70 g/kg per day of loxtidine did not produce a significant further rise in plasma gastrin concentration in germ-free rats (178 ± 11 pmol/l), but did result in a further increase in plasma gastrin concentrations in conventional rats (278 ± 27 pmol/l).

Histological studies revealed significantly more eosinophils present in the gastric mucosa of conventional rats than germ-free rats during infusion of high-dose, but not low-dose, loxtidine. Whether gastric bacteria including *Helicobacter* species were present in the stomach was not reported. Calam *et al.* suggested that gastric bacterial overgrowth contributes to the increased hypergastrinaemia seen in the absence of acid[23]. The results of their study are also consistent with the notion that gastric inflammatory cells may modulate gastrin release[23].

Dial *et al.*[17] have recently demonstrated that gastrin release is markedly augmented following a meal with high ammonia content in two animal models of gastric inflammation. Thus, luminal ammonia and mediators of gastric inflammation may act synergistically to enhance meal-stimulated gastrin release in rats, and possibly in patients infected with *H. pylori*[17].

SUMMARY

In summary, it is well known that *H. pylori* is associated with hypergastrin-aemia in humans, and that eradication of the bacterium decreases gastrin levels. A variety of studies have demonstrated that ammonia and amines are capable of inducing secretion of gastrin from G cells both *in vivo* (from normal and inflamed gastric mucosa) and *in vitro*. Further, soluble factors produced by *H. pylori* can stimulate secretion of gastrin from isolated G cells. However, there are two major deterrents to acceptance of the theory that production of ammonia or amines by *H. pylori* is responsible for hypergastrinaemia: (1) experimental manipulation of gastric pH, urea concentration and urease activity in *H. pylori*-infected individuals fails to affect gastrin secretion appreciably; and (2) to date, no studies documenting the ability of *H. pylori* to produce amines either *in vitro* or *in vivo* have yet appeared. Regarding the first point, perhaps longer follow-up periods are needed prior to measurement of gastrin levels after specific experimental manipulations. Further, gastric luminal pH and urea concentration may not reflect the environment immediately subjacent to the gastric mucus layer in such experimental studies.

In conclusion, currently there is insufficient information either to prove or disprove whether *H. pylori*-associated hypergastrinaemia is dependent upon production and secretion of bacterial ammonia or amines. This area should prove fertile for further research.

References

1. Marshall BJ. *Campylobacter pylori*: its link to gastritis and peptic ulcer disease. Rev Infect Dis. 1990;12:S87–93.
2. Peterson WL. *Helicobacter pylori* and peptic ulcer disease. N Engl J Med. 1991;324:1043–8.
3. Graham DY, Go MF. *Helicobacter pylori*: current status. Gastroenterology. 1993;105: 279–82.
4. Axon ATR. *Helicobacter pylori* therapy: effect on peptic ulcer disease. J Gastroenterol Hepatol. 1991;6:131–42.
5. Dunn BE. Pathogenic mechanisms of *Helicobacter pylori*. Gastroenterol Clin N Am. 1993;22:43–57.
6. Smoot DT, Mobley HLT, Chippendale GR, Lewison JF, Resau JH. *Helicobacter pylori*

urease activity is toxic to human gastric epithelial cells. Infect Immun. 1990;58:1992–6.

7. Cover TL, Dooley CP, Blaser MJ. Characterization of and human serologic response to proteins in *Helicobacter pylori* broth culture supernatants with vacuolizing cytotoxin activity. Infect Immun. 1990;58:603–10.

8. Langton SR, Cesareo SD. *Helicobacter pylori* associated phospholipase A_2 activity: a factor in peptic ulcer production? J Clin Pathol. 1992;45:221–4.

9. Dixon M. Acid, ulcers, and *H. pylori*. Lancet. 1993;342:384–5.

10. Denizot Y, Sobhani I, Rambaud J-C, Lewin M, Thomas Y, Benveniste J. Paf-acether synthesis by *Helicobacter pylori*. Gut. 1990;31:1242–5.

11. Mai UEH, Perez-Perez GI, Wahl LM, Blaser MJ, Smith PD. Soluble surface proteins from *Helicobacter pylori* activate monocytes/macrophages by lipopolysaccharide-independent mechanism. J Clin Invest. 1991;87:894–900.

12. Negrini R, Lisato L, Zanella I et al. *Helicobacter pylori* infection induces antibodies cross-reacting with human gastric mucosa. Gastroenterology. 1991;101:437–45.

13. Levi S, Beardshall K, Playford R, Ghosh P, Haddad G, Calam J. *Campylobacter pylori* and duodenal ulcers: the gastrin link. Lancet. 1989;1:1167–8.

14. Graham DY, Opekun A, Lew GM, Evans DJ Jr, Klein PD, Evans DG. Ablation of exaggerated meal-stimulated gastrin release in duodenal ulcer patients after clearance of *Helicobacter (Campylobacter) pylori* infection. Am J Gastroenterol. 1990;85:394–8.

15. Levi S, Beardshall K, Swift I et al. Antral *Helicobacter pylori*, hypergastrinaemia, and duodenal ulcers: effect of eradicating the organism. BMJ. 1989;299:1504–7.

16. Prewett EJ, Smith JTL, Nwokolo CU, Hudson M, Sawyer AM, Pounder RE. Eradication of *Helicobacter pylori* abolishes 24-hour hypergastrinaemia: a prospective study in healthy subjects. Aliment Pharmacol Ther. 1991;5:283–90.

17. Dial E, Tatsumi Y, Hall L, Romero J, Lichtenberger L. Synergistic interaction of gastric inflammation and luminal ammonia in gastrin release. Poster 14, Proceedings of *Helicobacter pylori*: basic mechanisms to clinical cure, Amelia Island, FL, 3–6 Nov. 1993.

18. Hunt RH. pH and Hp – Gastric acid secretion and *Helicobacter pylori*: implications for ulcer healing and eradication of the organism. Am J Gastroenterol. 1993;88:481–3.

19. Kelly SM, Crampton J, Hunter JO. *Helicobacter pylori* increases the pH of the gastric mucosa *in vivo*. Gut. 1990;31:A1177.

20. Blaser MJ. Hypotheses on the pathogenesis and natural history of *Helicobacter pylori*-induced inflammation. Gastroenterology. 1992;102:720–7.

21. Chittajallu RS, Howie CA, McColl KEL. Effect of *Helicobacter pylori* on parietal cell sensitivity to pentagastrin in duodenal ulcer patients. Scand J Gastroenterol. 1992;27:857–62.

22. Golodner EH, Territo MC, Walsh JH, Soll AH. Stimulation of gastrin release from cultured canine G cells by *Helicobacter pylori* and mononuclear cells. Gastroenterology. 1992;102:A630.

23. Calam J, Goodlad RA, Lee CY et al. Achlorhydria-induced hypergastrinaemia: the role of bacteria. Clin Sci. 1991;80:281–4.

24. Moss SF, Legon S, Bishop AE, Polak JM, Calam J. Effect of *Helicobacter pylori* on gastric somatostatin in duodenal ulcer disease. Lancet. 1992;340:930–2.

25. Kaneko H, Nakada K, Mitsuma T et al. *Helicobacter pylori* infection induces a decrease in immunoreactive-somatostatin concentrations of human stomach. Dig Dis Sci. 1992;37:409–16.

26. Wu V, Sumii K, Tari A, Sumii M, Walsh JH. Regulation of rat antral gastrin and somatostatin gene expression during starvation and after refeeding. Gastroenterology. 1991;101:1552–8.

27. Morrison RT, Boyd RN. Organic chemistry, 3rd edn. Boston: Allyn & Bacon; 1973: 727–44.

28. D'Amato RF, Bottone EJ, Amsterdam D. Substrate profile systems for the identification of bacteria and yeasts by rapid and automated approaches. In: Balows A, Hausler WJ Jr, Herrmann K, Isenberg HD, Shadomy HJ, editors. Manual of clinical microbiology. Washington, DC: American Society for Microbiology; 1991:128–36.

29. Lichtenberger LM, Graziani LA, Dubinsky WP. Importance of dietary amines in meal-induced gastrin release. Am J Physiol. 1982;243:6341–7.

30. Lichtenberger LM, Nelson AA, Graziani LA. Amine trapping: physical explanation for the

inhibitory effect of gastric acidity on the postprandial release of gastrin. Gastroenterology. 1986;90:1223–31.

31. DelValle J, Yamada T. Amino acids and amines stimulate gastrin release from canine antral G-cells via different pathways. J Clin Invest. 1990;85:139–43.

32. Dial EJ, Cooper LC, Lichtenberger LM. Amino acid- and amine-induced gastrin release from isolated rat endocrine granules. Am J Physiol. 1991;260:6175–81.

33. Graham DY, Go MF, Evans DJ Jr. Review article: urease, gastric ammonium/ammonia, and *Helicobacter pylori* – the past, the present and recommendations for future research. Aliment Pharmacol Ther. 1992;6:659–69.

34. Bromberg PA, Robin ED, Forkner CE. The existence of ammonia in blood *in vivo* with observations of the significance of the NH_4^+-NH_3 system. J Clin Invest. 1960;39:332–41.

35. Graham DY, Opekune A, Lew GM, Klein PD, Walsh JH. *Helicobacter pylori*-associated exaggerated gastrin release in duodenal ulcer patients. The effect of bombesin infusion and urea ingestion. Gastroenterology. 1991;100:1571–5.

36. Hazell SL, Mendz GL. The metabolism and enzymes of *Helicobacter pylori*: function and potential virulence factors. In: Goodwin GC, Worsley BW, editors. *Helicobacter pylori*: biology and clinical practice. Boca Raton: CRC Press; 1993:115–41.

37. Beardshall K, Adamson D, Gill J, Unwin R, Calam J. *Helicobacter pylori* raises the pH of the juxta epithelial region of the mucus layer of the gastric antrum and body. Gut. 1991;32:A569.

38. El Nujumi AM, Dorian CA, Chittajallu RS, Neithercut WD, McColl KE. Effect of inhibition of *H. pylori* urease activity by acetohydroxamic acid on serum gastrin in duodenal ulcer patients. Gut. 1991;32:866–9.

39. Chittajallu RS, Neithercut WD, Ardill JES, McColl KEL. *Helicobacter pylori*-related hypergastrinemia is not due to elevated antral surface pH. Scand J Gastroenterol. 1992;27:218–22.

40. Moss SF, Playford RJ, Ayesu K, Li SK, Calam J. pH-dependent secretion of gastrin in duodenal ulcer disease: effect of suppressing *Helicobacter pylori*. Digestion. 1992;52:173–8.

25
Do gastric mucosal nerves remodel in *H. pylori* gastritis?

R. H. STEAD, B. R. HEWLETT, S. LHOTAK, E. C. C. COLLEY, M. FRENDO and M. F. DIXON

INTRODUCTION

The gastrointestinal mucosa has a dense network of nerve fibres arising from intrinsic and extrinsic neuronal cell bodies[1]. In the pyloric antrum, mucosal nerves are involved in the regulation of gastrin (G) and somatostatin (D) cell function[1]. Cholinergic nerves inhibit D cell production of somatostatin, and gastrin release is stimulated by gastrin-releasing peptide[2]. Luminal factors (e.g. pH) and distension also regulate G and D cell function. Thus, the release of gastrin is modulated by luminal, paracrine and neurocrine mechanisms. *Helicobacter pylori* infection results in disruption of the G and D cell regulatory pathways, and can lead to increased basal and meal-stimulated serum gastrin levels[3,4]. Since gastrin acts in an endocrine fashion on the corpus mucosa[5], increasing acid release, the increased level of this hormone is thought to be an important factor in the pathogenesis of peptic ulcers.

G and D cell numbers/densities in the antral mucosa in gastritis and duodenal ulcer disease have been determined in several histological studies. Although there are conflicting reports[6], it appears that there is a net reduction in D cells and somatostatin levels in the antrum of patients with duodenal ulcer[7,8], without G cell hyperplasia. However, G cells may have an increased gastrin content, at least in *H. pylori* gastritis[9]. Various mechanisms have been proposed for the altered G and D cell densities, including altered luminal acidity and the action of cytokines on G cells[2-4]. However, we are not aware of any microanatomical studies on mucosal nerves in *H. pylori*-associated gastric disorders.

There are reports of nerve degeneration in other inflammatory diseases of the gut[10], most notably Crohn's disease[11,12]. These include ultrastructural features of 'axonal necrosis'[10,11] and the demonstration of reduced nerve densities in the mucosa using immunocytochemistry[12]. Stead *et al.* reported remodelling of intestinal mucosal nerve fibres in the jejuna of *Nippostrongylus brasiliensis*-infected rats[13]. Mucosal nerve fibres were found to degenerate

281

during the acute inflammatory phase (between 1 and 2 weeks post *N. brasiliensis* infection) and nerve regeneration occurred during the recovery phase. Such effects are likely to be mediated by the activation of specific cell types as part of the inflammatory process, rather than in response to a specific agent. Accordingly, we hypothesize that nerve degeneration should accompany other forms of mucosal inflammation, including *H. pylori*-associated antral gastritis.

Therefore, we examined *H. pylori*-positive antral biopsies and *H. pylori*-negative controls, to determine if nerve degeneration occurs during *H. pylori*-associated inflammation. In parallel, we examined a number of biopsies from chemical gastropathies (due to bile reflux and NSAID) which are known to exhibit a different histopathological appearance to *H. pylori* gastritis: these types of gastropathy have minimal, if any, inflammatory cell infiltrates.

MATERIALS AND METHODS

Biopsies

Formalin-fixed, paraffin-embedded antral biopsies were retrieved from the files of the Departments of Pathology at the University of Leeds and McMaster University. The cases included *H. pylori*-positive gastritis ($n = 21$), controls that were *H. pylori*-negative and showed no specific pathological abnormality ($n = 27$), biopsies from patients with bile reflux (fasting gastric juice bile acid concentrations of > 0.5 mmol/l (2.52 ± 3.38, mean $\pm$ SD); $n = 5$)[14], and frequent NSAID users (aspirin and/or other NSAID several times a week or daily; $n = 6$). All biopsies in both reflux and NSAID groups were *H. pylori*-negative.

Staining techniques

Sections were cut from all biopsies at $3\,\mu$m and stained with H&E for the assessment of inflammatory features; and with an immunocytochemical technique to localize PGP 9.5 for the determination of nerve densities[15]. To localize PGP 9.5 we employed polyclonal rabbit anti-PGP 9.5 (Ultraclone, Cambridge, UK), diluted 1:500, using a biotin/streptavidin-peroxidase technique[13]. Sections were then counterstained with eosin, dehydrated, cleared and coverslipped with Permount. To assess the presence of *H. pylori* organisms, H&E and Warthin-Starry stains were employed.

Histological assessment

The following features were assessed on a scale of 0 to 3 (0: normal, 1: mild, 2: moderate, 3: severe): acute inflammatory cells, chronic inflammatory cells, glandular atrophy, vasodilatation and congestion, oedema and foveolar hyperplasia. To determine an overall 'gastritis' score, the acute and chronic scores were added.

Table 1 Results of histological assessment

	Controls (n = 27)	H. pylori positive (n = 21)	Reflux (n = 5)	NSAID (n = 5)	Kruskal-Wallis
Acute score	0.00 ± 0.00	1.24 ± 0.77	0.20 ± 0.45	0.17 ± 0.41	p < 0.001
Chronic score	0.26 ± 0.45	1.90 ± 0.62	0.80 ± 0.84	0.17 ± 0.41	p < 0.001
Gastritis score*	0.26 ± 0.45	3.14 ± 1.28	1.00 ± 1.22	0.33 ± 0.82	p < 0.001
Foveolar hyperplasia	0.33 ± 0.48	0.57 ± 0.75	1.20 ± 0.84	1.67 ± 0.52	p < 0.005
Oedema	0.56 ± 0.58	0.33 ± 0.58	1.60 ± 0.55	1.50 ± 0.55	p < 0.005
Congestion, vasodilatation	1.30 ± 0.67	1.19 ± 0.75	1.60 ± 1.14	2.33 ± 0.52	p < 0.05
Atrophy	0.00 ± 0.00	0.43 ± 0.51	0.20 ± 0.45	0.67 ± 0.82	p < 0.05

*Gastritis scores represent the combined acute and chronic inflammation scores
Data are presented as mean ± SD

Quantitation

Nerve volume densities (area/unit area), integrated nerve areas per millimetre of muscularis mucosa, nerve feature densities, numbers of nerve features per millimetre of muscularis mucosa and nerve feature areas were determined in the PGP 9.5/eosin preparations using a Quantimet 570 (true-colour) Image Analysis System. The entire mucosa of each biopsy was measured (screen magnification × 1600), with editing to exclude non-mucosal tissue, stain deposits and, in some biopsies, PGP 9.5-immunoreactive endocrine cells. The mean mucosal thickness for each biopsy was calculated by dividing the measured mucosal area by the length of muscularis mucosa (or basal lamina propria).

Statistical analysis

Data were analysed using Minitab Version 8. One-way analysis of variance (ANOVA) was employed, with Tukey's and Dunnett's tests ($\alpha = 0.05$) for pairwise comparison of different groups or comparison of inflamed and non-inflamed biopsies, respectively. Statistical normality for these data was determined using Rootogram analysis of the residuals from ANOVA. Overall differences between the histological features were assessed using Kruskal-Wallis analysis. To determine the relationships between inflammation scores and nerve parameters, we also did rank correlations.

RESULTS

Histopathological assessment

The presence of acute and chronic inflammatory cells, foveolar hyperplasia, oedema, congestion/vasodilatation and atrophy is presented in Table 1. Statistically significant differences were determined for all parameters, using Kruskal-Wallis analysis. Controls did not contain acute inflammatory cells, although occasional chronic inflammatory cells were noted. Both Reflux and

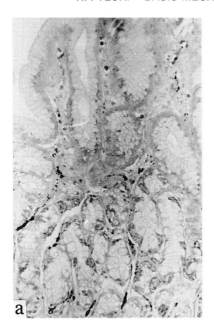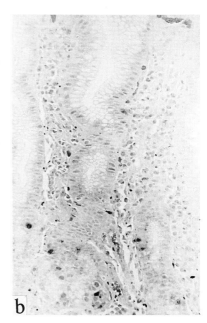

Fig. 1 PGP 9.5-immunostained sections from control and *H. pylori* positive biopsies. A relative lack of PGP 9.5-immunoreactive nerve is apparent in *H. pylori* positive biopsies (**b**) compared with controls (**a**). (Original magnification × 240)

NSAID groups also contained occasional acute and chronic inflammatory cells. However, the most dense inflammatory infiltrates were observed in the *H. pylori*-positive group. Foveolar hyperplasia and oedema were increased in both Reflux and NSAID groups, compared with controls and *H. pylori*-positive biopsies. Congestion/vasodilatation scores were apparently increased in both Reflux and NSAID groups. Atrophy was not present in control biopsies but was increased in all other groups (NSAID > *H. pylori* positive > Reflux).

Assessment of PGP 9.5-stained slides

Visual assessment of the PGP 9.5/eosin-stained preparations revealed differences in the densities and distributions of the diaminobenzidine reaction product (Fig. 1). Quantitation of these slides confirmed the visual appearances. The nerve feature densities, numbers of features per unit length of muscularis mucosa, nerve volume densities and integrated nerve areas per unit length of muscularis mucosa are shown in Fig. 2, with statistical analyses in Table 2. The nerve volume and profile densities were significantly increased in *H. pylori*-positive biopsies, compared with controls. NSAID biopsy nerve densities were similar to *H. pylori*-positive biopsies but Reflux samples had increased nerve parameters. When expressed per unit length of muscularis mucosa, the same patterns were observed, but statistical significance was not

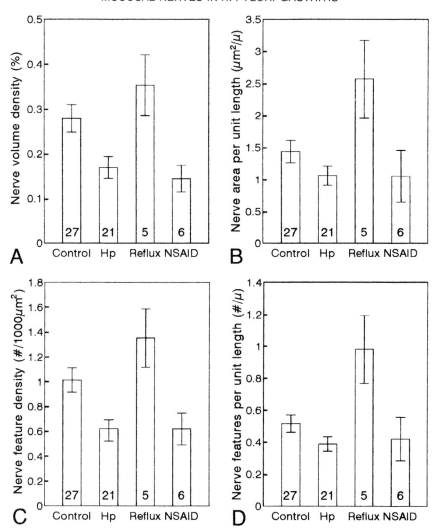

Fig. 2 Nerve volume densities (**A**), integrated nerve areas per unit length of muscularis mucosa (**B**), nerve feature densities (**C**) and numbers of nerve features per unit length of muscularis mucosa (**D**). Means ± SE for control, *H. pylori* positive, Reflux and NSAID biopsies are shown. The number of biopsies studied is shown at the base of each bar. Statistical analyses are presented in Table 2

determined. This could be accounted for by increased mucosal thickness in pathological samples (Controls: 0.52 ± 0.11 mm, *H. pylori* positive: 0.64 ± 0.20 mm, Reflux: 0.71 ± 0.08 mm, NSAID 0.71 ± 0.40 mm; mean ± SD; $p = 0.02$). Nerve profile areas did not differ significantly between groups (Controls: $2.68 \pm 0.52 \, \mu m^2$, *H. pylori*-positive: $2.60 \pm 0.50 \, \mu m^2$, Reflux: $2.59 \pm 0.17 \, \mu m^2$, NSAID: $2.36 \pm 0.40 \, \mu m^2$; mean ±SD, $p = 0.55$).

Table 2 Results of statistical analyses on nerve parameters

	ANOVA	Control vs. H. pylori	Control vs Reflux	Control vs NSAID	H. pylori vs Reflux	H. pylori vs NSAID	Reflux vs NSAID
Nerve volume densities	$p = 0.006$	$p < 0.05$	n.s.	n.s.	$p < 0.05$	n.s.	n.s.
Nerve feature densities	$p = 0.001$	$p < 0.05$	n.s.	n.s.	$p < 0.05$	n.s.	$p < 0.05$
Integrated nerve areas per mm muscularis mucosa	$p = 0.010$	n.s.	n.s.	n.s.	$p < 0.05$	n.s.	$p < 0.05$
Numbers of nerve features per mm muscularis mucosa	$p = 0.010$	n.s.	$p < 0.05$	n.s.	$p < 0.05$	n.s.	$p < 0.05$

Results of one-way analysis of variance (ANOVA), using Tukey's wholly significant difference allowance to compare pairs of experimental groups

Relationships between nerve and histological parameters

The moderate and severe inflammation scores for *H. pylori* positive and *H. pylori* negative controls were combined for these analyses, to reduce the number of groups having low sample numbers. In general, we found decreased mean nerve parameters with increasing acute or chronic inflammatory cell scores (Table 3) and that these were moderately negatively correlated. We also determined a general decrease in nerve parameters with increasing atrophy, but this was not statistically significant (data not shown).

DISCUSSION

We report a reduction in the densities of PGP 9.5-immunoreactive nerves in the mucosae of antral biopsies from patients with *H. pylori* positive gastritis, compared with non-inflamed controls. This can be accounted for by reductions in the numbers of stained nerve profiles but not by changes in nerve profile areas. When expressed as nerve volume and feature densities these reduced nerve parameters are statistically significant ($p < 0.05$). In relationship to the length of muscularis mucosa, the integrated nerve areas and numbers of nerve features in *H. pylori*-positive biopsies are 20–25% lower than controls, although not statistically significant. The mucosal thickness was found to be increased in *H. pylori*-positive compared with *H. pylori*-negative biopsies ($\sim 25\%$); therefore, the reduced densities can partly be accounted for by thickening of the mucosae. Antral biopsies from patients with bile reflux and frequent NSAID users were included in our study. These chemical gastropathies exhibit similar histopathological appearances[16] and both groups had thickened mucosae. The NSAID and *H. pylori* positive groups had similar nerve densities but the Reflux group had increased nerve parameters. Our data do not provide an explanation for this difference, although glandular atrophy was more pronounced in the NSAID group.

It could be argued that the nerves penetrating the mucosa are supplied by a fixed number of neuronal cell bodies, which would suggest that our data expressed per unit length of muscularis mucosa are more representative of the actual nerve fibre differences. However, this does not take into account that, for mucosal innervation to be maintained, the nerve fibres supplying

Table 3 Nerve density parameters in control and *H. pylori* positive biopsies classified by acute and chronic inflammation scores

	Acute inflammation score*			Statistics†		Chronic inflammation score*			Statistics†	
	0 (n = 30)	1 (n = 11)	2/3 (n = 7)	ANOVA	r	0 (n = 20)	1 (n = 12)	2/3 (n = 16)	ANOVA	r
Mucosal thickness (mm)	0.54 ± 0.13	0.66 ± 0.24	0.58 ± 0.12	F = 2.41 p = 0.101	0.160	0.50 ± 0.10	0.60 ± 0.15	0.64‡ ± 0.21	F = 3.43 p = 0.041	0.333
Nerve volume density (%)	0.27 ± 0.16	0.19 ± 0.13	0.14 ± 0.07	F = 2.76 p = 0.074	−0.330	0.28 ± 0.15	0.22 ± 0.16	0.17‡ ± 0.12	F = 2.83 p = 0.069	−0.335
Nerve feature density (no./mm²)	971 ± 507	671 ± 374	557 ± 244	F = 3.40 p = 0.042	−0.350	1004 ± 470	849 ± 557	634‡ ± 347	F = 2.92 p = 0.064	−0.336

*Data presented as mean ± SD. Acute inflammation scores of 2 (n = 6) and 3 (n = 1), and chronic inflammation scores of 2 (n = 13) and 3 (n = 3) are combined.
†Results of one-way analysis of variance (ANOVA) and rank correlation. The latter were performed on raw data, using separate moderate (2) and severe (3) acute and chronic inflammation scores.
‡$p < 0.05$ compared with '0' score using Dunnett's test.

287

the epithelium and lamina propria must be of greater length in thickened mucosae. Therefore, nerve volume and feature densities are likely to be better indicators of functional nerve changes than data expressed per unit length of muscularis mucosa. Since the nerves appeared to follow somewhat tortuous paths (see Fig. 1), the numbers of nerve profiles we measured actually represent fragments of nerve fibres. Increased tortuosity and apparent fragmentation might be predicted in inflamed mucosae but we observed fewer profiles, which further supports a reduction of nerve densities in the *H. pylori* positive cases.

We analysed our data from *H. pylori* positive biopsies and *H. pylori* negative controls according to the extent of inflammatory cell infiltration, and found that all of the nerve parameters were reduced in the presence of increased numbers of acute or chronic inflammatory cells. For those biopsies with moderate to severe chronic inflammation, both nerve volume and feature densities were significantly reduced, compared with controls ($p < 0.05$). Rank correlation analysis revealed a negative, albeit moderate relationship between inflammatory cells and nerve densities, which suggests some other contributory factor(s). Interestingly, the Reflux group had relatively high chronic inflammation scores and increased nerve parameters, which indicates that increased mononuclear cellular infiltration *per se* is not related to loss of nerve. Specifically which factors are responsible for the presumed nerve degeneration remains to be elucidated.

In this study we did not take into account the duration of gastropathy. In the *N. brasiliensis* model of jejunal inflammation we previously demonstrated sequential changes in the mucosal nerve fibres[13]. Nerve degeneration occurred during the acute inflammatory phase (approximately 1–2 weeks post-infection). Over the following weeks, small-diameter fibres were observed and interpreted to represent a phase of reinnervation. Seven weeks post-*N. brasiliensis* infection there was a net 30% increase in the density of mucosal nerve fibres. Functional data support this pattern of nerve changes in the same animal model[17]. Thus, following nerve damage during an inflammatory episode, mucosal innervation appears to be restored. However, the extent of nerve remodelling during an ongoing inflammatory process is not known. After an initial phase of degeneration, both damage and regrowth of fibres may occur concurrently. This is of obvious importance in the context of the current study, since we do not know the duration of disease in the *H. pylori* positive biopsies, nor the nature of any previous gastropathies in any of our samples. It will not be easy to derive complete time-course data from studies on *H. pylori*-associated gastritis in humans, although repeated biopsies over a period of months following eradication of *H. pylori* will reveal if the mucosal innervation recovers at the structural level. Animal models will provide useful tools for more detailed investigations.

It is important to note that PGP 9.5 (a ubiquitin hydroxylase[18], found in most nerves, including a high density of nerves in the gastrointestinal lamina propria)[15,19] might not be present in detectable amounts in all antral mucosal nerves, especially during the inflammatory process. Our data may not, therefore, be representative of the entire antral mucosal nerve population. It is possible that certain fibre types (e.g. intrinsic vs extrinsic) are more susceptible to inflammation-induced damage, although we suspect that this is unlikely. However, it is not wise to assume that nerve fibres in inflamed antral mucosae are functionally the same as those in normal tissues. In fact there is accumulating evidence for phenotypic neuroplasticity during inflammation[20–25]. These might be connected, since the extensively studied cytokine regulators of immune responses are now known to affect nerve growth; and some of these have effects on nerve differentiation[26–30]. Furthermore, nerve fibres growing into a previously inflamed mucosa might arise ectopically, i.e. from neuronal somata not originally supplying that tissue. If the intrinsic nerves are irreversibly damaged, these could be replaced by fibres of extrinsic origin, or by collaterals arising from different populations of intrinsic neurons.

Mucosal nerve degeneration during antral gastritis has several implications. This might contribute to gastric nociception, the mechanisms of which are poorly understood[31,32]. Damage to mucosal nerve fibres may be a (or the) pain stimulus in dyspepsia. It is also likely that disruption of the mucosal nerve network results in dysregulation of endocrine (as well as other cell) function. Cholinergic nerves inhibit D cell activity and gastrin-releasing peptide containing nerves promote G cell function[1,2]. If there is non-specific nerve degeneration during the early stages of inflammation, one would predict increased somatostatin and decreased gastrin release; and consequent hypochlorhydria. This has been described in the early stages of *H. pylori* infection[4]. Since mucosal nerve fibres represent terminations of direct and indirect extrinsic neural inputs, mucosal nerve degeneration must affect the cephalic phase of gastric acid secretion and disrupt nerve-mediated reflex responses. It will not be possible to define the importance of neuroplasticity in the pathogenesis of peptic ulcers until we fully understand the extent of nerve remodelling during the inflammatory process in the gastrointestinal mucosa.

SUMMARY

It was recently shown that mucosal nerve fibres remodel in the jejuna of rats infected with *Nippostrongylus brasiliensis*. This is composed of nerve degeneration during the acute inflammatory phase and regeneration during the recovery phase. Other studies have revealed changes in the levels of neurotransmitters during inflammatory episodes, suggesting that both structural and phenotypic plasticity of nerves occurs during intestinal inflammation. Accordingly, we examined antral biopsies from *Helicobacter pylori*-infected patients and *H. pylori*-negative controls. We also included antral biopsies from reflux and NSAID gastropathies. Inflammatory features were assessed in H&E-stained slides and parallel sections were immuno-stained for PGP 9.5, to reveal the mucosal nerve network. The areas and numbers of PGP 9.5-immunoreactive nerve profiles, as well as mucosal areas and lengths of muscularis mucosae, were determined on a Quantimet 570C image analysis system. Both the volume and feature densities of PGP 9.5-immunoreactive nerves were reduced in *H. pylori*-positive compared with

H. pylori-negative biopsies ($0.17 \pm 0.02\%$ vs $0.28 \pm 0.03\%$, $p < 0.05$ and 622 ± 70 mm^{-2} vs 1013 ± 98 mm^{-2}, $p < 0.05$; mean $\pm$ SE, Tukey's tests). There was also a 25% reduction of the number of nerve features or sum of nerve areas per millimetre of muscularis mucosa in *H. pylori*-positive biopsies, although these were not statistically significant, indicating that the increased mucosal thickness ($\sim 25\%$) in inflamed biopsies partly accounted for the reduced nerve densities. Similar reductions were observed in the NSAID biopsies but the reflux group had increased numbers of nerve features and nerve areas per millimetre. These data suggest a loss of PGP 9.5-positive mucosal nerves during *H. pylori*-associated antral gastritis. Since these fibres are involved in the regulation of antral G and D cells, we speculate that inflammation-induced disruption of antral mucosal nerves may contribute to the hormonal disturbances and pathogenesis of peptic ulcer disease.

Acknowledgements

The authors would like to thank George Sobala for clinical data, and Janice Butera for typing the manuscript. This work was supported by the Medical Research Council of Canada and the Crohn's and Colitis Foundation of Canada.

References

1. Furness JB, Costa M. The enteric nervous system. Edinburgh: Churchill Livingstone, 1987.
2. Blaser MJ. Hypotheses on the pathogenesis and natural history of *Helicobacter pylori*-induced inflammation. Gastroenterology. 1992;102:720–7.
3. Dunn BE. Pathogenic mechanisms of *Helicobacter pylori*. Gastroenterol Clin N Am. 1993;22:43–57.
4. Moss S, Calam J. *Helicobacter pylori* and peptic ulcers: the present position. Gut. 1992;33:289–92.
5. Wolfe MM, Soll AH. The physiology of gastric acid secretion. N Engl J Med. 1988;319:1707–15.
6. Graham DY, Lew GM, Lechago J. Antral G-cell and D-cell numbers in *Helicobacter pylori* infection: effect of *H. pylori* eradication. Gastroenterology. 1993;104:1655–60.
7. Moss SF, Legon S, Bishop AE, Polak JM, Calam J. Effect of *Helicobacter pylori* on gastric somatostatin in duodenal ulcer disease. Lancet. 1992;340:930–2.
8. Kaneko H, Nakada K, Mitsuma T *et al*. *Helicobacter pylori* infection induces a decrease in immunoreactive-somatostatin concentrations of human stomach. Dig Dis Sci. 1992;37:409–16.
9. Sankey EA, Helliwell PA, Dhillon AP. Immunostaining of antral gastrin cells is quantitatively increased in *Helicobacter pylori* gastritis. Histopathology. 1990;16:151–5.
10. Riemann JF, Schmidt H. Ultrastructural changes in the gut autonomic nervous system following laxative abuse and in other conditions. In: Polak JM, Bloom SR, Wright NA, Oaly MN, editors. Basic science in gastroenterology: structure of the gut. London: Glaxo Research Group; 1982:289–302.
11. Dvorak AM, Osage JE, Monahan RA, Dickersin GR. Crohn's disease: transmission electron microscopic studies. III. Target tissues. Proliferation of and injury to smooth muscle and the autonomic nervous system. Hum Pathol. 1980;11:620–34.
12. Kubota Y, Petras RE, Ottaway CA, Tubbs RR, Farmer RG, Fiocchi C. Colonic vasoactive intestinal peptide nerves in inflammatory bowel disease. Gastroenterology. 1992;102:1242–51.
13. Stead RH, Kosecka-Janiszewska U, Oestreicher AB, Dixon MF, Bienenstock J. Remodelling

of B-50(GAP-43)- and NSE-immunoreactive mucosal nerves in the intestines of rats infected with *Nippostrongylus brasiliensis*. J Neurosci. 1991;11:3809–21.
14. Sobala GM, O'Connor HJ, Dewar EP, King RFG, Axon ATR, Dixon MF. Bile reflux and intestinal metaplasia in gastric mucosa. J Clin Pathol. 1993;46:235–40.
15. Stead RH, Dixon MF, Bramwell NH, Riddell RH, Bienenstock J. Mast cells are closely apposed to nerves in the human gastrointestinal mucosa. Gastroenterology. 1989;97: 575–85.
16. Sobala GM, King RFG, Axon ATR, Dixon MF. Reflux gastritis in the intact stomach. J Clin Pathol. 1990;43:303–6.
17. Perdue MH, Marshall J, Masson S. Ion transport abnormalities in inflamed rat jejunum: involvement of mast cells and nerves. Gastroenterology. 1990;98:561–7.
18. Wilkinson KD, Lee K, Deshpande S, Duerksen-Hughes P, Boss JM, Pohl J. The neuron-specific protein PGP 9.5 is a ubiquitin carboxyl-terminal hydrolase. Science. 1989;246: 670–3.
19. Stead RH, Franks AJ, Goldsmith CH, Bienenstock J, Dixon MF. Mast cells, nerves and fibrosis in the appendix: a morphological assessment. J Pathol. 1990;161:209–19.
20. Swain MG, Agro A, Blennerhassett P, Stanisz A, Collins SM. Increased levels of substance P in the myenteric plexus of *Trichinella*-infected rats. Gastroenterology. 1992;102:1913–19.
21. Collins SM, Hurst SM, Main C *et al.* Effect of inflammation of enteric nerves: cytokine-induced changes in neurotransmitter content and release. Ann NY Acad Sci. 1992;664: 415–24.
22. Collins SM, Blennerhassett PA, Blennerhassett MG, Vermillion DL. Impaired acetylcholine release from the myenteric plexus of *Trichinella*-infected rats. Am J Physiol. 1989;257: G898–903.
23. Eysselein VE, Reinshagen M, Cominelli F *et al.* Calcitonin gene-related peptide and substance P decrease in the rabbit colon during colitis. A time study. Gastroenterology. 1991;101:1211–19.
24. Goldin E, Karmeli F, Selinger Z, Rachmilewitz D. Colonic substance P levels are increased in ulcerative colitis and decreased in severe constipation. Dig Dis Sci. 1989;34:754–7.
25. Koch TR, Carney JA, Go VLW. Distribution and quantitation of gut neuropeptides in normal intestine and inflammatory bowel disease. Dig Dis Sci. 1987;32:369–76.
26. Mehler MF, Rozental R, Dougherty M, Spray DC, Kessler JA. Cytokine regulation of neuronal differentiation of hippocampal progenitor cells. Nature. 1993;362:62–5.
27. Araujo DM, Cotman CW. Trophic effects of interleukin-4, -7 and -8 on hippocampal neuronal cultures: potential involvement of glial-derived factors. Brain Res. 1993;600: 49–55.
28. Haugen PK, Letourneau PC. Interleukin-2 enhances chick and rat sympathetic, but not sensory, neurite outgrowth. J Neurosci Res. 1990;25:443–52.
29. Kamegai M, Niijima K, Kunishita T *et al.* Interleukin 3 as a trophic factor for central cholinergic neurons *in vitro* and *in vivo*. Neuron. 1990;4:429–36.
30. Kamegai M, Konishi Y, Tabira T. Trophic effect of granulocyte–macrophage colony-stimulating factor on central cholinergic neurons *in vitro*. Brain Res. 1990;532:323–5.
31. Cervero F. Neurophysiology of gastrointestinal pain. Bailliere's Clin Gastroenterol. 1988;2:183–99.
32. Grundy D. Speculations on the structure/function relationship for vagal and splanchnic afferent endings supplying the gastrointestinal tract. J Auton Nerv Syst. 1988;22:175–80.

Section V
Immunological response to
H. pylori

26
Overview of the immune response to *H. pylori*

P. B. ERNST, Y. JIN, J. NAVARRO, V. REYES and S. CROWE

INTRODUCTION

Since *Helicobacter pylori* has been recognized as a key factor in the pathogenesis of an array of gastric disorders, several investigators have explored the host response to this pathogen. In order to understand the role of the immune/inflammatory response in the prevention or pathogenesis of disease associated with *H. pylori*, one must consider the state of the immune system in the normal stomach. However, our current understanding of gastric immunology has been obtained primarily from a limited number of reports in control patients that are defined in the course of studies of the same parameters in patients infected with *H. pylori*. This review will summarize some of the information that is now available regarding the host response to *H. pylori*, and how it may alter the course of the disease.

THE RELATIONSHIP OF GASTRIC IMMUNOLOGY TO OTHER MUCOSAL TISSUES

In simple terms the epithelial layer is the primary cellular barrier between the outside world and the host. The countless interactions with environmental antigens, toxins and irritants require an effective local immune response. However, the challenge to the immune response in these sites is to confer protection without destroying the fragile epithelium or adversely perturbing the very specialized functions they perform[1].

Like the specialized epithelia they protect, immune responses are highly adapted to function in the specific environment in which the various immune and inflammatory cells are found. This is most evident when the properties of the vastly different systemic immune responses are compared to those in mucosal tissues. The similarities in the mechanisms conferring immunity amongst the mucosal sites have in fact nurtured the concept of a common mucosal immune system. However, the direct examination of the cells and factors produced in the lung, intestine or the uterus during pregnancy show even more specialized responses to cope with the peculiarities of these different sites. Thus, our understanding of the role of the immune response in interactions between *H. pylori* and the host must be viewed in the context of mucosal immunity in general, and gastric responses in particular.

Microbial invasion is, in part, prevented by the epithelial tight junctions, and is complemented by mucus production and various antibacterial proteins such as lysozyme, lactoferrin, interferon and defensin/cryptdin. The latter are of particular interest since they have recently been shown to be produced by the Paneth cells at the base of the intestinal crypts[2], which suggests they will bathe the epithelium in a protective paint. In general, the expression of these defence molecules in the stomach is more pronounced in the antrum than the body, suggesting they defer to gastric acid in other regions of the stomach to protect against infection from the lumen. However, their presence suggests that the harsh luminal conditions are not always sufficient, particularly in the antral region where there is more antigenic stimulation[3].

In response to epithelial stress, inflammatory changes are initiated by the release of cytokines and possibly products of the arachidonic acid metabolism pathway, which recruit and activate polymorphonuclear cells, monocytes and mast cells. This response by the epithelium reflects its need to deal with luminal challenge, and points to the role of the epithelium as the first line of active defence against infection. Some of the responses by the epithelium may be protective while others, when chronically activated, may lead to disruption of function, epithelial cell death and erosions. These will be covered in the discussion later.

Complementing the non-specific mechanisms of protection are the antigen-specific, adaptive responses, although these are relatively sparse in uninfected stomachs. Of note, IgA is the predominant antibody in mucosal secretions and is produced in greater quantities than the immunoglobulin in all other tissues combined[4]. This reflects the adaptation of the local immune responses because IgA is selectively transported across epithelial surfaces by the polymeric immunoglobulin receptor (secretory component)[5], resists acid hydrolysis or proteolysis and can provide immunity without inducing much inflammation[6]. The latter property is due to its inability to efficiently activate complement, which is highly desirable in view of the numerous antigen–antibody complexes formed in mucosal sites such as the stomach or the intestine. Although much less frequent, IgG-producing cells can also be detected in mucosal tissues; however, they do increase during infection with *H. pylori*[7]. IgG_2 and IgG_4 subclasses, which are less efficient at activating complement, may play a role in protecting the lamina propria. Local IgG may reach the lumen in small amounts by passive intercellular diffusion and mediate some effect against infections that are immediately adjacent to the lumen under the protective umbrella of the mucus gel layer.

Cell-mediated immune responses in the intestinal epithelium and lamina propria are also quite specialized, and discussed in more detail by Dr Croitoru elsewhere in this publication. The recent explosion of literature documenting the unique, thymus-independent nature of the intestinal intra-epithelial T cells attests to the excitement the immunological world is now feeling with respect to these cells[8]. In short, all dogma based on studies of systemic T cells can be challenged, as these paradigms may not predict the biology of intestinal lymphocytes. For example, CD8[+] intraepithelial lymphoctes (IEL) in mice produce substantial levels of cytokines[9]. Further evidence suggests the IEL rearrange their T cell receptors in the gut epithelium[10] and not the thymus. Both lamina proprial and epithelial lymphocytes appear to be highly activated, and yet few antigen-specific functions have been demonstrated for most enteric T cell subsets. This, in part, is due to their relative anergy which, when broken, is undoubtedly involved in local inflammation and disruption of epithelial function and/or integrity.

The conclusion from these observations is that immune responses have adapted significantly amongst species as well as within the different tissues of an individual host. Thus, no single element is sufficient or perhaps necessary for immunity, but the collection of different immune mechanisms provides layers of protection that greatly favour the host. In addition to the well-recognized immunological mediators, the 'biomatrix' selecting for the most appropriate responses includes luminal factors as well as contributions by the epithelium, neuroendocrine system and tissue fibroblasts. By altering this environment, for example, during infection, the normal response changes and a cascade of potentially deleterious effects can occur.

THE INITIATION OF INFLAMMATORY RESPONSES BY THE GASTRIC EPITHELIUM

As the front line in defence, the epithelium is the first to see and respond to infection. *H. pylori* binds to gastric epithelial cell lines[11,12] and can induce activation of the cell, as evidenced by actin polymerization[11] and the increase in inositol triphosphate[12]. It is logical that this evidence for cell activation may lead to signals which initiate inflammation. Besides the act of infection, some isolates of *H. pylori* cause vacuolization of the epithelium[13] which also may contribute to the epithelial stress and activation of mediator production. *H. pylori* induces the production of IL-8 in patients with gastritis[14] and within hours of infection *in vitro*[15]. IL-8 is also produced by paracrine factors released during *H. pylori* infection including IL-1 and TNF-α, the latter of which may activate transcription factors[16]. Since these transcription factors can modulate several cytokine genes, the total contribution of the gastric epithelium to cytokine production is not yet completely documented. The epithelium also has the ability to respond to local damage, such as ulceration, by undergoing differentiation to produce EGF/urogastrone[17]. Through the production of these autocrine factors it can participate in the healing process.

H. PYLORI INDUCED NEUTROPHIL ACTIVATION

It is clear that infection with *H. pylori* leads to the production of IL-8, a potent chemoattractant and activation signal for neutrophils[18], and possibly

T cells[19]. This is based on independent reports showing that IL-8 is increased during infection with *H. pylori*[14,15]. Moreover, other factors, including activated complement fragments or leukotriene production, could also contribute to neutrophil recruitment. Others have shown that *H. pylori* produces a molecule which is also a potent chemoattractant for neutrophils[20,21]. In addition other stress, for example, leaked neutrophil elastase, gastric acid or local ischaemia, on the epithelium could increase the production of IL-8. This view is consistent with the appearance of neutrophils in the mucosa of patients infected with *H. pylori*.

Gastric epithelial cell lines also produce ICAM-1, the counterreceptor for the CD11b/CD18 adhesion molecule on neutrophils and T cells, which suggests that the production of IL-8 and ICAM-1 by the infected epithelium will focus the neutrophil, and possibly the T cell response, at the site of the bacteria[15]. This is somewhat controversial, as there is one report that ICAM-1 is not expressed on the gastric epithelium during infection with *H. pylori*[22]. Perhaps novel adhesion molecules exist in the neutrophil–epithelial cell interaction that are analogous to the 'epithelial form' of class II MHC molecules in the intestinal epithelium (D. Kaiserlain, personal communication).

Although T cells and basophils have been reported to be activated by IL-2, neutrophils appear to be the major target for IL-8 based on the literature examining the expression of the known IL-8 receptors. There are two forms of IL-8 receptor that differ in their extracellular region. One form appears to be specific for IL-8 while the other can also bind other immediate-early gene products including GRO or NAP2[23]. The significance of expressing one form more than the other is unknown. In either case, binding the receptor by IL-8 leads to substantial activation of the neutrophil. Changes include the induction of cytokine production by the neutrophil, increased oxidative burst, as well as increased expression of CD11b/CD18. *H. pylori* also seems to produce factors which can augment oxidative burst of neutrophils directly, likely through the release of *N*-formyl methionyl-leucyl-phenylalanine[24].

By co-culturing neutrophils with intestinal epithelial cell lines, Madara has shown that neutrophils can migrate across the epithelium to the lumen. Moreover, activation of the neutrophil can alter the permeability of the tight junctions and the secretory function of the T84 cell line[25-27]. Thus, it is reasonable to speculate that the neutrophil has good access to the gastric epithelium, and possibly the bacteria. They could be helpful but may also damage the epithelium by the leakage of their potent intracellular enzymes and reactive products. It is not obvious whether the neutrophil has a protective or aggressive role during infection with *H. pylori*. Probably, in small amounts, a local neutrophil response is desirable but when stimulated to extreme levels, it is unlikely to be beneficial.

LYMPHO-EPITHELIAL INTERACTIONS IN THE STOMACH

Studies by Engstrand and co-workers[28] suggest that infection with *H. pylori* leads to an increase in T cells bearing the γ/δ T cell receptor in association with an increased expression of the groEL stress protein homologue. Like the bowel, the inflamed gastric epithelial cells express class II MHC molecules and cathepsin E[29] (E. Solcia, personal communication) which may contribute to local antigen processing and presentation[30–32]. Class II MHC molecules are induced by interferon-γ or TNF-α in other epithelia[33] and these factors may be increased during infection with *H. pylori*[34,35]. Using immunoprecipitation, the gastric epithelial cell line KATO III has been shown to constitutively express class II and invariant chain (Ii), both of which are increased in expression after exposure to interferon-γ[36]. Interferon-γ concomitantly increases IL-8 production by KATO III and produces even more IL-8 in the presence of TNF-α[16]. Thus, paracrine factors associated with inflammation induced by *H. pylori* can modulate epithelial gene expression to produce several proteins needed for the initiation of inflammation and antigen presentation.

Antigen presentation by epithelial cells may be more theoretical than practical in light of the massive surface area of epithelia that could assume this role in inflammation therefore making additional immunological stimulation undesirable. It is possible that the purpose of class II MHC molecules expressed by the epithelium is to induce tolerance and not immunity. This is supported by observations that epithelial cells preferentially stimulate CD8$^+$ T cells[31,37]. Moreover, these T cells recognize the epithelial using novel ligands[38] and class II may even preferentially stimulate CD8$^+$ cells[32,37]. Furthermore, there are relatively few CD4$^+$ T cells within the epithelium, which again supports the hypothesis that the class II-bearing epithelial cells may stimulate CD8$^+$ cells. However, in disease, activation of a response in lieu of inhibiting a response may occur due to an undesirable effect of these cells on antigen presentation[39,40]. It is also possible that antigen reaches the lamina propria where it can drive local immune responses using more conventional antigen-presenting cells that are designed to present antigen to helper T cells.

In summary, the epithelium expresses a number of molecules that are extremely important in *initiating* immune or inflammatory processes. While there is good evidence that they can initiate inflammation, their role in T cell activation is less clear. It is obvious that they are the front line and likely manifest the earliest host response to infection or other epithelial stress.

CHANGES IN MUCOSAL ANTIBODY DURING INFECTION WITH *H. PYLORI*

B cell responses to *H. pylori* include local responses as well as those disseminated throughout the body. The latter may be found in serum or saliva and have proven useful in diagnosis or monitoring for eradication. Local responses are far more relevant to pathogenesis or prevention. We have observed an increase in IgA and even IgG in the gastric juice of patients infected with *H. pylori* (J. Rademaker, unpublished observations). This would be consistent with the increase in IgA- and IgG-producing cells in the gastric mucosa during gastritis[5]. Others have also reported an increase in local IgA and IgG in the gastric mucosa, some of which is specific for *H. pylori*[7,41,42]. These antibodies function primarily in the protected mucus gel layer which is less acidic than the lumen, and would still allow them to prevent the adherence of pathogens.

Since 70–90% of the B cells in the mucosa of the stomach and intestine of humans and laboratory animals normally produce IgA[6], the increase in IgG could lead to a mucosal model of an 'Arthus reaction' where chronic stimulation of the B lymphocytes finally leads to a destructive crescendo and the eventual onset of symptoms. One would predict that activated complement fragments will be found in this tissue, as has been observed in association with the increase in IgG in the mucosa of patients with inflammatory bowel disease[43]. The role of antibodies in the pathogenesis is supported by reports that antibodies to *H. pylori* can recognize human or murine gastric epithelium and induce gastritis in mice[44]. Moreover, a mucosal IgA to a 120 kDa protein from *H. pylori* appears to be associated with duodenal ulcer[45]. The site of induction of these responses, and the pathway leading to their dissemination throughout the body, are unclear. This remains a key question if one is interested in understanding the initiation of local immune responses which may contribute to the pathogenesis of gastritis or its prevention through immunization. Thus, local responses to specific antigens on *H. pylori* should be characterized and the segregation of these responses to different gastric diseases established.

As is typical of most epithelia, the polymeric immunoglobulin receptor is also expressed on the gastric epithelium, particularly in the isthmus zone of the antral mucosa[3,5]. Confusing the issue somewhat is the presence of IgA-producing B cells in the body of the stomach which lacks the polymeric immunoglobulin receptor except in more severe gastritis[3]. Presumably, these B cells would be important for protecting the lamina propria if not the lumen.

THE EFFECT OF T CELL CYTOKINES ON ANTIBODY REGULATION

The local cell-mediated immune response will be key for the generation of pro-inflammatory antibodies, perturbation of epithelial differentiation/function and possibly the initiation of epithelial damage. Cytokine production by gastric T cells needs to be considered in the context of current understanding of helper T cell (Th) biology. It has been observed that Th clones can be divided into two types, Th1 and Th2, based on the panel of cytokines they produce. Th1 cells were associated with delayed hypersensitivity and some IgG responses and produce IFN-γ and IL-2[46]. Th2 cells preferentially select for IgE, mastocytosis and the eosinophilia associated with parasite infestations due to their production of IL-3, IL-4 and IL-5 for example[47]. IL-4, IL-5 and IL-6 from Th2 cells can also contribute to IgA responses[48].

In humans the regulation of isotype is less clear. T cell clones from the intestine selectively enhance IgA through isotype switch and expansion of IgA committed B cells[49]. This may be due to IL-5 and other B cell differentiating factors. The cytokine profile and regulatory T cell function may be altered, which could contribute to the increase in IgG/IgA ratio seen in inflammatory conditions such as periodontal disease, gastritis, coeliac disease and inflammatory bowel disease.

The increase in gastric IgG during infection with *H. pylori* plus the changes in the expression of class II molecules and secretory component on the epithelium, are consistent with an increase in IFN-γ, possibly from Th1 cells, but this remains to be confirmed and the contribution of TNF-α or IL-4 to these changes must be considered[50]. Moreover, acute gastric mucosal injury has been reported in patients treated with recombinant IL-2 and IL-4[51]. The report that IL-10 can inhibit Th1 proliferation and cytokine production[52] suggests that an absence of IL-10 may lead to the increased T cell involvement in *H. pylori* infection.

In evaluating the mechanisms by which immune responses contribute to the health of gastric tissue, one must consider some novel observations suggesting that immune function itself is governed by gastrin, histamine or acetylcholine[53]. For example, does the hypergastrinaemia associated with *H. pylori* alter cytokine production? If so, does this directly affect epithelial integrity, cytoprotection or acid secretion in addition to any deleterious effects on local immune responses? To date, very few studies have addressed the regulation of gastric antibody responses through conventional means, let alone the role of these novel interactions which may be important in the pathogenesis of gastric disease during infection with *H. pylori*.

IMPACT OF CYTOKINES ON PHYSIOLOGICAL FUNCTION

The traditional view of the extracellular control of acid secretion may be shattered by a recent report which suggests that receptors for regulatory factors controlling acid secretion may be expressed to a greater degree on cells of the immune system[53]. This observation implies that factors from immune cells, perhaps released following stimulation by gastrin, histamine or carbachol, may regulate acid secretion as supported by several studies[54–60].

Studies suggesting a link between the immune system and non-immune elements in the stomach have shown that antigen presented orally to a sensitized dog leads to an increase in gastrin release and changes in transport function[61,62]. This may be quite significant when one considers that macromolecules can be taken up by the gastric mucosa and trigger sensitized immune cells within the mucosa[63]. It has also been shown that IL-1 can increase gastrin release[64]. Since IL-1, IL-6, TNF-α and IL-8 are increased during infection with *H. pylori*[35], these mediators may alter acid secretion directly or indirectly by an effect on gastrin. Interestingly, IL-1 inhibits acid secretion[58] and has a sparing effect on gastric ulceration[65,66]. These observations, combined with the report that acute gastric mucosal injury occurs in patients treated with recombinant IL-2 or IL-4[51], support the notion that an imbalance in the local immune response during infection with *H. pylori* plays a key role in the pathogenesis of peptic ulcers.

CONCLUSIONS AND FUTURE DIRECTIONS

Many of the reports to date would support the hypothesis that the stomach behaves like other mucosal tissues in health and disease. Despite the parallels to other tissues, however, one cannot ignore the specialization of immune responses in this site. Future research should identify the significant features of T and B cell lineage or repertoire that could be important in health or disease. In addition, the processes that initiate immune and inflammatory pathways have to be characterized, as well as the functional interactions among physiological transmitters, cytokines and inflammatory mediators that are perturbed during infection with *H. pylori*. This approach will most likely succeed at identifying key elements that improve our understanding of why only some people that carry the infection succumb to certain clinical manifestations. Perhaps more importantly, the ease of access to the stomach, combined with the growing understanding of the aetiologic agent, may help us understand basic mechanisms of host responses to infection that will enhance our understanding of the pathogenesis of other chronic inflammatory disorders in the gastrointestinal tract.

References

1. Marshall JS, Bienenstock J, Perdue MH, Stanisz AM, Stead RH, Ernst PB. Novel cellular interactions and networks involving the intestinal immune system and its microenvironment. Acta Pathol Microbiol Immunol Scand. 1989;97:383–94.
2. Ouellette AJ, Lualdi JC. A novel mouse gene family coding for cationic, cysteine-rich peptides. J Biol Chem. 1990;265:9831–7.
3. Valnes K, Brandtzaeg P, Elgjo K, Stave R. Specific and nonspecific humoral defense factors in the epithelium of normal and inflamed gastric mucosa. Gastroenterology. 1984;86:402–12.
4. Brandtzaeg P, Halstensen TS, Kett K *et al.* Immunobiology and immunopathology of human gut mucosa: humoral immunity and intraepithelial lymphocytes. Gastroenterology. 1989;97:1562–84.
5. Brandtzaeg P, Valnes K, Scott H, Rognum TO, Bjerke K, Baklien K. The human gastrointestinal secretory immune system in health and disease. In: Polak JM, Bloom SR, Wright NA, Butler AG, editors. Basic science in gastroenterology: diseases of the gut. Norwich: Page Bros, 1986:179–200.
6. Bienenstock J, Befus AD. Some thoughts on the biologic role of immunoglobulin A. Gastroenterology. 1983;84:178–85.
7. Witt CS. The mucosal immune response to *Helicobacter pylori*. In: Cripps AW, editor. Mucosal immunology. Newcastle: Newey & Beath, 1991:149–53.
8. Lefrancois L. Extrathymic differentiation of intraepithelial lymphocytes: generation of a separate and unequal T cell repertoire. Immunol Today. 1991;12:436–8.
9. Taguchi T, McGhee JR, Coffman RL *et al.* Analysis of Th1 and Th2 cells in murine gut-associated tissues. Frequencies of CD4+ and CD8+ cells that secrete IFN gamma and IL-5. J Immunol. 1990;145:68–77.
10. Mosley RL, Styre D, Klein JR. Differentiation and functional maturation of bone marrow-derived intestinal epithelial T cells expressing membrane T cell receptor in athymic radiation chimeras. J Immunol. 1990;145:1369–75.
11. Smoot DT, Resau JH, Naab T *et al.* Adherence of *Helicobacter pylori* to cultured human gastric epithelial cells. Infect Immun. 1993;61:350–5.
12. Dytoc M, Gold B, Louie M *et al.* Comparison of *Helicobacter pylori* and attaching–effacing *Escherichia coli* adhesion to eukaryotic cells. Infect Immun. 1992;61:448–56.
13. Cover TL, Blaser MJ. Purification and characterization of the vacuolating toxin from *Helicobacter pylori*. J Biol Chem. 1992;267:10570–5.

14. Crabtree JE, Peichl P, Wyatt JI, Stachl U, Lindley IJD. Gastric interleukin-8 and IgA IL-8 autoantibodies in *Helicobacter pylori* infection. Scand J Immunol. 1993;37:65–70.
15. Crowe SE, Hunt RH, Jordana M *et al*. Interleukin 8 secretion by gastric epithelial cells infected with *H. pylori in vitro*. Gastroenterology. 1993;105:A303(abstract).
16. Yasumoto K, Okamoto S, Mukaida N, Murakami S, Mai M, Matsushima K. Tumor necrosis factor α and interferon γ synergistically induce interleukin 8 production in a human gastric cancer cell line through acting concurrently on AP-1 and NF-kappaB-like binding sites of the interleukin 8 gene. J Biol Chem. 1992;267:22506–11.
17. Wright NA, Pike C, Elia G. Induction of a novel epidermal growth factor-secreting cell lineage by mucosal ulceration in human gastrointestinal stem cells. Nature. 1990;343:82–5.
18. Baggiolini M, Walz A, Kunkel SL. Neutrophil-activating peptide-1/interleukin 8, a novel cytokine that activates neutrophils. J Clin Invest. 1989;84:1045–9.
19. Larsen CG, Anderson AO, Appellia E, Oppenheim JJ, Matsushima K. The neutrophil-activating protein (NAP-1) is also chemotactic for T lymphocytes. Science. 1989;243: 1464–6.
20. Mai UEH, Perez-Perez GI, Allen JB, Wahl SM, Blaser MJ, Smith PD. Surface proteins from *Helicobacter pylori* exhibit chemotactic activity for human leukocytes and are present in gastric mucosa. J Exp Med. 1992;175:517–25.
21. Nielsen H, Andersen LP. Chemotactic activity of *Helicobacter pylori* sonicate for human polymorphonuclear leukocytes and monocytes. Gut. 1992;33:738–42.
22. Scheynius A, Engstrand L. Gastric epithelial cells in *Helicobacter pylori*-associated gastritis express HLA-DR but not ICAM-1. Scand J Immunol. 1991;33:237–41.
23. LaRosa GJ, Thomas KM, Kaufmann ME *et al*. Amino terminus of the interleukin-8 receptor is a major determinant of receptor subtype specificity. J Biol Chem. 1992;267:25402–6.
24. Mooney C, Keenan J, Munster D *et al*. Neutrophil activation by *Helicobacter pylori*. Gut. 1991;32:853–7.
25. Nash S, Stafford J, Madara JL. Effects of polymorphonuclear leukocyte transmigration on the barrier function of cultured intestinal epithelial monolayers. J Clin Invest. 1987;80: 1104–13.
26. Parkos CA, Colgan SP, Delp C, Arnaout MA, Madara JL. Neutrophil migration across a cultured epithelial monolayer elicits a biphasic resistance response representing sequential effects on transcellular and paracellular pathways. J Cell Biol. 1992;117:757–64.
27. Madara JL, Parkos C, Colgan S *et al*. Cl⁻ secretion in a model intestinal epithelium induced by a neutrophil-derived secretagogue. J Clin Invest. 1992;89:1938–44.
28. Engstrand L, Scheynius A, Pahlson C. An increased number of gamma/delta T cells and gastric epithelial cell expression of the groEL stress-protein homologue in *Helicobacter pylori*-associated chronic gastritis of the antrum. Am J Gastroenterol. 1991;86:976–80.
29. Finzi G, Cornaggia M, Capella C *et al*. Cathepsin E in follicle associated epithelium of intestine and tonsils: localization to M cells and possible role in antigen processing. Histochemistry. 1993;99:201–11.
30. Mayer L, Eisenhardt D. Lack of induction of suppressor T cells by gut epithelial cells from patients with inflammatory bowel disease. The primary defect? Gastroenterology. 1987;92:1524.
31. Mayer L, Shlien R. Evidence for function of Ia molecules on gut epithelial cells in man. J Exp Med. 1987;166:1471–83.
32. Bland PW, Warren LG. Antigen presentation by epithelial cells of the rat small intestine I. Kinetics, antigen specificity and blocking by anti-Ia antisera. Immunology. 1986;58:1–7.
33. Sollid LM, Kvale D, Brandtzaeg P, Markussen G, Thorsby E. Interferon gamma enhances expression of secretory component, the epithelial receptor for polymeric immunoglobulins. J Immunol. 1987;138:4303–6.
34. Engstrand L, Scheynius A, Pathlson C, Grimelius L, Schwan A, Gustavsson S. Association of *Campylobacter pylori* with induced expression of class II transplantation antigens on gastric epithelial cells. Infect Immun. 1989;57:827–32.
35. Crabtree JE, Shallcross TM, Heatley RV, Wyatt JI. Mucosal tumour necrosis factor α and interleukin-6 in patients with *Helicobacter pylori* associated gastritis. Gut. 1991;32:1473–7.
36. Crowe SE, Espejo R, Jin Y *et al*. The potential role of gastric epithelium in neutrophil recruitment, attachment and antigen presentation during *Helicobacter pylori* infection. J Immunol. 1993;150:10(abstract).

37. Bland PW, Warren LG. Antigen presentation by epithelial cells of the rat small intestine. II. Selective induction of suppressor T cells. Immunology. 1986;58:9–14.
38. Mayer L, Panja A, Li Y. Antigen recognition in the gastrointestinal tract: death to the dogma. Immunol Res. 1991;10:356–9.
39. Mayer L, Eisenhardt D, Salomon P, Bauer W, Plous R, Piccinini L. Expression of class II molecules on intestinal epithelial cells in humans. Differences between normal and inflammatory bowel disease. Gastroenterology. 1991;100:3–12.
40. Mayer L, Eisenhardt D. Lack of induction of suppressor T cells by intestinal epithelial cells from patients with inflammatory bowel disease. J Clin Invest. 1990;86:1255–60.
41. Wyatt JI, Rathbone BJ, Heatley RV. Local immune response to gastric Campylobacter in non-ulcer dyspepsia. J Clin Pathol. 1986;39:863–70.
42. Stacey AR, Hawtin PR, Newell DG. Local immune responses to Helicobacter pylori infections. In: Malfertheiner P, Ditschuneit H, editors. Helicobacter pylori, gastritis and peptic ulcer. New York: Springer-Verlag; 1990:162–6.
43. Halstensen TS, Mollnes TE, Garred P, Olav F, Brandtzaeg P. Epithelial deposition of immunoglobulin G1 and activated complement (C3b and terminal complement complex) in ulcerative colitis. Gastroenterology. 1990;98:1264–71.
44. Negrini R, Lisato L, Zanella I et al. Helicobacter pylori infection induces antibodies cross-reacting with human gastric mucosa. Gastroenterology. 1991;101:437–45.
45. Crabtree JE, Taylor JD, Wyatt JI et al. Mucosal IgA recognition of Helicobacter pylori 120 kDa protein, peptic ulceration, and gastric pathology. Lancet. 1991;338:332–5.
46. Romagnani S. Human Th1 and Th2 subsets: doubt no more. Immunol Today. 1991;12:256–7.
47. Del Prete GF, De Carli M, Mastromauro C et al. Purified protein derivative of Mycobacterium tuberculosis and excretory-secretory antigen(s) of Toxocara canis expand in vitro human T cells with stable and opposite (Type 1 T helper or Type 2 T helper) profile of cytokine production. J Clin Invest. 1991;88:346–50.
48. McGhee JR, Mestecky J, Dertzbaugh MT, Eldridge JH, Hirasawa M, Kiyono H. The mucosal immune system: from fundamental concepts to vaccine development. Vaccine. 1992;10:75–88.
49. Benson EB, Strober W. Regulation of IgA secretion by T cell clones derived from the human gastrointestinal tract. J Immunol. 1988;140:1874–82.
50. Phillips JO, Everson MP, Moldoveanu Z, Lue C, Mestecky J. Synergistic effect of IL-4 and IFN-gamma on the expression of polymeric Ig receptor (secretory component) and IgA binding by human epithelial cells. J Immunol. 1990;145:1740–4.
51. Rubin JT, Lotze MT. Acute gastric mucosal injury associated with the systemic administration of interleukin-4. Surgery. 1992;111:274–80.
52. Del Prete GP, De Carli M, Almerigogna F, Giudizi MG, Biagiotti R, Romagnani S. Human IL-10 is produced by both type 1 helper (Th1) and type 2 helper (Th2) T cell clones and inhibits their antigen-specific proliferation and cytokine production. J Immunol. 1993;150:353–60.
53. Mezey E, Palkovits M. Localization of targets for anti-ulcer drugs in cells of the immune system. Science. 1992;258:1662–4.
54. Robert A, Olafsson AS, Lancaster C, Zhang W-R. Interleukin-1 is cytoprotective, anti-secretory, stimulates PGE2 synthesis by the stomach and retards gastric emptying. Life Sci. 1991;48:123–34.
55. Saperas ES, Yang H, Rivier C, Tache Y. Central action of recombinant interleukin-1 to inhibit acid secretion in rats. Gastroenterology. 1990;99:1599–606.
56. Uehara A, Okumura T, Sekiya C, Okaura K, Takasugi Y, Namiki M. Interleukin-1 inhibits the secretion of gastric acid in rats: possible involvement of prostaglandin. Biochem Biophys Res Commun. 1989;162:1578–84.
57. Uehara A, Okumura T, Kitamori S, Takasugi Y, Namiki M. Interleukin-1: a cytokine that has potent antisecretory and anti-ulcer actions via the central nervous system. Biochem Biophys Res Commun. 1990;173:585–90.
58. Wallace JL, Cucula M, Mugridge K, Parente L. Secretagogue-specific effects of interleukin 1 on gastric acid secretion. Am J Physiol Gastrointest Liver Physiol. 1991;261:559–64.
59. Nompleggi D, Beinborn M, Wolfe M. The effect of cytokines on [^{14}C]aminopyrine accumulation in isolated canine parietal cells. Gastroenterology. 1992;102:A-748 (abstract).

60. Modlin IM, Tsunoda T, Coffey RJ, Goldenring JR. Structure–activity relationship of transforming growth factor-alpha (TGF-α) in the inhibition of parietal cell secretion. Gastroenterology. 1992;102:A-746(abstract).
61. Teichmann RK, Andress HJ, Gycha S, Seifert J, Brendel W. Immunologic mediated gastrin release. Gastroenterology. 1983;84:1333–9.
62. Catto-Smith AG, Patrick MK, Scott RB, Davison JS, Gall DG. Gastric response to mucosal IgE-mediated reactions. Am J Physiol. 1989;257:G704–8.
63. Curtis GH, Gall DG. Macromolecular transport by rat gastric mucosa. Am J Physiol Gastrointest Liver Physiol. 1992;262:G1033–40.
64. Kramling H-J, Enders G, Teichman RK, Demmel T, Merkle R, Brendel W. Antigen-induced gastrin release: an immunologic mechanism of gastric antral mucosa. Adv Exp Med Biol. 1987;216A:427–9.
65. Wallace JL, Keenan CM, Mugridge KG, Parente L. Reduction of the severity of experimental gastric and duodenal ulceration by interleukin-1β. Eur J Pharmacol. 1990;1860:279–84.
66. Uehara A, Okumura T, Kitamori S *et al.* Gastric antisecretory and antiulcer actions of interleukin-1: Evidence for the presence of an 'immune-brain–gut' axis. J Clin Gastroenterol. 1992;14(Suppl. 1):S149–55.

27
Specific *H. pylori* immune response

U. E. H. MAI

Epidemiological, clinical, and pathological evidence implicates *Helicobacter pylori* in the aetiology of human chronic mucosal inflammation. However, the pathophysiology of *H. pylori*-induced inflammation is widely unknown.

In *H. pylori*-infected patients the microorganisms are located within or beneath the mucus layer closely associated with the epithelium. Although *H. pylori* is a non-invasive bacterium, the presence of *H. pylori* is associated with a mucosal inflammatory response that consists of large numbers of polymorphonuclear and mononuclear inflammatory cells. These observations suggest that *H. pylori* recruits inflammatory cells by actively releasing or passively shedding cellular components which, after absorption into the mucosa, serve as chemo-attractants for mononuclear phagocytes and polymorphonuclear leukocytes.

To investigate this hypothesis we assessed the ability of material released by *H. pylori* as well as extracted *H. pylori* surface proteins and *H. pylori* urease to induce chemotaxis by human leukocytes *in vitro*[1]. Additionally, gastric biopsy specimens from *H. pylori*-infected patients were evaluated for the existence of *H. pylori* chemotactic products within the antral mucosa.

It could be shown that *H. pylori in vitro* releases products with chemotactic activity for monocytes and neutrophils. This chemotactic activity was inhibited by antisera to either *H. pylori* whole bacteria or *H. pylori*-derived urease. Moreover, surface proteins extracted from *H. pylori* and purified *H. pylori* urease, which is a major component of the surface proteins, exhibited dose-dependent, antibody-inhibitable chemotactic activity. In addition, a synthetic 20-amino acid peptide from the NH_2-terminal portion of the 61-kDa subunit, but not the 30-kD subunit, of urease exhibited chemotactic activity for monocytes and neutrophils, localizing the chemotactic activity, at least in part, to the NH_2-terminus of the 61-kDa subunit of urease. The ability of leukocytes to be attracted to *H. pylori* surface proteins despite formyl-methionyl-leucyl-phenylalanine (FMLP) receptor saturation, selective inhibition of FMLP-mediated chemotaxis, or preincubation of the surface proteins with antiserum to FMLP, indicated that the chemotaxis was not FMLP-mediated.

Finally, *H. pylori* surface proteins and urease could be identified by

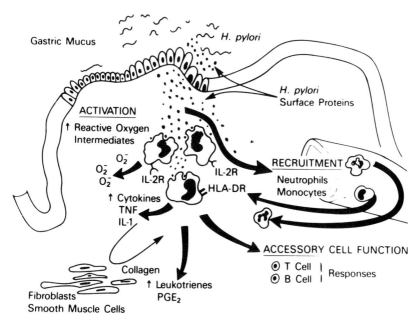

Fig. 1 Initiation of an inflammatory response in the human gastrointestinal mucosa by *H. pylori*

immunoperoxidase staining in the lamina propria of biopsies from the gastric antrum of patients with *H. pylori*-associated gastritis but not from uninfected subjects. Deposits of peroxidase-positive material were detected throughout the lamina propria in close proximity to the crypt epithelium within monocytes/macrophages beneath the basal membrane.

To elucidate the potential role of monocytes/macrophages in the inflammatory response to *H. pylori*, we investigated the interaction between soluble *H. pylori* surface proteins, which are enriched for urease and do not contain lipopolysaccharides, and highly purified human monocytes *in vitro*[2]. These studies provided evidence that *H. pylori* is capable of activating human monocytes. This activation is reflected for example in the increased expression of the surface molecules HLA-DR and interleukin 2-receptor, enhanced synthesis of interleukin-1 and tumour necrosis factor mRNA and peptide, and the secretion of the reactive oxygen intermediate superoxide anion. Moreover, both non-lipopolysaccharide containing surface constituents and purified lipopolysaccharide from *H. pylori* stimulated phenotypic, transcriptional, and functional changes in monocytes. Taken together, these results indicate that *H. pylori* activates monocytes by both a lipopolysaccharide-dependent and a novel lipopolysaccharide-independent mechanism.

These findings suggest the following sequence of events (Fig. 1): After ingestion of the bacteria and colonization of the gastric mucosa, *H. pylori*, like many other microorganisms, sheds cellular components, including surface proteins such as urease. The bacterial products become solubilized in the gastric mucus and are absorbed across the antral epithelium into the lamina propria where the urease recruits monocytes and neutrophils. Resident and recruited mononuclear phagocytes consequently phagocytize the foreign material and become activated. For example, since *H. pylori* can induce HLA-DR expression by monocytes *in vitro*, it is possible that the microorganism can stimulate HLA-DR expression on mucosal monocytes/macrophages *in vivo*. In view of the requirement that antigens be presented to lymphocytes in the context of class II molecules, increased HLA-DR expression may facilitate presentation of the relevant *H. pylori* antigens. This is a critical step in the production of *H. pylori*-specific antibodies. Interleukin 1 and tumour necrosis factor, also produced by *H. pylori*-activated monocytes/macrophages, are important mediators of inflammation, including mucosal destruction. Both cytokines exhibit potent pro-inflammatory activities which likely amplify the recruitment and activation of leukocytes. In addition, interleukin-1 secretion by activated monocytes/macrophages is an essential cytokine signal to elicit an antigen specific immune response by B and T cell lymphocytes. Finally, *H. pylori*-induced secretion of superoxide anion, a reactive oxygen intermediate, which is capable of inducing cell and mucosal injury and serves as a precursor for other toxic oxygen species, also contributes to the mucosal inflammation. These cell products and possibly other factors released by the newly recruited monocytes and neutrophils, may induce and perpetuate the tissue inflammatory lesions associated with *H. pylori*.

Acknowledgement

I thank my coworkers, especially P. D. Smith and M. J. Blaser, for their valuable contributions.

References

1. Mai UEH, Perez-Perez GI, Allen JB *et al*. Surface proteins from *Helicobacter pylori* exhibit chemotactic activity for human leukocytes and are present in gastric mucosa. J Exp Med. 1992;175:517–25.
2. Mai UEH, Perez-Perez GI, Wahl LM *et al*. Soluble surface proteins from *Helicobacter pylori* activate monocytes/macrophages by lipopolysaccharide-independent mechanism. J Clin Invest. 1991;87:894–900.

28
B cell responses in *H. pylori* infection

D. G. NEWELL and A. R. STACEY

INTRODUCTION

In the past the main impetus for investigating host B cell responses during *H. pylori* infection has been the need to develop accurate, non-invasive serodiagnostic tests. More recently the role of antibodies in the disease process, and the possibility of immunotherapy or vaccination, have become important research areas. In addition *H. pylori* has provided a unique opportunity for the immunologist to study immune responses to an infection at this unusual mucosal site.

CHARACTERISTICS OF THE HOST CIRCULATING ANTIBODY RESPONSE

Most adult patients colonized with *H. pylori* elicit a measurable systemic antibody response which comprises predominantly IgG. IgA antibodies are detectable in 30–40% of seropositive patients, but IgM antibodies are rarely seen[1,2]. This isotype profile is consistent with a prolonged chronic mucosal infection. In children the antibody responses seem to be different as circulating IgA antibodies are infrequent[3,4], which may reflect either an immaturity of the immune response or, more likely, the acute nature of the disease.

Because of the chronic nature of the normal adult infection the kinetics of the antibody response during the acute phase are unknown. In one volunteer study, IgG seroconversion occurred between 22 and 33 days post-infection[5]. Subsequent studies showed that there was also an initial, short-lived IgM response and a seroconversion of specific IgA[6]. These observations have recently been confirmed during a naturally acquired *H. pylori* infection[7].

The constant level of circulating antibodies throughout the chronic phase of infection[8] suggests a long-term balance between antigen load and host immunity. Following successful treatment there is a detectable fall in both serum IgA and IgA antibody levels. However, this decline in response is

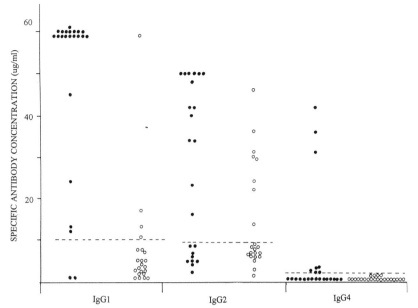

Fig. 1 ELISA of the serum IgG subclass responses to *H. pylori* acid extractable surface antigens: ●, *H. pylori*-positive patients; ○, *H. pylori*-negative patients

remarkably slow, and return to seronegativity may take months or even years after eradication. Recent studies indicate that this antibody longevity is, in part, an antigen-specific effect[9].

Because the profile of IgG subclasses induced during infection is a consequence of antigen type, exposure time and host genetic factors, such information may contribute to our understanding of the disease process. The IgG subclass response, as detected by ELISA using subclass-specific monoclonal antibodies, also varies significantly between patients (Fig. 1). Circulating IgG1 are generally raised, while IgG2 and IgG4 antibodies are frequent. Not surprisingly, serum IgG3 antibodies, which are generally indicative of acute infections, are not detected[2,10]. The predominant subclass of serum IgA antibodies is IgA1[11].

It might be expected that as severity of gastritis increases, the enhanced epithelial damage would allow more systemic access to bacterial antigens and, therefore, circulating antibodies would be increased. Some studies indicate that IgG antibodies increase with severity of gastritis in adults[12] and children[3]. However, this is inconsistent, and certainly may not be extended to other isotypes in adults[2], although specific IgG2 may increase in duodenal ulcer patients[10].

ANTIBODY PRODUCTION AT THE GASTRIC MUCOSA

Because of stomach acidity, the rapidity of food passage and the viscosity of the mucous layer, the gastric mucosa is exposed to relatively few bacterial antigens under normal conditions. Lack of antigenic stimulation is reflected in the relative paucity of immunoglobulin-producing cells in normal gastric mucosa. However, during *H. pylori*-associated gastritis there is a massive recruitment of immune competent mononuclear cells into the gastric mucosa. Many of these are T cells but a large proportion of the infiltrating lymphocytes are of the B cell lineage[13]. Immunoglobulins of all isotypes are expressed by these infiltrating B cells during histologically defined gastritis (not specifically *H. pylori*-related), with IgA predominating but IgG showing the greatest increase over normal[14].

There seems to be a close relationship between mucosal B cells and disease. The ratio of IgA:IgG cells decreases with increasing severity of histological gastritis. Most of these increased IgG immunocytes are IgG1-producing, though the proportion of these cells decreases with severity of gastritis while IgG2- and IgG3-producing cells increase[15]. IgE-producing cells have also been observed in gastritis, though the importance of these in any disease process is unknown[14].

H. pylori-associated chronic superficial gastritis is now generally accepted as the natural host response to antigen load. Although *H. pylori* is non-invasive, antigenic material, including urease, is constantly lost from the bacterial surface[16]. These bacterially derived antigens penetrate into the gastric lamina propria as detected by immunohistology with monoclonal antibodies (Newell, unpublished data). This probably involves endocytosis by the gastric epithelial cells and/or passive transport across leaky tight junctions. This antigen penetration is probably enhanced by the local production of IgG which can increase epithelial permeability[14]. Sometimes even whole organisms will penetrate damaged junctions, and this may be more frequent in the acute phase of infection[17].

Undoubtedly the isotype and specificity of the local antibody response reflects the amount and type of antigen penetrating the gastric epithelium. From the tissue culture of gastric biopsy tissue the local antibody response is shown to be primarily of the IgA isotype (Fig. 2). Immunoglobulin G, mainly IgG1 (Fig. 3), and some IgM antibodies are also produced. Some of these antibodies, mainly IgA and some IgM but not IgG, can be found in gastric juice[1]. It seems likely that the short half-life of most IgG subclasses in the gastric environment accounts for this discrepancy.

The specific IgA produced at the gastric mucosal surface is primarily sIgA1[10]. Interestingly, epithelial expression of secretory component, especially by the mucous neck cells, and uptake of IgA for epithelial transport is enhanced during gastritis[18]. Not all infected patients produce mucosal IgA antibodies[19] though, in general, specific mucosal IgA is a better indicator of infection than serum IgG (Stacey, unpublished data).

It would appear that antigen responsiveness is not confined to those sites adjacent to the gastric mucosa as antibody-producing B cells are also present in the draining lymph nodes[20]. There is a continuous traffic of antigen-stimulated lymphocytes recirculating within the mucosal-associated lymphoid system (MALT). Lymphocyte homing mechanisms mean that antigen stimulation at the gastric mucosa should elicit antibody responses at other mucosal sites. Consistent with such a mechanism sIgA anti-*H. pylori* antibodies are

OD(450nm)

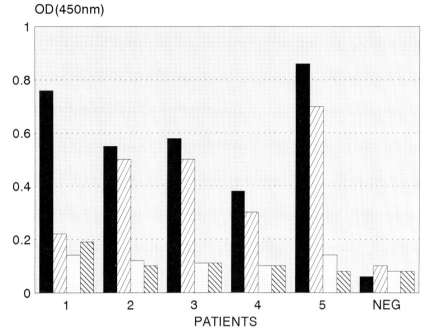

Fig. 2 Comparison of the serum and local IgG and IgA antibody levels of five *H. pylori*-positive patients (1–5) and an *H. pylori*-negative patient (neg). ■, Serum IgG; ▨, serum IgA; ▧, local IgG; ▨, local IgA.

detectable in saliva[21] and breast milk of infected patients (Stacey, unpublished data). However, the commonality of the MALT may not be complete, as regions of the gut, slightly distant from the site of colonization, have significantly lower antibody production[22], indicating either some compartmentalization of the antibody-producing cells to antigen-loaded areas or induced tolerance at other mucosal sites.

THE ANTIGENIC SPECIFICITY OF ANTI-*H. PYLORI* ANTIBODIES

The specificities of the serum and mucosal antibodies are directed by a variety of host and bacterial factors. As the infection is primarily mucosal, exposure to intracellular bacterial antigens is limited. Exposure to shed bacterial surface antigens, on the other hand, will be chronic, inducing a very mature immune response with high-affinity antibodies. On the host side the extent of epithelial damage, the massive infiltration of immunocompetent cells and genetic factors will all affect the specificity of the response.

The host circulating antibody response to *H. pylori* infection is remarkably variable[23]. This variability also occurs within local antibodies (Fig. 4). Nevertheless a number of *H. pylori* antigens appear to be consistently immunogenic during infection.

Most *H. pylori*-positive patients produce circulating antibodies that react

OD (450nm)

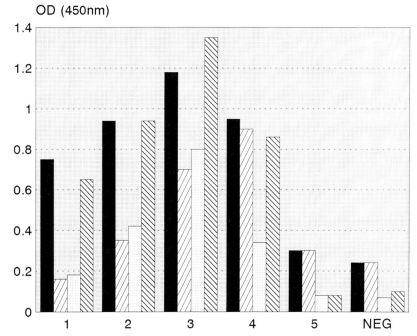

Fig. 3 Production of local IgG subclass anti-*H. pylori* antibodies from the gastric biopsies of five *H. pylori*-positive patients (1–5) and an *H. pylori*-negative patient (neg). ■, Total IgG; ▨, IgG1; ▦, IgG2; ▩, IgG4. Note that no specific IgG3 was detectable

against the 61 kDa and 28 kDa polypeptides which are subunits of urease[24,25]. This specificity has been confirmed using variants apparently lacking the urease subunits[26].

A 56 kDa protein copurifies with the urease, but is not essential for enzymic activity[25]. This protein is also highly immunogenic during infection, and is a homologue of the heat-shock protein Hsp60[27–29]. Purified native *H. pylori* Hsp60 is detectable by about 50% of human sera[29].

Most sera from *H. pylori*-positive patients also contain antibodies directed against a 120 kDa protein[30,31]. Local antibodies are also produced against this antigen[19] which is expressed on the surface of only 80% of *H. pylori* strains[31] and is associated with the vacuolating cytotoxic activity of *H. pylori*[32]. This 120 kDa antigen has some interesting antigenic properties. In particular the presence of local antibodies has a strong association with severity of disease[19]. Moreover, antibodies directed against this antigen are remarkably persistent following eradication of infection[9]. The mechanisms to this persistence are unknown. It seems unlikely that the antigen is retained in the tissue for any length of time, or that these antibodies have an unexpectantly long half-life. It is more likely that the 120 kDa antigen possesses epitopes cross-reactive with other, possibly self, antigens, to which the host is continually exposed.

Circulating antibodies are also detectable against a number of other *H.*

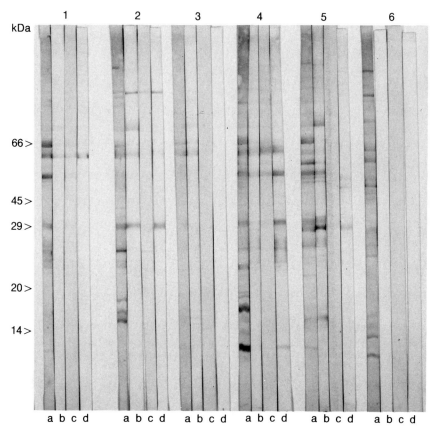

Fig. 4 The variation in the specificity of systemic and local antibody responses from six *H. pylori*-positive patients (1–6) against the acid-extractable surface a antigens of *H. pylori*: serum IgG (**a**), serum IgA (**b**), local IgG (**c**) and local IgA (**d**)

pylori antigens including several series of medium (87 000–86 000, 63 000–50 000) and low (20 000–22 000, 14 000–16 000) molecular weight proteins which are largely uncharacterized[23,33,34]. However, some of these antigens are associated with the flagella. By immunogold electron microscopic labelling techniques all sera and local antibodies from *H. pylori*-positive patients react with the sheathed flagella of *H. pylori* (Fig. 5). The antigenic composition of the flagellin sheath has been difficult to establish, but is apparently similar to that of the outer membrane[35]. It would seem that this sheath is not always intact, because most patient sera react with the 53 kDa major flagellin (flagellin A) protein[36]. In addition the flagellins of *H. pylori* have significant cross-reactivity with those of *Campylobacter jejuni* which is detectable with sera from patients infected with either organism[23].

Another antigenic polypeptide with approximately the same apparent mobility is the 54 kDa catalase subunit. This polypeptide has also recently

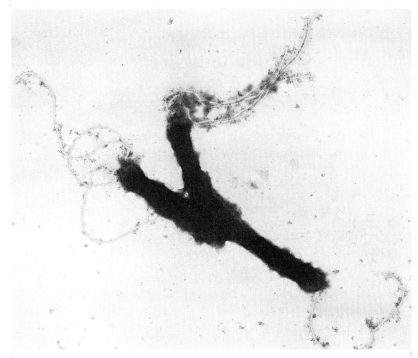

Fig. 5 Immunogold TEM labelling of *H. pylori in vitro* by local IgA antibodies produced by the gastric biopsies of an *H. pylori*-positive patient

been partly cloned and sequenced[37] and about 30% of sera from *H. pylori*-positive patients recognize the N-terminal portion of the recombinant catalase protein.

Some antigens appear to elicit isotype-specific responses. The antigen profiles detectable by serum and local IgG antibodies have a narrower spectrum than those of local IgA antibodies (see Fig. 4). Surprisingly, most patients had a broader pattern of reactivity in the serum IgG antibodies than in the gastric mucosal IgG antibodies (see Fig. 4), though this difference was not as striking between the local and serum IgA responses. This anomaly can be explained if serum IgA antibodies truly reflect the host response to those antigens seen at the mucosal surface while serum IgG antibodies are largely derived from both intracellular and extracellular bacterial antigens, possibly as a result of antigen uptake in the lower gut.

THE ROLE OF ANTIBODIES IN *H. PYLORI*-ASSOCIATED GASTRITIS

The role of local antibodies in the disease process is debatable. Although organisms attached to the gastric epithelium are coated with human immunoglobulin[38] the specificity of this binding has not been demonstrated. However, local antibodies can bind to surface antigens of H. pylori in vitro (Fig. 5). These local antibodies neither eliminate the colonization of the gastric mucosa, prevent the recrudescence of infection after temporary clearance[39] nor protect from iatrogenic reinfection[40]. The reasons for this ineffectiveness are unclear.

H. pylori is sensitive in vitro to both antibody-dependent and -independent complement-mediated serum bactericidal activity[41,42]. Nevertheless, mucosal antibodies are unable to generate bactericidal activity in vitro[43] even in the presence of additional complement.

H. pylori also elicits a chemotaxic activity for polymorphonuclear cells[44]. Despite their mucosal location the bacteria remain accessible to these professional phagocytes, which can traverse the gastric epithelium and phagocytose colonizing bacteria[45]. The isotypes of antibodies, produced in the tissue adjacent to the site of colonization, should enable any antibody-mediated phagocytosis by these cells. Moreover, complement alone can opsonize these H. pylori[46]. The absence of invading bacteria or systemic infections indicates that these defence mechanisms are, at the least, effective within host tissue.

Eradication of this infection from the gastric mucosa would probably necessitate a mucosal antibody response which would effectively inhibit colonization. Serum antibodies are directed against a number of putative bacterial colonization factors, in particular the fibrillar haemagglutinin[47] and the urease[48]. Certainly some anti-urease antibodies can inhibit enzyme activity[49]. Although it can be assumed that mucosal antibodies reflect a similar specificity, infection, once acquired, persists lifelong. Nevertheless, these antibodies may contribute to limiting the extent of colonization. Certainly serum antibodies can neutralize the vacuolating cytotoxin[50], although there is little evidence that such neutralizing antibodies reduce the effects of the toxin.

Prevention of initial infection, by the host immune response, may be more likely. Most recently experimental mouse models of H. felis infections[51,52] indicate that antibody-mediated protection from infection can be induced following either oral vaccination or passive immunization. This demonstrates that mucosal antibodies can have some protective capacity at the gastric mucosal surface.

The capacity of bacterium to survive in this immunologically hostile host environment suggests that the organism has evolved mechanisms to avoid host defences. The molecular basis of such mechanisms is unknown, but the shedding of antibody/antigen complexes and the blocking of antibody activity with soluble antigen are possible, given the nature of the bacterial surface.

The localized immune response is so extensive that immunopathological events may play a significant role in the disease processes[53–55]. Several B cell-dependent mechanisms may be involved in such immunopathological events. The antibody-mediated activation of complement in the gastric mucosa should induce polymorphonuclear cell infiltration and subsequent tissue damage. Many of the isotypes produced during this infection mediate strong complement activating capacities. In addition, the increased specific

IgG4 detectable in mucosal secretions, although not complement binding, is consistent with prolonged antigenic stimulation[56] and is thought to have a role in hypersensitivity reactions.

There is increasing evidence for an autoimmune component to the immune response. Mice immunized with *H. pylori* produce antibodies which cross-react with gastric mucosa[57,58]. Moreover the 56 kDa protein of *H. pylori*, a homologue of Hsp60, induces significant antibody responses[28]. Antibodies directed against heat-shock proteins are known to have a role in the hypersensitivity reactions and immunopathological responses in a variety of diseases, including chlamydial and mycobacterial infections and Lyme's disease.

In view of the potential immunopathological component of this disease the potential of vaccination must be questioned. Interestingly, in two experimental models, *H. mustelae* in the ferret[59] and *H. pylori* in the pig[60], oral vaccination was not only unable to prevent colonization, but induced a more severe pathology than expected in unvaccinated animals.

CONCLUSION

The majority of people colonized with *H. pylori* elicit strong, specific circulating and gastric mucosal antibody responses of appropriate isotypes. Nevertheless this immune response appears to be generally ineffective in eliminating natural infections. Immunochemical techniques have shown that the antibody response to *H. pylori* is not only complex but extremely variable. Increasingly evidence indicates that the way the host responds to this infection, in terms of antibody isotype and specificity, is an important factor in the pathogenesis of *H. pylori*-associated diseases. In view of the evidence for immunopathological events, within the gastric mucosa and as a consequence of antigen load, the design and application of vaccines against *H. pylori* should be tempered with caution.

References

1. Rathbone BJ, Wyatt JI, Worsley BW *et al.* Systemic and local antibody responses to gastric *Campylobacter pyloridis* in non-ulcer dyspepsia. Gut. 1986;27:642–7.
2. Steer HW, Hawtin PR, Newell DG. An ELISA technique for the serodiagnosis of *Campylobacter pyloridis* infection in patients with gastritis and benign duodenal ulceration. Serodiagn Immunotherapy. 1987;1:253–9.
3. Czinn SJ, Carr HS, Speck WT. Diagnosis of gastritis caused by *Helicobacter pylori* in children by means of an ELISA. Rev Infect Dis. 1991;13(Suppl.8):S700–3.
4. Crabtree JE, Mahony MJ, Taylor JD, Heatley RV, Littlewood JM, Tompkins DS. Immune responses to *Helicobacter pylori* in children with recurrent abdominal pain. J Clin Pathol. 1991;44:768–71.
5. Morris A, Nicholson G. Ingestion of *Campylobacter pyloridis* causes gastritis and raised fasting pH. Am J Gastroenterol. 1987;82:192–9.
6. Morris A, Nicholson G. *Campylobacter pylori*: human ingestion studies. In: Rathbone, BJ, Heatley RV, editors. *Campylobacter pylori* and gastroduodenal disease. Oxford: Blackwell Scientific Publications; 1989:185–9.
7. Sobala GM, Crabtree JE, Dixon MF. Acute *Helicobacter pylori* infection: clinical features,

local and systemic immune responses, gastric mucosal histology and gastric juice ascorbic acid concentrations. Gut. 1991;32:1415–18.

8. Langenberg W, Rauws EAJ, Houthoff HJ *et al.* Follow-up of individuals with untreated *Campylobacter pylori*-associated gastritis and of non-infected persons with non-ulcer dyspepsia. J Infect Dis. 1988;157:1245–8.

9. Stacey AR, Bell GD, Newell DG. The value of class and subclass ELISAs and antibody specificity in monitoring treatment of *H. pylori*. In: Gasbarrini G, Pretolani S, editors. Basic and clinical aspects of *Helicobacter pylori* infection. Berlin, Springer-Verlag; 1993:159–63.

10. Bonktes HJ, Veenend RA, Pena AS *et al.* IgG subclass response to *Helicobacter pylori* in patients with chronic active gastritis and duodenal ulcer. Scand J Gastroenterol. 1992;27: 129–33.

11. Van der Est MMC, Veenendaal RA, Pena AS, Van Duijn W, Kuiper I, Lamers CBHW. ELISA analysis of IgA subclass antibodies to *Helicobacter pylori*. Elevated serum IgA1 antibodies in *Helicobacter pylori* infected patients. J Clin Nutr Gastroenterol. 1990;5: 185–90.

12. Faulde M, Schroder JP, Sobe D. Serodiagnosis of *Helicobacter pylori* infections by detection of immunoglobulin G antibodies using an immunoblot technique and enzyme immunoassay. Eur J Clin Infect Dis. 1992;11:589–94.

13. Kirchner T, Melber A, Fischbach W, Heilmann KL, Muller-Hermelink HK. Immunohisto-chemical patterns of the local immune response in *Helicobacter pylori* gastritis. In: Malfertheiner P, Ditschuneit H, editors. *Helicobacter pylori*, gastritis and peptic ulcer. Berlin, Springer-Verlag; 1990:213–22.

14. Valnes K, Brandtzaeg P, Elgjo K, Stave R. Quantitative distribution of immunoglobulin-producing cells in gastric mucosa: relation to chronic gastritis and glandular atrophy. Gut. 1986;27:505–14.

15. Valnes K, Brandtzaeg P. Subclass distribution of mucosal IgG-producing cells in gastritis. Gut. 1989;30:322–6.

16. Mai UI, Perez-Perez GI, Allen JB, Wahl SM, Blaser MJ, Smith PD. Surface proteins from *Helicobacter pylori* exhibit chemostatic activity for human leukocytes and are present in gastric mucosa. J Exp Med. 1992;175:517–25.

17. Tytgat GNT. Does the stomach adapt to *Helicobacter pylori*? Scand J Gastroenterol. 1992;27(Suppl.193):28–32.

18. Isaacson P. Immunoperoxidase study of the secretory immunoglobulin system and lysozyme in normal and diseased gastric mucosa. Gut. 1982;23:578–88.

19. Crabtree JE, Taylor JD, Wyatt JI *et al.* Mucosal IgA recognition of *Helicobacter pylori* 120 kDa protein, peptic ulceration and gastric pathology. Lancet. 1991;338:332–5.

20. Newell DG, Stacey AR. Isotype and specificity of local and systemic anti-*Helicobacter pylori* antibodies. In: Menge H, Gregor M, Tytgat GNJ, Marshall BJ, McNulty CAM, editors. *Helicobacter pylori* 1990. Berlin: Springer-Verlag; 1991:83–9.

21. Wirth HP, Vogt P, Ammann R, Altorfer J. IgA antikorper gegan *Helicobacter pylori* in magensekret; gastrische sekretorische immunantwork oder specihelverunreinigung? Schweiz Med Wochschr. 1993;123:1106–10.

22. Crabtree JE, Shallcross TM, Wyatt JI *et al.* Mucosal humoral immune response to *Helicobacter pylori* in patients with duodenitis. Dig Dis Sci. 1991;44:768–71.

23. Newell DG. Human antibody responses to the surface protein antigens of *Campylobacter pyloridis*. Serodiagn Immunother. 1987;1:209–17.

24. Hu LT, Mobley HLT. Purification and N-terminal analysis of urease from *Helicobacter pylori*. Infect Immun. 1990;58:992–8.

25. Hawtin PR, Stacey AR, Newell DG. Investigation of the structure and localization of the urease of *Helicobacter pylori* using monoclonal antibodies. J Gen Microbiol. 1990;136: 1995–2000.

26. Perez-Perez GI, Olivares AZ, Cover TL, Blaser MJ. Characteristics of *Helicobacter pylori* variants selected for urease deficiency. Infect Immun. 1992;60:3658–63.

27. Evans DJ, Evans DG, Engstrand L, Graham DY. Urease-associated heat shock protein of *Helicobacter pylori*. Infect Immun. 1992;60:2125–7.

28. Dunn BE, Roop RM, Sung C-C, Sharma SA, Perez-Perez GI, Blaser MJ. Identification and purification of a cpn60 heat shock protein homolog from *Helicobacter pylori*. Infect Immun. 1992;60:1046–1051.

29. Macchia G, Massone A, Burroni D, Covacci A, Censini S, Rappuoli R. The Hsp60 protein of *Helicobacter pylori*: structure and immune response in patients with gastroduodenal diseases. Mol Microbiol. 1993;9:645–52.
30. Von Wulffen H, Grote HJ. Enzyme-linked immunosorbent assay for detection of immunoglobulin A and G antibodies to *Campylobacter pylori*. Eur J Clin Microbiol Infect Dis. 1988;7:559–65.
31. Apel I, Jacobs E, Kist M, Bredt W. Antibody response of patients against a 120 kDa surface protein of *Campylobacter pylori*. Zentralbl Bakteriol Microbiol Hyp. 1988;268:271–6.
32. Crabtree JE, Figura N, Taylor JD, Bugnoli M, Armellini D, Tompkins DS. Expression of 120 kilodalton protein and cytotoxicity in *Helicobacter pylori*. J Clin Pathol. 1992;45: 733–4.
33. Jones DM, Eldridge J, Fox AJ, Sethi P, Whorwell PJ. Antibody to the gastric Campylobacter-like organism ('*Campylobacter pyloridis*') – clinical correlations and distribution in the normal population. J Med Microbiol. 1986;22:57–62.
34. Von Wulffen H, Grote HJ, Gaterman S, Loning T, Berger B, Buhl C. Immunoblot analysis of immune response to *Campylobacter pylori* and its clinical associations. J Clin Pathol. 1988;41:653–9.
35. Geis G, Suerbaum S, Forsthoff B, Leying H, Opferkuch W. Ultrastructure and biochemical studies of the flagellar sheath of *Helicobacter pylori*. J Med Microbiol. 1993;38:371–7.
36. Suerbaum S, Josenhans C, Labigne A. Cloning and genetic characterisation of the *Helicobacter pylori* and *Helicobacter mustelae* flaB flagellin genes and construction of mutants by electroporation-mediated allelic exchange. J Bacteriol. 1993;175:3278–88.
37. Newell DG, Nuijten PJM, Stacey AR, Hazell SL. The cloning and partial sequence analysis of the catalse gene of *Helicobacter pylori*. In: Gasbarrini G, Pretolani S, editors. Basic and clinical aspects of *Helicobacter pylori* infection. Berlin: Springer-Verlag; 1993:223–6.
38. Wyatt JI, Rathbone BJ, Heatley RV. Local immune response to gastric *Campylobacter* in non-ulcer dyspepsia. J Clin Microbiol. 1986;39:86370.
39. Langenberg W, Rauws EAJ, Widjojokusumo A, Tytgat GNJ, Zanen HC. Identification of *Campylobacter pyloridis* isolates by restriction endonuclease DNA analysis. J Clin Microbiol. 1986;24:414–17.
40. Langenberg W, Rauws EAJ, Oudbier JH, Tytgat GNJ. Patient-to-patient transmission of *Campylobacter pylori* infection by fiber optic gastroduodenoscopy and biopsy. J Infect Dis. 1990;167:507–11.
41. Das SS, Karin QN, Easmon CSF. Opsonophagocytosis of *Campylobacter pylori*. J Med Microbiol. 198;27:125–30.
42. Pruul H, Lee PC, Goodwin CS, McDonald PJ, Interaction of *Campylobacter pyloridis* with human immune defence mechanisms. J Med Microbiol. 1987;23:233–8.
43. Stacey AR, Hawtin PR, Newell DG. Local and systemic antibody responses during *Helicobacter pylori* infections. In: Pajares JM, et al., editors. *H. pylori* and gastro duodenal pathology. Berlin: Springer Verlag; 1993:in press.
44. Neilsen N, Andersen LP. Chemotactic activity of *Helicobacter pylori* sonicate for human polymorphonuclear leucocytes and monocytes. Gut. 1992;33:738–42.
45. Steer HW. Ultrastructure of *Helicobacter pylori* in vivo. In: Rathbone BJ, Heatley RV, editors. *Helicobacter pylori* and gastroduodenal disease, 2nd edn. Oxford: Blackwell Scientific Publications; 1992:42–50.
46. McKinlay AW, Young A, Russell RI, Gemmell CG. Opsonic requirements of *Helicobacter pylori*. J Med Microbiol. 1993;38:209–15.
47. Evans DJ, Evans DG, Smith KE, Graham DY. Serum antibody responses to the *N*-acetylneuraminyllactose-binding hemagglutinin of *Campylobacter pylori*. Infect Immun. 1989;57:664–7.
48. Stacey AR, Hawtin PR, Newell DG. Antigenicity of fractions of *Helicobacter pylori* prepared by fast protein liquid chromatography and urease captured by monoclonal antibodies. Eur J Clin Microbiol Infect Dis. 1990;9:732–7.
49. Hawtin PR, Stacey AR, Newell DG. Investigation of the structure and localization of the urease of *Helicobacter pylori* using monoclonal antibodies. J Gen Microbiol. 1990;136: 1995–2000.
50. Cover TL, Cao P, Murthy UK, Sipple MS, Blaser MJ. Serum neutralizing antibody response to the vacuolating cytotoxin of *Helicobacter pylori*. J Clin Invest. 1992;90:913–18.

51. Chen M, Lee A, Hazell S. Immunisation against gastric helicobacter infection in a mouse/*Helicobacter felis* model. Lancet. 1992;339:1120–1.
52. Czinn SJ, Cai A, Negrud JG. Protection of germ-free mice from infection by *Helicobacter felis* after active oral or passive IgA immunization. Vaccine. 1993;11:637–42.
53. Newell DG, Stacey AR. Isotype and specificity of local and systemic anti-*Helicobacter pylori* antibodies. In: Menge H, Gregor M, Tytgat GNJ, Marchall BJ, McNulty CAM, editors. *Helicobacter pylori* 1990. Berlin: Springer-Verlag; 1991:83–8.
54. Rautelin H, Kosunen TU. *Helicobacter pylori* and associated gastroduodenal diseases. APMIS. 1991;99:677–95.
55. Blaser MJ. Hypotheses on the pathogenesis and natural history of *Helicobacter pylori*-induced inflammation. Gastroenterology. 1992;102:720–7.
56. Aalberse RC, Van der Gaag R, Leeuwen J. Serologic aspects of IgG4 antibodies. 1. Prolonged immunization results in an IgG4 restricted response. J Immunol. 1993;130: 722–6.
57. Negrini R, Lisato L, Cavazzini L et al. Monoclonal antibodies for specific immunoperoxidase detection of *Campylobacter pylori*. Gastroenterology. 1989;96:414–20.
58. Rathbone BJ, Trejdosiewicz LK. A strain-restricted monoclonal antibody to *Campylobacter pyloridis*. In Kaijser B, Falsen E, editors. Campylobacter IV. Goteborg: University of Goteborg; 1988:426–7.
59. Palley LS, Murphy J, Yan L, Taylor N, Polidoro D, Fox J. The effects of an oral immunisation scheme using muramyl dipeptide as an adjuvant to prevent gastric *Helicobacter mustelae* infection of ferrets. Acta Gastroenterol Belg. 1993;56(Suppl.):54.
60. Eaton KA, Krakowka S. Chronic gastritis due to *Helicobacter pylori* in immunized gnotobiotic piglets. Gastroenterology. 1992;103:1580–6.

29
T cell subsets in *H. pylori*-associated gastritis

K. DEUSCH, C. SEIFARTH, K. REICH and M. CLASSEN

INTRODUCTION

The pathogenesis of chronic gastritis and the presumed causative role of *Helicobacter pylori* has led to considerable dispute in this field of research. However, a large number of studies involving self-inoculations[1,2], epidemiological assessments[3,4], histopathological evaluations[5-7] and the fact that after eradication of *H. pylori* the marked inflammatory lesions in the gastric mucosa disappear[8,9] have provided compelling evidence suggesting *H. pylori* as a principal causative agent in this form of gastritis. Furthermore, therapeutic trials showed that combined antibiotic and antacid therapy was more effective in preventing disease relapse than antacid therapy alone[10]. Mechanisms involved in the development of mucosal lesions include a variety of toxins[11-14] and enzymes secreted by *H. pylori* that destroy epithelial cells and digest the protective gastric mucus[14,15]. Moreover, mucosal lesions are characterized by a marked lymphocytic infiltrate, suggesting a specific immune reaction that may lead to considerable mucosal pathology[5,6,9]. Specifically, it has been claimed that CD4$^+$ T cells and $\gamma\delta$ T cells play a critical role in *H. pylori*-associated gastritis[16]. The presence of $\gamma\delta$ T cells in the mucosal lesions has implicated endogenous and bacterial heat-shock proteins as potential target antigens for the specific local immune reaction, as some investigators have reported that heat-shock proteins selectively stimulate $\gamma\delta$ T cells *in vitro*[17]. Heat-shock proteins are a group of proteins believed to function as chaperones in all prokaryotic and eukaryotic cells that are expressed at enhanced levels under conditions such as physical, thermal or chemical stress in order to prevent denaturation of proteins that are vital for cell function[18-20]. Importantly, enhanced heat-shock protein expression was observed in tissues stressed by chronic bacterial infection[19] in rheumatoid arthritis lesions in conjunction with local accumulation of $\gamma\delta$ T cells[17]. However, whether the accumulation of $\gamma\delta$ T cells in *H. pylori*-affected mucosal lesions represents a specific phenomenon is unclear at present, since to date the presence of $\gamma\delta$ T cells has not been evaluated in other forms of gastritis that are not associated with *H. pylori*. In addition to the marked lymphocytic infiltration epithelial cells within the mucosal lesions exhibit an increased expression of MHC class II molecules[21–23]. Therefore, in our study we comparatively analysed the T cell receptor usage of infiltrating lymphocytes in chronic gastritis with regard to the presence or absence of *H. pylori*. In addition, the functional status of the infiltrating inflammatory cells was assessed by determining the expression of IL-2 receptors and MHC class II molecules.

MATERIALS AND METHODS

Patients

Thirty-five adult patients (17 males and 18 females) aged from 19 to 68 with upper abdominal symptoms underwent gastroscopy to exclude gastrointestinal diseases. Some of the patients with chronic active gastritis received conservative treatment with H_2-receptor antagonists or antacids, but no patient took antibiotics, omeprazole or colloidal bismuth. The distribution of treated and untreated patients was similar in the *H. pylori*-positive and *H. pylori*-negative group (see below). The patients of the other two groups took no medication influencing the gastric mucosa.

Histopathology

Three biopsy specimens from a prepyloric region of the antrum were obtained from every patient. Two of the three biopsies were paraffin-embedded and serial sections were performed. Subsequently, sections were stained with haematoxylin/eosin and analysed by two independent pathologists to assess the degree of gastritis. In addition, sections were Warthin Starry silver stained to search for the presence of *H. pylori* in the biopsy specimen. Cryostat serial sections of the third biopsy were immunohistochemically analysed (see below) and assessed for *H. pylori* colonization.

According to the presence or absence of infiltrating neutrophils and the colonization with *H. pylori*, four groups were defined:

Group 1: The mucosa was normal and no *H. pylori* could be found ($n = 5$).
Group 2: Chronic inactive gastritis without *H. pylori* colonization ($n = 7$).
Group 3: Chronic active gastritis without *H. pylori* colonization ($n = 5$).
Group 4: Chronic active *Helicobacter*-associated gastritis ($n = 18$).

Immunohistochemistry

Biopsy specimens obtained endoscopically from antrum mucosa were snap-frozen in isopentane liquid nitrogen and stored at $-70°C$. Serial cryostat sections were mounted on poly-L-lysine coated glass slides, air-dried and stored at $-70°C$ until use. Sections were examined for the expression of

CD3, CD4, CD8 (Becton Dickinson, Heidelberg, Germany), $\alpha\beta$TCR (βF1, T Cell Sciences, Cambridge, MA, USA), $\gamma\delta$TCR (TCRδ1), HLA-DR, HLA-DQ (Dianova, Hamburg, Germany) and control antibody (absorbed normal mouse IgG, Dianova, Hamburg, Germany). Immunohistochemical staining was performed as described in the manual to the Vectastain ABC Kit (Vectastain ABC Kit: Vector, Burlingame, CA, USA). Briefly, serial sections were acetone-fixed, washed and blocked with normal horse serum. The sections were incubated for 30 min with the respective antibodies and subsequently washed and incubated with biotin-conjugated horse anti-mouse antibody. Next, the sections were washed again and incubated with avidin–biotin–peroxidase complex (ABC). Finally antibody-labelled cells were stained with 9-amino-3-ethylcarbazole (AEC) and counterstained with Mayer's haemalaun. The relative distribution of lymphocyte subsets was determined by counting the number of cells immunostained by the respective subset-specific antibody in relation to the number of cells stained by CD3 antibody. To determine the frequency of T cell subsets within the epithelium the number of CD3$^+$ cells per 500 epithelial cells was enumerated. Next, the total number of cells per 500 epithelial cells expressing the respective subset specific marker in the same region of the adjacent section was divided by the total number of CD3$^+$ cells. The resulting fraction represents the relative frequency of each subset within the CD3$^+$ cell population.

In the lamina propria the frequency of T cell subsets was expressed as the fraction of the CD3$^+$ population in adjacent sections within the same tissue region. For the enumeration of cells within each section a counting grid was used that consisted of one large square encompassing an area of $0.0567 \, mm^2$ (at $40\times$ magnification). The large square was subdivided into 10 small squares. In each section 10 large squares were evaluated, i.e. an area of $0.567 \, mm^2$ was analysed. For the evaluation of MHC class expression qualitative scores were employed. A distinction was made between the staining of singular epithelial cells (grade 1), groups of epithelial cells (grade 2) and confluent staining of epithelial cells (grade 3), i.e. the intense staining does not allow distinction between individual cells.

RESULTS

Selective accumulation of CD4$^+$ T cells in *H. pylori*-positive gastritis

To obtain information about the function of the infiltrating lymphocytes in the mucosal lesions observed with *H. pylori*-positive gastritis, tissue sections were immunostained with monoclonal antibodies directed towards the CD4 and CD8 molecules, respectively. First, the numerical relation between CD4$^+$ and CD8$^+$ T cells contained within the entire mucosal layer (epithelium and lamina propria) was determined. In patients with histologically normal antral mucosa (group 1) the CD4/CD8 ratio was 0.5, whereas those with chronic inactive gastritis without *H. pylori* (group 2) and those with chronic active *H. pylori*-negative gastritis (group 3) had a slightly increased number of CD4 cells in the lesions (CD4/CD8 ratio = 0.6). Most importantly, patients within the group having chronic active *H. pylori*-positive gastritis (group 4) showed a markedly increased number of CD4$^+$ cells, resulting in a CD4/CD8 ratio of 2.5 ($p < 0.02$). When a distinction was made between lymphocytes contained in the lamina propria and the epithelium it became evident that the increase in mucosal CD4 cells in *H. pylori*-positive lesions was largely due to a selective accumulation of these cells in the lamina propria: normal mucosa CD4/CD8 ratio = 0.7 (group 1); *H. pylori*-negative gastritis, CD4/CD8 ratio = 1.0 (group 2 and group 3); *H. pylori*-positive gastritis, CD4/CD8 ratio = 2.2 (group 4) (Fig. 1a). Analysis of the total number of T cells revealed that the increase of the CD4/CD8 ratio was due to an absolute increase in the number of CD4$^+$ cells. In contrast, in the epithelium CD4$^+$ T cells were only rarely found in normal mucosa, and slightly increased in active gastritis. However, the total number of intraepithelial lymphocytes remained constant in all groups (Fig. 1b).

Increased CD25-Expression on T cells in *H. pylori*-positive gastritis

To determine the fraction of activated T cells in the lamina propria (LPL) and the epithelium (IEL) the expression of the IL-2 receptor (CD25) was evaluated by immunohistochemistry. In normal gastric mucosa and in chronic inactive gastritis the fraction of CD25$^+$ T cells was always less than 1%, whereas in chronic active *H. pylori*-negative gastritis the fraction of these cells was 3.25%. In chronic active *H. pylori*-positive gastritis (group 4) the fraction of CD25$^+$ T cells was significantly increased (12.5%) (Fig. 2). Interestingly, in this group intraepithelial lymphocytes expressed IL-2 receptors.

MHC class II expression in chronic gastritis

To further characterize the nature of the inflammatory changes in the gastric mucosa MHC class II expression (HLA-DR) was immunohistochemically analysed. In order to compare the degree of MHC class II expression between the individual patient groups the intensity of immunohistochemical staining was graded from 0 to 3, where the staining pattern in the epithelium and the lamina propria was used as a parameter (Fig. 3). The degree of epithelial HLA-DR expression correlated well with the activity of the chronic inflammation with the most intense and widespread staining in *H. pylori*-positive lesions ($p = 0.02$). In contrast, HLA-DR expression in the lamina propria did not correlate with the activity of the inflammatory reaction.

The number of $\gamma\delta$ T cells in chronic active gastritis does not correlate with the presence of *H. pylori*

Next, we were intrigued to find out whether the presence or absence of *H. pylori* in chronic active gastritis would have any influence on the number of

T CELL SUBSETS IN *H. PYLORI*-ASSOCIATED GASTRITIS

percent of CD3+ cells

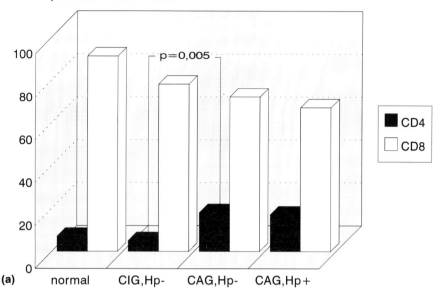

(a)

percent of CD3+ cells

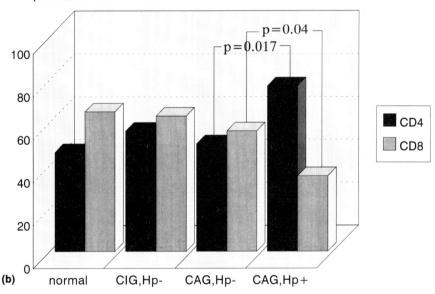

(b)

Fig. 1 Percentage of CD4$^+$ and CD8$^+$ cells compared to the number of CD3$^+$ cells in chronic gastritis. A distinction was made between cells localized in the epithelium (**a**) and in the lamina propria (**b**). Note the inversion of the CD4/CD8 ratio in the lamina propria of *H. pylori*-positive chronic active gastritis. Normal ($n = 5$), CIG; chronic inactive gastritis ($n = 7$), CAG; chonic active gastritis *H. pylori*-negative ($n = 5$) and *H. pylori*-positive ($n = 18$).

percent of CD3+ cells

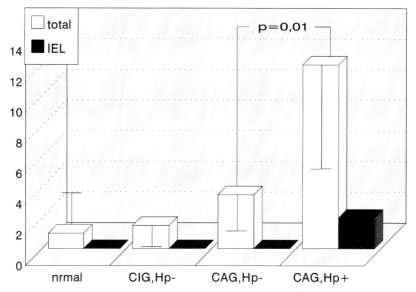

Fig. 2 CD25 expression in chronic gastritis. The fraction of CD3$^+$ T cells expressing the IL-2-R (CD25) was determined by immunostaining of serial sections obtained from gastric mucosa. There is a marked increase of activated LPL in *H. pylori*-positive gastritis. Mean percentages are indicated. Normal ($n = 5$), CIG: chronic inactive gastritis ($n = 7$), CAG; chronic active gastritis, *H. pylori*-negative ($n = 5$) and *H. pylori*-positive ($n = 18$)

$\gamma\delta$ T cells in the mucosal lesions. To this end, serial sections were immuno-stained with monoclonal antibodies directed against the CD3 and the $\gamma\delta$ T cell receptor. As shown in Fig. 4, $\gamma\delta$ T cells are infrequent in normal antral mucosa. In contrast, in chronic gastritis the number of mucosal $\gamma\delta$ T cells is significantly increased ($p = 0.01$). In the epithelium this increase was most pronounced in active gastritis. In the lamina propria the number of $\gamma\delta$ T cells correlated with the degree of activity of the gastritis. However, the presence or absence of *H. pylori* had no influence on the number of $\gamma\delta$ T cells. The fraction of $\alpha\beta$ T cells in the mucosa remained constant regardless of the activity of gastritis or the presence of *H. pylori*.

DISCUSSION

In this study, immunohistochemical characterization of the inflammatory cells in various forms of chronic gastritis employing a panel of monoclonal antibodies directed to markers identifying the differentiation and functional status of T lymphocytes revealed a number of most intriguing findings that implicate T cells as a major component of the local immune response, and therefore suggests that these cells may play an immunopathogenetic role in the development particularly of *H. pylori*-associated gastritis. Taken together our results revealed that in normal gastric mucosa CD8$^+$ T cells represent

degree of HLA DR expression

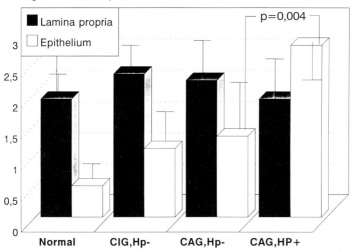

Fig. 3 Pattern of epithelial HLA DR expression in chronic gastritis. Serial sections from gastric mucosa were immunostained with HLA-DR antibodies and the intensity of HLA-DR expression evaluated by light microscopy in the four patient groups: (a) normal mucosa ($n = 5$), (b) chronic inactive gastritis, *H. pylori*-negative (CIG, H.p.⁻) ($n = 7$), (c) chronic active gastritis, *H. pylori*negative (CAG, H.p.⁻) ($n = 5$); (d) chronic active gastritis, *H. pylori*-positive (CAG, H.p.⁺) ($n = 18$). A qualitative score for HLA-DR expression was developed in order to assess the degree of HLA-DR expression and to compare the results between the individual patient groups (for details see material and methods): (0 = no epithelial HLA DR expression; 1 = weak epithelial HLA-DR expression; 2 = moderate epithelial HLA-DR expression; 3 = strong epithelial HLA-DR expression)

the major fraction of T lymphocytes in both the epithelium and the lamina propria. In *H. pylori*-negative forms of gastritis the number of CD4⁺ T cells is slightly increased; however, in *H. pylori*-positive forms this increase is much more pronounced. Moreover, in chronic active gastritis a large fraction of infiltrating CD4⁺ cells express the IL-2 receptor on their surface, and in the epithelium MHC class II expression is markedly enhanced. In chronic active gastritis the absolute number of $\gamma\delta$ T cells was increased irrespective of the presence or absence of *H. pylori*. Rather, the increase in $\gamma\delta$ T cell number correlated solely with the degree of activity of the mucosal lesions. From these data we conclude that the selective accumulation of activated CD4⁺ T cells in *H. pylori*-associated chronic active gastritis may be the consequence of specific recognition of *H. pylori* antigens by the T cell receptors expressed on these cells. For example, bacterial heat-shock proteins could serve as a specific antigen to infiltrating T cells. In this regard, Ottenhoff *et al.* and van Eden *et al.* could induce proliferation and differentiation of cytotoxic CD4⁺ T cells specific for bacterial heat-shock proteins *in vitro*[17,24]. Furthermore, it is conceivable that these cells are stimulated to secrete pathogenetically relevant cytokines such as IFN-γ and TNF[25,26]. Increased secretion of the former could be responsible for the observed increased expression of MHC class II molecules on epithelial cells and the latter could

% of CD3+ cells

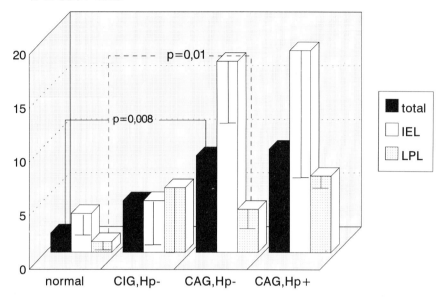

Fig. 4 $\gamma\delta$ T cell receptor expression in chronic gastritis. The percentage of CD3$^+$ T cells in the antral mucosa (IEL and LPL, respectively) expressing the $\gamma\delta$ T cell receptor was determined by immunohistochemistry on serial section employing antibodies against CD3 and the $\gamma\delta$ TCR, respectively. The increase of $\gamma\delta$ T cells correlates with the severity of gastritis but not with the presence or absence of *H. pylori*. In the epithelium there is a marked increase of $\gamma\delta$ T cells in both types of active gastritis. Normal ($n = 5$), CIG: chronic inactive gastritis ($n = 7$), CAG: chronic active gastritis, *H. pylori*-positive ($n = 5$) and *H. pylori*-negative ($n = 18$)

be, besides many other pro-inflammatory effects, directly toxic to epithelial cells and thereby aggravate mucosal tissue destruction by interfering with the production of acid-protective mucus. The increased MHC class II expression would lead to more effective presentation of putative ligands for cytotoxic class II restricted CD4$^+$ T cells, and thereby lead to a vicious cycle of mucosal destruction. Furthermore, local activation of mononuclear cells could lead to increased IL-8 secretion, which results in the recruitment of neutrophils and additional mononuclear cells to the site of inflammation. A similar model involving bacterial heat-shock specific CD4$^+$ T cells as orchestrators of the local immune response was suggested by Kiessling *et al.* for the pathogenesis of lesions in rheumatoid arthritis and leprosy[26]. Another possibility could be the induction of secondary autoimmune responses by a molecular mimicry between bacterial and autologous heat-shock protein expressed by gastric epithelial cells. A recent report by Brenner *et al.*[38] shows that CD4-CD8-$\alpha\beta$- and $\gamma\delta$ T cells specific for microbial antigens are restricted by the CD1b molecule that belongs to a family of antigen-presenting molecules separate from those encoded by the MHC. These molecules are structurally non-polymorphic and exhibit a limited tissue distribution such as the skin and intestine[27,28]. Notably, a number of microbial antigens such as heat-shock proteins are highly conserved molecules and thereby obviate the need for highly polymorphic antigen-presenting molecules. In consequence, CD1 molecules may be particularly suitable as antigen-presenting molecules for antigens that are non-polymorphic themselves. The preferential expression of CD1 molecules at sites where microbial antigens are abundantly present may offer some advantage to the host. It is conceivable that presentation of a restricted spectrum of antigens by non-polymorphic CD1 molecules may secure the host's immune response towards most microbials. However, this would render the local intraepithelial lymphocytes 'anergic' towards the large variety of luminal antigens that bear in themselves the potential of eliciting a detrimental immune reaction towards food antigens that are vital for the host's survival. The down side of this could be the lack of polymorphism favouring cross-reaction between conserved antigens such as bacterial and mammalian heat-shock proteins.

The observed increase in $\gamma\delta$ T cell number in *H. pylori*-associated gastritic lesions by Engstrand *et al.*[16] would suggest specific recognition of *H. pylori* antigens. However, in our experiments we observed an accumulation of $\gamma\delta$ T cells in both forms of chronic active gastritis lesions, i.e. there was no correlation between the $\gamma\delta$ T cell number and presence of *H. pylori*. The key factor was the presence of active gastritis. One explanation for this discrepancy could be that these investigators did not examine biopsy specimens from *H. pylori*-negative chronic active gastritis as was performed in our study[16]. Together with the observed altered pattern of HSP expression[29] these data support the notion that, instead of reacting towards *H. pylori*-specific antigens, in chronic gastritis, mucosal $\gamma\delta$ T cells may specifically respond to either bacterial or autologous heat-shock proteins. However, other, hitherto unknown autologous or heterologous stress proteins could be targeted by the mucosal immune reaction. Nevertheless, the role of the infiltrating $\gamma\delta$ T cells remains unclear, since the functional *in vivo* properties of these cells have not been elucidated. That the increase in $\gamma\delta$ T cell number is not simply due to the mere presence of bacteria in the gastric lumen is supported by the observations of Bandeira *et al.* which clearly show that the number of $\gamma\delta$ T cells within the intestinal mucosa is not influenced by bacterial colonization[30]. Earlier studies by some investigators have documented specific stimulation of $\gamma\delta$ T cells by mycobacterial heat-shock proteins[31]; however, others failed to observe specific stimulation of $\gamma\delta$ T cells towards heat-shock proteins *in vitro* or in cells obtained from synovial arthritis lesions[32,33]. Finally, in concordance with our data, Trejdosievicz *et al.* did not find any increase of $\gamma\delta$ T cells in *H. pylori*-associated gastritis[34].

In conclusion, our data suggest that $\gamma\delta$ T cell accumulation in the mucosal lesions is due to their specific recognition of possible cross-reacting autologous antigens expressed in response to inflammatory stress imposed upon the tissue by cytokines and toxic endogenous or bacterial pro-inflammatory mediators. In immunological terms the chronicity of the *H. pylori*-associated chronic gastritis and peptic ulcer disease remains enigmatic. Even though the local cellular immune response described in this report and by others[16], and a humoral immune response against *H. pylori* antigens, can be regularly observed, the clearing of the infection appears to be a problem. These observations do not support the concept of a general immunosuppressive

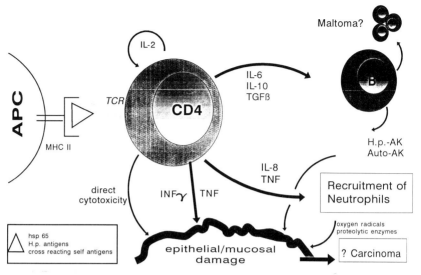

Fig. 5 Presumable consequence of the involvement of the immune system *H. pylori*-associated chronic gastritis (see text for details)

effect of *H. pylori*-derived substances, but rather a more selective immunomodulating effect resulting in a qualitatively less efficient response. As a result of this, the infection would become locally confined and does not lead to strong tissue destruction. However, the response is inefficient insofar as it allows the bacteria to persist in the epithelium. Conceivably, this may have some advantage to the host. Nevertheless, the persistence of the local immune reaction may lead to an undesirable recruitment of by-stander autoimmune cells or cross-reactive autoimmune cells (Fig. 5). Alternatively, the chronicity of the *H. pylori* infection and ensuing cellular immune response could simply be the result of its resistance to killing by phagocytosis. Whatever the mechanism, the chronicity of the local immune reaction in *H. pylori* infection may lead to a continuous presence of cytokines that drive B-cell growth or epithelial regeneration differentiation. The former may be related to the observed increased incidence of T-cell dependent low grade maltomas[35,36] and the latter to gastric carcinoma[37], respectively (Fig. 5). Therefore, the eradication of this bacterium may become a most critical issue with regard to public health.

SUMMARY

During recent years the infectious aetiology of the majority of cases of chronic active gastritis and peptic ulcers has become increasingly evident. The chronicity of clinical symptoms and histopathological features such as numerous mucosal lymphocytic aggregates have implied a role of the specific cellular immune system. Whereas in autoimmune chronic gastritis a pathogenetic role of lymphocytes and their target structures has been amply documented, in non-autoimmune chronic active gastritis, particularly that associated with *H. pylori* infection, the nature of a specific immune response and its role in the pathogenesis of the epithelial and mucosal lesion has remained obscure. Here we report that CD4$^+$ mucosal lymphocytes appear to selectively accumulate in *H. pylori*-associated chronic active antral gastritis. Moreover, lamina propria $\gamma\delta$ T lymphocytes were found to be more frequent in chronic active gastritis irrespective of the presence or absence of *H. pylori*.

References

1. Marshall B, Armstrong J, McGechie D *et al.* Attempt to fulfill Koch's postulates for *pyloric* campylobacter. Med J Aust. 1985;142:436–9.
2. Morris A, Nicholson G. Ingestion of *Campylobacter pyloridis* causes gastritis and raised fasting gastric pH. Am J Gastroenterol. 1987;82:192–9.
3. Maroos HI, Kekki M, Villako K, Sipponen P, Tamm A, Sadeniemi L. The occurrence and extent of *Helicobacter pylori* colonization and antral and body gastritis profiles in an Estonian population sample. Scand J Gastroenterol. 1990;9(4):1010–17.
4. Loffeld RJLF, Potters HVPJ, Arends JW, Stobberingh E, Flemdrig JA, Van Spreeuwel JP. *Campylobacter*-associated gastritis in patients with nonulcer dyspepsia. J Clin Pathol. 1988;41:85–8.
5. Jones DM, Lessels AM, Eldridge J. *Campylobacter*-like organisms on the gastric mucosa: Culture, histological and serological studies. J Clin Pathol. 1984;37:1002–6.
6. Girdwood R, Fricker CR, Forrest JAH *et al. Campylobacter*-like organisms in biopsy samples of normal and diseased human stomachs: pathological, serological and bacteriological findings. In Pearson AD, Skirrow MB, Lior H *et al.*, editors. *Campylobacter*, III. London: Public Health Laboratory Service; 1985:180.
7. Ormand JE, Talley NJ, Shorter RG *et al.* Prevalence of *Helicobacter pylori* in specific forms of gastritis. Further evidence supporting a pathogenic role of *H. pylori* in chronic nonspecific gastritis. Dig Dis Sci. 1991;36(2):142–5.
8. Marshall BJ, Goodwin CS, Warren JR *et al.* Prospective double blind trial of duodenal ulcer relapse after eradication of *Campylobacter pylori*. Lancet. II. 1988;(8625/8627): 1437–41.
9. Tytgat GNJ, Rauws EAJ, De Koster E. *Campylobacter pylori*: Scand J Gastroenterol. 1988;23(Suppl.155):68–79.
10. Marshall BJ, Armstrong JA, Francis GJ, Nokes NT, Wee SH. The antibacterial action of bismuth in relation to *Campylobacter pyloridis* colonization and gastritis. Digestion. 1987;37(Suppl.2):16–30.
11. Bode G, Malfertheiner P, Lehnhardt G, Ditschuneit H. Virulence factors of *Helicobacter pylori* – ultrastructural features. In Malfertheiner P, Ditschuneit H, editors. *Helicobacter pylori*, gastritis and peptic ulcer. Berlin: Springer-Verlag; 1990:63–73.
12. Hupertz V, Czinn S. Demonstration of a cytotoxin from *Campylobacter pylori*. Eur J Clin Microbiol Infect Dis. 1988;7:576–8.
13. Leunck RD, Johnson PT, David BC, Kraft WG, Morgan DR. Cytotoxic activity in broth-culture filtrates of *Campylobacter pylori*. J Med Microbiol. 1988;26:93–9.
14. Marshall BJ. Virulence and pathogenicity of *Helicobacter pylori*. J. Gastroenterol Hepatol. 1991;6:121–4.
15. Raedsch R, Stiehl A, Pohl S, Plachky J. Quantification of phospholipase A2-activity of *Campylobacter pylori*. Gastroenterology. 1989;96:A405.
16. Engstrand L, Scheynius A, Pahlson C. An increased number of $\gamma\delta$ T-cells and gastric epithelial cell expression of the groE1 stress-protein homologue in *Helicobacter pylori*-associated chronic gastritis of the antrum. Am J Gastroenterol. 1991;86:976–80.
17. van Eden W, Thole JER, van der Zee R, Noodzij A, van Embden JDA, Hensen EJ, Cohen IR. Cloning of the mycobacterial epitope recognized by T lymphocytes in adjuvant arthritis. Nature. 1988;331:171.

18. Ottenhoff T, Haanen J, Geluk A *et al.* Regulation of mycobacterial heat-shock protein-reactive T cells by HLA class II molecules: lessons from leprosy. Immun Rev. 1991;121: 171–91.
19. Kaufmann S, Schoel B, v. Embden DA *et al.* Heat shock protein 60: implications for pathogenesis of and protection against bacterial infections. Immun Rev. 1991;121:67–88.
20. Karlsson-Parra A, Söderström K, Ferm M, Invanyi J, Kiessling R, Klareskog L. Presence of human 65 kD heat shock protein (hsp) in inflamed joints and subcutaneous nodules of RA patients. Scand J Immunol. 1990;31:283.
21. McDonald GB, Jewell DP. Class II antigen (HLA-DR) expression by intestinal epithelial cells in inflammatory bowel disease of colon. J Clin Pathol. 1987;40:312–17.
22. Pallone F, Fais S, Capobianchi MR. HLA-D region antigens on isolated human colonic epithelial cells; enhanced expression in inflammatory bowel disease and *in vitro* induction by different stimuli. Clin Exp Immunol. 1988;74:75–9.
23. Zschaler U, Weber P, Jedrychowski A, Wiedmann KH. Immunohistologische Untersuchungen zur differentiellen HLA-Expression bei Patienten it verschiedenen Darmerkrankungen. Z Gastroenterol. 1991;29:92–100.
24. Ottenhoff THM, Kaleab B, van Embden JDA, Thole JER, Kiessling R. The recombinant 65 kilodalton heat shock protein of *Mycobacterium bovis* BCG/M. *tuberculosis* is an important target molecule for CD4$^+$ HLA DR restricted cytotoxic T lymphocytes that lyse human monocytes. J Exp Med. 1988;168:1947.
25. Kaleab B, Kiessling R, van Embden JDA, Thole JFR, Kumararatne DS, Vondimu A, Ottenhoff THM. Induction of antigen specific CD4$^+$ HLA-DR restricted cytotoxic T lymphocytes as well as nonrestricted killer cells by the recombinant mycobaterial 65 kilodalton heat shock protein. Eur J Immunol. 1990;20:369.
26. Kiessling R, Grönberg A, Ivanyi J *et al.* Role of hsp60 during autoimmune and bacterial inflammation. Immun Rev. 1991;121:91–111.
27. Porcelli S, Morita CT, Brenner M. CD1b restricts the response of human CD4-8-T lymphocytes to a microbial antigen. Nature. 1991;360:593–7.
28. Balk SP, Ebert EC, Blumenthal L *et al.* Oligoclonal expansion and CD1 recognition by human intestinal intraepithelial lymphocytes. Science. 1991;253:1411–15.
29. Deusch K, Seifarth C, Funk A, Dähne I, Reich K, Classen M. Selective increase of CD4+ and CD25+ T cells but not of $\gamma\delta$ T cells in *H. pylori* associated gastritis. 1992. Proceedings of the V Workshop on gastruoduodenal pathology and *Helicobacter pylori* (In press).
30. Bandeira A, Mota-Santos T, Itohara S *et al.* Localization of $\gamma\delta$ T cells to the intestinal epithelium is independent of normal microbial colonisation. J Exp Med. 1990;172:239–44.
31. Holoshitz J, Koning F, Coligan JE, De Bruyn J, Strober S. Isolation of CD4- CD8-mycobacteria reactive T lymphocyte clones from rheumatoid arthritis synovial fluid. Nature. 1989;339:226.
32. Kabelitz D, Bender A, Schondelmaier S, Schoel B, Kaufmann SHE. A large fraction of human peripheral blood gd T cells is activated by *Mycobacterium tuberculosis* but not by its 65-kD heat shock protein. J Exp Med. 1990;171:667.
33. Fisch P, Malkovsky M, Kovats S *et al.* Recognition by human Vγ9/Vδ2 T cells of a GroE1 homolog on Daudi Burkitt's lymphoma cells. Science. 1990;250:1269.
34. Trejdosiwicz LK, Calabrese A, Smart CJ *et al.* $\gamma\delta$ T cell receptor-positive cells of the human gastrointestinal mucosa: occurrence and V region gene expression in *Helicobacter pylori*-associated gastritis, coeliac disease and inflammatory bowel disease. Clin Exp Immunol. 1991;84:440–4.
35. Hussell T, Isaacson P, Crabtree JE, Spencer J. The response of cells from low grade B-cell gastric lymphomas of mucosa-associated lymphoid tissue to *Helicobacter pylori*. Lancet. 1993;342:571.
36. Wotherspoon AC, Ortitz-Hidalgo C, Falzon MR, Isaacson P. *Helicobacter pylori*-associated gastritis and primary B-cell gastric lymphoma. Lancet. 1991;338:1175.
37. The Eurogast Study Group. An international association between *Helicobacter pylori* infection and gastric cancer. Lancet. 1993;341:1359.
38. Porcelli S, Brenner MB, Greenstein JL, Balk SP, Terhost C, Bleicher TA. Recognition of cluster of differentiation antigens by human CD4$^-$ CD8$^-$ cytolytic lymphocytes. Nature. 1989;341:447–50.

30
Down-regulation of the immune response to *H. pylori*

K. CROITORU

INTRODUCTION

Infection of the human stomach by *Helicobacter pylori* results in a chronic inflammatory response associated with an apparent inactivation of the immune system. This immune response is characterized in part, by the production of *H. pylori*-specific IgA and IgG antibodies (Ab). Case reports of invasive *H. pylori* infection in children with X-linked agammaglobulinaemia suggest that the humoral response is critically important in restricting the infection[1]. Nonetheless, *H. pylori* infection of the stomach is a chronic infection in spite of stimulation of this immune response. The reason for this is not clear. Studies of mice infected with *Salmonella* indicate that protection from this bacterial infection requires both Ab and T cell responses[2]. It is reasonable, therefore, to speculate that the persistence of *H. pylori* in the human stomach reflects a down-regulation of the local T cell response. To explore this possibility it is helpful to first review the role of mucosal T cells, highlighting the differences that exist between the intestinal and gastric mucosa. This will lay the groundwork necessary to address three questions: (1) How can mucosal T cells be down-regulated? (2) What purpose would be served by T cell down-regulation? and (3) Is down-regulation of the T cell response a characteristic of *H. pylori* gastritis?

MUCOSAL IMMUNE RESPONSE

As reviewed elsewhere in these proceedings, the gut-associated lymphoid tissue or GALT refers to the organized lymphoid tissue found in the intestine. This includes the Peyer's patches, the mesenteric lymph nodes and the lymphoid follicles in the lamina propria. In addition the lymphoid populations that occupy the lamina propria, the lamina propria lymphocytes (LPL) and epithelium, the intraepithelial lymphocytes (IEL), can also be considered part of the GALT. This is because the make-up of both the LPL and IEL populations is unique in phenotype and function and contributes to the local immune response[3]. The lamina propria contains macrophages, eosinophils, mast cells and lymphoid cells. The lymphocytes here are mostly B cells and IgA-secreting plasma cells, and the T cells are mostly CD4[+] helper T cells with fewer CD8[+] T cells represented. The epithelium, on the other hand, contains a heterogeneous collection of mononuclear cells which include mast cell precursors, natural killers and lymphocytes. The majority of lymphocytes express the CD3/T cell receptor (TcR) complex and CD8; although a large proportion lack expression of pan-T cell markers such as Thy1 and CD5[4]. The functions of the T cells within these different compartments include cytokine production, cytotoxicity reactions and regulatory influences on antibody responses in the lamina propria[4-6]. In addition, T cells in both the lamina propria and epithelium can function in an antigen-specific manner[4,7]. Questions remain as to the biological function of the IEL compartment in the host response or in disease pathogenesis[4,8].

STOMACH-ASSOCIATED LYMPHOID TISSUE

In contrast to the intestine, the immune system of the stomach has not been well studied. The inclusion of the stomach as part of the circuit of the 'common mucosal immune system' has not been formally demonstrated[3]. Specifically, it remains to be determined whether antigen-specific lymphocytes immigrate into the stomach, as part of the lymphocyte trafficking that occurs between mucosal sites, or are generated in the gastric mucosa. The organization of the stomach-associated lymphoid tissue, or SALT, clearly differs from that of the GALT. Firstly, the SALT lacks organized lymphoid follicles, Peyer's patches and M cells. In humans, IEL are present in the stomach and contain both α/β and γ/δ TcR expression lymphocytes[9,10]. In the stomach the lamina propria contains B and T cells in a manner analogous to that in the small intestine, although the number and density of these cells are less in the gastric mucosa. Furthermore, the presence of acid-producing cells and the low pH of gastric juice will have important influences on the local immune response. It is in this context that the gastric immune system encounters a pathogen or a foreign antigen.

DOWN-REGULATION OF MUCOSAL T CELL RESPONSES

There are several levels at which T cell responses to foreign antigens or pathogens can be down-regulated. Tolerance or T cell down-regulation can be induced, at the level of the induction of the immune response, i.e. during antigen presentation; at the level of the T cell itself; at the level of the microenvironment; or finally at the level of the pathogen itself. In *H. pylori* infection of the stomach one or a combination of these mechanisms can serve potentially to down-regulate the T cell response to *H. pylori*.

Induction of mucosal immune responses

The organization of the GALT provides a road map for the encounter between a foreign Ag and the local immune system. Overlying the Peyer's patches are a specialized epithelium referred to as M cells. These M cells are involved in the uptake of foreign proteins and pathogens, e.g. reovirus and *Salmonella*, via specific receptors, transporting them across via pinocytosis to the underlying lymphocytes[11-13]. The Ag-stimulation of B and T cells within the Peyer's patch results in the production of IgA antibodies. Since there are no Peyer's patches or M cells in the stomach, alternative routes of antigen presentation must exist if an immune response is to be initiated at the gastric mucosa.

In the intestine the epithelium expressed MHC class II molecules that can be involved in antigen presentation. Intestinal epithelial cells from humans or laboratory rodents function in Ag presentation *in vitro*. The important distinction between the M cell/Peyer's patch route and the epithelial cell route of antigen presentation is that the epithelial cell induces predominantly a CD8[+] T cell response[14-16]. It has been argued that this is part of the normal down-regulation of the local immune response, preventing chronic inflammation that might occur if the local immune response were unbridled.

In the non-inflamed stomach the gastric epithelial cells do not express MHC class II molecules, suggesting that the stomach is not equipped to initiate immune responses under normal conditions. However, in *H. pylori* gastritis MHC class II is expressed on epithelial cells[17,18]. This raises the possibility that, under conditions of inflammation, the gastric epithelial cell can function in antigen presentation. The nature of the resulting T cell response still needs to be defined since, in the inflamed intestine of patients with ulcerative colitis, epithelial cells lead to a CD4 response[19].

Mucosal T cells

In the intestine the functional abilities of the T cell populations in the lamina propria and IEL are diverse. The ability of the T cell to recognize antigen via the TcR would permit antigen-directed or antigen-specific responses. Classically, the restriction that T cells recognize foreign antigen in the context of self-MHC molecules, while not recognizing self-antigens, is the result of repertoire selection processes that occur in the thymus[20]. In addition to the selection processes that delete self-reactive T cell clones, T cell tolerance to self-antigen can also occur via the induction of anergy or the suppression of function by antigen-specific suppressor T cells. Recently, it has been suggested that the selection of the T cell repertoire can occur in extrathymic tissues such as the gut[21-24]. The induction of anergy in mucosal T cells bearing self-reactive TcR was first suggested in experiments using a transgenic mouse carrying a self-reactive γ/δ TcR. In these mice the T cells bearing the transgenic TcR were deleted in the thymus and spleen, yet IEL bearing the self-reactive TcR were present[25,26]. These mice did not show inflammation in their intestine, suggesting that these cells were functionally anergic. We have shown that in mice with Mls-1ᵃ phenotype the IEL expressing the self-reactive Vβ6 TcR are functionally anergic. This subset failed to proliferate in response to crosslinking of the TcR with anti-Vβ6 monoclonal antibodies. Similar unresponsiveness was evident in IEL bearing the γ/δ TcR and was reversed by the addition of exogenous IL-2[27]. These studies suggest that mucosal lymphocytes can be anergized in response to self-antigens. This may reflect the unique fashion in which self-antigens are presented to the mucosal T cells. There is evidence that the MHC class I-like molecule CD1d, expressed on intestinal epithelial cells, can act as a ligand for CD8 T cells[28,29]. The exact manner in which this molecule serves in antigen presentation and selectively stimulates CD8 T cells remains to be elucidated. As the cellular and molecular components of such interactions are dissected we will begin to understand the role epithelial cells play in presenting antigen, particularly bacterial and food antigens, to the local immune system. It is not difficult to imagine how autoreactive lymphocytes that have escaped the processes that regulate self-tolerance can cause autoimmune disease.

There may be other mechanisms that serve to down-regulate mucosal T cell responsiveness. The IEL, for example, are particularly unresponsive to mitogenic signals including crosslinking of the TcR. Interestingly, activation of IEL through the CD2 surface protein is preserved, and suggests a role for epithelial cell ligands that specifically interact with CD2[30].

The intestinal microenvironment

A feature unique to the gastric microenvironment is the presence of acid-producing epithelial cells and the acidic pH of gastric secretions. The ability of IgA to elude acid degradation makes it ideally suited for its role in protecting the gastric mucosa. In the inflamed stomach there is expression of secretory component (the polymeric immunoglobulin receptor) on epithelial cells that transport IgA across epithelial cells into the lumen[8]. Therefore, locally produced secretory IgA should be able to function in the protection of the gastric mucosa. The effect of the low pH on the function of other cells of the immune system is not known.

In addition to the acid environment, other microenvironmental factors could influence local T cell function. Supernatants from cultured human intestinal mucosa can, for example, alter T cell reactivity to TcR-mediated activation. This appears to be due to a low molecular weight soluble factor that is a non-peptide possessing oxidative functions[31,32]. This and other factors present in the gastric mucosa may serve to down-regulate the local T cell response.

The gastrointestinal tract is also highly innervated, and changes that occur in the intrinsic nerves during inflammation may alter the levels of neurotransmitters such as substance P and VIP, both of which can influence mucosal lymphocyte functions[33–35]. Furthermore, there is evidence that histamine may influence lymphocyte function, inducing suppressor activity[36]. Therefore, a number of microenvironmental factors could influence the local T cell response in normal and inflamed gastric mucosa.

The role of the pathogen

Lastly, one must consider the possibility that the pathogen itself may influence the T cell response. Such a role has not been defined for *H. pylori* as yet. The ability of *H. pylori* to persist in the human stomach in spite of an ongoing inflammatory or immune response, suggests that the organism may well have learned to take advantage of some of the unique features of the environmental niche it occupies, e.g. urease activity, and/or it has acquired the ability to modulate the immune response to prevent elimination. For example, *H. pylori* can directly augment natural killer activity in PBL, probably through the stimulation of interferon-γ production[37]. It is possible that *H. pylori* can also induce other cytokines.

There are many examples in humans, as well as in animal models, of how immunodeficiencies or down-regulation of the immune response can lead to chronic infections; cryptosporidiosis in patients with AIDS and chronic giardiasis in mice deficient in T and B cell populations[38,39]. Some insight into how pathogens evade the host response is provided by studies of intestinal parasites, such as the intestinal nematode, *Heligmonoides polygyrus*. Certain strains of mice develop a chronic infection with *H. polygyrus* and are unable to mount the mastocytosis usually associated with elimination of the worm. *H. polygyrus* appears to secrete an immunomodulatory factor, IMF, that inhibits the mast cell response[40]. Furthermore, while the parasite appears to stimulate IL-4 release, it fails to stimulate IL-9 and IL-10, another factor contributing to chronic infection. When susceptible mice are co-infected with *Trichinella spiralis* and *H. polygyrus*, both parasites are eliminated[41,42]. The possibility that *H. pylorus* can exert similar influences on the host response needs to be explored.

CONSEQUENCES OF DOWN-REGULATING THE MUCOSAL IMMUNE RESPONSE

The most predictable outcome of inhibiting the local immune response is that the pathogen escapes elimination. If the infection is not rapidly fatal, then the pathogen has set up a long-term occupancy of a well-furnished dwelling. T cell activation not only helps direct the immune response in pathogen elimination, it also influences other physiological functions of the intestine[43,44]. The changes in the normal function of epithelial cells, smooth muscle and nerves can lead to fluid and ion secretion, altered intestinal motility and changes in the neural and coordinated functions of the intestine. We have shown that specific T cell activation can alter permeability, and fluid and ion secretion of an intestinal epithelial cell line monolayer *in vitro*[45]. Such changes in gut physiology can explain many of the symptoms associated with intestinal infections. It is possible that T cell responses are down-regulated in the intestine specifically to minimize the disruption of the normal physiological processes.

In the stomach similar phenomena are being identified. Using an isolated mouse mucosal gastric gland, Muller and Hunt have shown that interferon-γ

can alter the histamine- and carbachol-stimulated acid secretion of isolated mouse mucosal gastric gland preparations[46]. Therefore, changes in acid or pepsinogen secretion may result from the local inflammatory or immune response. In addition to providing a link with ulcerogenesis, such a mechanism may help explain how the parasite enhances its local environment to promote its survival.

T CELL ALTERATIONS IN PATIENTS WITH *H. PYLORI* GASTRITIS

How is the gastric immune system altered in *H. pylori* infection or, more specifically, is there down-regulation of the T cell response to *H. pylori*? Surprisingly little is known about this. Associated with *H. pylori* infection and the concomitant inflammation are several important changes. In *H. pylori* gastritis the gastric epithelial cells express MHC class II antigens[17,18], and there are increases in the level of cytokines locally, including TNF-α, IL-6[47] and IL-8[48]. A number of studies show increases in local T cell number[49], including CD8$^+$ T cells in both LPL and IEL[10,50]. The change in γ/δ T cells, and the increase in the expression of heat shock proteins (HSP), has led to the suggestion that a crossreactive T cell response is initiated in *H. pylori* gastritis[10,51]. However, in IBD, where a similar hypothesis has been suggested, there is little evidence to support this notion. We have shown that HSP65 expression can be detected in normal non-inflamed bowel as well as inflamed bowel[52].

The *H. pylori*-specific response of gastric T cells has not been well delineated. Peripheral blood T cells proliferate when cultured with *H. pylori* antigen *in vitro*; however, when *H. pylori*-antibody positive patients with dyspepsia are compared to Ab-negative patients, the former respond less well, suggesting that infection is associated with a down-regulation of this response[53,54]. Perhaps more important is the state of T cell responsiveness to *H. pylori* in the gastric mucosa. This is a difficult question to answer, because access to sufficient numbers of freshly isolated cells is limited and therefore the studies require *in vitro* expansion of T cells. This introduces a bias that is difficult to control for. Nonetheless, early attempts have shown that T cells from *H. pylori*-positive individuals proliferate to *H. pylori* antigen, but again the response is less than that seen in *H. pylori*-negative individuals. Similar results are described for interferon-γ production by mucosal T cells from these patients. It is indeed possible that these gastric T cells have been anergized or tolerized during the exposure to *H. pylori* and in the process of inflammation.

ENIGMA OF CHRONIC *H. PYLORI* INFECTION

We are left, therefore, with an enigma. In the face of a measurable immune response how does *H. pylori* in the stomach persist as a chronic infection? Since it is not clear whether patients can be reinfected once cured of their *H. pylori* infection, we cannot be sure that the immune response is protective.

In the mouse model of *H. pylori*, vaccination with *H. felis* seems to provide protection against infection[55,56], yet mice cured of their *H. felis* can be reinfected (A. Lee, personal communication). On the other hand, in AIDS patients there is an apparent decrease in the incidence of *H. pylori* gastritis as compared to age-matched controls; yet there is a report of invasive *H. pylori* in an AIDS patient[57,58]. This implies that the mucosal immune response may help limit the invasiveness of *H. pylori* infection but also serves to promote colonization. It remains possible that there is an autoimmune response generated by *H. pylori* that is responsible, in part, for the tissue inflammation. The understanding of these apparently incongruous observations will require further efforts directed at exploring the immunology and microbiology of this unique pathogen.

References

1. Shirley LR, Marsh WH. *Campylobacter pylori* gastritis in children with X-linked agammaglobulinemia. (Abst). J Allergy Clin Immunol. 1989;83:287.
2. Mastroeni P, Villarreal-Ramos B, Hormaeche CE. Adoptive transfer of immunity to oral challenge with virulent salmonellae in innately susceptible BALB/c mice requires both immune serum and T cells. Infect Immun. 1993;61:3981–4.
3. Croitoru K, Bienenstock J. Characteristics and function of mucosa-associated lymphoid tissue. In: Ogra PL, Maestecky J, Lamm ME, Strober W, McGhee J, Bienenstock J, editors. Handbook of mucosal immunology. San Diego: Academic Press; 1993:141–9.
4. Croitoru K, Ernst PB. Leukocytes in the intestinal epithelium: an unusual immunological compartment revisited. Regional Immunol. 1992;4:63–9.
5. Lefrancois L. Extrathymic differentiation of intraepithelial lymphocytes: generation of a separate and unequal T-cell repertoire? Immunol Today. 1991;124:36–8.
6. Fujihashi K, Taguchi T, McGhee JR et al. Regulatory function for murine intraepithelial lymphocytes: two subsets of CD3$^+$, T cell receptor-1$^+$ intraepithelial lymphocyte T cells abrogate oral tolerance. J Immunol. 1990;145:2010–19.
7. Elson CO, Kagnoff MF, Fiocchi C, Befus AD. Intestinal immunity and inflammation: recent progress. Gastroenterology. 1986;91:746–68.
8. Brandtzaeg P, Sollid LM, Thane PS et al. Lymphoepithelial interactions in the mucosal immune system. Gut. 1988;29:1116–30.
9. Trejdosiewicz LK, Calabrese A, Smart CJ et al. Γ/δ T cell receptor-positive cells of the human gastrointestinal mucosa: occurrence and V region gene expression in *Helicobacter pylori*-associated gastritis, coeliac disease and inflammatory bowel disease. Clin Exp Immunol. 1991;84:440–4.
10. Engstrand L, Scheynius A, Påhlson C. An increased number of γ/δ T-cells and gastric epithelial cell expression of the groEL stress-protein homologue in *Helicobacter pylori*-associated chronic gastritis of the antrum. Am J Gastroenterol. 1991;86:976–80.
11. Wolf JL, Rubin DJ, Finberg R et al. Intestinal M cells: a pathway for entry of reovirus into the host. Science. 1981;212:471–2.
12. Grützkau A, Hanski C, Hahn H, Riecken EO. Involvement of M cells in the bacterial invasion of Peyer's patches: a common mechanism shared by *Yersinia enterocolitica* and other enteroinvasive bacteria. Gut. 1990;31:1011–15.
13. Owen RL. Sequential uptake of horseradish peroxidase by lymphoid follicle epithelium of Peyer's patches in the normal unobstructed mouse intestine: an ultrastructural study. Gastroenterology. 1977;72:440–51.
14. Mayer L, Shlien R. Evidence for function of Ia molecules on gut epithelial cells in man. J Exp Med. 1987;166:1471–83.
15. Bland PW, Warren LG. Antigen presentation by epithelial cells of the rat small intestine. II. Selective induction of suppressor T cells. Immunology. 1986;58:9–14.
16. Kaiserlian D. Murine gut epithelial cells express Ia molecules antigenically distinct from

those of conventional antigen-presenting cells. Immunol Res. 1991;10:360–4.

17. Papadimitrou CS, Ioachim-Velogianni EE, Tsianos B, Moutsopoulos HM. Epithelial HLA-DR expression and lymphocyte subsets in gastric mucosa in type B chronic gastritis. Virchows Arch. [A] 1988;413:197–204.

18. Wee A, Teh M, Kang JY. Association of *Helicobacter pylori* with HLA-DR antigen expression in gastritis. J Clin Pathol. 1992;45:30–3.

19. Mayer L, Eisenhardt D. Lack of induction of suppressor T cells by intestinal epithelial cells from patients with inflammatory bowel disease. J Clin Invest. 1990;86:1255–60.

20. Fowlkes BJ, Pardoll DM. Molecular and cellular events of T cell development. Adv Immunol. 1989;44:207–64.

21. Mosley RL, Klein JR. Peripheral engraftment of fetal intestine into athymic mice sponsors T cell development: direct evidence for thymopoietic function of murine small intestine. J Exp Med. 1992;176:1365–73.

22. Poussier P, Edouard P, Lee C, Binnie M, Julius M. Thymus-independent development and negative selection of T cells expressing T cell receptor α/β in the intestinal epithelium: evidence for distinct circulation patterns of gut- and thymus-derived T lymphocytes. J Exp Med. 1992;176:187–99.

23. Lefrançois L. Extrathymic differentiation of intraepithelial lymphocytes: generation of a separate and unequal T-cell repertoire. Immunol Today. 1991;12:436–8.

24. Rocha B, Vassalli P, Guy-Grand D. The extrathymic T-cell development pathway. Immunol Today. 1992;13:449–54.

25. Barrett TA, Delvy ML, Kennedy DM et al. Mechanisms of self-tolerance of γ/δ T cells in epithelial tissue. J Exp Med. 1992;176:65–70.

26. Barrett TA, Tatsumi Y, Bluestone JA. Tolerance of T cell receptor γ/δ cells in the intestine. J Exp Med. 1993;177:1755–62.

27. Croitoru K, Bienenstock J, Ernst PB. Phenotypic and functional assessment of IEL bearing a 'forbidden' α/β T cell receptor. (submitted).

28. Bleicher PA, Balk SP, Hagen SJ, Blumberg RS, Flotte TJ, Terhorst C. Expression of murine CD1 on gastrointestinal epithelium. Nature. 1990;250:679–82.

29. Panja A, Blumberg RS, Balk SP, Mayer L. CD1d is involved in T cell-intestinal epithelial cell interactions. J Exp Med. 1993;178:1115–19.

30. Ebert EC. Proliferative responses of human intraepithelial lymphocytes to various T-cell stimuli. Gastroenterology. 1989;97:1372–81.

31. Qiao L, Schürmann G, Betzler M, Meuer SC. Activation and signaling status of human lamina propria T lymphocytes. Gastroenterology. 1991;101:1529–36.

32. Qiao L, Schürmann G, Autschbach F, Wallich R, Meuer SC. Human intestinal mucosa alters T-cell reactivities. Gastroenterology. 1993;105:814–19.

33. Stanisz AM, Befus D, Bienenstock J. Differential effects of vasoactive intestinal peptide, substance P, and somatostatin on immunoglobulin synthesis and proliferation by lymphocytes from Peyer's patch, mesenteric lymph node and spleen. J Immunol. 1986;136:152–6.

34. Croitoru K, Ernst PB, Stanisz AM, Stead RH, Bienenstock J. Neuroendocrine regulation of the mucosal immune system. In: Targan SR, Shanahan F, editors. Immunology and immunopathology of the liver and gastrointestinal tract. New York: Igaku-Shoin; 1989: 183–201.

35. Croitoru K, Ernst PB, Bienenstock J, Padol I, Stanisz AM. Selective modulation of the natural killer activity of murine intestinal intraepithelial leukocytes by the neuropeptide substance P. Immunology. 1990;71:196–201.

36. Beer DJ, Rocklin RE. Histamine-induced suppressor cell activity. J Allergy Clin Imunol. 1984;73:439–52.

37. Tarkkanen J, Kosunen TU, Saksela E. Contact of lymphocytes with *Helicobacter pylori* augments natural killer cell activity and induces production of γ interferon. Infect Immun. 1993;61:3012–16.

38. Carlson JR, Heyworth MF, Owen RL. T-lymphocyte subsets in nude mice with *Giardia muris* infection. Thymus. 1987;9:189–96.

39. Snider DP, Gordon J, McDermott MR, Underdown BJ. Chronic *Giardia muris* infection in anti-IgM-treated mice. I. Analysis of immunoglobulin and parasite-specific antibody in normal and immunoglobulin-deficient animals. J Immunol. 1985;134:4153–62.

40. Dehlawi MS, Wakelin D, Behnke JM. Suppression of mucosal mastocytosis by infection

with the intestinal nematode *Nematospiroides dubius*. Parasite Immunol. 1987;9:187–94.

41. Behnke JM, Cabaj W, Wakelin D. Susceptibility of adult *Heligmosomoides polygyrus* to intestinal inflammatory responses induced by heterologous infection. Int J Parasitol. 1992;22:75–86.

42. Kirberg J, Bruno L, von Boehmer H. CD4$^+$8$^-$ help prevents rapid deletion of CD8$^+$ cells after a transient response to antigen. Eur J Immunol. 1993;23:1963–7.

43. Perdue MH, McKay DM. Immunomodulation of the gastrointestinal epithelium. In: Wallace JL, editor. Immunopharmacology of the gastrointestinal system. London: Academic Press; 1992:15–39.

44. Collins SM, Croitoru K. The pathophysiology of inflammatory bowel disease: the effect of inflammation on intestinal function. In: Targan S, Shanahan F, editors. Inflammatory bowel disease: from bench to bedside. Baltimore: Williams & Wilkins; 1993:in press.

45. McKay DM, Croitoru K, Perdue MH. Activation of T lymphocytes causes increased permeability of T84 epithelial monolayers and reduces responses to secretagogues. Gastroenterology. 1993;104:A741(abstract).

46. Muller MJ, Padol I, Ernst PB, Croitoru K, Hunt RH. Interferon-γ inhibits secretagogue-mediated acid secretion in isolated murine gastric glands. Gastroenterology. 1993;104:A151(abstract).

47. Crabtree JE, Shallcross TM, Heatley RV, Wyatt JI. Mucosal tumour necrosis factor α and interleukin-6 in patients with *Helicobacter pylori*-associated gastritis. Gut. 1991;32:1473–7.

48. Crabtree JE, Peichl P, Wyatt JI, Stachl U, Lindley IJ. Gastric interleukin-8 and IgA IL-8 autoantibodies in *Helicobacter pylori* infection. Scand J Immunol. 1993;37:65–70.

49. Jaskiewicz K, Louw JA, Marks IN. Local cellular and immune response by antral mucosa in patients undergoing treatment for eradication of *Helicobacter pylori*. Dig Dis Sci. 1993;38:937–43.

50. Rubio CA, Ost A, Larsson B. The lymphoepithelial phenomenon of the stomach. Acta Pathol Microbiol Scand. 1988;96:898–900.

51. Dunn BE, Roop RM, Sung C, Sharma SA, Perez-Perez GI, Blaser MJ. Identification and purification of a cpn60 heat shock protein homolog from *Helicobacter pylori*. Infect Immun. 1992;60:1946–51.

52. Baca-Estrada ME, Gupta RS, Stead RH, Croitoru K. Intestinal expression and cellular immune responses to human heat-shock protein 60 in Crohn's disease. Dig Dis Sci. 1994:in press.

53. Karttunen R, Andersson G, Poikonen K et al. *Helicobacter pylori* induces lymphocyte activation in peripheral blood cultures. Clin Exp Immunol. 1990;82:485–8.

54. Karttunen R. Blood lymphocyte proliferation, cytokine secretion and appearance of T cells with activation surface markers in cultures with *Helicobacter pylori*. Comparison of the responses of subjects with and without antibodies to *H. pylori*. Clin Exp Immunol. 1991;83:396–400.

55. Czinn SJ, Nedrud JG. Oral immunization against *Helicobacter pylori*. Infect Immun. 1991;59:2359–63.

56. Chen M, Lee A, Hazell S. Immunization against gastric helicobacter infection in a mouse/*Helicobacter felis* model [letter]. Lancet. 1992;339:1120–1.

57. Edwards PD, Carrick J, Turner J, Lee A, Mitchell H, Cooper DA. *Helicobacter pylori*-associated gastritis is rare in AIDS: antibiotic effect or a consequence of immunodeficiency? Am J Gastroenterol. 1991;86:1761–4.

58. Meiselman MS, Miller-Catchpole R, Christ M, Randall E. *Campylobacter pylori* gastritis in the acquired immunodeficiency syndrome. Gastroenterology. 1988;95:209–12.

31
The clinical value of a saliva diagnostic assay for antibody to *H. pylori*

R. L. CLANCY, A. W. CRIPPS, D. C. TAYLOR, L. McSHANE and V. J. WEBSTER

INTRODUCTION

The link between colonization of the gastric mucosa with *Helicobacter pylori* and dyspepsia-associated disease has been established[1,2], and at least for those with peptic ulcer disease an attempt to eradicate the infection is recommended[3]. The use of non-invasive tests to identify infection and to validate eradication of *H. pylori* by antimicrobial therapy is important, both to ensure cost-effective referral for endoscopy[4], and to determine management strategies. The recommendation of initial empirical treatment of dyspepsia in general practice[5] would be strengthened by knowledge of *H. pylori* status given the value of antimicrobial therapy. The reports that infection with *H. pylori* is a risk factor for gastric cancer[6,7] can best be further epidemiologically defined with a cheap and sensitive non-invasive test. Detection of circulating *H. pylori* antibody is a sensitive and specific assay for infection with practical advantages over the urea breath tests[8,9], which are the currently available alternatives to serology. Serological assay is reported to be sufficient to detect *H. pylori* infection and to be an acceptable primary diagnostic test, replacing endoscopy as a first-up test in patients under the age of 45 years with dyspepsia[4]. In addition, serology has been shown to be a cheap and reliable means of monitoring the success of eradication of *H. pylori*[11]. Serological assay has, however, several practical problems in monitoring eradication therapy, including technical difficulties such as inaccuracies caused by dilutions, and a period of at least 6 months before most successfully treated patients have antibody levels of less than half pretreatment values[10]. This period is considerably in excess of the 6-week period used for repeat biopsy to show clearance of bacteria[3]. We therefore have developed a saliva assay for *H. pylori* antibody, with the aim of having a simple and cheap non-invasive test of infection with *H. pylori*, whose results closely reflect infection status following antimicrobial therapy. The objective of this study was primarily to compare the saliva assay with a serum test as the standard of current infection.

METHODS

Patients were recruited to the study with symptoms or history of upper gastrointestinal disease. Patients were endoscoped and biopsy specimens of the gastric antrum assessed with regard to histopathology and urease testing for *H. pylori* at the commencement of the study, 4 and 20 weeks after eradication chemotherapy. The eradication treatment consisted of colloidal bismuth subcitrate (2 × 108 mg), metronidazole (400 mg), and amoxycillin trihydrate (500 mg). Bismuth was administered every 12 h for 4 weeks, while metronidazole and amoxycillin trihydrate were administered every 8 h for 2 weeks. In addition mixed, unstimulated saliva and serum were collected at the commencement of the study and at each of the post-treatment visits. IgG antibody to *H. pylori* was measured by an enzyme-linked immunoabsorbent assay (ELISA). Separate assay systems have been developed for serum and saliva[11]. These assays used a purified high molecular weight antigen, and the saliva assay has been commercially developed by Cortecs Diagnostics, Deeside, UK as HELISAL™ (patent pending). Gastritis was defined histologically as 'acute' when the dominant cell was the neutrophil granulocyte, and 'chronic' when the mononuclear cells dominated.

RESULTS

Distribution analysis

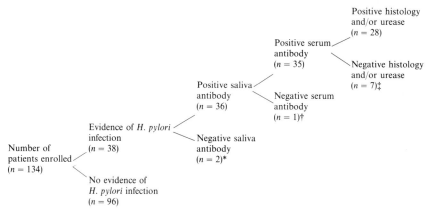

*Patient 1 – healed duodenal ulcer with negative *H. pylori* and urease but positive serum test; patient 2 – diagnosis 'normal' with negative *H. pylori* and urease but positive serum test
†Patient 1 – diagnosis 'normal', with negative *H. pylori* and urease
‡Six of seven patients had histological chronic gastritis, two of whom also had acute changes

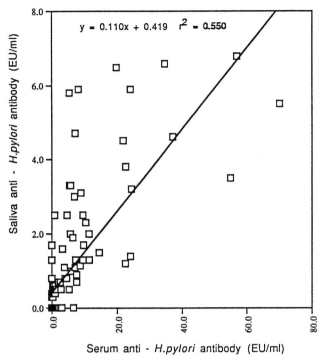

Fig. 1 Correlation of saliva and serum anti-*H. pylori* antibody in patients with gastrointestinal symptoms (*n* = 134)

Comparison of saliva ELISA for anti-*H. pylori* antibody with the serum ELISA assay

The database obtained from the 134 patients was used to determine the clinical value characteristics of salivary antibody detection compared to the serological results. The sensitivity of the saliva assay was 89%, the specificity 94%, accuracy was 93%, positive predictive value 89% and the negative predictive value was 94%. Regression analysis of IgG anti-*H. pylori* antibody from paired serum and saliva samples (Fig. 1) ($r^2 = 0.55$) was most consistent with a contribution to antibody in saliva from local synthesis.

The effect of eradication treatment on saliva anti-*H. pylori* antibody at 4 weeks post-treatment

Twenty-four patients with evidence of *H. pylori* infection were given eradication therapy and reassessed 4 weeks after completion of treatment. Half of those patients with a positive saliva test became negative (Table 1, Fig. 2), more than twice the percentage that became seronegative. If a reduction in antibody titre of more than 50% was assessed (Table 2), less than half the serum test results reduced by $\geq 50\%$ while the result for saliva (83%) was

344

Table 1 Patients with pretreatment positive saliva anti-*H. pylori* antibody becoming negative 1 month post-treatment

Patient number	Saliva antibody* (EU/ml) Pre-	Serum antibody† (EU/ml) Pre-	Serum antibody† Post-	Serum antibody† <50%‡	Urease Test Pre-	Urease Test Post-	H. pylori present Pre-	H. pylori present Post-	Acute Pre-	Acute Post-	Chronic Pre-	Chronic Post-	Endoscopic diagnosis Pre-	Endoscopic diagnosis Post-
1	1.1	+	+	−	+	−	+	−	+	−	+	+	Gastritis	Normal
2	1.1	+	−	+	+	−	+	−	+	−	+	+	Gastritis	Normal
3	2.2	+	+	+	+	−	+	−	−	−	+	+	Gastritis	Normal
4	0.9	+	+	−	+	−	+	−	+	−	+	−	GU	GU
5	1.3	+	+	+	−	−	+	−	+	−	−	−	Gastritis	Normal
6	1.3	+	+	+	+	−	+	−	−	−	−	−	GU	Gastritis
7	1.2	+	+	−	+	−	+	−	+	−	+	+	EO	Oesophagitis
8	3.1	+	+	+	+	−	+	−	+	−	+	+	GU	Normal
9	1.5	+	+	−	+	−	+	−	−	−	+	+	Gastritis	Normal
10	0.8	+	−	+	+	+	+	+	−	−	+	+	Gastritis	Gastritis
11	2.0	+	−	+	−	−	−	−	−	−	+	+	DU	Normal
12	1.4	+	+	+	+	−	+	−	−	−	+	+	Gastritis	Gastritis

*Positive saliva ≥ 0.70 ELISA units/ml
†Positive serum ≥ 2.50 ELISA units/ml
‡ <50% of pretreatment level
+, Positive; −, negative; DU, duodenal ulcer; GU, gastric ulcer; EO, erosive oesophagitis.

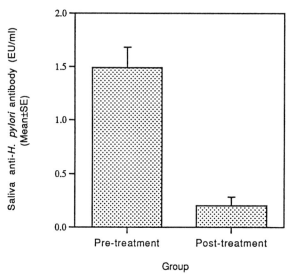

Fig. 2 Decrease in saliva anti-*H. pylori* IgG antibody post-eradication treatment (*n* = 12)

Table 2 Conversion from positive to negative results for anti-*H. pylori* antibody at 1 month post-treatment

		One month post-eradication treatment	
	Pretreatment positive (no. of patients)	*Negative (%)*	*<50% of pretreatment level (%)*
Saliva antibody	23	52	83
Serum antibody	24	21	46
Urease test	23	91	—
Histopathology: *H. pylori* present	22	86	—
Histopathology: Acute inflammation	9	89	—

of the same order as that found for the standard parameters used to monitor elimination. Thus sections were negative for *H. pylori* (86%) and urease tests became negative (89%). The high frequency (89%) of reversal of histological evidence of acute inflammation is consistent with eradication of *H. pylori*. The pretreatment level of salivary antibody was a major determinant of the time taken to fall in response to antimicrobial treatment (Tables 3 and 4). Thus for 4-week post-treatment negative saliva tests the mean pretreatment antibody level was 1.5 EU/ml, compared to a value for those reducing to less than 50% of pretreatment values of 3.3 EU/ml, with a value of 5.0 EU/ml for those not falling below the 50% level. Three patients in this last group showed levels <50% (*n* = 2) or negative (*n* = 1) for saliva antibody at the 6-month follow-up visit.

Eradication was not achieved by 4 weeks in three patients (Table 1: patient

Table 3 Patients with pretreatment positive saliva anti-*H. pylori* antibody who at 1 month post-treatment have positive saliva antibody and saliva antibody less than 50% pretreatment level

Patient number	Saliva antibody* (EU/ml) Pre-	Serum antibody† (EU/ml)			Antral mucosa biopsy										Comment
		Pre-	Post-	<50%‡	Urease test		Histopathology						Endoscopic diagnosis		
					Pre-	Post-	H. pylori present		Inflammation				Pre-	Post-	
							Pre-	Post-	Acute		Chronic				
									Pre-	Post-	Pre-	Post-			
1	4.6	+	+	+	+	−	+	−	−	−	+	+	Gastritis	Normal	Previous DU
2	3.8	+	+	+	+	−	+	−	−	−	+	+	Gastritis	Normal	Symptoms persist
3	3.5	+	+	+	+	−	+	−	−	−	+	+	DU	Normal	Asymptomatic
4	2.3	+	+	+	+	−	+	−	−	−	+	−	Gastritis	Normal	Symptoms improved
5	2.5	+	+	−	+	−	+	+	+	+	−	+	Gastritis	Normal	Symptoms improved
6	5.9	+	+	−	+	+	+	+	−	+	+	+	Gastritis	Gastritis	Symptoms persist
7	3.3	+	+	−	+	−	+	−	−	−	+	+	Gastritis	Normal	Reduced symptoms

*Positive saliva ≥ 0.70 ELISA units/ml
†Positive serum ≥ 2.50 ELISA units/ml
‡<50% of pretreatment level
+, Positive; −, negative; DU, duodenal ulcer

347

Table 4 Patients with pretreatment positive saliva anti-*H. pylori* antibody who at 1 month post-treatment have positive saliva antibody and saliva antibody not less than 50% pretreatment level

Patient number	Saliva antibody* (EU/ml) Pre-	Serum antibody† (EU/ml)			Antral mucosa biopsy								Endoscopic diagnosis		Comment
		Pre-	Post-	<50%‡	Urease test		Histopathology								
					Pre-	Post-	H. pylori present		Inflammation				Pre-	Post-	
							Pre-	Post-	Acute		Chronic				
									Pre-	Post-	Pre-	Post-			
1	6.8	+	+	–	+	–	+	–	–	–	+	–	DU	Healed	(6m) Sal <50% Ser >50%
2	1.2	+	+	–	+	–	+	–	+	–	+	+	Normal	Normal	(6m) Sal and Ser Neg Previous GU
3	5.5	+	+	–	+	–	+	–	–	–	+	+	Gastritis	Normal	
4	6.5	+	+	–	+	–	–	–	–	–	–	–	DU	Normal	(6m) Sal <50% Ser <50%

*Positive saliva ≥ 0.70 ELISA units/ml
†Positive serum ≥ 2.50 ELISA units/ml
‡<50% of pretreatment level
+, Positive; –, negative; DU, duodenal ulcer; GU, gastric ulcer

10, Table 3: patients 5 and 6). Reviewing these three patients, the fall in saliva antibody probably reflects a sensitive response to partial eradication as seroconversion, reversal of positive urease test and improvement of symptoms (in various combinations) in these patients is most consistent with that explanation.

DISCUSSION

Anti-*H. pylori* IgG antibody has been detected in the saliva of patients infected with *H. pylori*. The concordance with serum antibody confirmed its value as a diagnostic assay for *H. pylori* infection in patients with dyspepsia. Reassessment 4 weeks after completing a 4-week eradication programme demonstrated the saliva assay to have advantages over the serum test as a practical monitor of successful therapy. A level of independence of IgG antibody levels in saliva was consistent with a component of local secretion from B lymphocytes migrating from the gut mucosa.

The saliva assay for anti-*H. pylori* antibody contained a high molecular weight antigen which has been validated against a serum test[11]. The high level of performance indices against serum antibody may even underestimate its value in reflecting contemporary infection statistics as, in the two instances of seropositivity with a negative saliva test, *H. pylori* infection was doubtful. Practical advantages in both the collection of samples, and in the laboratory performance of the assay, especially the ability to quantitate all saliva samples with the one dilution, provides further support for the clinical value of the saliva test.

Successful eradication of *H. pylori* can be confirmed by repeat endoscopy 6 weeks after completion of a 2-week course of combination antimicrobial agents[3]. Serological tests are a reliable and relatively non-invasive means of confirming the success of eradicating *H. pylori*, but significant reduction of antibody level in most patients is delayed by months[10]. The current study confirmed the success of eradication therapy in the majority of patients with no *H. pylori* in biopsies taken at 4 weeks following completion of therapy. The fall in the level of salivary antibody was noted in a proportion of patients, which was similar to that found for the classic parameters of infection found with antral biopsies. In contrast, the rate of disappearance of serum antibody was about half of saliva antibody levels. The rate of fall in serum antibody concentration, however, was faster than rates previously reported using tests that contained crude bacterial extract for antigen[10]. Patients with high saliva (and serum) antibody levels took longer to revert to negative following successful eradication therapy. On standard criteria, three patients failed to eradicate *H. pylori* at 4 weeks post-therapy. The three patients had a fall in salivary antibody. Two of these patients had histological, serological and clinical evidence of a partial response to antimicrobial therapy. An early 'dip' in serum antibody occurs following eradication therapy[10], probably reflecting a partial response to therapy. A longer period of observation is needed to define the kinetics of salivary antibody response to eradication treatment.

The source of the IgG antibody in saliva is not clear, but is consistent with previous demonstrations of IgG antibody following mucosal stimulation with microbial antigens[12,13]. In animal models, secretory IgG antibody correlates with the kinetics of local IgA secretion and does not closely follow serum levels[14], suggesting that local synthesis from gut-derived lymphocytes may contribute to the IgG antibody pool in secretions. Further support for local secretion of IgG was gained from the observation of IgG-containing plasma cells within the respiratory mucosa following intestinal immunization[15]. This concept is consistent with observations in the current study of a poor correlation between IgG antibody levels in saliva and serum, and a difference in elimination kinetics between serum and saliva.

It is considered that the saliva ELISA antibody assay should prove useful in the clinical assessment of patients with dyspepsia, and in monitoring the results of eradication treatment. Saliva anti-*H. pylori* antibody appears to be a more reliable index of current infection than serological assessment. A modification of this ELISA assay has been developed which provides the physician with an immediate 'yes/no' read-out facilitating management discussions.

References

1. Marshall BJ, Warren JR. Unidentified curved bacilli in the stomach of patients with gastritis and peptic ulceration. Lancet. 1984;1:1311–14.
2. Rauws EAJ, Langenberg W, Houthoff HJ, Tytgat GNJ. *Campylobacter pyloridis*-associated chronic active antral gastritis. Gastroenterology. 1988;94:33–40.
3. Graham DY. Treatment of peptic ulcers caused by *Helicobacter pylori*. N Engl J Med. 1993;328:349–50.
4. Sobala GM, Crabtree JE, Pentith JA *et al*. Screening dyspepsia by serology to *Helicobacter pylori*. Lancet. 1991;338:94–6.
5. Brown C, Rees WDW. Dyspepsia in general practice. BMJ. 1990;300:829–30.
6. Nomura A, Stemmermann GN, Chyou P-H, Kato I, Perez-Perez GI, Blaser MJ. *Helicobacter pylori* infection and gastric carcinoma among Japanese Americans in Hawaii. N Engl J Med. 1991;325:1132–6.
7. Parsonnet J, Friedman GD, Vandersteen DP *et al*. *Helicobacter pylori* infection and the risk of carcinoma. N Engl J Med. 1991;325:1127–31.
8. Bell GD, Weil J, Harrison G *et al*. ^{14}C-urea breath analysis, a non-invasive test for *Campylobacter pylori* in the stomach. Lancet. 1987;1:1367–8.
9. Graham DY, Klein PD, Evans DR Jr *et al*. *Campylobacter pylori* detected noninvasively by the ^{13}C-urea breath test. Lancet. 1987;1:1174–7.
10. Kosunen TU, Seppala K, Sarna I, Sipponen P. Diagnostic value of decreasing IgG, IgA, and IgM antibody titres after eradication of *Helicobacter pylori*. Lancet. 1992;1:893–5.
11. Cripps AW, Clancy RL, Taylor D, McShane L. A salivary ELISA for the detection of *Helicobacter pylori* infection. Proceedings; *Helicobacter pylori*: basic mechanisms to clinical cure. 3–6 November, Amelia Island, USA
12. Clancy R, Cripps AW, Husband AJ, Buckley D. Specific immune response in the respiratory tract following an oral polyvalent bacterial vaccine. Infect Immun. 1983;39:491–6.
13. Cripps AW, Clancy RL, Murree-Allen K, Engel MB, Pang G, Yeung S. Quantitation of isotype specific *Haemophilus influenzae* antibody in serum and saliva of normal subjects and chronic bronchitics. Asian Pacific J Allergy Immunol. 1986;4:5–11.
14. Pang G, Clancy RL, O'Reilly S, Cripps AW. A novel particulate form of influenza virus vaccine stimulates durable and broad-based protection in mice following oral immunisation. J Virol. 1992;66:1162–70.
15. Scicchitano R, Husband AJ, Clancy RL. Antigen-specific response among T lymphocytes following intestinal administration of alloantigens. Immunology. 1984;53:375–84.

Section VI
Gastroduodenal inflammation in *H. pylori* infection

32
Spectrum and implications of inflammation with *H. pylori*

M. F. DIXON

The acute phase of *Helicobacter* infection is uncommon in gastric biopsies because the initial illness is trivial in its symptomatology or goes unnoticed by the patient. Usually the presence of an acute phase is inferred from serological findings. The published accounts are largely confined to human ingestion studies[1,2], or from 'naturally' acquired infection in endoscopy personnel[3].

ACUTE *HELICOBACTER*-ASSOCIATED GASTRITIS

Following ingestion, the organism penetrates through the viscid mucous layer and multiplies close to the apical membranes of the surface epithelial cells. Some organisms become adherent and attach to the plasma membrane while others penetrate between epithelial cells and may enter the lamina propria. Attachment is likely to be followed by endocytosis[4], but this has not been fully documented *in vivo* in the human. Tissue invasion and the elaboration of chemical mediators provokes an intense polymorph response. The epithelium responds to infection by marked degenerative changes including mucin depletion, cellular exfoliation and syncytial regenerative changes. The latter changes may be sufficiently bizarre to mimic premalignant dysplasia. Polymorph infiltration into foveolar and surface epithelium can be conspicuous, in which case one can find 'pit abscess' formation and adherent polymorph exudation on the surface. This histological picture is termed *acute neutrophilic gastritis*.

The acute phase is short-lived. In a minority of people the organisms may be spontaneously cleared, the polymorph infiltrate resolves and appearances return to normal. In most people, however, the host immune response fails to eliminate the infection, and over the next 3–4 weeks there is a gradual accumulation of chronic inflammatory cells, which come to dominate the histological picture. Consequently the diagnosis of acute neutrophilic gastritis gives way to that of an active chronic gastritis.

CHRONIC *HELICOBACTER*-ASSOCIATED GASTRITIS

The histological features of chronic gastritis have long been recognized, but their significance regarding disease progression and functional consequences has had to await recognition of its aetiology. Now that *Helicobacter pylori* has been firmly established as the major cause of chronic gastritis, we can assess the part that infection plays in the development of these histological changes.

Surface epithelial degeneration

Damage to the surface epithelium is a conspicuous feature of *Helicobacter*-associated chronic gastritis. Such degeneration is manifest as mucin depletion and a cuboidal appearance of the cells with a high nucleo-cytoplasmic ratio. Exfoliated cells are seen in the adherent mucus, or gaps may be evident in the surface layer where cell 'drop-out' has occurred[5]. A curious feature is the appearance of 'budding' where a protuberance is formed by a syncytia-like collection of cells. These appearances are usually associated with marked polymorph infiltration of adjacent epithelium and are related to the colonization density of *H. pylori*. The surface epithelium rapidly recovers after eradication of infection, and we have recently documented the increase in cell height found in post-treatment biopsies. Prior to treatment patients with *H. pylori*-positive gastritis had a mean cell height of $7.98 \pm 0.88\,\mu$m (compared to $9.02 \pm 0.95\,\mu$m in uninfected normal controls) which increased to $8.99 \pm 0.86\,\mu$m 5 weeks after successful eradication treatment ($p = 0.0056$)[6]. However, we have found no significant differences in the grade of epithelial degeneration between groups of patients with duodenal ulcer, gastric ulcer and age-matched controls with functional dyspepsia (mean grades; DU = 1.16, controls = 1.04; GU = 1.6; controls = 1.32)[7].

Surface epithelial degeneration is positively correlated with the proportion of *H. pylori* in intimate contact with the plasma membrane[8], a finding that supports a direct toxic effect of bacterial products on epithelial cells. Certain strains of *H. pylori* produce a vacuolating cytotoxin that is demonstrable *in vitro* by observing its effects on cultured cell lines[9]. However, the pathological importance of this cytotoxin *in vivo* is controversial. Interest has also centred on the possibility that ammonia production via bacterial urease activity may be a potent cellular toxin. Graham *et al.*[10] have argued against ammonia as a gastric toxin, and have suggested that other ammonium products may be more important. Notable among these is the production of mono-N-chloramine formed by the interaction of ammonia with hypochlorous acid produced by activated neutrophils.

Phospholipases produced by *H. pylori* might also exert damaging effects on the surface epithelium. Phospholipase A_2 and C could disrupt the normal phospholipid bilayer of the epithelial cell membrane and affect cellular integrity. They also liberate arachidonic acid which is then converted into leukotrienes and other eicosanoids[11]. These compounds can produce altered membrane permeability and mucus discharge in addition to their pro-inflammatory effects. Another way in which phospholipases affect epithelial integrity is by degradation of the mucous layer. *H. pylori*-infected mucus is less hydrophobic than normal mucus, and this may be partly mediated by phospholipases.

H. pylori synthesizes or causes mast cells to release a platelet-activating factor (PAF)[12]. Release of PAF might lead to occlusion in the microcirculation and affect epithelial integrity by ischaemic damage. Likewise, the production of endotoxin could have deleterious effects on capillary endothelium with similar consequences.

Neutrophil activity

Infiltration by polymorphs is an almost invariable, if not constant, feature of *Helicobacter*-associated chronic gastritis. Conventionally their presence is used to indicate 'active' chronic inflammation, but the use of *active* and *inactive* to describe chronic inflammation is not universally accepted. At least it forms a useful abbreviation for 'chronic gastritis with neutrophil infiltration', and there is evidence to suggest that polymorph activation is a critical factor in tissue injury and thus in progression of the disease process.

The closeness of the association between polymorph infiltration and current *H. pylori* infection has been underestimated in many studies because of different criteria for the diagnosis of 'activity' and an inadequate number of biopsies. While two antral biopsies are considered adequate to establish the *H. pylori* status, four or more biopsies are required to confirm the presence (or absence) of activity with >95% confidence[13]. On the basis of two antral biopsies we found activity in 85% of patients with *H. pylori*-positive chronic gastritis, but the evidence of Bayerdorffer *et al.*[13] indicates that this figure would be 100% if sufficient biopsies had been examined. If carefully sought, activity is found in a high proportion of adult cases of chronic gastritis – 82% in our experience. The great majority of these will prove to be *H. pylori*-positive. However, activity is much less marked in chronic gastritis in childhood even when this is associated with *H. pylori* infection.

Neutrophil polymorphs are seen either in the lamina propria or infiltrating the epithelium of the foveolae or mucosal surface. Infiltration is frequently concentrated around the pit-isthmus region, and in more severe cases may fill the pit-lumen forming a 'pit-abscess', or give rise to a surface exudate. Such infiltration is topographically related to *H. pylori* colonization, and is not seen, for example, in areas of intestinal metaplasia where the organisms fail to colonize. Likewise activity is absent in the severely atrophic stomach from which *H. pylori* have been eliminated, and polymorphs disappear rapidly after successful eradication therapy.

The presence of polymorphs in the mucosa is generally attributed to the mucosal immune response to *H. pylori* antigens. Complement activation consequent upon specific antibody production, liberation of interleukins, especially IL-8, and leukotriene formation could all contribute to polymorph chemotaxis[14]. However, the presence of polymorphs in the acute phase of infection without the intervention of lymphocytes and plasma cells suggests that non-immune mechanisms such as complement activation via the alternative pathway are important.

Chronic inflammation

The normal antral mucosa does not contain chronic inflammatory cells. The corpus mucosa contains an occasional small lymphoid aggregate close to the muscularis mucosa but none in the superficial lamina propria. It is self-evident that chronic inflammatory cell infiltration is a prominent feature of chronic gastritis, but the infiltrate may be sparse in gastritis with severe glandular atrophy and metaplasia. The infiltrate comprises lymphocytes, plasma cells and small numbers of eosinophils.

There is a good correlation between the density of the chronic inflammatory cell infiltrate and the extent and degree of H. pylori colonization. This has been demonstrated both in subjective grading studies[15] and morphometric investigations[16,17]. The degree of colonization is overall more marked in the antrum than the corpus, which accords with the generally greater degree of inflammatory cell infiltration seen in the antrum; for the same degree of H. pylori colonization in the corpus, one will often see a lesser degree of chronic gastritis. This indicates that either the organism loses virulence in the corpus part of the stomach, or that this region is more resistant to infection despite the presence of organisms in the overlying mucus layer.

Chronic inflammation is seen first in the antrum but gradually extends along the lesser curve and spreads to give diffuse involvement of the corpus[18]. Thus most patients eventually exhibit a pan-gastritis. In a minority, however, inflammation remains much more pronounced in the antrum and the degree of inflammation in the corpus is minimal. Such a pattern of chronic gastritis is found in patients with DU and pre-pyloric ulcers. The extension and increasing severity of chronic inflammation is followed by glandular atrophy.

While the presence of chronic inflammatory cells is entirely non-specific, at a cellular level the infiltrating cells may be serving specific roles. Thus there is an increase in $CD4^+$ helper T-lymphocytes[19], increased numbers of B lymphocytes with lymphoid follicle formation[20] and an increase in plasma cells secreting specific IgM, IgA and IgG anti-H. pylori antibodies. While secretory IgA plays an important role in blocking bacterial adhesion, these immunoglobulins may also be responsible for intracellular neutralization following bacterial endocytosis, and for the transport of potential harmful immune complexes through the surface epithelium. Opsonization and complement activation by IgG forms the main arm of the mucosal immune response. IgG antibodies promote complement-dependent phagocytosis and killing of H. pylori by polymorphs, although catalase production by the organism offers some protection against polymorph attack. Certainly in the large majority of people the antibody response does not lead to successful eradication of infection.

Other inflammatory mediators produced by activated monocytes and polymorphs include prostaglandins (PGE_2), leukotrienes, proteases and reactive oxygen metabolites such as superoxide radicals. Polymorph and monocyte release of proteases and reactive oxygen metabolites is likely to be important in causing tissue damage, particularly where there is a relative deficiency of antioxidants such as vitamins C^{21} and E^{22}. The tendency for polymorphs to congregate around the proliferative compartment of the pit-isthmus may cause lethal damage to stem cells and result in glandular atrophy.

The finding of follicles (aggregations of lymphocytes with germinal centres) is of particular interest as it is virtually restricted to *H. pylori*-associated gastritis, and if sufficient biopsies and sections are examined it is claimed that follicles will be found in all *H. pylori*-positive cases[23]. Lymphoid follicles are sufficiently prominent in childhood infection to produce a distinctive nodularity in the gastric antrum.

Atrophy

Atrophy can be defined as loss of glandular tissue from repeated mucosal injury. Atrophy leads to thinning of the gastric mucosa, and is a common denominator in all pathological processes causing severe or progressive mucosal damage. Thus, loss of glands may follow erosion or ulceration of the mucosa with destruction of the glandular layer, or as a result of a prolonged inflammatory process where individual glands undergo destruction in a 'piecemeal' fashion. When such loss occurs it is followed by fibrous replacement so that connective tissue stains such as a reticulin or Masson trichrome stain are helpful in assessing minor degrees of atrophy. It appears that destruction of the glandular basement membrane and the immediately surrounding sheath of supporting cells prevents orderly regeneration. Indeed, if any regeneration occurs it usually follows a divergent differentiation pathway and gives rise to metaplastic glands of 'pseudo-pyloric' appearance.

The prevalence and severity of atrophy among patients with chronic gastritis increases steadily with age. This is not an effect of ageing *per se*; there is no evidence that atrophy occurs as a physiological ageing phenomenon, and elderly subjects without gastritis have a normal acid output[24]. It is believed that there is a transition from non-atrophic to atrophic gastritis according to the duration of inflammation. In the main this is explained by the duration of infection with *H. pylori*, but any long-standing gastritis will have the same effect. A cohort follow-up study by Correa *et al.*[25] supports this conclusion. These investigators showed that when 780 people with normal mucosa or chronic superficial gastritis were re-biopsied after an average of 5.1 years, 284 had developed atrophic gastritis, a rate of transition of 7.5/100 person-years.

As well as an increase in prevalence, glandular atrophy becomes more extensive with increasing age. This has been long recognized in terms of the progression of antral-type mucosa at the expense of body-type mucosa so that the antral–corpus border moves proximally with age[26]. The sequence of events appears to be chronic inflammation, loss of body-type glands and replacement by metaplastic pyloric glands occurring either on a broad front or, as others argue, in a diffuse or multi-focal fashion throughout the stomach. Such atrophy is generally maximal on the lesser curve in the region of the incisura.

The prevalence of *H. pylori*-positivity in the stomach declines with increasing glandular atrophy. There are two main reasons for the loss of organisms. Firstly, *H. pylori* only colonizes gastric epithelium; thus the organisms are absent from areas of intestinal metaplasia. Secondly, the hypochlorhydric stomach is inimical to *H. pylori*. The organism requires a partially acidic environment in which to thrive, because the ammonia which is released in its vicinity as a consequence of bacterial urease activity remains un-neutralized and accumulates. This leads to ingress of ammonia into the organism with protonation of intracellular proteins, failure of intermediary metabolism, and death of the bacterium by autodestruction[27]. Therefore the failure to demonstrate *H. pylori* in the atrophic stomach does not deny a role for infection in the causation of the underlying gastritis.

Atrophy in *Helicobacter*-associated gastritis could result from direct bacterial effects or alternatively to consequences of the inflammatory reaction. Thus, cellular destruction by cytotoxins, ammonia products or proteases and reactive oxygen metabolites released by polymorphs and other inflammatory cells may be involved. A further possibility is that the immune reaction mounted against *H. pylori* cross-reacts with antigens on glandular epithelial cells and destroys them[28]. It is also likely that other factors such as a high-salt diet or bile reflux accelerate the development of atrophy in *Helicobacter*-associated gastritis. Our findings, based on 350 patients in whom intragastric bile acids were measured, indicate that there exists synergism between bile-induced damage and *H. pylori* colonization in the production of glandular atrophy[29]. On the other hand, certain dietary factors may exert a protective influence against the development of atrophy; vitamin C, vitamin E, β-carotene and trace elements may play some part.

Intestinal metaplasia

Intestinal metaplasia is a common finding in chronic gastritis of all causes, and appears to increase in prevalence according to the duration. There are therefore wide variations in the incidence of metaplasia between countries according to the peak age of acquisition of *H. pylori* infection.

Intestinal metaplasia (IM) can be divided into three main types according to its mucin content and morphology; a 'complete' type (type I) where the epithelium resembles that of the normal small intestine, and two 'incomplete' types, type II where goblet cells appear between the normal gastric mucous cells and type III where goblet cells and intervening diffuse mucus-containing cells stain for sulphomucins more like colonic epithelium. IM is found more frequently in *H. pylori*-positive than negative cases – despite the tendency for stomachs with extensive metaplasia to become negative[30]. Likewise it has been shown that *H. pylori* is an additional independent risk factor for intestinal metaplasia separate from bile reflux[31]. It seems likely therefore that, as with atrophy, there is some synergy between *H. pylori* and bile in the production of intestinal metaplasia such that epithelium already sustaining damage from *H. pylori* is more likely to be eroded by bile reflux and be substituted by intestinal type cells during the regenerative process. Such 'regenerative' intestinal metaplasia is likely to be transient, but repetitive injury leads to more extensive and permanent type I, or in a small minority, type III intestinal metaplasia.

In so far as *H. pylori* does not adhere to intestinal epithelium, it is possible to view intestinal metaplasia as a defence response in which gastric epithelium is substituted by an epithelium better suited to counteract two adverse factors which operate either independently or synergistically to produce chronic injury to the gastric mucosa, namely bile reflux and *H. pylori* infection. Interestingly, when well-developed intestinal metaplasia is present in *H. pylori*-associated gastritis, there is an appreciable decline in inflammatory cells in the underlying lamina propria[32], an observation which indicates that the inflammatory infiltrate is closely related to sites of bacterial adhesion and not simply a diffuse response to *H. pylori* in the stomach.

CONCLUSIONS

From the foregoing it is clear that *H. pylori* gastritis begins as an acute neutrophilic inflammatory response which in the majority of individuals progresses to chronic gastritis. The key features of *Helicobacter*-associated chronic gastritis are the infiltrate of lymphocytes and plasma cells as mediators of the mucosal immune response, surface epithelial degeneration indicating direct cytotoxic effects by bacterial products, and continuing polymorph 'activity' provoked by bacterial products, complement activation or cytokine release. Long-standing chronic gastritis is characterized by the development of glandular atrophy and intestinal metaplasia. The former could be due to polymorph-mediated damage or other cytotoxic injury to stem cells, and a failure to replenish glandular epithelial cells. Metaplasia is likely to be an adaptive phenomenon to persistent infection or to other injurious agents operating on a susceptible mucosa. With increasing atrophy the hypochlorhydric (and metaplastic) stomach becomes hostile to *H. pylori* and the organisms disappear. Loss of organisms is accompanied by a gradual waning of the chronic inflammatory cell infiltrate so that the end-stage atrophic gastric mucosa appears largely devoid of inflammatory cells.

The tissue and immune response to *H. pylori* infection can satisfactorily explain all the histological aspects of the associated chronic gastritis. A spectrum of changes is seen which matches the duration and severity of infection. Starting as a classical acute inflammatory response, the infection progresses through chronic inflammation to a quiescent stage with atrophy and intestinal metaplasia, a stage by which the organism has usually been eliminated. Thus, in this terminal phase *H. pylori* departs the battlefield but the field never recovers. Whether or not lesser degrees of atrophy and metaplasia can be reversed by eradication of *H. pylori* must await the outcome of current intervention trials.

References

1. Marshall BJ, Armstrong JA, McGechie DB, Glancy RJ. Attempt to fulfil Koch's postulates for pyloric campylobacter. Med J Aust. 1985;142:436–9.
2. Morris A, Nicholson G. Ingestion of *Campylobacter pyloridis* causes gastritis and raised fasting gastric pH. Am J Gastroenterol. 1987;82:192–9.
3. Sobala GM, Crabtree J, Dixon MF *et al.* Acute *Helicobacter pylori* infection: clinical features, local and systemic immune response, gastric mucosal histology and gastric juice ascorbic acid concentrations. Gut. 1991;32:1415–18.
4. Graham DY. Pathogenic mechanisms leading to *Helicobacter pylori*-induced inflammation. Eur J Gastroenterol Hepatol. 1992;4(Suppl. 2):s9–16.
5. Chan WY, Hui PK, Leung KM, Thomas TMM. Modes of *Helicobacter* colonization and gastric epithelial damage. Histopathology. 1992;21:521–8.
6. Hassan F, Clarke A, Sobala GM, Axon ATR, Dixon MF. Epithelial recovery after *H. pylori* eradication. Acta Gastroenterol Belg. 1993;56:S124.
7. Dixon MF, Sobala GM, Wyatt JI. Surface epithelial degeneration in *H. pylori* gastritis: relationship to coexistent peptic ulcer. Ir J Med Sci. 1992;161(Suppl. 10):13.
8. Hessey SJ, Wyatt JI, Axon ATR, Sobala GM, Rathbone BJ, Dixon MF. The relationship between adhesion sites and disease activity in *C. pylori* associated gastritis. Gut. 1990;31:134–8.
9. Leunk RD, Johnson PT, David BC, Kraft WG, Morgan DR. Cytotoxic activity in broth-culture filtrates of *Campylobacter pylori*. J Med Microbiol. 1988;26:93–9.
10. Graham DY, Go MF, Evans DJ. Urease, gastric ammonium/ammonia, and *Helicobacter pylori* – the past, the present, and recommendations for future research. Aliment Pharmacol Ther. 1992;6:659–69.
11. Marshall BJ. Virulence and pathogenicity of *Helicobacter pylori*. J Gastroenterol Hepatol. 1991;6:121–4.
12. Denizot Y, Sobhani I, Rambaud JC, Lewin M, Thomas Y, Benveniste J. PAF-acether synthesis by *Helicobacter pylori*. Gut. 1990;31:1242–5.
13. Bayerdörffer E, Oertel H, Lehn N *et al.* Topographic association between active gastritis and *Campylobacter pylori* colonisation. J Clin Pathol. 1989;42:834–9.
14. Dixon MF. Pathophysiology of *H. pylori* infection. Scand J Gastroenterol. 1993:in press.
15. Stolte M, Eidt S, Ohnsmann A. Differences in *Helicobacter pylori* associated gastritis in the antrum and body of the stomach. Z Gastroenterol. 1990;28:229–33.
16. Collins JSA, Sloan JM, Hamilton PW, Watt PCH, Love AHG. Investigation of the relationship between gastric antral inflammation and *Campylobacter pylori* using graphic tablet planimetry. J Pathol. 1989;159:281–5.
17. Steininger H, Schneider U, Bartz K, Simmler B. *Campylobacter pylori* and gastritis – colonization density and degree of inflammation. A semiquantitative and morphometric study. Leber, Magen, Darm. 1989;19:70–8.
18. Ihamaki T, Saukkonen M, Siurala M. Longterm observation of subjects with normal mucosa and with superficial gastritis. Results of 23–27 years follow-up examination. Scand J Gastroenterol. 1978;13:771–6.
19. Wyatt JI, Rathbone BJ. Immune response of the gastric mucosa to *Campylobacter pylori*. Scand J Gastroenterol. 1988;23(Suppl. 142):44–9.
20. Stolte M, Eidt S. Lymphoid follicles in antral mucosa: immune response to *Campylobacter pylori*? J Clin Pathol. 1989;42:1269–71.
21. Sobala GM, Schorah CJ, Sanderson M *et al.* Ascorbic acid in the human stomach. Gastroenterology. 1989;97:357–63.
22. Phull PS, Gower JD, Price AB, Green CJ, Jacyna MR. α-Tocopherol (vitamin E) antioxidant levels in chronic gastritis; correlation with mucosal neutrophil infiltration. Gut. 1993;34(Suppl. 1):S34.
23. Genta RM, Hamner HW, Graham DY. Gastric lymphoid follicles in *Helicobacter pylori* infection. Hum Pathol. 1993;24:577–83.
24. Katelaris PH, Seow F, Lin B, Napoli J, Ngu MC, Jones DB. The effect of age, *Helicobacter pylori* infection and gastric atrophy on serum gastrin and gastric acid secretion in healthy men. Gut. 1993;34:1032–7.
25. Correa P, Haenszel W, Cuello C *et al.* Gastric precancerous process in a high risk population: cohort follow-up. Cancer Res. 1990;50:4737–40.

26. Fujishima K, Misumi A, Akagi M. Histopathologic study on development and extension of atrophic change in the gastric mucosa. Gastroenterol Jpn. 1984;19:9–17.
27. Neithercut WD, Grieg MA, Hossack M, McColl KEL. Suicidal destruction of *Helicobacter pylori*: metabolic consequence of intracellular accumulation of ammonia. J Clin Pathol. 1991;44:380–4.
28. Negrini R, Lisato L, Zanella I *et al. Helicobacter pylori* infection induces antibodies cross-reacting with human gastric mucosa. Gastroenterology. 1991;101:437–45.
29. Sobala GM, Wyatt JI, Dixon MF. Histologic aspects of atrophic gastritis. In Holt PR, Russell RM, editors. Chronic gastritis and hypochlorhydria in the elderly. Boca Raton: CRC Press; 1993:49–68.
30. Craanen ME, Dekker W, Blok P, Ferwerda J, Tytgat GNJ. Intestinal metaplasia and *Helicobacter pylori*: an endoscopic bioptic study of the gastric antrum. Gut. 1992;33:16–20.
31. Sobala GM, O'Connor HJ, Dewar EP, King RFG, Axon ATR, Dixon MF. Bile reflux and intestinal metaplasia in gastric mucosa. J Clin Pathol. 1993;46:235–40.
32. Wyatt JI, Dixon MF. *Campylobacter*-associated chronic gastritis. In: Rosen PP, editor. Pathology annual. New York: Year Book Publishers; 1990 (Part 1):75–98.

33
'Hypertrophic' gastritis in *H. pylori* infection

M. STOLTE, C. BÄTZ, S. EIDT and E. BAYERDÖRFFER

INTRODUCTION

Giant folds of the gastric mucosa may be due to foveolar hyperplasia, glandular hyperplasia as in Zollinger–Ellison syndrome, tumorous infiltration, or inflammatory processes[1-5]. They may be focal or diffuse, in various regions of the stomach, and are defined by a thickening of the gastric rugae to more than 10 mm.

Diffuse foveolar hyperplasia with giant folds in the fundus and corpus, coupled with gastrointestinal protein loss, is known as Ménétrier's disease[6,7]. In earlier reports, inflammatory giant folds have been termed gastritis hypertrophica gigantica[8]. With the exception of a number of granulomatous inflammatory processes associated with giant folds[1-4] and CMV gastritis[9,10] the aetiopathogenesis of hypertrophic gastritis is usually not clear. In recent years, it has been shown in individual cases that giant fold formation can occur in lymphocytic gastritis[11] and in colonization of the gastric mucosa with *Helicobacter pylori*[12-17] as confirmed by the disappearance of the giant folds following successful eradication of the organism[13,17]. In an earlier study, we were able to demonstrate that hypertrophic gastritis may be a special form of *H. pylori* associated gastritis[18]. We have continued and expanded the earlier studies, and have additionally tested the effect of the eradication of *H. pylori*.

MATERIAL AND METHODS

Patients with giant folds

Biopsies obtained from the gastric mucosa of 235 patients in whom the endoscopist had detected giant folds in the corpus/fundus, were submitted to histological investigation. The information on the extent and degree of the giant folds was often too unspecific to permit an accurate analysis of the giant fold formation. The spectrum of giant folds described in this study therefore ranges from localized to generalized giant fold formation affecting the whole of the fundus and corpus.

The period covered by the study extended from 1987 to June, 1992. Admission to the study was conditional on the removal of at least two biopsies from the corpus mucosa. In 158 patients, at least two biopsies were additionally obtained from the antral mucosa. The sex ratio of the 235 patients was 1.1 men : 1.0 women; their average age was 60.5 years.

Control patients with *H. pylori* gastritis but no giant folds

A group of 1196 patients (m : f ratio: 1.1 : 1.0; average age 51.9 years) with *H. pylori* gastritis but no giant folds or other lesions of the gastric mucosa, served as a control group. The admission criterion for this group was the removal of at least two biopsy specimens each from antrum and corpus.

Patients with giant folds receiving *H. pylori* eradication treatment

In 47 patients diagnosed as having *H. pylori* gastritis with giant fold formation, *H. pylori* eradication treatment was initiated, usually in the form of amoxicillin and omeprazole[19]. The effect of this treatment was investigated both endoscopically and histologically at least 4 weeks after conclusion of therapy. One woman in this group had suffered from giant fold gastritis with protein loss of 8 years standing, thus meeting the criteria for the diagnosis of Ménétrier's disease.

Histological methodology and grading

Histological work-up was done after prior fixation of the biopsy specimens in 4% formalin, embedding in paraffin, and staining of the sections with haematoxylin and eosin and the Warthin Starry silver stain. Helicobacter colonization and gastritis were graded in accordance with the Sydney System for the classification of gastritis[20]. The three parameters: density of *H. pylori* colonization, degree of gastritis and activity of gastritis were graded semiquantitatively and separately for the antrum and corpus, applying criteria described elsewhere[21]: 1 = minimal, 2 = low grade, 3 = medium grade, 4 = high grade.

For further evaluation, grades 1 and 2 were pooled in a 'low-grade' category and grades 3 and 4 in a 'high-grade' category. In addition, the grade and activity of gastritis were expressed in a numerical score of between 1 and 4, and a summed score of between 1 and 8.

Statistical analysis

Statistical significance was tested using the χ^2 test and the K2 field test described by Brandt and Snedekor[22].

RESULTS

Frequency of *H. pylori* colonization in cases of giant folds

Colonization with *H. pylori* was found in 219 out of 235 patients (93.2%). The relationships between the degree of colonization with *H. pylori* and the degree and activity of gastritis in the antrum and corpus are shown in Figs. 1 and 2. A statistical analysis of these data revealed a highly significant correlation between the individual variables ($p < 0.001$).

Comparison of the giant fold group and the group with *H. pylori* gastritis but no giant folds

(a) Antrum
A comparison of the degree of *H. pylori* colonization, the degree, and the activity of gastritis in the antrum, is shown in Fig. 3. The differences in the three parameters in the groups with and without giant folds are not statistically significant.

(b) Corpus
A comparison of the degree of *H. pylori* colonization, and the degree and activity of gastritis in the corpus is shown in Fig. 4. In the group with giant fold formation, all three parameters show higher grades than in the group with *H. pylori* gastritis but no giant folds. The differences are highly significant ($p < 0.001$).

(c) Comparison of the gastritis scores
A comparison of the scores for the degree and activity of gastritis in the antrum and corpus (Fig. 5) again shows that the gastritis of the corpus mucosa in patients with giant folds is significantly more severe and more active than in patients with *H. pylori* gastritis but no giant folds ($p < 0.001$).

Effect of *H. pylori* eradication treatment

In 8 out of 47 patients, treatment aimed at eradicating *H. pylori* was unsuccessful. The follow-up examinations revealed no changes in the endoscopic appearance of giant folds or in the histological parameters.

In the other 39 patients, *H. pylori* eradication therapy was successful. In two of these patients, however, giant folds nevertheless persisted. Here, follow-up biopsies revealed the cause of the condition to be a diffusely growing carcinoma. In one patient, the giant folds almost completely regressed, while in 36 patients normal endoscopic findings were found after eradication of *H. pylori*. These correlated well with the histological findings, since successful eradication treatment was associated with elimination of gastritis activity and a marked reduction in the degree of gastritis. In the patient with Ménétrier's disease, the course of which has already been described elsewhere[17], eradication of *H. pylori* resulted in healing.

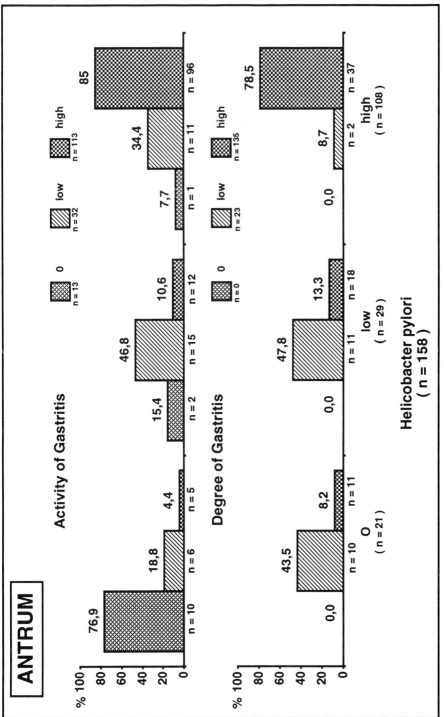

Fig. 1 Relationships between the degree of colonization with *H. pylori* and the degree and activity of gastritis in the antrum

365

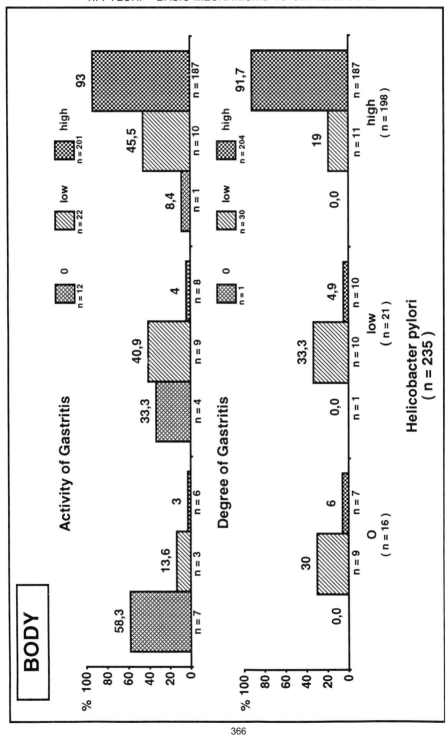

Fig. 2 Relationships between the degree of colonization with *H. pylori* and the degree and activity of gastritis in the corpus

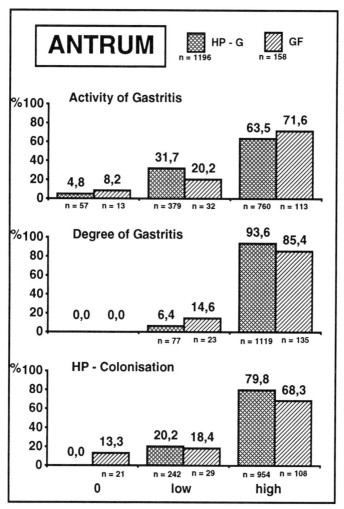

Fig. 3 Comparison of the degree of *H. pylori* (HP) colonization, the degree of gastritis, and the activity of gastritis in the antrum in patients with giant folds (GF) and in patients with *H. pylori* gastritis (HP-G) without giant folds

DISCUSSION

Our comparative analysis together with the results of *H. pylori* eradication therapy, confirm the findings of our earlier study in which we showed that the formation of giant folds in the fundic and corpus mucosa could very often be traced back to *H. pylori* infection with very severe and highly active gastritis of the oxyntic mucosa[18] – a finding to which we first drew attention in 1988[15]. The spectrum of our knowledge of the effects of *H. pylori* on the gastric mucosa can, thus, now be expanded to include this very rare variant of gastritis. Some 80 to 90% of all cases of gastritis can be attributed to an

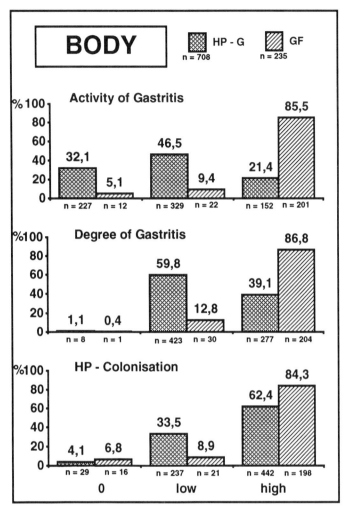

Fig. 4 Comparison of the degree of *H. pylori* (HP) colonization, the degree of gastritis, and the activity of gastritis in the corpus in patients with giant folds (GF) and in patients with *H. pylori* gastritis (HP-G) without giant folds

infection of the gastric mucosa by *H. pylori*[21,23–25]. This organism also induces the formation of mucosal-associated lymphatic tissue (MALT) in the stomach[26,27], which can form the basis for the development of a MALT lymphoma[28,29]. Other possible consequences of *H. pylori* infection are chronic erosions of the antral mucosa[30], duodenal ulcer[31,32], gastric ulcer[33], and intestinal metaplasia[15,27,34]. There is now no doubt that *H. pylori* gastritis is a precancerous condition[35–38]. The degree of colonization of gastric mucosa by *H. pylori* determines the degree and activity of gastritis[23]. Usually, *H. pylori* gastritis in the antrum is more pronounced and more

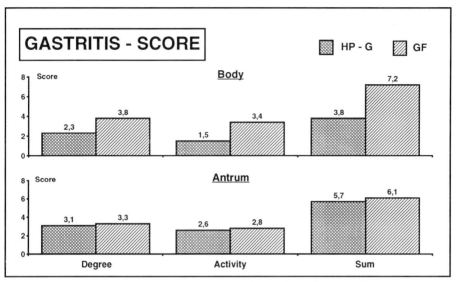

Fig. 5 Comparison of the scores for the degree and the activity of the gastritis in the antrum and body in patients with giant folds (GF) and in patients with *H. pylori* gastritis (HP-G) without giant folds

active than in the corpus, which may be due to neutralization of the ammonia produced by *H. pylori* by the acid produced by the corpus mucosa[39]. *H. pylori* giant fold gastritis is apparently the rare exception to this rule. Our comparative analysis of the cases with giant fold formation and a large group of patients with *H. pylori* gastritis with no giant folds, reveals that the inflammatory reaction in the antrum is similar in both groups. In contrast, highly significant statistical differences are found in the corpus: in patients with giant folds, the density of *H. pylori* colonization is greater than in those with *H. pylori* gastritis but no giant folds. Accordingly, the degree and the activity of gastritis in the corpus are significantly more pronounced. The 'weak point' in our study is the endoscopic appearance. In many cases, the information provided was not specific, so that accurate topographic classification and grading of the giant folds were not possible. Further prospective studies will be needed to show whether, depending on the extent of the giant folds, there may be differences in terms of the degree of *H. pylori* colonization and the degree and activity of gastritis.

Colonization by *H. pylori* in the group with giant fold formation is the determining factor in the development of the latter as shown by the results of *H. pylori* eradication therapy, which was successful in 82.9% (39 cases) of the 47 patients. In 36 of these 39 cases, the giant folds cleared up completely, and in another case almost completely, while in the two cases in which they persisted, repeat biopsy showed the underlying cause to be diffuse carcinoma. In one case, this treatment resulted in complete healing of Ménétrier's disease – as reported elsewhere[17]. So far, no plausible explanation for the rare giant fold formation in *H. pylori* gastritis has been advanced. The more dense colonization of *H. pylori* does not suffice as the sole explanation. Possibilities that need to be considered and examined are (1) whether an especially virulent strain of *H. pylori* is involved; (2) whether, as a result of reduced gastric acid secretion, buffering of ammonia is impaired resulting in aggravation of the inflammatory reaction; or (3) whether other host-related factors may be responsible for the very pronounced inflammatory reaction.

In conclusion, our studies show that

- the formation of giant folds in the oxyntic mucosa may be a rare reaction to *H. pylori* infection,
- in the individual case, Ménétrier's disease might even develop,
- giant folds and the protein loss syndrome resolve when *H. pylori* is eradicated and,
- persistence of giant folds following eradication of *H. pylori* may represent a further factor in the differential diagnosis of other causes of this condition.

References

1. Seifert E. Riesenfalten des Magens. In: Demling L (Hrsg). Klinische Gastroenterologie; 2. Aufl. Stuttgart, New York, Thieme, 1984; Bd. 1, 342–48.
2. Fenoglio-Preiser CM. Gastrointestinal pathology – an atlas and text. Raven Press, New York; 1989:162–70.
3. Wanke M. Magen. In: Doerr W, Seifert G, Uehlinger E (Hrsg). Spezielle pathologische Anatomie. Springer, Berlin, Heidelberg; 1971: Bd. 2, 273–9.
4. Whitehead R. Gastrointestinal and oesophageal pathology. Livingstone, Edinburgh, London, Melbourne, New York; 1989:421–4.
5. Stamm B, Saremaslami P. Coincidence of fundic glandular hyperplasia and carcinoma of the stomach. Cancer. 1989;63:354–9.
6. Ménétrier P. Des polyadenomes gastriques et de leurs rapports avec le cancer de l'estomach. Arch Physiol Norm Pathol. 1888;1:32–55,236–62.
7. Stamm B. Pathologie der idiopathischen hyperplastischen Gastropathie. Morbus Ménétrier. Thieme, Stuttgart, New York; 1988.
8. Palmer ED. Gastritis. A reevaluation. Medicine (Baltimore). 1954;33:199.
9. Rodgers VD, Kagnoff MF. Gastrointestinal manifestations of the acquired immunodeficiency syndrome. West J Med. 1987;146–57.
10. Stillmann AE, Sieber O, Manther U, Pinnas J. Transient protein losing enteropathy and enlarged rugae in childhood. Am J Dis Child. 1981;135:23–33.
11. Wolber RA, David A, Anderson FH, Freemann JH. Lymphocytic gastritis and giant gastric folds associated with gastrointestinal protein loss. Mod Pathol. 1991;4:13–15.
12. Choloupka JC, Gay BB, Caplan D. Campylobacter gastritis simulating Menetrier's disease by upper gastrointestinal radiography. Pediatr Radiol. 1990;20:200–1.
13. Herz R, Lombardi E, Wipping F, Stolte M. *Helicobacter pylori*-assoziierte Riesenfalten-gastritis mit gastralem Eiweissverlust (Imitation eines Morbus Ménétrier). In: Schmidt W, Ottenjann R (Hrsg). Der seltene gastroenterologische Fall. Demeter, Gräfelfing; 1991: Bd 3, 24–8.
14. Morrison S, Beverly BD, Hoffenberg R, Steven JC. Enlarged gastric folds in association with *Campylobacter pylori* gastritis. Radiology. 1989;171:819–21.
15. Stolte M, Eidt S, Ohnsmann A. *Helicobacter pylori*: Unterschiedliche Auswirkungen auf die Magenschleimhaut. In: Ottenjann R, Schmidt W (Hrsg). *Helicobacter pylori* – Konsequenzen für die Klinik und Praxis. Thieme, Stuttgart, New York; 1990:38–50.
16. Salmeron M, Desplaces N, Lavergne A, Houdart R. *Campylobacter pylori* hypertrophic erosive gastritis and hyperalbuminemia healed by cephalexin. Gastroenterol Clin Biol. 1989;13:109–10.

17. Bayerdörfer E, Ritter MM, Hatz R, Brooks W, Stolte M. Ménétrier's disease and *Helicobacter pylori*. N Engl J Med. 1993;329:60.
18. Stolte M, Bätz Ch, Eidt S. Giant fold gastritis – A special form of *Helicobacter pylori* associated gastritis. Z Gastroenterol. 1993;31:289–93.
19. Bayerdörffer E, Mannes GA, Sommer A, Höchter W, Weingart J, Hatz R, Lehn N, Ruckdeschel G, Dirschedl P, Stolte M. Long-term follow-up after eradication of *Helicobacter pylori* with a combination of omeprazole and amoxycillin. Scand J Gastroenterol. 1993;28(Suppl 196):19–25.
20. Price AB. The Sydney System: histological division. J Gastroenterol Hepatol. 1991;6:209–2.
21. Stolte M, Eidt S, Ritter M, Bethke B. *Campylobacter pylori* und Gastritis-Assoziation oder Induktion. Pathologe. 1989;10:21–6.
22. Sachs L. Angewandte Statistik. Springer, Berlin, Heidelberg, New York; 1984.
23. Stolte M, Bethke B, Ritter M, Lauer E, Eidt H. Praxis der Gastritis-Klassifikation. Endoskopie heute. 1990;4:228–30.
24. Stolte M, Heilmann KL. Neue Klassifikation und Graduierung der Gastritis. Leber Magen Darm. 1989;19:220–6.
25. Weineck G, Steininger H, Mollenkopf C. *Helicobacter pylori* and B-Gastritis: unspezifische und spezifische Abwehrmechanismen. Pathologe. 1990;11:336–41.
26. Stolte M, Eidt S. Lymphoid follicles in the antral mucosa-immun response to *Campylobacter pylori*? J Clin Pathol. 1989;42:1269–71.
27. Hauke C, Graber W, Große M, Stolte M. Zur Frage der Lymphfollikelbildung und der Entstehung der intestinalen Metaplasie in der Antrumschleimhaut als Reaktion auf eine *Helicobacter pylori*-Infektion. Leber Magen Darm. 1990;20:156–60.
28. Wotherspoon AC, Ortitz-Hidalgo C, Falzon MR, Isaacson PG. *Helicobacter pylori*-associated gastritis and primary B-cell gastric lymphoma. Lancet. 1991;338:1175–6.
29. Eidt S, Stolte M. *Helicobacter pylori* gastritis and primary gastric non-Hodgkin's lymphomas. J Clin Pathol. 1993;submitted.
30. Stolte M, Eidt S. Chronic erosions of the antral mucosa: a sequela of *Helicobacter pylori*-induced gastritis. Z Gastroenterol. 1992;30:846–50.
31. Wyatt JI, Rathbone BJ, Sobala GM, Shallcross T, Heatley RV, Axon ATR. Gastric epithelium in the duodenum: its association with *Helicobacter pylori* and inflammation. J Clin Pathol. 1990;43:981–6.
32. Axon ATR. *Helicobacter pylori* therapy: effect on peptic ulcer disease. J Gastroenterol Hepatol. 1991;6:131–7.
33. Graham DY, Lew GM, Klein PD, Evans DJ, Saeed ZA, Malty HM. Results of treatment of *Helicobacter pylori* infection on the recurrence of gastric or duodenal ulcers: A randomized single blind single center study. Gastroenterology. 1991;100:A431.
34. Eidt S, Stolte M. Antral intestinal metaplasia in *Helicobacter pylori* gastritis. Digestion. 1994;55:13–18.
35. Parsonnet J, Friedman GD, Vandersteen DP, Chang Y, Vogelman JH, Orentreich H, Sibley R. *Helicobacter pylori* infection and the risk of gastric carcinoma. N Engl J Med. 1991;325:1127–31.
36. Nomura A, Stemmermann GN, Chyou PH, Kato I, Perez-Perez GI, Blaser MJ. *Helicobacter pylori* infection and gastric carcinoma among Japanese Americans in Hawaii. N Engl J Med. 1991;325:1132–6.
37. Forman D, Jewell DG, Fullerton F, Yarnell JWG, Stacey AR, Wald N, Sitas F. Association between infection with *Helicobacter pylori* and risk of gastric cancer: evidence from a prospective investigation. Br Med J. 1991;302:1302–5.
38. Forman D and the Eurogast Group. An international association between *Helicobacter pylori* infection and gastric cancer. Lancet. 1993;341:1359–62.
39. Stolte M, Eidt S, Ohnsmann A. Difference in *Helicobacter pylori* associated gastritis in the antrum and body of the stomach. Z Gastroenterol. 1990;28:229–33.

34
Long-term consequences of *H. pylori* infection: time trends in *H. pylori* gastritis, gastric cancer and peptic ulcer disease

P. SIPPONEN and K. SEPPÄLÄ

INTRODUCTION

Peptic ulcer (PU) diseases and gastric cancer (GCA) are most important clinical outcomes of the *Helicobacter pylori* gastritis. Aetiological fraction (attributable risk) of *H. pylori* gastritis is 80–90% in PU disease and 60–70% in GCA. From this standpoint gastritis and prior *H. pylori* acquisition are important epidemiological parameters: elimination of *H. pylori* acquisition and subsequent gastritis from the population could result in a remarkable decline in morbidity and mortality to GCA and PU diseases.

The significance of *H. pylori* gastritis in PU diseases has been shown by demonstrating a reduction in recurrence rate of ulcers if the bacterium is successfully eradicated[1-3], after which the stomach will also be healed[4]. In addition, the cumulative rate of PU is shown to be extremely low in subjects with normal, non-gastritic and non-infected stomach[5,6], supporting the view that PU (after exclusion of ulcers of specific aetiology, such as those induced by NSAID or corticosteroids) appear only in patients with *H. pylori* gastritis; i.e. the ulcers are secondary outcomes of a morbid stomach.

The epidemiology of PU and GCA shows features which support the view that infectious mechanisms may play a role in the pathogenesis of these disorders[7]. The causative association of PU and GCA with *H. pylori* gastritis assumes, however, that the epidemiology of *H. pylori* gastritis should show features similar to those of PU and GCA. Otherwise, these assumptions of causality between *H. pylori* gastritis and GCA or PU diseases are incorrect, and the relations could be epiphenomena at most. In this respect, for instance, a marked decrease in the incidence of GCA in most Western countries would imply that *H. pylori* gastritis should also have decreased in prevalence. Correspondingly, this could also be anticipated to be the case in PU disease.

Table 1 Change in incidence of gastric carcinoma in Finland in a period of 15 years. Data from Finnish Cancer Registry[10]

Age group (years)	Incidence of gastric cancer per million		
	1970–74	1985–89	Change (%)
Males			
35–39	50	33	−34
45–49	172	119	−31
55–59	640	465	−27
65–69	1639	1090	−33
75–79	2711	2251	−17
85–	5017	3355	−33
Total	274	189	−31
Females			
35–39	45	35	−34
45–49	107	105	−2
55–59	249	221	−11
65–69	700	493	−30
75–79	1360	1167	−14
85–	3432	1974	−42
Total	140	104	−26

Reliable registry-based data on GCA incidence, and our knowledge of occurrence of gastritis in various populations and in different time periods, give some possibilities to test the hypothesis of an epidemiological relationship between *H. pylori* gastritis and GCA. Such studies on gastritis and PU diseases are, however, more problematic, or even impossible, mainly because of lack of reliable data on epidemiology and time trends of PU diseases in the populations.

In this review we briefly describe some recent observations on time trends of gastritis in consecutive hospital-based series of endoscopized patients, and we try to give some answers to the question of whether the epidemiological features of *H. pylori* gastritis fit with those of GCA. Some comments and suggestions are also given regarding PU diseases.

TIME TRENDS IN GASTRIC CANCER

The incidence of GCA has declined markedly in many Western countries in recent years[8-12]. In this respect the epidemiology of GCA has been very dissimilar to that of many other forms of malignant tumour: the decline in GCA incidence has been an unplanned triumph without any explanation or reasons[8].

The decrease has been particularly great in Finland, where the incidence of GCA has dropped by 60–70% in the past three or four decades[10,12]. Earlier Finland was among the countries with a typically high incidence, but now it is among those of moderate incidence at most.

Interestingly, although GCA incidence is exponentially related to age (Table 1), the decrease of GCA incidence has been roughly of the same magnitude in percentage in all age groups, in different time periods (reliable registry data exist since the early 1950s), but possibly slightly greater in males than in females[10]. Correspondingly, the mean and median ages of GCA patients have risen slightly with time. All these trends have been surprisingly coherent over the years. Similar conclusions on time trends and other epidemiological features of GCA, as seen in Finland, also seem to be valid relating to those in other countries[8,9].

The decrease of GCA incidence, which is independent of age or time period (or of gender), indicates some important conclusions on the relationship of GCA to gastritis and its atrophic sequelae.

First, the decline in incidence must relate to all histological GCA types – not only some of the subgroups of GCA tumour. The GCA of intestinal (IGCA) and diffuse (DGCA) subtypes have earlier been seen to represent different epidemiological entities[13–16]. Correspondingly, it has been thought that IGCA, but not DGCA, has decreased in incidence with time, or that the major differences in GCA incidence between different countries are due to a dissimilar epidemiology of IGCA and DGCA tumours[13–15]. This cannot be the case, however. If only IGCA had decreased with time an age-independent decline in total GCA incidence would be impossible – simply because of the dissimilar age distribution of IGCA and DGCA tumours in the population[12,16].

Secondly, GCA incidence has decreased most extensively in populations and countries which now are developed, whereas the incidence remains high in those that are still developing[8,11]. Some exceptions to this rule exist, however. For unknown reasons GCA incidence is high, e.g. in Japan, which can hardly be considered a developing country[9,17].

Thirdly, the main aetiological factor in the genesis of GCA must be environmental[18]; furthermore, this factor (or factors) must be extremely common in nature, otherwise the decline in GCA incidence would not be so rapid and worldwide as is the case. In addition, a uniform decline in GCA incidence cannot be easily explained by changes in some exotic habits that are related, for instance, to eating and drinking, etc. Habits of such 'exotic' nature are usually local, and often deal with a limited number and specific age groups of people.

The above conclusions very much favour the view that gastritis and earlier *H. pylori* acquisition could be the missing environmental factor in the worldwide pathogenesis of GCA: the background features in *H. pylori* gastritis and GCA seem to be very similar indeed[18]. It is easily understood that rapid changes in epidemiology of a globally common bacterial infection result also in changes in the epidemiology of related disorders, such as gastritis or atrophic gastritis (and intestinal metaplasia), and subsequently in the occurrence of GCA or PU diseases. Correspondingly, these changes could be globally uniform.

TIME TRENDS IN GASTRITIS

Recent studies from Finland indicate that the prevalence of chronic gastritis has markedly decreased in the past 15 years (from 1977 to 1992)[19]. This

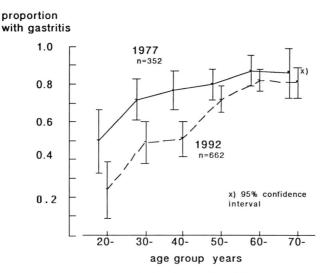

Fig. 1   Decrease of proportion of males with chronic gastritis in different age groups in Finland from 1977 to 1992. Consecutive series of outpatients in Jorvi Hospital (Espoo, Finland). The vertical lines indicate 95% confidence intervals of the proportions

seems to be the case in both non-atrophic and atrophic gastritis, in both sexes, and in all age groups, as is the case with the decrease of GCA incidence.

The decrease has been surprisingly great and corresponds in extent to the decrease in GCA incidence. From 1977 to 1992 the prevalence of chronic gastritis (including cases of both chronic non-atrophic and atrophic gastritis) has dropped by 18% on average, and by 38% in young age groups (the prevalence has decreased from 66% to 41% in the age group 20–49 years)[19]. The proportions of gastritis in six age groups in consecutive male outpatients in Jorvi Hospital in 1977 and 1992 are shown in Fig. 1.

Figures on the age-specific proportion of gastritis suggest that the occurrence of gastritis in the population is a cohort phenomenon; i.e. the population consists of birth cohorts with dissimilar, 'specific' prevalence of gastritis[19]. Patients having the same prevalence of gastritis in 1977 and 1992 are approximately 15–20 years older in 1992 than in 1977. Further, by estimating the prevalences of gastritis for defined birth cohorts, it appears that the prevalence of gastritis has remained practically unchanged in the same birth cohorts over the period of 15 years (data on males: see Table 2). Thus, it seems that the prevalence of gastritis has stayed at a high stable level in the elderly, but at a low stable level in younger generations during the period of 15 years. In people born in 1948–57 (both sexes included), the prevalence was 48% in 1977 (the people were 20–29 years old at that time) and 43% in the same cohort in 1992. The corresponding figures were 79% and 76% in the birth cohort born in 1918–27, respectively[19].

Considering that chronic gastritis is infectious (*H. pylori*) in origin in a great majority of cases, it is likely that the decrease in prevalence of gastritis is a result of a decline in *H. pylori* acquisitions with time, and, correspondingly,

Table 2 Prevalence of gastritis in males in different birth cohorts in 1977 and 1992. Total number of cases is in parentheses. Data from consecutive series of outpatients endoscopized in Jorvi Hospital, Espoo, Finland[19]

Cohort born	Prevalence (%) of chronic gastritis	
	1977	1992
1918–27	80 ($n = 86$)	82 ($n = 101$)
1928–37	77 ($n = 75$)	77 ($n = 167$)
1938–47	72 ($n = 67$)	62 ($n = 173$)
1948–57	50 ($n = 34$)	50 ($n = 114$)

that the cohort phenomenon of the gastritis is based on acquisition of people particularly at a young age. Regarding time trends, new acquisitions must have been more infrequent in children and young adults in recent decades than before. Correspondingly, it seems that a persisting ('old') infection has remained relatively common in generations that are old now, and in which the infection rate in childhood has obviously been very high.

The above conclusions suggest that the rate and risk of *H. pylori* gastritis has been dissimilar in childhood in different generations with time, and that these rates have gradually decreased. This 'cohort-specific rate' of *H. pylori* gastritis seems to be an important epidemiological parameter that determines the prevalence of gastritis in the population at large. It seems likely that the people are infected mainly in childhood or adolescence, after which new infections are rare[20]. Being a chronic disease with a low likelihood of healing spontaneously[21–23], the *H. pylori* infection and subsequent gastritis, if obtained in childhood, may remain stable in prevalence in the cohort for decades (or for the rest of the subject's life).

Based on observations in serology, the epidemiology of *H. pylori* infection has been emphasized to be a cohort effect in recent studies of Parsonnet *et al.*[24] and Banatvala *et al.*[25]; these observations being in line with the present histological results and views of the cohort effect of chronic gastritis. These are, in addition, in concordance with other earlier serological studies which suggest that the socioeconomic conditions, especially in childhood, are factors that determine the prevalence of *H. pylori* gastritis in the population. Poor environmental hygiene in households, absence of fixed hot-water supply, and dense housing in childhood are some of the factors that seem to favour a high rate of acquisition, and predict *H. pylori* seropositivity in adulthood[26–29]. Direct follow-up studies also support these views. Seroconversion seems to be a rather rare event in adulthood[29], suggesting that the rate of new *H. pylori* infections, and the risk of contracting gastritis subsequently, is obviously lower above the age of 20 years than we have believed so far.

TIME TRENDS IN GASTRITIS AND GASTRIC CANCER – HOW DO THEY FIT?

The observations on epidemiology and time trends of chronic gastritis are in good concordance with those of GCA. The epidemiological features are very much alike. By looking at the time trends of GCA and gastritis in

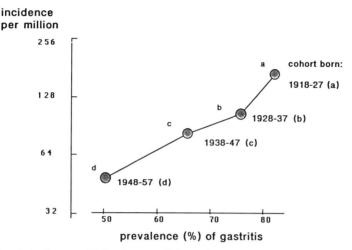

Fig. 2 Correlation between 'birth cohort-specific' prevalence rate of gastritis and incidence of gastric cancer (cancer at age of 35–44 years). The prevalence rate of gastritis indicates the mean of the prevalence of gastritis in the cohort in 1977, 1985 and 1992 (see Table 2). Different birth cohorts are indicated by symbols *a–d*. Data from Finnish Cancer Registry[10] and from ref. 19

generations born after the Second World War, the decrease of prevalence of gastritis has been up to 38% in 15 years (Fig. 1), thereby corresponding well with the mean decrease (Table 2) of GCA incidence by 26–31% in a period of 15 years[10,12].

The available data of prevalences of gastritis at two or three time points[19] give the possibility of extrapolating the 'specific' prevalence of gastritis for different birth cohorts of people in the population. Correlation of these 'cohort-specific' prevalence rates of gastritis to incidence of GCA gives interesting results. The cohort-specific prevalence of gastritis correlates positively with the log of incidence of GCA at a fixed age (Fig. 2). Thus, an increase or decrease in prevalence of gastritis will respectively increase or decrease the incidence of GCA in the cohort exponentially (logarithmically). The data (Fig. 2) further indicate that the time is also exponentially related to incidence of GCA; i.e. when the age of the cohort rises, the risk of GCA increases exponentially in those with gastritis (Fig. 3).

PEPTIC ULCER DISEASES

The above-described features in epidemiology and time trends should also occur in the relationship between PU diseases and *H. pylori* gastritis. No unbiased registry-based data are, unfortunately, available on time trends of PU diseases, either in Finland or other countries. However, the PU diseases are claimed to have decreased in prevalence with time, even before the time of fibreoptic endoscopy or usage of H_2 receptor antagonists. In the USA and Europe, for example, the incidence of elective surgery for PU disease is

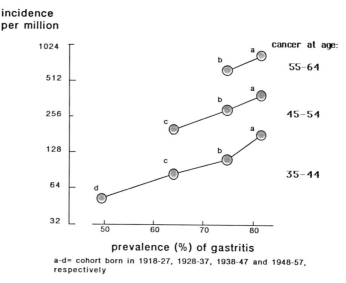

Fig. 3 Correlation between birth cohort-specific prevalence rate of gastritis and the incidence of gastric cancer (cancer at age of 55–64 years, 45–54 years or 35–44 years). The prevalence rate of gastritis indicates the mean of the prevalence of gastritis in the birth cohort in 1977, 1985 and 1992 (see Table 2). Different birth cohorts are indicated by symbols *a–d*, and correspond to those in Fig. 2. Data from Finnish Cancer Registry[10] and from ref. 19

reported to have declined by 30–40% between 1956 and 1976[31–34], and further thereafter. This decrease, if proven to be true and unbiased, corresponds to the decline of GCA incidence, and parallels the decrease in prevalence of gastritis.

ATROPHIC GASTRITIS

Recent observations in outpatients from Jorvi Hospital indicate that the prevalence of atrophic gastritis has also decreased in the past 15 years in a similar way to non-atrophic gastritis, or to gastritis in general[19]. This is a logical result if we take into account the natural history of chronic gastritis[7]. Atrophic gastritis (and intestinal metaplasia) appears with time (years, decades) in a proportion of patients with non-atrophic *H. pylori* gastritis. This development is obviously multifactorial in nature[7,23], but results gradually in a loss of normal mucosal glands (atrophy), and in the appearance of metaplasia (intestinal and pseudopyloric metaplasia) in antrum, corpus, or both. A high rate of *H. pylori* infection in childhood, and a subsequent high prevalence of gastritis in the population (cohort) on average, would correspondingly indicate a high prevalence rate of atrophic gastritis and metaplasia. On the other hand, a decrease of these rates would result in a decrease in prevalence of atrophic gastritis (and intestinal metaplasia) in the specific birth cohort of people, as the case seems to be.

378

SUMMARY

Peptic ulcer (PU) and gastric cancer (GCA) are most important outcomes of the *H. pylori*-positive chronic gastritis. Assumption of causative relation of *H. pylori* gastritis to PU or GCA implies that the epidemiology and time trends of these diseases should be alike. Recent observations indicate that this could be the case, regarding at least the association of *H. pylori* gastritis to GCA. The incidence of GCA has declined in Finland by 26–31% in the past 15 years, as has the age-specific prevalence of gastritis. The prevalence of gastritis has decreased most in young people (20–49 years), among whom the prevalence has dropped by 38% (from 66% to 41%) from 1977 to 1992. The observations on time trends indicate, furthermore, that the occurrence of gastritis and GCA are cohort phenomena in the population; i.e. there are differences in prevalences of gastritis and GCA between different birth cohorts, the prevalences are higher in people born at the beginning of the century and lower in those born after the Second World War. Regarding gastritis it seems, in addition, that the people in the cohort are infected by *H. pylori*, and have contracted gastritis consequently, at a young age (< 20 years), after which the prevalence of gastritis seems to remain unchanged in the cohort.

Unfortunately, reliable data for comparison of epidemiology and time trends between *H. pylori* gastritis and PU diseases do not exist. It has been assumed, however, that the incidence rate of PU diseases has declined with time and could also thereby parallel the time trends of *H. pylori* gastritis.

References

1. Rauws EAJ, Tytgat GNJ. Cure of duodenal ulcer associated with eradication of *Helicobacter pylori*. Lancet. 1990;335:1233–5.
2. Graham DY, Lew GM, Klein PD, Evans DJ Jr, Saeed ZA, Malaty HM. Effect of treatment of *Helicobacter pylori* infection on the long-term recurrence of gastric and duodenal ulcer. A randomized controlled study. Ann Intern Med. 1992;116:705–8.
3. Seppälä K, Färkkilä M, Nuutinen H *et al.* Triple therapy of *Helicobacter pylori* infection in peptic ulcer. A 12-month follow-up study of 93 patients. Scand J Gastroenterol. 1992;27:973–6.
4. Valle J, Seppälä K, Sipponen P, Kosunen T. Disappearance of gastritis after eradication of *Helicobacter pylori*: a morphometric study. Scand J Gastroenterol. 1991;26:1057–65.
5. Sipponen P, Varis K, Fräki O, Korri U-M, Seppälä K, Siurala M. Cumulative 10-year risk of symptomatic duodenal and gastric ulcer in patients with or without chronic gastritis. Scand J Gastroenterol. 1990;25:966–73.
6. Sipponen P, Seppälä K, Äärynen M, Helske T, Kettunen P. Chronic gastritis and gastroduodenal ulcer: a case control study on risk of coexisting duodenal or gastric ulcer in patients with gastritis. Gut. 1989;30:922–9.
7. Sipponen P, Kekki M, Siurala M. The Sydney System: epidemiology and natural history of chronic gastritis. J Gastroenterol Hepatol. 1991;6:244–51.
8. Howson CP, Hiyama T, Wynder EL. The decline in gastric cancer: epidemiology of an unplanned triumph. Epidemiol Rev. 1986;8:1–27.
9. Muir C, Waterhouse J, Mack T *et al.* Cancer incidence in five continents, Vol. V. Lyon: IARC; 1987.
10. Pukkala E, Rimpelä A, Läärä E. Cancer in Finland. Cancer Society in Finland publication No. 36. Helsinki; 1987.

11. Coggon D, Acheson ED. The geography of cancer of the stomach. Br Med Bull. 1984;40: 335–41.
12. Sipponen P, Järvi O, Kekki M, Siurala M. Decreased incidence of intestinal and diffuse types of gastric carcinoma in Finland during a 20-year period. Scand J Gastroenterol. 1987;22:865–71.
13. Munoz N, Asvall J. Time trends of intestinal and diffuse types of gastric cancer in Norway. Int J Cancer. 1971;6:144–57.
14. Munoz N, Correa P, Cuello C, Duque E. Histologic types of gastric carcinoma in high- and low-risk areas. Int J Cancer. 1968;3:809–18.
15. Correa P. Clinical implications of recent developments in gastric cancer pathology and epidemiology. Semin Oncol. 1985;12:2–10.
16. Siurala M, Varis K, Sipponen P. Carcinogenesis in the foregut. Part 2. Gastric carcinoma. In: Baron JH, Moody FG, editors. Foregut. London: Butterworths; 1981:276–312.
17. Hiroyama T. The epidemiology of gastric cancer in Japan. In: Pfeiffer CJ, editor. Gastric cancer. New York: Gerhard Witztrock; 1979:60–82.
18. Sipponen P. *Helicobacter pylori* infection – a common worldwide environmental risk factor of gastric cancer? Endoscopy. 1992;24:424–7.
19. Sipponen P, Helske T, Järvinen P, Hyvärinen H, Seppälä K. Decrease in prevalence of chronic gastritis in a period of 15 years: analysis of outpatient series in Finland in 1977, 1985, 1992. Gut. 1994:in press.
20. Mitchell HM, Li YY, Hu PJ et al. Epidemiology of *Helicobacter pylori* in southern China: identification of early childhood as a critical period of acquisition. J Infect Dis. 1992;166:149–53.
21. Siurala M, Sipponen P, Kekki M. Chronic gastritis: dynamic and clinical aspects. Scand J Gastroenterol. 1985;20(Suppl. 109):69–76.
22. Ihamäki T, Kekki M, Sipponen P, Siurala M. The sequelae and course of chronic gastritis during a 30–40-year bioptic follow-up study. Scand J Gastroenterol. 1985;20:485–91.
23. Correa P. Chronic gastritis. In: Whitehead R, editor. Gastrointestinal and oesophageal pathology. London: Churchill Livingstone; 1989:402–20.
24. Parsonnet J, Blaser MJ, Perez-Perez GI, Hargett B, Tauxe RV. Symptoms and risk factors of *Helicobacter pylori* infection in a cohort of epidemiologists. Gastroenterology. 1992;102:41–6.
25. Banatvala N, Mayo K, Megraud F, Jennings R, Decks JJ, Feldman RA. The cohort effect and *Helicobacter pylori*. J Dig Dis. 1993;168:219–21.
26. Mendall MA, Goggin PM, Molineaux N et al. Childhood living conditions and *Helicobacter pylori* seropositivity in adult life. Lancet. 1992;339:896–7.
27. Jones DM, Eldridge J, Whorwell PJ. Antibodies to *Campylobacter pyloridis* in household contacts of infected people. BMJ. 1987;294:615.
28. Drumm B, Perez-Perez G, Blaser MJ, Sherman PM. Intrafamilial clustering of *Helicobacter pylori* infection. N Engl J Med. 1990;322:359–63.
29. Hazell SL, Mitchell HM, Hu PJ et al. Gastric cancer – is childhood acquisition of *H. pylori* the key? Ir J Med. 1992;161:22.
30. Kuipers EJ, Pena AS, Hamp van G, Roosendaal R, Meuwissen SGM. Seroconversion for *Helicobacter pylori*; an 11 year follow-up study. VI Int Workshop on gastroduodenal pathology and *Helicobacter pylori*. 23–25 September 1993; Brussels.
31. Gustavsson S, Nyren O. Time trends in peptic ulcer surgery, 1956 to 1986. A nation-wide survey in Sweden. Ann Surg. 1989;210:704–9.
32. Sonnenberg A. Changes in physician visits for gastric and duodenal ulcer in the United States during 1958–1984 as shown by National Disease and Therapeutic Index (NDTI). Dig Dis Sci. 1987;32:1–7.
33. Bloom BS. Cross-sectional changes in the effects of peptic ulcer disease. Ann Intern Med. 1991;114:558–62.
34. Kurata JH. Ulcer epidemiology: an overview and proposed research framework. Gastroenterology. 1989;96:569–80.

35
Determinants of gastritis phenotype in *H. pylori* infection

P. CORREA, D. ZAVALA, E. FONTHAM, B. RUIZ,
T. RAMAKRISHNAN, F. T. GARCIA, T. COLLAZOS and H. RAMIREZ

INTRODUCTION

There seems to be general agreement in assigning a major role to *Helicobacter pylori* in the causation of chronic gastritis. However, the definition and nomenclature of the types of chronic gastritis are controversial issues. Most pathologists agree that there are two main types, namely non-atrophic and atrophic. For the purposes of this chapter atrophy is equivalent to gland loss, a purely histopathological parameter. In the populations providing the material for this report, the types of non-atrophic gastritis are predominantly either superficial gastritis (SG) or diffuse antral gastritis (DAG), while all of the atrophic gastritis cases belong to the multifocal atrophic gastritis (MAG) previously described[1].

Epidemiological methodology can be used to explore the determinants of the different types of gastritis, but only a few studies are available addressing this issue. One of the major difficulties encountered in carrying out this type of study has to do with the scarcity of subjects with documented normal gastric histology. Such subjects are needed to represent the baseline of epidemiological parameters to be compared with subjects with abnormal gastric histology.

We have conducted two separate case–control studies addressing the issue under discussion. One study was carried out in the gastroenterology service of the University Hospital in Cali, Colombia. In that group of patients the prevalence of gastritis is so high that there were not enough subjects with normal gastric histology, and therefore the only comparison possible is that of patients without atrophy vs patients with atrophy. The other study was conducted in New Orleans Charity Hospital, whose clientele is predominantly black and of low socioeconomic strata. In such populations it is also difficult to find gastric biopsies with normal histology, but enough were accumulated to establish a comparison group of individuals with normal gastric histology. The results presented below should be considered as separate studies, in different populations, addressing similar issues. Although direct comparisons require cautious interpretation, any similarity in the results favours the notion that the effect is generalizable.

MATERIALS AND METHODS

Colombian study

The investigation in Cali dealt with patients attending the gastroenterology clinic of the University Hospital, primarily of middle and low socioeconomic strata, seeking services for gastrointestinal symptoms from December 1990 to December 1991. Eligible patients were between 15 and 75 years of age who were not taking antibiotics or bismuth compounds and were scheduled for gastroscopy because of gastrointestinal symptoms. All patients gave written informed consent and the study was approved by the Institutional Review Board. Before gastroscopy, an experienced social worker administered a questionnaire with information on demographic characteristics (e.g. current residential address, place of birth, marital status), hygienic conditions at home, tobacco and alcohol use and diet. Current residence was used to classify into high, medium or low socioeconomic strata utilizing standards set previously by surveys conducted by the municipality.

A urine sample was taken before gastroscopy to measure sodium and creatinine concentrations and calculate sodium/creatinine ratios as a surrogate measure of salt ingestion.

The patients were examined after an overnight fast. A minimum of four biopsies were taken: three antral (lesser and greater curves and posterior wall) and one corpus biopsy from the posterior wall. Each biopsy was placed in a separate container, fixed in 10% buffered formalin, embedded in paraffin and stained with haematoxylin and eosin. Two experienced pathologists (H.R. and B.R.) interpreted the biopsies independently and made a global diagnosis, as well as a detailed evaluation of histopathological parameters of acute and chronic inflammation, atrophy, metaplasia and other lesions. *H. pylori* was evaluated by means of the Giemsa and the modified Steiner silver stain[2].

The dietary questionnaire was developed following a format similar to the Block (NCI) questionnaire, enquiring about specific food items and usual portion size. A total of 73 food items of specific relevance to the Cali population as determined by previous surveys constituted the foods in the food-frequency list. Two questions related to salt consumption were asked: preference for salty foods and adding salt to the food on the table. Recent dietary changes were recorded. Three dietary exposure variables were created based on the frequency and usual size of consumption of: (a) all fruits and vegetables; (b) fruits and vegetables rich in vitamin C, and (c) fruits and vegetables rich in carotenoids.

The Student's test and the Wilcoxon's rank test were used to compare means or medians[3]. Odds ratios and 95% confidence intervals were calculated for the parameters of interest. In all comparisons cases were defined as having the diagnosis of MAG; and controls were subjects with normal histology, SG or DAG.

New Orleans study

All patients scheduled for gastroscopy at Charity Hospital between January 1991 and July 1993, between 18 and 70 years of age, mentally alert, English-speaking, not previously treated at the clinic, were eligible for the study. They were predominantly black, female and of low socioeconomic strata. All participants gave written consent. The study was approved by the Institutional Review Board. Two hundred and eighty (86% of those eligible) agreed to participate. All patients were interviewed prior to gastroscopy by experienced personnel. The interview included the 60-item version of the Block (NCL) questionnaire. This semi-quantitative food-frequency instrument was used to estimate the average daily food and nutrient intake[4]. Nutrient composition values are derived from NHANES II as population use-weighted median values. Salt intake was self-reported as light, moderate or heavy. In addition to the dietary and lifestyle questions the Social Readjustment Scale (SRRS) of Holmes and Rahe was used to quantify stressful life events[5].

Prior to gastroscopy a urine specimen was obtained to determine sodium and creatinine concentrations. Patients were examined after an overnight fast. Four antral biopsies were obtained: one from the lesser curvature was used to perform a rapid urease test[6] and another one for Gram's stain. Two additional antral biopsies taken from the area of the incisura angularis and the greater curvature, as well as a biopsy from the corpus (mid-portion of the anterior wall) were fixed in buffered 10% formalin, paraffin-embedded and stained with haematoxylin-eosin, PAS-Alcian blue and the modified Steiner technique. The histopathological interpretation was as described for the Colombian study. Odds ratios and the chi-square statistics were used to estimate the association between risk factors and histopathological diagnosis.

RESULTS

Colombian study

A total of 221 patients were available for analysis: 90 cases of MAG (cases) and 131 controls who on histological examination had no evidence of atrophy (eight normal, 46 SG, and 73 DAG). Odds ratios and 95% confidence intervals are shown in Table 1. Ten per cent of the patients were negative for *H. pylori*. The mean age for the cases was 49.1 years, compared to 37.1 for the controls. Seventy-one per cent of the subjects were females, with no significant differences between cases and controls. The cases had fewer years of education than the controls. There were no significant differences in current residence (equivalent to census tracts) between cases and controls, indicating no gross differences in socioeconomic stratification as far as place of residence was concerned. There were, however, other parameters indicating lower socioeconomic status of the cases: 84% of them reported availability of

Table 1   Estimated relative risk of atrophic gastritis in Cali, Colombia

Factors	Crude OR (95% CI)	Adjusted[a] OR (95% CI)
Age	4.17 (2.26, 7.74)	3.50 (1.76, 6.97)
Education	4.17 (2.26, 7.74)	2.88 (1.47, 5.64)
Sewerage service	8.0 (2.12, 44.47)	17.26 (3.87, 76.91)
Smoking	2.23 (1.18, 4.24)	2.34 (1.15, 4.77)
Fresh fruits and vegetables[b]	0.79 (0.44, 1.39)	0.47 (0.24, 0.91)

OR = Odds ratio, CI = confidence interval
[a]Each factor adjusted for all others: age (39 years old or younger vs >39 years old), education (≥ 6 years of formal education vs <6), sewage service (yes vs no), smoking (never vs ever)
[b]High in pro-vitamin A

residential sewage service, compared to 98% of the controls.

Questions on smoking status revealed that the group of current smokers and ex-smokers had an increased risk of atrophic gastritis when compared to non-smokers. The results indicate a tendency for smoking to increase the risk of atrophic gastritis, and they also suggest that the effects of smoking persist over time. No significant differences between cases and controls in the use of salt were observed, as evaluated by preference for salty foods, adding salt at the table or sodium/creatinine ratios in the urine.

Crude analysis of the dietary questionnaire showed a protective effect of total fruits and vegetables. After adjusting for other relevant factors, as shown in Table 1, a significant protective effect was associated with items with a high content of pro-vitamin A carotenoids.

New Orleans study

Table 2 shows the age-adjusted odds ratios for the patients with different histological diagnoses. Ten cases with superficial biopsies insufficient for diagnosis and four cases of superficial gastritis are not included in these tabulations. Increasing age results in a non-statistically significant decrease in risk of DAG (which requires absence of atrophy in its histological diagnosis) and in a significant increase of risk of MAG. In this clinic population blacks have a significantly higher risk of both types of gastritis than whites. Gender has no apparent effect on risk of gastritis. Smoking increases the risk with borderline significance for DAG and significance for MAG. Alcohol use has no significant effect for either type of gastritis. Stress has no effect on MAG but increases the risk of DAG, although the result is not statistically significant. Subjects who classify themselves as 'light' consumers of salt appear to have a decreased risk of both types of gastritis, but the results are not statistically significant. The sodium to creatinine ratio did not differ significantly by histological diagnosis.

Further analysis of the aetiological factors specifically related to atrophic changes in New Orleans is ongoing. Preliminary results suggest that frequent consumption of fresh fruits and vegetables reduces the risk of atrophy by approximately one-half. Contrary to the Cali results, the protection in New Orleans is more clearly linked to vitamin C than to vitamin A.

Table 2   Estimated relative risk (OR) of diffuse antral gastritis (DAG) and multifocal atrophic gastritis (MAG) in New Orleans

Factors	Controls n	DAG		MAG	
		n	OR (95% CI)[a]	n	OR (95% CI)[a]
Age (years)					
<30	5	7	1.0	9	1.0
30–45	17	12	0.5 (0.1, 1.9)	70	2.3 (0.6, 7.0)
45+	13	10	0.5 (0.1, 2.2)	108	4.6 (1.3, 15.0)
Race					
White	14	3	1.0	32	1.0
Black	21	26	6.2 (1.5, 25.2)	155	2.9 (1.3, 6.3)
Smoking status					
Non-smokers	26	15	1.0	103	1.0
Current smokers	9	4	2.6 (0.9, 7.5)	84	2.8 (1.2, 6.6)
Stress					
<199	12	7	1.0	73	1.0
200+	23	22	1.5 (0.5, 4.7)	114	0.9 (0.6, 1.9)
Salt intake					
Light	29	18	1.0	135	1.0
Moderate/heavy	6	11	2.8 (0.8–9.3)	52	2.1 (0.8, 5.5)
Vitamin A					
Q1	4	7	1.0	51	1.0
Q2–Q3	25	11	0.3 (0.1, 1.2)	89	0.2 (0.1, 0.7)
Q4	6	11	1.3 (0.2, 7.3)	47	0.4 (0.1, 1.7)
Vitamin C					
Q1	5	6	1.0	52	1.0
Q2–Q3	16	14	0.7 (0.2, 2.9)	88	0.5 (0.2, 1.4)
Q4	14	9	0.6 (0.1, 2.5)	47	0.3 (0.1, 0.8)*
Vitamin E					
Q1	6	8	1.0	48	1.0
Q2–Q3	20	10	0.7 (0.1, 1.2)	92	0.2 (0.1, 0.7)
Q4	9	11	1.3 (0.2, 7.3)	47	0.4 (0.1, 1.7)
Carotenoids					
Q1	6	7	1.0	48	1.0
Q2–Q3	20	13	0.6 (0.1, 1.4)	97	0.5 (0.2, 1.5)
Q4	9	9	0.9 (0.2, 3.6)	42	0.7 (0.2, 2.3)

[a]Odds ratio (OR) for all factors (except age) are age-adjusted, with 95% confidence intervals (CI)
[b]Q1–Q4: Quartiles of consumption with Q1 representing the lowest level of intake and Q4 the highest
*p for trend <0.05

In the New Orleans study *Helicobacter* infection is positively associated with atrophic changes in the mucosa.

DISCUSSION

A decade after the introduction of *H. pylori* in the modern medical literature[7], a consensus has been reached that this bacterium is the major cause of chronic active gastritis[8]. Most pathologists and gastroenterologists recognize the fact that there are several phenotypic variants of chronic gastritis. In affluent populations of Europe, the United States and Oceania, where the risk of gastric cancer is low, the type of gastritis has a predominantly antral localization and is not usually accompanied by gland loss (atrophy). In the case series reported in this chapter, such cases have been classified as diffuse antral gastritis (DAG). In populations with high gastric cancer risk the predominant type of chronic gastritis is characterized by gland loss (atrophy) following a multifocal pattern involving antrum and corpus. This type of gastritis is frequently accompanied by intestinal metaplasia, and for the purposes of this chapter is called multifocal atrophic gastritis (MAG). In the Sydney system these variants would correspond to 'antral predominant' and 'pangastritis', respectively[9].

H. pylori plays a major role in both DAG and MAG. There is also agreement that causation of chronic gastritis is multifactorial, and it is therefore important to explore the aetiological factors that determine which of the two main types of gastritis will be observed in patients with *H. pylori* infection.

There is also a strong possibility that in some subjects these two types of gastritis are sequential in nature, namely that DAG will be transformed into MAG with time. This is supported by the fact that most cases of gastritis in children are predominantly antral and non-atrophic[10,11]. In our studies, patients with MAG were about 10 years older than those with non-atrophic gastritis. If a transition from DAG to MAG is postulated, that step does not seem to be of an obligatory nature. This is supported by reports that *H. pylori* infection is very prevalent in populations at low gastric cancer risk. This is the case in the coast of Costa Rica, in Africa and in Japan (Okinawa)[11–14]. In other areas of Costa Rica and Japan, with high gastric cancer risk, MAG and *H. pylori* infection are very prevalent[11,13,15,16].

Although previous epidemiological studies have implicated excessive salt intake in the aetiology of gastric cancer[17,18] the present results do not provide support for its role in chronic gastritis. Previous studies, in the Nariño region of Colombia, have shown that the excessive intake measured in terms of sodium:creatinine ratios is associated with atrophic gastritis, which is much more prevalent than in Cali[19]. The sodium:creatinine ratio in Nariño was 2.10, compared to 1.06 for Cali. There is therefore other evidence of an effect of excessive salt intake as a determinant of atrophic gastritis.

A protective role of fresh fruits and vegetables in chronic atrophic gastritis has been reported in Colombia, New Orleans and Japan[13,20,21]. The protection linked to these items has always been stronger than individual indexes of vitamin C, carotenoids or tocopherols. The main sources of antioxidant micronutrients in human nutrition are fresh fruits and vegetables. Other substances in these food items may participate in the protective role, but not enough information on them is available at the present time.

In the Cali population foods rich in carotenoids have a statistically significant protective role against atrophic gastritis. In the New Orleans population it is vitamin C which appears to convey the protective effect. The diets of these two populations are very different. In Colombia the supply of vitamin C is abundant, but that of carotenoids is not[22]. In Louisiana the supply of vitamin C is less than optimal[21]. These observations lend support to the notion that the important protection against gastritis may come from the antioxidants as a group, with international variations as to the relevant specific items.

Smoking has been considered a factor in chronic gastritis, and its role in both non-atrophic and atrophic gastritis is supported by the present report. Emotional stress has been mentioned as a factor in gastritis. Our results suggest that it may play a role in DAG but not in MAG, but the results are not statistically significant and the difficulties in evaluating this factor are generally recognized.

Our preliminary results in the New Orleans study indicate a strong role of *H. pylori* infection in the causation of atrophy. This could not be evaluated in the Colombian study because approximately 90% of the patients were infected. In both populations (Cali and New Orleans) the subjects studied were from lower socioeconomic strata, a homogeneity that hinders the evaluation of *H. pylori* and other factors associated with lower socioeconomic status.

In conclusion, our study in Colombia points to a protective role of fresh fruits and vegetables in atrophic gastritis, more marked for vitamin A precursors. Additionally, a modest positive association with smoking is reported.

In New Orelans the protective role of fresh fruits and vegetables is also observed, but more clearly seen for their vitamin C content. Smoking is also found as a factor, especially related to atrophic gastritis. Emotional stress is suggested as a factor only for non-atrophic types of gastritis, but this finding needs further evaluation.

Other factors are involved in determining gastritis in general and atrophy in particular. We have previously reported genetic susceptibility to atrophic gastritis by segregation analysis in Nariño, Colombia. An autosomal recessive gene of high prevalence in the community may be modulated by environmental factors[24].

Bile reflux has also been postulated as a factor determining atrophy[25,26]. The determinants of bile reflux are poorly understood.

Dietary factors not yet identified by the currently available epidemiological studies may also be involved. They could be toxicants or irritants of the gastric mucosa or they may act as protective substances.

Finally, the characteristics of the *H. pylori* infection may vary considerably. The density of colonization could be greater in patients with atrophy. The presence of vacuolating cytotoxins has been identified as a determinant of tissue injury[27]. The associated gene, cag A, appears to play a role in tissue injury, and it could be postulated that strains with prominent expression of this gene are determinant forces in the outcome of gastritis phenotypes[28].

SUMMARY

Factors that may be involved in the causation of non-atrophic and atrophic gastritis were investigated in two independent epidemiological case–control studies. One study carried out in the city of Cali, Colombia, shows a protective role for frequent consumption of fresh fruits and vegetables, especially those rich in carotenoids. For the other study, carried out in New Orleans, Louisiana, only preliminary results are available. They also show a protective effect of fresh fruits and vegetables, especially those rich in vitamin C. Smoking increased the risk of gastritis in both studies.

Acknowledgements

This work was supported by NIH grant no. P01-CA-28842 from the National Cancer Institute.

References

1. Correa P. Chronic gastritis: a clinico-pathological classification. Am J Gastroenterol. 1988;83:504–9.
2. Garvey W, Fathi A, Bigelow F. Modified Steiner for the demonstration of spirochetes. J Histotechnol. 1985;8:15–17.
3. Armitage PB. Methods in medical research. Oxford: Blackwell Scientific Publications; 1980:394–407.
4. Block G, Harman AM, Naughton D. A reduced dietary questionnaire: Development and validation. Epidemiology. 1990;1:58–64.
5. Holmes TH, Rahe RH. The social readjustment rating scale. J Psychosom Res. 1967;11: 213–18.
6. Ruiz B, Janney A, Diavolitsis S, Correa P. One-minute test for *Campylobacter pylori*. Am J Gastroenterol. 1989;84:202.
7. Marshall BJ, Warren JR. Unidentified curved bacilli in the stomach of patients with gastritis and peptic ulceration. Lancet. 1984;1:1311–15.
8. Blaser MJ. Hypothesis on the pathogenesis and natural history of *Helicobacter pylori*-induced inflammation. Gastroenterology. 1992;102:720–7.
9. Price AB. The Sydney system: histologic division. J Gastroenterol Hepatol. 1991;6:209–22.
10. Czin SJ, Carr HS, Speck WT. Diagnosis of gastritis caused by *Helicobacter pylori* in children by means of ELISA. Rev Infect Dis. 1991;13(Suppl. 18):700–3.
11. Sierra R, Muñoz N, Peña AS *et al*. Antibodies to *Helicobacter pylori* and pepsinogen levels in children from Costa Rica: comparison of two areas with different risk for stomach cancer. Cancer Epid Biomarkers Prev. 1992;1:449–54.
12. Megraud F. Epidemiology of *Helicobacter pylori* infection. Gaastroenterol Clin N Am. 1993;22:73–88.
13. Kabuto M, Imai H, Gey F *et al*. *Helicobacter pylori*, dietary factors and atrophic gastritis in Japanese populations with different gastric cancer mortality. Cancer Causes Control. 1993;4:297–305.
14. Shousa S, El Sherif AM, El Guneid A, Arnaout AH, Murray-Lyon IM. *Helicobacter pylori* and intestinal metaplasia: comparison between British and Yemeni patient. Am J Gastroenterol. 1993;88:1373–6.
15. Fukao A, Hisamichi S, Ohato N, Fumino N, Endo N, Iha M. Correlation between the prevalence of gastritis and gastric cancer in Japan. Cancer Causes Control. 1993;4:17–20.
16. Salas J. Metaplasia intestinal de la mucosa gastrica. Patología (Mexico). 1971;9:127–42.
17. Joossen J, Geboers J. Nutrition and gastric cancer. Nutr Cancer. 1981;2:250–61.
18. Correa P. Human gastric carcinogenesis: a multistep and multifactorial process. First American Cancer Society Award Lecture on Cancer Epidemiology and Prevention. Cancer Res. 1992;52:6735–40.
19. Chen VW, Abu-Elyazeed R, Zavala D *et al*. Risk factors of gastric precancerous lesions in a high-risk Colombian population. I. Salt. Nutr Cancer. 1990;13:59–65.
20. Nomura A, Yamakawa H, Ishidate T. Intestinal metaplasia in Japan: association with diet.

J Natl Cancer Inst. 1982;68:401–5.

21. Fontham E, Zavala D, Correa P *et al.* Diet and chronic atrophic gastritis: a case–control study. J Natl Cancer Inst. 1986;76:621–7.
22. Correa P, Cuello C, Fajardo LF, Haenszel W, Bolaños O, Ramirez B. Diet and gastric cancer. Nutrition survey in a high risk area. J Natl Cancer Inst. 1983;70:673–8.
23. Block G. Vitamin C and gastric prevention: the epidemiologic evidence. Am J Clin Nutr. 1991;53(Suppl.):270S–80S.
24. Bonney Ce, Elston RC, Correa P *et al.* Genetic etiology of gastric carcinoma. I. Chronic gastritis. Genet Epidemiol. 1986;3:213–24.
25. Miller LJ, Malagelada JR, Longstreth GF, Go VL. Dysfunctions of the stomach with gastric ulceration. Dig Dis Sci. 1980;25:857–64.
26. Ortiz P, Calvo C. Concentración de ácidos biliares en pacientes con distinta capacidad secretora de acido. Anales Medicos (Chile). 19899;26:59–62.
27. Fox JG, Correa P, Taylor NS *et al.* High prevalence and persistence of cytotoxic positive *Helicobacter pylori* strains in a population with high prevalence of atrophic gastritis. Am J Gastroenterol. 1992;87:1554–60.
28. Crabtree JE, Taylor JD, Wyatt JI *et al.* Mucosal recognition of *Helicobacter pylori* 120 kDa protein, peptic ulceration and gastric pathology. Lancet. 1991;338:332–5.

36
The ulcer-associated cell lineage (UACL); a newly recognized pathway of gastrointestinal differentiation of importance in the natural healing of peptic ulcer disease

N. A. WRIGHT

INTRODUCTION

For many years pathologists have remarked on the emergence, in chronic intestinal ulcers in the human gut, of tubular structures containing mucin-producing cells which are quite dissimilar from the indigenous cell lineages[1–4]. These complex structures are confined to the lamina propria, usually close to the ulcer margins, and the contained cells produce neutral mucin staining positively with the diastase periodic acid Schiff (D/PAS) method, unlike the acid mucin-producing, alcianophilic intestinal goblet cells[4]; they were usually explained away as 'pyloric' or 'pseudopyloric' metaplasia[1,2], or even as 'Brunner's gland' metaplasia because of morphological similarities with these cells[1], and the suggestion was made that the production of these cells in some way 'protected' the mucosa. But Kawel and Tesluk[1] were quick to point out that, until the function of these cells was established, it would be fruitless to speculate on their nature.

Recent morphological, immunohistochemical and *in situ* hybridization studies have shown that, far from being an inert metaplasia, these cells do in fact have novel functional properties: they have a definable life history during which they sequentially acquire differentiation antigens constituting a distinct phenotype, and synthesize and secrete large amounts of regulatory peptides of considerable interest; the presence of these cells in the ulcerated mucosa also appears to induce peptide gene expression in the local intestinal cells. They also develop their own proliferative organization[4–8]. For these reasons we propose that these cells, while differentiation progeny of intestinal stem cells, constitute a cell lineage in their own right: the 'ulcer-associated cell lineage' (UACL).

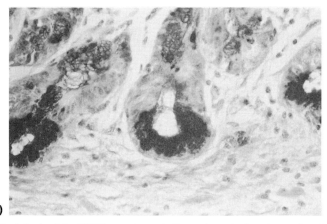

(a)

Fig. 1 (a) Early buds of the UACL growing out of parent crypts close to an ulcerated area of the mucosa in Crohn's disease. Note the abrupt origin of the UACL cells, from the stem cell zone, and the absence of mitotic activity in the UACL cells; (b) a more developed acinar complex, growing as a newly formed gland in the lamina propria; (c) a mature UACL complex, showing the acinar area, the duct, and the UACL cells clothing the surface of a villus, displacing the indigenous cell lineages; note the single goblet cell in the duct region; (d) the 'pore' by which the duct emerges onto the mucosal surface; (e) a higher-power view of the surface cells on the villus. All sections are stained with the Alcian blue/diastase PAS method

THE ORIGINS AND LIFE HISTORY OF THE UACL

The UACL has so far been found only in conditions which cause chronic intestinal ulceration, or indeed ulcerative disease in endodermal derivatives such as the pancreas, biliary system and salivary glands. It appears first as a small, intensely D/PAS-positive bud at the base of the intestinal crypts adjacent to the ulcer (Fig. 1a). These buds push outwards into the surrounding stroma of the lamina propria as small tubules, which quickly coalesce with tubules from other crypts to form a more or less complex acinar arrangement (Fig. 1b). They also lie within a distinctive, immature, acid mucopolysaccharide-rich stroma. It is interesting to note that, at this stage, the buds and acini are devoid of mitotic figures, or indeed of proliferative activity as assessed by Ki67[4] or proliferating cell nuclear antigen (PCNA)[5] staining. In larger gland formations a single duct is formed by the joining of two or more smaller ductules, and this duct grows upwards through the core of an adjacent villus towards the epithelial surface (Fig. 1c). At the epithelial surface the duct emerges through a distinct pore (Fig. 1d). While secretions can readily be seen within the tubules and the duct system, and emerging onto the surface in histological sections (Fig. 1c), the UACL itself also moves out of the tubule and onto the villous surface, where it replaces the indigenous surface cell lineages (Fig. 1e). The entire villous surface can thus become covered with the UACL cells.

While most commonly seen in the small intestine, particularly in duodenal ulcer disease, the UACL also appears in the colon, although by no means as commonly, but is also readily seen in peptic ulcer disease in the stomach.

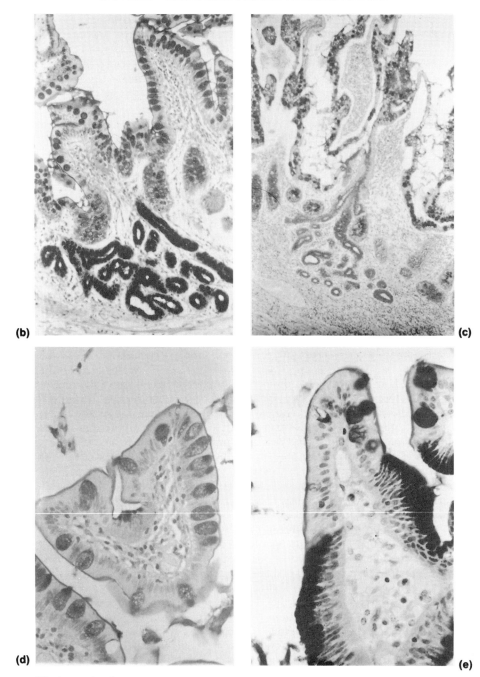

(b)

(c)

(d)

(e)

Fig. 1 *continued*

Nor is the UACL confined to the luminal gastrointestinal tract; its presence has been detected in pancreatic ducts in chronic pancreatitis, frequently in the gall bladder in chronic cholecystitis, and even in the Fallopian tube in chronic salpingitis and in inflammatory nasal polyps[9]. It could therefore be that the UACL is a newly defined pathway of *endodermal* differentiation, induced in response to chronic inflammation in mucosal surfaces.

THE MORPHOGENESIS AND PROLIFERATIVE ORGANIZATION OF THE UACL

It is singular that mitotic figures, and indeed cycling cells as indicated by Ki67 or PCNA staining, are not found in the buds or acini of the UACL (Fig. 2a). Since the tubules clearly bifurcate, it is interesting to speculate how this occurs in the absence of cell division. However, once the duct is formed then the UACL develops its own proliferative architecture: about two-thirds of the way up the duct a clearly defined zone of PCNA-positive cells appears (Fig. 2b), in which mitotic figures can also sometimes be seen. This zone is quite discrete, and ends well before the duct emerges onto the surface. This pattern, with the proliferative compartment towards the top of the duct, is similar to that found in the gastric glands in the antral part of the stomach. However, this mode of histogenesis is not unique. It is not generally appreciated that Brunner's gland primordia begin as small buds which grow out of the duodenal crypts at about 16 weeks of intrauterine life in the human, grow as tubules in the submucosa, and by 36 weeks achieve the familiar adult tubuloalveolar pattern[6]. But in the adult Brunner's gland there is no defined proliferative organization in contrast to the UACL. It thus appears as if the UACL reiterates the histogenetic programme of the Brunner's glands, but then develops the proliferative organization of gastric gland tubules[6].

The life history of the UACL is complex: certainly, in the absence of cell division, the buds and early tubules appear to be direct differentiation progeny of the stem cells from the parent crypts and migrate downwards into the evolving tubule, whose structure may be dictated by the newly formed mesenchyme. This proposal is supported by the presence, within the UACL tubules and even the duct, of other stem cell derivatives – Paneth, goblet and neuroendocrine cells (Fig. 1c). This concept of downward migration in the intestinal crypt is not novel – the stem cell zone hypothesis of Bjerknes and Cheng[10] states that beneath cell position 5 in the crypt, cells which are destined to differentiate into all lineages migrate downwards into the base of the crypt, and that the only cells which divide in this zone are the crypt stem cells. In the case of the UACL, once differentiation to this pathway is triggered, most stem cell production destined for downward migration is directed into the UACL with, however, an admixture of other intestinal cell lineages.

Once the duct is formed, however, a defined proliferative zone develops. In the paradigm of the gastric gland, cells born in the isthmus–neck region migrate upwards to renew the foveolar and surface mucous cells, and

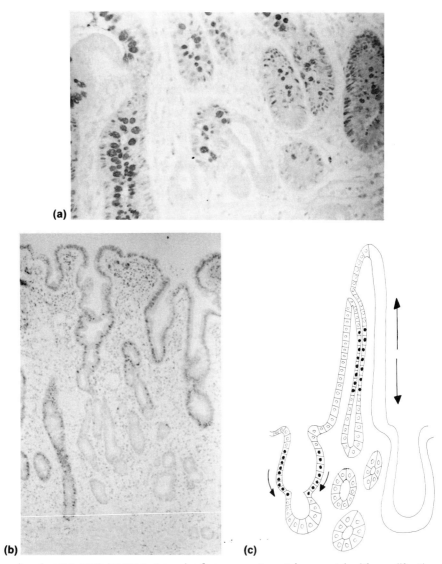

Fig. 2 (a) A newly formed bud growing from a parent crypt, immunostained for proliferating cell nuclear antigen to show proliferating cells. While the parent crypt contains many cycling cells, the bud is devoid of staining; (b) a mature UACL complex, showing the proliferative zone staining positively for PCNA in the duct; (c) a diagrammatic representation of the proliferative zone in the duct of the UACL, with the possible pathways of migration indicated

downwards to replace the parietal and chief cell populations, i.e. there is a bidirectional flux of cells. If this were to happen in the UACL, then the proliferative zone would take over replacement of the entire UACL, producing the surface cells and also cells to migrate downwards to expand the acinar cell population (Fig. 2c). If this is the case, how the proliferative zone interrelates with the parent crypts is obscure, but is likely to be complex.

GENE EXPRESSION IN THE UACL

Genes related to differentiation

The UACL itself is a differentiating cell lineage: that is to say, cells express different proteins depending on their position within the UACL. All parts of the UACL secrete neutral mucin, which is intensely D/PAS-positive. However, the pattern of immunostaining with monoclonal antibodies which recognize different but overlapping epitopes in the polymorphic epithelial mucin core protein varies; thus the acinar cells show membrane staining only with HMFG1, while the surface cells express membrane and cytoplasmic staining with HMFG2[4]. The positivity with these antibodies indicates that the UACL shows aberrant expression of the MUC1 gene, which is not constitutively expressed in the intestine. Moreover, the surface cells stain intensely with *Lens culinaris* lectin (which recognizes binding sites for α-mannose, α-galactose and N-acetylgalactosamine, in that order of preference), while the acinar cells are negative[4]. The surface cells also stain with PR3B10, a monoclonal antibody which recognizes a 150 kDa glycoprotein related to carcinoembryonic antigen, but the acinar cells are negative[4].

Regulatory peptide gene expression in the UACL

The UACL also expresses different secretory proteins; again there is a very distinctive pattern of synthesis within the organized structure. The acinar portion contains abundant immunoreactive epidermal growth factor/uro-gastrone (EGF/URO), which is also seen in the secretions[4]. It is significant that EGF/URO should be produced locally around ulcers in the intestine, for several reasons. EGF/URO is a very potent stimulator of cell proliferation in the rodent and human gastrointestinal mucosa[11,12], and also modulates intestinal epithelial cell differentiation[13]. In normal conditions EGF/URO is produced by gut-associated salivary and Brunner's glands, but not by other cell lineages in the gut[14]. The location of EGF/URO receptors (EGFR) in gastrointestinal cells is currently under dispute: there is evidence that EGFR in the gut are polarized to the laterobasal membranes in the rat[15], but Thompson et al.[16] have shown apically sited EGFR in the neonate; however, these EGF receptors in the microvillar membrane are apparently not associated with phosphorylation of membrane proteins after ligand : receptor binding[17]. Radiolabelled EGF/URO given orally to normal rats does not bind to the intact mucosa, but readily binds locally when a mucosal defect is present[9]; moreover, EGF/URO has been reported to be mitogenically active parenterally, but not when given directly into the intestine[18], although this too has been disputed[19]. Whatever the exact binding mechanism, the secretion of EGF/URO by the UACL ensures that the peptide is available locally to stimulate repair and regeneration in the local ulcer environment, and we have suggested that this is an important *in vivo* role for EGF/URO[4].

Other regulatory peptide genes are also expressed by the UACL in a site-specific manner. Human spasmolytic polypeptide (hSP) and pS2 mRNA expression can be readily demonstrated by hybridization *in situ* using ^{35}S-labelled riboprobes: hSP mRNA is found in the acini and lower duct cells, whereas pS2 mRNA and protein are localized in large amounts in the upper duct and all surface cells (Figs 3a,b,c). hSP and pS2 are members of the trefoil peptide family, a growing group of proteins which share the unique 'trefoil' motif, a three-leafed domain held by disulphide bonds based on cysteine residues[20]. The canonical molecule is pS2, a 60 amino acid secretory protein which was originally found by differentially screening a cDNA library from the human breast carcinoma cell line MCF-7[21]. The function of pS2 is as yet unknown, but it is highly homologous with spasmolytic polypeptide (SP), a known gastrointestinal regulatory peptide, in which the trefoil domain is tandemly repeated[22]. Porcine spasmolytic polypeptide inhibits gastric acid secretion and also intestinal motility[23,24] and is mitogenic for MCF-7 and colorectal carcinoma cells *in vitro*[25], and ligand : receptor binding results in inhibition of adenylate cyclase[23]. In normal stomach, pS2 and hSP are secreted and are co-expressed by the foveolar and surface cells[26], although they are products of different genes[27]. Moreover, hSP is expressed in large amounts in the pyloric glands of the gastric antrum and in Brunner's gland acini. In the UACL, however, expression of these genes is evidently defined by position in the UACL. Moreover, it has recently been shown that the UACL expresses a third member of the trefoil peptide family, intestinal trefoil factor (ITF), a single trefoil domain peptide[17], constitutively expressed by intestinal goblet cell, but not by gastric mucous cells[28]. ITF is expressed throughout the UACL; addition of recombinant rat ITF to the basolateral surface of rat small intestine results in an increase in short-circuit current, associated with increased chloride secretion (H. Cox, in preparation) and binding sites have been demonstrated on the surface of the rat small intestinal mucosa[28]. Thus the UACL secretes at least four peptides with potentially important biological effects. A further protein of significance is produced by the UACL: lysozyme, which has antibacterial and putative immunoregulatory function, is also secreted. Both lysozyme mRNA and protein are found in abundance in the UACL[9].

In addition, it is becoming clear that the UACL is also associated with trefoil peptide gene expression in the indigenous cell lineages in the adjacent mucosa[8]. The normal cell lineages in the intestine include the mucin-producing goblet cells, neuroendocrine cells and enterocytes; the mucous cells in the vicinity of the UACL express abundant immunoreactive pS2 in the basal parts of the cytoplasm in formalin-fixed paraffin-embedded sections (Fig. 4a). In glutaraldehyde-fixed, resin-embedded sections, in addition to labelling in the Golgi area, pS2 is seen within the theca also (Fig. 4b). *In situ* hybridization with an ^{35}S-labelled antisense riboprobe shows pS2 mRNA localized in considerable concentration in the cytoplasm beneath the mucus-filled theca (Fig. 4c). Ultrastructural immunocytochemistry confirms that immunoreactive pS2 is found in the RER of these cells, and is also co-packaged via the Golgi into the mucous granules (Figs 4d and 4e). Thus the

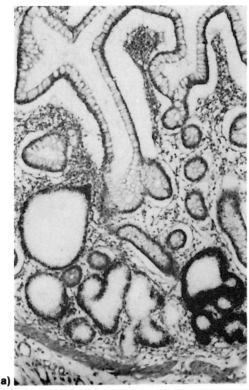

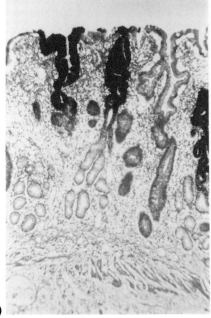

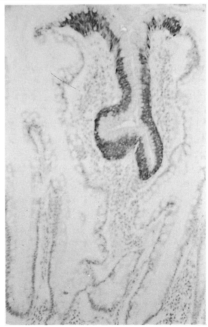

mucous cells adjacent to peptic ulcers where the UACL is seen show pS2 expression, and also co-secrete pS2 with the liberated mucus into the intestinal lumen.

These observations cast some light on the possible function of pS2, and also indicate a new functional role for intestinal mucous cells: they indicate that pS2 is co-secreted with mucin into the viscoelastic layer which covers the intestinal epithelium. That pS2 is induced in goblet cells only in disease states[8] suggests that pS2 has a role in cytoprotection or regeneration; this hypothesis is reinforced by the constitutive secretion of pS2 by the foveolar and surface cells of the gastric mucosa, where of course cytoprotection is a constant need[26]. There is also indirect evidence that the association of trefoil peptides and mucus is not merely coincidental, since the *Xenopus* mucin gene product has trefoil sequences on either side of the protein[29].

Hitherto, intestinal goblet cells were regarded solely as a source of mucin. It is now clear that they are a major source of trefoil peptides if conditions are appropriate. It appears that pS2 is processed and packaged by the Golgi apparatus: the mucous granules are also processed here, and the two secretory products are packaged together. pS2 is in fact not the only trefoil peptide expressed in the goblet cell theca: Suemori *et al.*[30] have demonstrated intestinal trefoil factor (ITF) in the theca of normal rat goblet cells; ITF mRNA has been localized to small and large intestinal goblet cells in the rat[28], and the human homologue is also found in small intestinal and colonic goblet cells[29]. It thus appears as if intestinal goblet cells are a rich source of potentially active regulatory peptides, especially in damaged tissues.

In addition, neuroendocrine cells adjacent to the UACL also express pS2 protein; Fig. 5a shows typically shaped pyramidal neuroendocrine cells stained with an antibody against chromagranin A. Figure 5b shows morphologically defined endocrine cells which stain positively with pS2. Figure 5c shows neuroendocrine cells stained with the immunogold method for pS2 at the ultrastructural level, while Fig. 5d shows that neuroendocrine granules contain abundant immunoreactive pS2. The finding of the same peptide co-packaged in both mucous granules and neuroendocrine granules is highly unusual: mucous granules are secreted into the lumen, whereas neuroendocrine granules are released into the basal and lateral membranes. The functions of these granules are of course very different. Mucus has lubricating and protective functions in the gut, but endocrine secretions release various regulatory peptides which act via paracrine or autocrine mechanisms to produce manifold effects on the gut[31]. Thus pS2 may be involved in the secretory mechanism itself, or may be presented to receptors on both apical and basolateral membranes. However, it is as yet unclear where the cells responsive to pS2 lie in the ulcerated environment.

But why should the mere presence of the UACL induce trefoil peptide gene expression in the mucous and endocrine cells? It is well known that

Fig. 3 Opposite: (a) Location of hSP mRNA in the acini and lower duct of the UACL, using an ^{35}S-labelled riboprobe for hSP; (b) pS2 mRNA in the upper duct and surface UACL cells; (c) the UACL immunostained for pS2 protein, confirming its synthesis

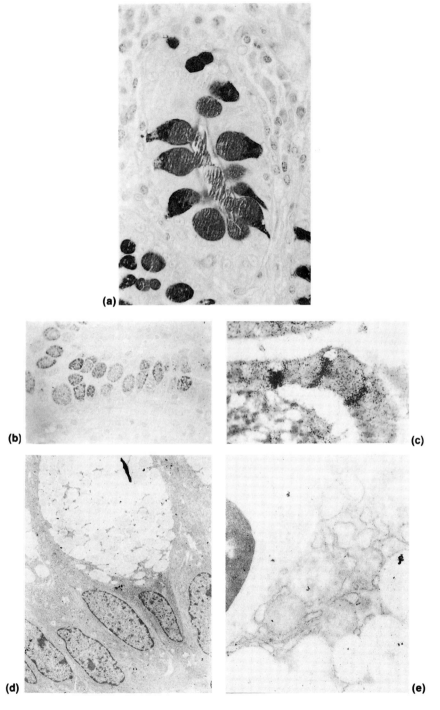

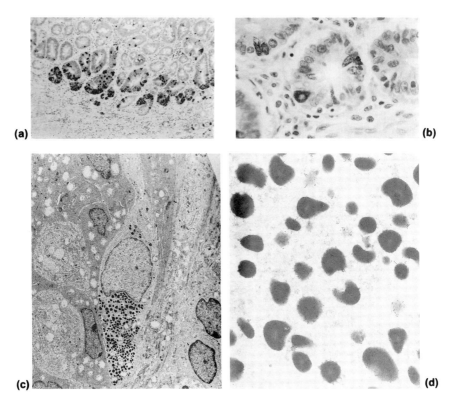

Fig. 5 (**a**) Neuroendocrine cells around the UACL, immunostained for chromogranin A (pancreastatin); (**b**) typical pyramid-shaped neuroendocrine cells immunostained with pS2; (**c**) neuroendocrine cells immunostained for pS2 using the immunogold method at the ultrastructural level; (**d**) showing that the neurosecretory granules contain pS2 protein

EGFR are readily detectable in gut epithelial cells; indeed, immunoreactive EGFR are present on the *apical surface* of the epithelial cells in the small intestine in Crohn's disease[8]. The 5′ upstream sequences of the pS2 gene contain a complex enhancer sequence, responsive, *inter alia*, and most powerfully, to EGF/URO[32]. Thus the EGF/URO secreted locally by the UACL could induce pS2 expression in the adjacent mucosa. But why the enterocytes do not express pS2, when they do bear EGFR, is not explained by this hypothesis. In this respect it is possible that there is a mechanism controlling phosphorylation which is overriden in the chronically inflamed environment, which might explain the presence of non-functional EGF

Fig. 4 Opposite: (**a**) pS2 protein localized in the subnuclear Golgi of goblet cells adjacent to the UACL; (**b**) in thin sections, embedded in methacrylate, pS2 protein can be seen co-packaged in the mucous granules; (**c**) pS2 mRNA can also be seen in the goblet cells beneath the mucin-filled theca; (**d**) a goblet cell immunostained at the ultrastructural level for pS2; (**e**) a higher-power view showing pS2 protein in the Golgi stacks

receptors on the enterocytes[17].

The pattern of peptide expression in the UACL also points to its histogenesis: Brunner's gland primordia begin as bud-like outgrowths from the bases of duodenal crypts, which form tubules which, by 28 weeks of intrauterine life, show the familiar tubuloalveolar pattern of the adult Brunner's glands. At 18 weeks immunoreactive EGF/URO is present in abundance, while pS2 peptide *is confined to the developing ducts.* However, hSP mRNA is present in considerable concentration throughout Brunner's gland acini and ducts. This pattern of trefoil gene expression is maintained throughout fetal life, and moreover, in the adult, pS2 peptide and transcripts are expressed by the ductal cells, and large amounts of hSP protein and mRNA are present in the acini[6,9]. These observations indicate that the UACL reiterates the developmental programme of Brunner's glands; however, it then acquires the proliferative organization of gastric gland tubules (see above).

THE NATURE OF THE UACL

The UACL shows several features which are novel for differentiating gastrointestinal cell lineages. It appears as direct differentiation progeny of crypt stem cells; it appears in response to injury, growing to form new glandular formations which make their own communication with the surface of the mucosa; in histogenesis it appears to follow the differentiation programme of Brunner's glands primorida; it develops a proliferative organization very similar to that of the gastric gland; the UACL shows regional differences in phenotype and function; it also shows a unique pattern of regulatory peptide gene expression, producing EGF/URO and the two trefoil peptides pS2 and hSP, again produced in specific parts of the UACL, and finally the presence of the UACL modifies the behaviour of the indigenous cell lineages in the vicinity – goblet cells actively synthesize and secrete pS2, while neuroendocrine cell granules also contain co-packaged pS2.

These observations indicate that the UACL is not a metaplasia, which formally can be defined as a change from one defined differentiated phenotype to another. The UACL, though sharing several phenotypic features with other cell lineages in the gut, does have a unique structure and function, and we are therefore justified in considering it a new pathway of gastrointestinal differentiation. Since it is induced only in chronic inflammatory and ulcerative conditions, it would certainly appear to be a primary defence reaction, producing a cocktail of active peptides and proteins, EGF/URO, hSP, pS2 and lysozyme, which would be expected to advance mucosal healing. There are also early indications that other peptides may be produced by the UACL and immunoreactive TGF-α has been detected, for instance[5].

CONCLUSIONS

The morphological organization and function of the UACL is now being worked out, and its phenotype more fully defined. But the above observations raise as many questions as they answer. What is the stimulus for the induction of the UACL? Possibly mesenchymal induction, since profound myofibroblast proliferation – cells usually confined to the pericryptal myofibroblast sheath – is seen around the early UACL buds. Stem cell differentiation certainly seems to be switched on directly, and wholly into the UACL pathway (Fig. 1a). How does growth of the bud continue in the absence of cell division? If cells are being directed downwards from the crypt stem cell compartment, then how does the tubule divide, in the absence of cell division, if not by mesenchymal direction, analogous to the situation in the developing salivary gland and lung? After the morphogenesis of the new gland and duct, the new proliferative compartment develops. What, then, are the migration pathways of the cells emerging from the new compartment, and what is the relationship between the new proliferative compartment and the parent crypts?

There also seems to be a very rigid positional organization of peptide gene expression, with cells changing expression as they migrate through the lineage. The abundance of message and protein for the trefoil peptides hSP and pS2, and the induction of pS2 in surrounding cells, possibly by the EGF/URO secreted by the UACL, indicates an important role for these molecules, possibly in mucosal defence. The discovery of their function in humans then becomes important in respect of novel therapeutic strategies for peptic ulcer disease.

The emergence of mucin-secreting cells in damaged mucosa has become topically very important, because of the ability of *H. pylori* to colonize cells of a foveolar–isthmus mucin-secreting phenotype. In duodenitis, cells of this phenotype are seen clothing the duodenal villi, and are often referred to as 'gastric metaplasia'. Far from being a metaplasia, it has been convincingly shown that 'gastric metaplastic' cells are in fact an overgrowth of Brunner's gland duct epithelium[34]; however, they do show trefoil peptide gene expression, but differ from that of the UACL. In this respect 'gastric metaplasia' resembles antral mucosa, in that the epithelium expresses both the pS2 and the hSP genes in the same cells[35].

To be teleological for a moment, we could speculate that, in acid-induced duodenal damage, Brunner's gland ducts undergo hyperplasia, leading to cells capable of secreting gastric-type mucin and gastric trefoil peptides; these help resist the damaging insult. However, there is a price to pay: *H. pylori* colonization. Why *H. pylori* has this predilection to colonize cells of this phenotype is a problem for the future.

SUMMARY

The main pathways of epithelial differentiation in the intestine, Paneth, mucous, endocrine and columnar cell lineages are well recognized; however, in abnormal circumstances, for example in mucosal ulceration, a cell lineage with features distinct from these emerges, which has often been dismissed in the past as 'pyloric' metaplasia, because of its morphological resemblance to pyloric mucosa in the stomach. However, this review concludes that this cell lineage has a defined phenotype unique within gastrointestinal epithelia, has a histogenesis which resembles that of embryonic Brunner's glands, but acquires a proliferative organization similar to that of the gastric gland. It expresses several peptides of considerable interest, including epidermal growth factor, three trefoil peptides – pS2, human spasmolytic polypeptide and intestinal trefoil factor – and also secretes lysozyme. The presence of the lineage also appears to cause altered gene expression in adjacent indigenous cell lineages. It is proposed that this cell lineage is induced in gastrointestinal stem cells as a result of mucosal ulceration, and plays an important role in ulcer healing. The name 'ulcer-associated cell lineage' is consequently coined, and should be added to the repertoire of intestinal stem cells.

Acknowledgements

I should like to thank Dennis Ahnen, Mark Carr, Pierre Chambon, Rebecca Chinery, George Elia, Paul Freemont, Andrew Hanby, Werner Hoffman, Rosemary Jeffrey, El-Nasir Lalani, Janet Longcroft, Bill Otto, Kirtika Patel, Christine Pike, Mary-Christine Rio, Richard Poulsom, Len Rogers, Catherine Sarraf and Gordon Stamp for contributions, theoretical and practical, towards making this review possible.

References

1. Kawel CA, Tesluk H. Brunner-type glands in regional enteritis. Gastroenterology. 1955;28:210–21.
2. Lee F. Pyloric metaplasia in the small intestine. J Pathol Bacteriol. 1964;87:257–79.
3. Liber AF. Aberrant pyloric glands in regional ileitis. Arch Pathol (Chicago). 1951;51: 205–19.
4. Wright NA, Pike C, Elia G. Induction of a novel epidermal growth factor-secreting cell lineage by mucosal ulceration in gastrointestinal stem cells. Nature. 1990;343:82–5.
5. Ahnen D, Gullick W, Wright NA. Expression of multiple growth factors by the ulcer-associated cell lineage in Crohn's disease. Gastroenterology. 1991;100:A512.
6. Ahnen DJ, Poulsom R, Stamp GWH et al. The ulceration associated cell lineage (UACL) reiterates the Brunner's gland differentiation program but acquires the proliferative organisation of the gastric gland. J Pathol. (submitted.)
7. Wright NA, Elia G, Pike C. Ulceration induces a novel epidermal growth factor-secreting cell lineage in the human gastrointestinal mucosa. Digestion. 1990;46(Suppl.2):125–33.
8. Wright NA, Poulsom R, Stamp GWH et al. Trefoil peptide gene expression in gastrointestinal epithelial cells in inflammatory bowel disease. Gastroenterology. 1993;104:12–20.
9. Wright NA, Poulsom R, Stamp GWH et al. Epidermal growth factor (EGF/URO) induces expression of regulatory peptides in damaged human gastrointestinal tissues. J Pathol. 1990;162:279–84.
10. Bjerknes R, Cheng H. The stem cell zone of the small intestinal epithelium. III. Evidence from columnar, enteroendocrine and mucous cells in the adult male mouse. Am J Anat. 1981;160:93–104.
11. Goodlad RA, Raja KP, Peters TJ, Wright NA. Effects of urogastrone/epidermal growth factor on intestinal brush border enzymes and mitotic activity. Gut. 1991;32:994–8.
12. Walker-Smith J, Phillips AD, Walford N et al. Intravenous epidermal growth factor increases small intestinal cell proliferation in congenital microvillous atrophy. Lancet. 1985;2:1239–40.
13. Goodlad R, Wilson G, Lenton W, Gregory H, McCullough K, Wright NA. Intravenous but not intragastric urogastrone/EGF is trophic to the intestine of parenterally-fed rats.

Gut. 1987;78:573–82.

14. Heitz P, Kasper M, Van Noorden S, Polak JM, Gregory H, Pearse AGE. Immunohistochemical localisation of urogastrone to human duodenal and submandibular glands. Gut. 1978;19:408–13.

15. Scheving LA, Shuirka RA, Nguyen TD, Gray GM. Epidermal growth factor receptor in the intestinal enterocyte. Localisation to laterobasal but not brush border membranes. J Biol Chem. 1989;264:1735–41.

16. Thompson JF. Specific receptors for epidermal growth factor on rat intestinal microvillus membranes. Am J Physiol. 1988;254:429–35.

17. Kelly D, Mcfadyen M, Morgan C, King TP. Growth factors in colostrum: receptor localisation and stimulation of phosphorylation in microvillar membranes of neonatal pigs. J Physiol. 1992;56:38.

18. Goodlad RA, Savage AP, Lenton W et al. Does urogastrone/EGF infusion have a synergistic effect on the intestine of parenterally-fed rats subject to small bowel resection? Clin Sci. 1988;75:121–6.

19. Ulshen MH, Lyn-Cook LE, Raasch RA. Effects of intraluminal epidermal growth factor on the small intestine of young rats. Gastroenterology. 1986;254:429–35.

20. Carr MD. ^{1}H NMR-based determination of the secondary structure of porcine pancreatic spasmolytic polypeptide: one of a new family of 'trefoil' motif containing cell growth factors. Biochemistry. 1992;31:1993–2004.

21. Masiakowski P, Breathnach R, Block J, Gannon F, Krust A, Chambon P. Cloning of cDNA sequences of hormone-related genes from the MCF-7 cancer cell line. Nucl Acids Res. 1982;10:7895–903.

22. Jorgensen KH, Thim L, Jacobsen HE. Pancreatic spasmolytic polypeptide 1. Preparation and initial chemical characterisation of a new polypeptide from porcine pancreas. Regul Pept. 1982;3:207–13.

23. Frandsen EK, Jorgensen KH, Thim L. Receptor binding of pancreatic spasmolytic polypeptide in rat intestinal mucosal cell membranes inhibits adenylate cyclase activity. Regul Pept. 1986;16:291–97.

24. Frandsen FK. Receptor binding of pancreatic spasmolytic polypeptide in intestinal mucosal cells and membranes. Regul Pept. 1988;20:645–52.

25. Hoosein WM, Thim L, Jorgensen KH, Brattain MG. Growth stimulatory effects of pancreatic spasmolytic polypeptide on cultured colon and breast tumour cells. FEBS Lett. 1989;247:303–6.

26. Rio M-C, Bellocq J-P, Daniel JU et al. Breast cancer-associated pS2 protein: synthesis and secretion by normal stomach mucosa. Science. 1988;50:705–8.

27. Tomasetto C, Rio M-C, Gautier C et al. hSP, the domain-duplicated homologue of pS2 protein, is co-expressed with pS2 in stomach but not in breast carcinoma. EMBO J. 1990;9:407–14.

28. Chinery R, Poulsom R, Jeffrey RE, Longcroft JM, Hanby A, Wright NA. Localisation of intestinal trefoil factor by in situ hybridisation. Biochem J. 1992;285:5–8.

29. Hauser F, Poulsom R, Chinery R et al. hP1.B, a human P-domain peptide homologous with rat intestinal trefoil factor, is expressed also in the ulcer-associated lineage and the uterus. Proc Natl Acad Sci USA. 1993;90:6961–5.

30. Suemori S, Lynch-Devaney K, Podolsky DK. Identification and characterisation of rat intestinal trefoil factor: tissue and cell specific member of the trefoil protein family. Proc Natl Acad Sci USA. 1991;88:11017–21.

31. Bloom SR, Polak JP (eds) Gut hormones. Edinburgh: Churchill Livingstone; 1981.

32. Nunez AM, Berry M, Kunar JZ, Chambon P. The 5' flanking region of the pS2 gene contains a complex enhancer sequence responsive to oestrogen, EGF, a tumour promoter (TPA), the c-ras oncoprotein and the c-fos oncoprotein. EMBO J. 1989;8:823–9.

33. Rio M-C, Chenard MP, Wolf C et al. Induction of pS2 and hSP genes as markers of mucosal ulceration in the digestive tract. Gastroenterology. 1991;100:375–9.

34. Liu KC, Wright NA. The migration pathway of epithelial cells on human duodenal villi: the origin and fate of 'gastric metaplastic' cells in duodenal mucosa. Epithelial Cell Biol. 1992;1:53–8.

35. Hanby AM, Poulsom R, Elia G, et al. The expression of the trefoil peptides pS2 and human spasmolytic polypeptide (hSP) in 'gastric metaplasia' of the proximal duodenum: implications for the nature of 'gastric metaplasia'. J Pathol. 1993;109:355–60.

Section VII
Determinants of clinical outcome of *H. pylori* infection

37
Acute infection with *H. pylori*

A. T. R. AXON

INTRODUCTION

Until Barry Marshall ingested the culture of *Helicobacter pylori* in an attempt to fulfil Koch's postulates[1] there had been no proof that an infectious organism was responsible for acute gastritis, a condition which had been recognized for many years. However, since that important experiment it has been possible to piece together and explain the previously confusing literature relating to epidemic hypochlorhydria, spontaneous hypochlorhydria and the clinical syndrome of acute gastritis.

HISTORICAL DATA

According to Marshall[2] the earliest description of acute *Helicobacter* gastritis is in the 1920 edition of Osler's *Textbook of Medicine*. It describes an acute gastritis affecting adults and children characterized by dyspepsia, flatulence and mucousy vomiting of hypochlorhydric gastric juice. This condition was thought to progress to a chronic form in some cases. The earliest well-documented description of the disease was made by Schiff and Tahl in 1938[3]. These workers had over a period of 4 years performed 433 gastric aspirations and had given 799 histamine injections to a 49-year-old paraplegic volunteer in a long-term study of gastric secretion. Over the period of experimentation four rigid endoscopies were carried out and one flexible gastroscopy (by Rudolf Schindler).

During the initial phase of experimentation in 1934 good volumes of gastric juice of high acidic content were obtained; however, in July of that year the patient developed a histamine-refractory achlorhydria and a decrease in the volume of gastric juice. The achlorhydria persisted until October when there was a return of free acid, gastric acidity reaching normal limits by July 1935. A similar period of hypochlorhydria occurred in February 1936 and continued for a month, when the acid reappeared.

In each case the relative achlorhydria was accompanied by almost complete disappearance of pepsin and the patient complained of epigastric distress immediately after meals with belching, diarrhoea, fatiguability and general malaise.

The gastroscopic examinations revealed no gross change in the appearance of the gastric mucosa, but mild superficial gastritis was encountered four times over the whole of the experimental period.

In retrospect it seems likely that this patient had had two episodes of acute *Helicobacter* infection.

In 1955[4] and 1956[5] Hirschowitz and colleagues, who had been investigating the effect of corticosteroids on gastric secretion, published two case reports of subjects who during the course of their studies became unwell, complaining of cramping epigastric pain, nausea, vomiting and profuse salivation. The gastric aspirate was hypochlorhydric with a low pepsin. Subsequently the juice became achlorhydric, totally lacking in pepsin and urinary excretion of pepsinogen increased to three to five times the previous concentration. In one patient radiography revealed a post-bulbar ulcer, and in the other a prepyloric ulcer, during the symptomatic period. Five to seven months later gastric secretion of acid in pepsin had returned to normal. These changes were attributed to the use of steroids.

In 1958[6] Spiro and Schwartz, who had also performed a series of experiments, demonstrated that spontaneous hypochlorhydria recovered, and for the first time obtained biopsies which suggested that the cause of transient hypochlorhydria was superficial gastritis.

The first personal experience of *Helicobacter*-associated gastritis was described by William Waterfall in 1969[7]. As a house surgeon in the Department of Surgery in the Royal Infirmary of Sheffield he had undertaken a series of pentagastrin tests. Both he and another subject who had a chronic duodenal ulcer developed hypochlorhydria between 1 and 5 weeks after their initial study. The acid and pepsin secretion fell, and in the case of Dr Waterfall there was no improvement in acid secretion over a period of 21 weeks. Gastric biopsies showed atrophy of the gastric mucosa and diffuse infiltration of mucosa by chronic inflammatory cells. This experiment is interesting for two reasons, firstly in the normal subject there were no symptoms during the period of hypochlorhydria. The second subject had a duodenal ulcer and should therefore have already been infected with *H. pylori*; it would appear that a second infection had induced hypochlorhydria and the ulcer symptoms which he was complaining of previously disappeared.

ACUTE INFECTION IN ZOLLINGER-ELLISON SYNDROME

As with the patient with the duodenal ulcer described in the previous experiment, acute infection with *H. pylori* has not always been disadvantageous. Three reports in the literature describe spontaneous cure of Zollinger-Ellison sydrome following intubation experiments. The first was described by Lawrie *et al.* in 1962[8] when a 48-year-old patient with Zollinger-Ellison syndrome developed achlorhydria 1 month after starting intubation studies. Five months later he remained hypochlorhydric and had become symptom-free. A similar case was described in 1969 by Desai and Antia[9]. A 53-year-old patient with Zollinger-Ellison underwent serial gastric intubations and 2 years later developed total achlorhydria with resolution of his symptoms. On this occasion, however, biopsies were taken and demonstrated atrophic gastritis with marked infiltration of lymphocytes and plasma cells. Again his symptoms resolved. These same workers went on to describe spontaneous hypochlorhydria in three further control subjects, and in seven patients with duodenal ulcer in whom there was an associated symptomatic improvement[10].

The third report in Zollinger-Ellison syndrome was from Wiersinga and Tytgat in 1977[11]. This patient was being investigated with intubation studies, and during the course of these became acutely ill with severe malaise, nausea, vomiting, perspiration and fever. Following his recovery the symptoms of his Zollinger-Ellison syndrome disappeared in association with a dramatic fall in gastric acid secretion. Histology in this case was taken before and after the illness. The second biopsy showed a severe inflammation with lymphocytes, plasma cells and polymorphonuclear leukocytes throughout the gastric mucosa with destruction of the glandular layer, crypt abscesses were present and severe inflammation was present from all areas of the stomach.

These early studies suggest that *H. pylori* infection is readily transmitted by intubation, and may or may not be associated with symptoms. There tends to be an associated gastritis with reduction in the volume of gastric secretion together with achlorhydria and a reduction in pepsin secretion. Pepsinogen excretion in the urine increases, presumably as the result of gastric damage and symptoms of peptic ulcer may decline. It is of particular interest that patients with duodenal ulcer (who are known to be infected with *H. pylori*) may develop a similar syndrome with achlorhydria, and that one individual may have been infected a second time in the experiment done in 1934.

EPIDEMIC HYPOCHLORHYDRIA AND VOLUNTEER EXPERIMENTS

The well-documented epidemics of hypochlorhydria described by Ramsey *et al.*[12,13] and Gledhill *et al.*[14] confirm that *H. pylori* is readily transmitted by intubation experiments and leads to characteristic symptoms and achlorhydria.

Since the identification of *H. pylori* two volunteers have taken the organism by mouth[1,15,16] and developed the clinical syndrome of *Helicobacter*-associated gastritis. In Marshall's case the condition resolved spontaneously, but Morris's infection became chronic and was eventually eradicated with the use of triple therapy. The latter case was studied serologically, IgM levels to *Helicobacter* rose and fell within weeks of the acute infection, and serial conversion in IgG occurred after IgM normalization. Initially when treated unsuccessfully serum IgG levels fell, but subsequently (presumably with recrudescence of infection) the IgM again rose, but rapidly fell followed again by a rise in IgG. Following the treatment which eventually eradicated *H. pylori* infection, and cleared the gastritis, IgG levels fell to normal.

SPONTANEOUS INFECTION

The immunological response to *Helicobacter* infection was studied in a research worker who was spontaneously infected by *H. pylori*[17]. Fourteen days after the onset of symptoms the supernatants from antral cultures were positive for *H. pylori* IgA and IgM by immunoblotting. IgM immunoblot positivity was slight on day 14, but by day 74 the supernatants were strongly positive for IgM and IgA antibodies. No mucosal IgG response, however, was evident at that stage.

Gastric pathology following acute infection has been well described in a number of case reports from patients thought to have been infected acutely by the organism[18–23]. Salmeron *et al.*[18] describe a 28-year-old female who developed a febrile infection with epigastric tenderness and at endoscopy had a purulent antral gastritis (*H. pylori* was detected histologically). Barbosa *et al.*[20] described antral erosions in an 8-year-old child who gave a 3-week history of epigastric pain and vomiting. This too was associated with *Helicobacter*. Frommer *et al.*[22] described a 46-year-old male who had had a haematemesis, endoscopy showed a raised irregular infiltrative lesion in the antrum, it was circumferential and associated with severe neutrophil infiltration with erosions, exudate and necrosis, *Helicobacter* organisms were present. A repeat endoscopy 3 days later showed resolution of the gross lesion, but a 1.5 cm diameter ulcer was present in the prepyloric area. At 6 months there was a 3 mm erosion present, and the biopsies showed chronic gastritis. There was seroconversion to *H. pylori* over a period of 21 months. Macroscopic lesions were also demonstrated by Graham *et al.*[23]; initially erosions and mucosal haemorrhage were present in body and antrum. Within 2 weeks the erosions had evolved into an antral ulcer which persisted for a further 2 weeks and then disappeared. Rocha *et al.*[21] described seven patients between the ages of 22 and 62, symptomatology was epigastric pain, vomiting and anorexia. Endoscopy showed oedema, multiple ulcerative irregular ulcerations with irregular edges and a red friable antral mucosa. Mitchell *et al.*[19] also described antral ulceration in an infant.

MACROSCOPIC PATHOLOGY

Acute infection with *H. pylori* may therefore cause macroscopic lesions usually in the antrum, but may also involve the corpus. The spectrum ranges from a purulent exudative gastritis to a pseudo-tumour appearance, erosions or ulcers; in other patients, however, there may be little to be seen. Resolution occurs over 2 weeks to a month.

MICROSCOPIC PATHOLOGY

The microscopic appearances of acute *Helicobacter* infection are characterized by an initial severe acute gastritis with infiltration of the lamina propria and surface epithelial cell degeneration. The pits are infiltrated and there is often a surface exudate and superficial erosion. These changes gradually resolve to be replaced by a mixture of chronic and acute inflammatory cells, the surface epithelium becomes less degenerate and the condition converts to the typical long-standing chronic, active gastritis which is well recognized.

CLINICAL SYNDROME

The incubation period for *Helicobacter* infection is less clearly defined because in the majority of cases infection has been diagnosed retrospectively; however, better data are available for the two volunteers who took cultures of the organism. In Marshall's case audible abdominal peristalsis was noted by the subject during the first 24 h, but no further symptoms arose for 1 week; on the seventh day, however, he had a feeling of fullness in the epigastrium; on the eighth day he vomited and symptoms persisted in milder form for 7 days. In Morris's case cramping epigastric pain occurred on day 2 after ingestion, became more severe on day 3, on day 4 vomiting and continued pain was present. The pains had subsided by the morning of the sixth day, and he was asymptomatic from day 12.

The clinical syndrome of acute *Helicobacter* infection appears to be one of epigastric cramping pain, nausea, vomiting, flatulence, malaise, in some cases there may be a fever, and mucousy vomiting may also be present. Characteristically these symptoms will last for about a week and then disappear, whether or not the organism has been spontaneously eliminated.

SUMMARY

The clinical and pathological characteristics of acute *H. pylori* infection are well recognized. The incubation period is from 1 to 7 days and may or may not be followed by a characteristic dyspeptic syndrome. The organism usually persists after initial infection, but may disappear spontaneously. The acute illness is characterized physiologically by hypochlorhydria and a reduction in gastric pepsin may persist for months. There is an initial IgM response which declines, to be followed by IgG conversion; this persists unless the organism is partially or completely eradicated. It is possible that individuals already infected with *H. pylori* may become superinfected with another strain, though the data suggesting this are indirect.

References

1. Marshall BJ, Armstrong JA, McGechie DB, Glancy RJ. Attempt to fulfil Koch's postulates for pyloric campylobacter. Med J Austral. 1985;142:436–9.

2. Marshall BJ. *Campylobacter pyloridis* and gastritis. J Infect Dis. 1986;153:4:650–7.
3. Schiff L, Dorrmann C, Tahl T. Gastric secretion in man. Arch Intern Med. 1938;61: 774–80.
4. Hirschowitz BI, Streeten DHP, Pollard HM, Boldt HA, Arbor A. Role of gastric secretions in activation of peptic ulcers by corticotropin (ACTH). JAMA. 1955;158(1):27–32.
5. Hirschowitz BI, Streeten DHP, London JA, Pollard HM. A steroid-induced gastric ulcer. Lancet. 1956;2:1081–3.
6. Spiro HM, Schwartz RD. A cause of temporary achlorhydria and hyperpepsinemia. N Engl J Med. 1958;259:682–4.
7. Waterfall W. Spontaneous decrease in gastric secretory response to humoral stimuli. BMJ. 1969;4:459–61.
8. Lawrie RS, Williamson AWR, Hunt JN. Zollinger-Ellison syndrome treated with poldine methyl methosulphate. Lancet. 1962;1:1002–4.
9. Desai HG, Antia FP. Spontaneous achlorhydria with atrophic gastritis in the Zollinger-Ellison syndrome. Gut. 1969;10:935–9.
10. Desai HG, Zaveri MP, Antia FP. Spontaneous and persisting decrease in maximal acid output. BMJ. 1971;2:313–15.
11. Wiersinga WM, Tytgat GN. Clinical recovery owing to target parietal cell failure in a patient with Zollinger-Ellison syndrome. Gastroenterology. 1977;73:1413–17.
12. Ramsey EJ, Carey KV, Peterson WL et al. Epidemic gastritis with hypochlorhydria. Gastroenterology. 1979;76:1449–57.
13. Peterson W, Lee E, Skoglund M. The role of *Campylobacter pyloridis* in epidemic gastritis with hypochlorhydria. Gastroenterology. 1987;92:5(2):1575.
14. Gledhill T, Leicester RJ, Addis B et al. Epidemic hypochlorhydria. BMJ. 1985;290:1383–6.
15. Morris A, Nicholson G. Ingestion of *Campylobacter pyloridis* causes gastritis and raised fasting gastric pH. Am J Gastroenterol. 1987;82(3):192–9.
16. Morris AJ, Ali MR, Nicholson GI, Perez-Perez GI, Blaser MJ. Long-term follow-up of voluntary ingestion of *Helicobacter pylori*. Ann Intern Med. 1991;114:662–3.
17. Sobala GM, Crabtree JE, Dixon MF et al. Acute *Helicobacter pylori* infection: clinical features, local and systemic immune response, gastric mucosal histology, and gastric juice ascorbic acid concentrations. Gut. 1991;32:1415–18.
18. Salmeron M, Desplaces N, Lavergne A, Houdart R. *Campylobacter*-like organisms and acute purulent gastritis. Lancet. 1986;2:975–6.
19. Mitchell JD, Mitchell HM, Tobias V. Acute *Helicobacter pylori* infection in an infant, associated with gastric ulceration and serological evidence of intra-familial transmission. Am J Gastroenterol. 1992;87:3:382–6.
20. Barbosa AJA, Queiroz DMM, Mendes EN, Rocha GA, St Carvalho A, Roquete MLV. *Campylobacter pylori* associated acute gastritis in a child. J Clin Pathol. 1989;42:779.
21. Rocha GA, Queiroz DMM, Mendes EN, Barbosa AJA, Lima GF, Oliveira CA. *Helicobacter pylori* acute gastritis: histological, endoscopical, clinical and therapeutic features. Am J Gastroenterol. 1991;86(11):1592–5.
22. Frommer DJ, Carrick J, Lee A, Hazell SL. Acute presentation of *Campylobacter pylori* gastritis. Am J Gastroenterol. 1988;83(10):1168–71.
23. Graham DY, Alpert LC, Smith JL, Yoshimura HH. Iatrogenic *Campylobacter pylori* infection is a cause of epidemic achlorhydria. Am J Gastroenterol. 1988;83(9):974–80.

38
H. pylori in asymptomatic people

C. A. O'MORAIN and M. BUCKLEY

INTRODUCTION

The local and systemic responses to the presence of *Helicobacter pylori* in the stomach demonstrate this organism is a pathogen rather than a commensal in the human stomach. This is underlined by its association with gastroduodenal pathology. Therefore asymptomatic people with *H. pylori* could be defined as individuals who are not receiving medical attention for a gastrointestinal disorder. Its role in asymptomatic people requires further clarification.

DYSPEPSIA

The symptoms of dyspepsia are varied, and it is difficult to know if individuals are truly asymptomatic. Dyspepsia or indigestion is a common complaint which many people consider trivial, and stoic individuals may suffer considerable discomfort before attending a doctor. The presence or absence of symptoms is subjective and a quantitative assessment is difficult. The individual's pain threshold, and fear of serious underlying pathology, will decide which symptoms are significant and warrant consultation. In addition, there is considerable overlap between dyspeptic symptoms and those of irritable bowel disease. Similar to the situation in regard to irritable bowel disease, only a minority of individuals with dyspepsia present to doctors. A recent survey of a business community in the City of London involving 854 employees of a single business indicated that 16.6% had irritable bowel disease symptoms but only 27% of these individuals had consulted a doctor. Many dyspeptic symptoms are also attributed to food intolerance. Epidemiological surveys have suggested specific food intolerance rates of 16–33%[1,2]. This diagnosis is often based on symptoms of postprandial nausea and vomiting, abdominal pain and bloating. However, Farah *et al.* demonstrated that only 13 of 49 patients suspected of having this diagnosis improved with a low-allergenicity diet[3]. Of these 13, 10 were shown to be strong 'placebo reactors' and only three (6.1%) were proven to have a specific food intolerance. Thus dyspeptic symptoms are often mistakenly attributed to, and wrongly explained by, other diagnoses.

Dyspeptic symptoms have been classified into four groups: (1) reflux-like dyspepsia, (2) ulcer-like dyspepsia, (3) dysmotility-like dyspepsia and (4) non-specific dyspepsia. Fifty per cent of patients with non-ulcer dyspepsia are *H. pylori*-positive. Dyspepsia accounts for 50% of gastrointestinal referrals and represents a substantial workload for the hospital specialist. The social and economic implications of functional dyspepsia have been studied in Sweden, where the cost of outpatient care and drugs for dyspepsia was estimated at $42 million per year for a population of about eight million people. When the cost of loss of earnings and sick-leave was taken into account, the annual cost was estimated as about $448 million[4]. Published prevalence rates of functional dyspepsia range from 19% in the USA[5] to 76% in Denmark[6]. However, this merely represents the tip of the iceberg as many, if not the majority of, individuals with dyspepsia do not present for medical attention. Over-the-counter sales of non-proprietary medications for dyspepsia are substantial, and there is extensive media advertisement of these products, suggesting that many individuals treat themselves. In addition, there is evidence that so-called asymptomatic *H. pylori*-positive individuals have more symptoms than age-matched *H. pylori*-negative controls (P. Malfertheiner, personal communication).

EFFECT OF *H. PYLORI* ERADICATION ON DYSPEPTIC SYMPTOMS

In our unit we have looked at the role of *H. pylori* in functional dyspepsia[7]. Patients with *H. pylori* gastritis and symptoms of dyspepsia were randomized to receive one of three treatment regimes: colloidal bismuth subcitrate (CBS), 1 g four times daily for 4 weeks ($n = 29$); CBS, 1 g four times daily for 4 weeks, amoxycillin, 500 mg three times daily for 1 week, and metronidazole, 400 mg three times daily for 1 week ($n = 28$); or amoxicillin, 500 mg three times daily for 1 week, plus metronidazole, 400 mg three times daily for 1 week ($n = 29$). Although gastritis scores improved significantly in patients in whom *H. pylori* had been eradicated, the mean symptom score, after short-term follow-up, was similar to that in patients in whom the organism had not been eradicated. Moreover, the mean symptom score improved whether or not there was an improvement in gastritis. However, after 1 year follow-up, the symptom score in patients with persistent *H. pylori* infection was significantly greater than in those who had been eradicated. In addition, 36 out of 38 (95%) patients in whom *H. pylori* persisted required additional treatment, compared with four out of 32 (12%) in whom *H. pylori* had been eradicated, suggesting that long-term remission in functional dyspepsia may be dependent upon eradication of *H. pylori*. In another study in our unit, 100 patients with functional dyspepsia and *H. pylori* were randomized to receive either CBS or triple therapy with CBS, metronidazole and tetracycline[8]; 14% of the former group were eradicated, as were 85% of the latter. Both groups had a similar short-term symptomatic response, suggesting a strong placebo

Table 1   One hundred patients with *H. pylori* and non-ulcer dyspepsia

No.	Treatment	Eradication rate (%)
50	Bismuth alone	14
50	Bismuth plus two antibiotics	85

Follow-up: significant decrease in symptoms with eradication; seven peptic ulcers developed in patients with persistent *H. pylori* infection[8]

response. However, those patients in whom eradication had occurred had a significantly lower symptom score at 1 year follow-up. This long-term reduction in symptoms was most pronounced in those who had had ulcer-like dyspeptic symptoms. This study demonstrates that *H. pylori* does have a role in functional dyspepsia, and that a subset of patients will benefit from eradication of the organism.

HELICOBACTER PYLORI AND THE CONTINUUM OF CHANGE

H. pylori binds only to the gastric epithelium, but must be present for some time before it elicits a significant inflammatory response. The inflammatory response may be limited and the host may only develop gastritis. However some will proceed to gastric or duodenal ulceration and, over a prolonged period of time, gastric cancer. A recent Eastern European study evaluated the frequency of development of peptic ulcer disease in patients with *H. pylori*-associated chronic gastritis and functional dyspepsia[9]. The study showed that there was a high probability of developing peptic ulceration; during a 5-year observation period, 21% of these patients developed gastric or duodenal ulceration. In contrast, in the *H. pylori*-negative patients, during the same period of observation, a peptic ulcer was found in only one patient (3.4%).

In our unit, in a long-term follow-up study of patients with *H. pylori*-associated chronic gastritis and functional dyspepsia, seven patients in whom the organism was not eradicated subsequently developed peptic ulcers[8] (Table 1). Earlier studies from Denmark demonstrated a high rate of peptic ulcers developing in patients originally diagnosed as having X-ray-negative dyspepsia[10]. In addition to progressing to peptic ulceration, a sequence of mucosal changes in *H. pylori*-infected gastric mucosa has been observed in populations with a high risk of developing gastric carcinoma[11]. This involves a progression of histological change from chronic active gastritis to chronic atrophic gastritis with intestinal metaplasia, and finally to dysplasia and invasive carcinoma. In a recent long-term follow-up study in our unit, 182 patients with an initial diagnosis of chronic active gastritis were assessed[12]. Of the 160 biopsies which were repeated at an interval of less than 2 years, all showed the original features of chronic active gastritis or had reverted to normal if the organism had been eradicated. Of the 22 biopsies which were repeated at an interval of greater than 2 years, 12 (54%) showed evidence of progression to chronic atrophic gastritis with intestinal metaplasia, while one patient (4.5%) showed evidence of dysplasia.

Table 2 Endoscopy in *H. pylori*-positive blood
donors (*n* = 121)[14]

Findings	Percentage
Gastric cancer	2.0
Duodenal ulcer	16.0
Gastric ulcer	5.0
Gastritis/erosions	45.0
Duodenitis/erosions	16.0
Normal	16.0

Thus *H. pylori* infection of the gastric mucosa leads to a continuum of changes which may ultimately lead to peptic ulceration or gastric cancer.

ASYMPTOMATIC GASTRODUODENAL PATHOLOGY

It is arguable that gastrointestinal diseases are sometimes asymptomatic. Peptic ulcer and gastric cancer are sometimes found in asymptomatic individuals. Symptoms related to gastric cancer usually develop late, and in countries where there are screening programmes, early lesions are detected long before symptoms develop. Japan has the highest age-adjusted mortality for gastric cancer. A mass screening for gastric cancer by mobile X-ray equipment was started in the Miyagi Prefecture, Japan in 1960, and was offered to all adults[13]. The total number of examinees in 1985 amounted to 5 161 876 and 6240 cases (0.12%) of gastric cancer were detected. The vast majority of these were asymptomatic.

In a recent Italian study, Vaira *et al.* investigated a large group of asymptomatic blood donors[14]. A high seroprevalence of IgG to *H. pylori* was found in 422/1010 (42%). Endoscopy was then offered to subjects with high levels of *H. pylori* IgG. Of the 288 who underwent endoscopy, only 39 were found to be macroscopically normal. Endoscopy in the remaining 247 asymptomatic subjects revealed one gastric cancer, one leiomyosarcoma, 50 duodenal ulcers, 19 gastric ulcers, 39 had erosive duodenitis, 30 had antral erosions and 109 had macroscopic antral gastritis (Table 2).

High levels of IgG to *H. pylori* may therefore have clinical relevance in asymptomatic populations. Screening for asymptomatic gastrointestinal pathology has been advocated in other situations; for example, faecal occult blood testing or colonoscopy for the early detection of colonic cancer. Serology could be a simple, inexpensive screening test for gastric cancer. The urea breath test could also be a screening test to detect current *H. pylori* infection, but may not be that useful for the early detection of gastric cancer as *H. pylori* may be an initiating event inducing a gastritis which progresses to atrophy and loss of the epithelial receptors for the bacterium.

PATHOGENIC STRAINS OF *H. PYLORI*

H. pylori has been associated with virulent factors. Firstly, there appear to be more adhesion pedestals between *H. pylori* and the gastric surface in patients with duodenal ulceration. It has been suggested that adhesion may be involved in tissue damage[15,16]. Only a small proportion of *H. pylori* adhere to the gastric epithelium while other helicobacters survive without adhering at all[17]. Thus it is possible to conclude that adhesion is not important for colonization. However, it is very possible that close attachment to the mucosa could be involved in cell damage. Data consistent with this hypothesis include the observation that the only adhering helicobacters are those associated with ulcers, i.e. *H. pylori* and *H. mustelae*[18]. This adhesion is very specific for gastric tissue; therefore many attempts have been made to define the adhesions[19]. A number of haemagglutinins have been identified and *n*-acetylneuraminyl lactose has been suggested as a major receptor for this molecule[20]. The glycolipid phosphatidyl ethanolamine has been reported to bind to *H. pylori*, as has the basement membrane component, laminin. The problem with all these studies is that they are involved in the sticking of *H. pylori* to any cell type, be it a red cell or HEp2 cell, and none of them provides any indication as to the existence of a gastric tissue specific adhesin.

The ability of *H. pylori* to produce phospholipases may be a factor determining the virulence of the organism. Phospholipases weaken the cell membrane and lead to cell damage. Since *H. pylori* is in close contact with the gastric mucosal cells, even small amounts of phospholipases could be harmful to the mucosal cells. In addition to a direct effect, phospholipases acting on lecithin can produce lysolecithin, which is cytotoxic. In ulcer patients there is an increased amount of lysolecithins in the gastric juice compared to normal individuals[21]. In a recent study in our unit, *H. pylori* strains were found to produce both phospholipase A and phospholipase C[22]. It was found that phospholipase C production was more variable among different strains of *H. pylori* than phospholipase A production. In addition, *H. pylori* strains isolated from patients with duodenal ulceration had a higher level of phospholipase C than those isolated from patients with gastritis, suggesting that this may be an important factor in determining the virulence of the organism.

The toxic product that is attracting most attention at present is the so-called vacuolating cytotoxin. Certain strains of *H. pylori* are capable of inducing a cytopathic effect in mammalian cells *in vitro* consisting in the formation of intracytoplasmic vacuoles. These strains contain proteins which are not present, or are present less frequently, in non-vacuolating strains. These proteins may be a marker for the vacuolating activity of *H. pylori*. In an Italian study, *H. pylori* strains isolated from patients with peptic ulcers, especially with duodenal ulcers, produced vacuolating toxin more frequently than did isolates from patients without ulcers (66.6% of strains, versus 30.1% of strains)[23]. Crabtree *et al.* examined the gastric mucosal IgA response to *H. pylori* of patients with chronic *H. pylori* gastritis: 75%, 83%, 97%, and 76%, respectively showed responses to the 120 kDa, 90 kDa, 61 kDa, and 31 kDa proteins[24]. None of the 19 patients with chronic gastritis who did not recognize the 120 kDa protein had peptic ulcers, whereas 25 of 57 patients with positive recognition had peptic ulcers. Mucosal recognition of the *H. pylori* 120 kDa protein was also positively associated with the activity of gastritis and the extent of surface degeneration. These findings suggest that

120 kDa-positive strains of *H. pylori* have pathogenic factors associated with active gastritis and peptic ulceration. However, the existence of hypervirulent strains has been doubted by some experts. A study of the *H. pylori* status of three generations of an ulcer-prone family in Coventry, UK, suggests that all strains of *H. pylori* have the ability to induce ulceration if other conditions are met[25]. Investigation of nine family members, spanning three generations, for *H. pylori* status showed eight to be positive for the bacterium and five to have duodenal ulcer disease. Using DNA fingerprinting it was found that three family members harboured almost identical strains of *H. pylori* but only two of these had ulcers. The remaining five individuals harboured distinct strains of *H. pylori*, yet three of these had ulcers. It was concluded in this study that the high proportion of ulcers in this family was not due to the sharing of a hypervirulent strain of *H. pylori* but was due to host factors that promoted ulceration in certain infected individuals.

HOST SUSCEPTIBILITY

If there are no distinct ulcerogenic strains of *H. pylori*, host factors must determine the consequences of *H. pylori* infection. A varying host response to *H. pylori* infection has been demonstrated by El-Omar *et al.*[26]. In this study the median acid output in response to intravenous infusion of gastrin-releasing peptide in asymptomatic *H. pylori*-positive volunteers was three times that of *H. pylori*-negative individuals. However, the median acid output in duodenal ulcer patients with *H. pylori* was three times that of *H. pylori*-positive asymptomatic individuals. Eradication of *H. pylori* in the duodenal ulcer patients lowered their acid secretion by a median of 66% and to values equivalent to the *H. pylori*-positive asymptomatic volunteers. Therefore *H. pylori* infection in certain individuals promotes an exaggerated acid response which leads to duodenal ulceration. The host factors that determine this response have not been elucidated.

The chronic gastritis accompanying duodenal ulceration is conventionally described as 'antral', and is claimed not to be associated with atrophy or intestinal metaplasia. This distinction from the gastritis found in gastric ulcer patients is overstated and corpus inflammation is a frequent finding in duodenal ulcer patients, albeit to a lesser degree than in the antrum, and atrophy and intestinal metaplasia are found in a substantial proportion of antral biopsies from duodenal ulcer patients. The relative sparing of the corpus could result from the high acid output in duodenal ulcer patients, as the higher local concentration of acid could overcome the ammonia-based buffering capacity of the organism and the usual spread of infection and inflammation from the antrum to the corpus would be halted or slowed. Thus one can speculate that the larger the host acid response to infection, the more *H. pylori*-associated gastritis would be restricted to the antrum. Conversely, hosts with a reduced acid response will lack acid 'protection' of the corpus region and will develop a pan-gastritis when they acquire *H. pylori* infection.

The age of the host at the time of infection may also be an important factor in determining subsequent pathology, as infection in infancy which commonly occurs in third world countries will result in a high prevalence of *H. pylori* and an increased incidence of gastric cancer.

TREATMENT

Treating symptomatic *H. pylori*-infected patients is justified, particularly those with peptic ulcer disease. *H. pylori* dyspepsia without ulceration may prove to be an indication for eradication therapy. It is difficult to justify eradication therapy in asymptomatic individuals at present, but the aforementioned data suggest that asymptomatic people are a link in the evolution of gastroduodenal pathology, including gastric cancer. There is no definitive treatment at present. The regime of choice is triple therapy with a bismuth preparation. However, there are limitations due to compliance and side-effects. Treatment with a proton pump inhibitor combined with antibiotics is promising, but eradication rates are variable. Two studies in our unit assessed the eradication rates of high-dose omeprazole and amoxicillin[27,28]. Eight of 18 patients (44%) and five of 13 patients (38%) were eradicated. More recently, favourable eradication rates of 89% have been reported in patients treated with omeprazole and other antibiotics, in particular, clarithromycin[29].

If future studies substantiate the link with gastric cancer, then the development of a vaccine may provide the most convenient way of treating populations at high risk.

CONCLUSION

Asymptomatic individuals with *H. pylori* infection may represent the base of an iceberg, so to speak, as many have symptoms which remain hidden from the medical profession. They may eventually develop pathology, or their pathology may in fact be asymptomatic. The bacterium may have different virulence factors or host factors may determine the consequences of infection. At present, treatment of *H. pylori* is recommended for symptomatic patients, but strong arguments can be made for treatment in asymptomatic individuals.

References

1. Barr ML, Merrett TG. Food intolerance: a community survey. Br J Nutr. 1883;4917–19.
2. Bender AE, Matthews DR. Adverse reactions to food. Br J Nutr. 1981;46:403–7.
3. Farah DA, Calder I, Benson L, MacKenzie JF. Specific food intolerance: its place as a cause of gastrointestinal symptoms. Gut. 1985;26:164–8.
4. Nyren O, Adami H, Gustavsson S *et al.* Social and economic effects of non-ulcer dyspepsia. Scand J Gastroenterol. 1985;209:(Suppl. 109)41–7.
5. Talley N, Phillips SF, Melton J *et al.* A patient questionnaire to identify bowel disease. Ann Intern Med. 1989;111:671–4.
6. Bonnevie O. The incidence and results of radiological examination of the stomach using a barium meal. Scand J Gastroenterol. 1976;11:839–47.

7. McCarthy C, Patchett S, Collins R *et al.* Long term prospective study of the role of *Helicobacter pylori* in non-ulcer dyspepsia. Lancet. 1993:in press.
8. Gilvarry J, Buckley M, Beattie S *et al.* Effects of eradicating *Helicobacter pylori* in non-ulcer dyspepsia. (Submitted for publication.)
9. Matysiak-Budnik T, Megraud F. *Helicobacter pylori* in Eastern countries: what is the current status? Gastroenterology. 1993:in press.
10. Krag E. The pseudo-ulcer syndrome: a clinical, radiographic and statistical follow-up study of patients with ulcer symptoms but no demonstrable ulcer in the stomach or duodenum. Dan Med Bull. 1969;16:6–9.
11. Correa P, Cuello C, Duque E. Gastric cancer in Columbia. Natural history of precursor lesions. J Natl Cancer Inst. 1976;57:1027–35.
12. Gilvarry J, Leen E, Sweeney E, O'Morain CA. The long-term effect of *Helicobacter pylori* on gastric ucosa. Eur J Gastroenterol Hepatol. (Submitted for publication.)
13. Hisamachi S. Screening for gastric cancer. World J Surg. 1989;13:31–7.
14. Vaira D, Miglioli M, Mule P *et al.* The prevalence of peptic ulcer in *Helicobacter pylori* positive blood donors. Gut. 1993:in press.
15. Chen XG, Correa P, Offerhaus J *et al.* Ultrastructure of the gastric mucosa harboring *Campylobacter*-like organisms. Am J Clin Pathol. 1986;86:575–82.
16. Steer HW. Ultrastructure of *Campylobacter pylori in vivo.* Oxford: Blackwell Scientific Publications; 1989:146–54.
17. Hessey SJ, Spencer J, Wyatt JI *et al.* Bacterial adhesion and disease activity in *Helicobacter* associated chronic gastritis. Gut. 1990;312:134–8.
18. O'Rourke JL, Lee A, Fox JG. An ultrastructural study of *Helicobacter mustelae* and evidence of a specific association with gastric mucosa. J Med Microbiol. 1992;36(In press.)
19. Wyatt JI, Rathbone BJ, Dixon MF, Heatley RV. *Campylobacter pyloridis* and acid induced gastric metaplasia in the pathogenesis of duodenitis. J Clin Pathol. 1987;40:841–8.
20. Evans DG, Evans Jr DJ, Moulds JJ, Graham DY. *N*-acetylneuraminyllactose-binding fibrillar hemagglutinin of *Campylobacter pylori*: a putative colonisation factor antigen. Infect Immun. 1988;5611:2896–906.
21. Rhodes J, Bernardo OE, Phillips SF *et al.* Increased reflux of bile into the stomach in patients with gastric ulcer. Gastroenterology. 1969;57:241–52.
22. Daw MA, Cotter L, Healy M *et al.* Phospholipases and the cytotoxic activity of *Helicobacter pylori.* Rev Esp Enferm Dig. 1990;78(Suppl.):78–9.
23. Figura N, Guglielmetti P, Rossolini A *et al.* Cytotoxin production by *Campylobacter pylori* strains isolated from patients with peptic ulcers and from patients with chronic gastritis only. J Clin Microbiol. 1989;27:225–6.
24. Crabtree JE, Taylor JD, Wyatt JI *et al.* Mucosal IgA recognition of *Helicobacter pylori* 120 kDa protein, peptic ulceration, and gastric pathology. Lancet. 1991;338:332–5.
25. Nwokolo CU, Bickley J, Attard AR *et al.* Evidence of clonal variants of *Helicobacter pylori* in three generations of a duodenal ulcer disease family. Gut. 1992;33:1323–7.
26. El-Omar E, Penman I, Dorrian CA *et al.* Eradicating *Helicobacter pylori* infection lowers gastrin mediated acid secretion by two thirds in patients with duodenal ulcer. Gut. 1993;34:1060–5.
27. Buckley M, Beattie S, Hamilton H, O'Morain CA. Omeprazole and amoxycillin in *Helicobacter pylori* associated duodenal ulceration. Irish Society of Gastroenterology, Summer meeting, 1993. (Presentation)
28. Collins R, Beattie S, Xia HX, O'Morain CA. Short report: high-dose omeprazole and amoxycillin in the treatment of *Helicobacter pylori*-associated duodenal ulcer. Aliment Pharmacol Ther. 1993;7:313–15.
29. Logan PPH, Gummett PA, Hegarty BT, et al. Clarithromycin and omeprazole for *Helicobacter pylori.* Lancet. 1992;340:239.

39
Determinants of clinical outcome of *H. pylori* infection: duodenal ulcer

M. F. GO and D. Y. GRAHAM

INTRODUCTION

Helicobacter pylori infection is the major acquired or environmental factor involved in the pathogenesis of a spectrum of gastroduodenal diseases including gastritis, duodenal ulcer, gastric ulcer, gastric carcinoma and gastric lymphoma[1]. Although *H. pylori* infection is present in the majority of patients with duodenal ulcer disease, duodenal ulcer is actually an uncommon outcome of *H. pylori* infection; investigators continue to be intrigued with why duodenal ulcer is such an infrequent manifestation of *H. pylori* infection. Possible explanations include differences in the host – for example, in host genetics, in social, dietary or other environmental factors; in the strain of *H. pylori*; or both host and bacterial factors.

THE ROLE OF THE HOST

Duodenal ulcer disease is often thought of as a heterogeneous set of disorders each resulting in a chronic and recurring ulcer in the duodenal mucosa[2]. There has been a long-standing and major interest in identifying host factors useful to predict development of ulcer disease, as well as factors which might play a role in the pathogenesis of disease. Evidence for important host genetic factors includes studies showing that ulcer disease tended to occur in families, and twin studies that showed a higher concurrence of ulcer disease in monozygotic twins compared to dizygotic twins[3,4]. Clues for a role in genetics also come from studies demonstrating an elevated serum pepsinogen I level in families with a high prevalence of ulcer[5].

Gastric physiology, especially acid and pepsin secretion, have been major interests because of their potential role as aggressive factors in the pathogenesis of ulcer disease. It has long been known that hypersecretion of acid is a common feature of duodenal ulcer disease. On average, patients with duodenal ulcer disease have elevated maximum acid secretion, and as maximum acid secretion is a reflection of parietal cell mass, patients with duodenal ulcer have a larger parietal cell mass than normal[2]. It remains unclear whether increased parietal cell mass precedes or follows the onset of duodenal ulcer. In the early 1970s increased meal-stimulated gastrin release was identified in duodenal ulcer patients, suggesting that acid hypersecretion might be a result of the trophic effects of increased gastrin secretion[6]. More recently it has become evident that both exaggerated meal-stimulated gastrin release and hyperpepsinogenaemia are actually epiphenomena and consequences of *H. pylori* infection; both serum gastrin and pepsinogen levels return to normal after cure of *H. pylori* gastritis[7–10]. Follow-up of ulcer patients after cure of *H. pylori* infection and return of gastrin secretion to normal has, with few exceptions, not been associated with return of acid secretion to normal, suggesting that acid hypersecretion predated the ulcer disease[11]. It has therefore been suggested that the outcome of *H. pylori* infection may be, in part, dependent on the level of acid secretion that was genetically determined[11,12]. This line of reasoning was strengthened by studies that showed that, although the infection was spread throughout the stomach in patients with duodenal ulcer disease, significant gastritis was largely confined to the antrum (an antral predominant form of gastritis)[11,12]. After vagotomy, gastritis rapidly advances into the gastric body, suggesting that hypersecretion of acid was the factor limiting *H. pylori* from causing significant damage to the gastric corpus[13,14]. This hypothesis remains.

There has been interest in identifying differences in acid secretion between individuals without *H. pylori* infection, *H. pylori* gastritis, and *H. pylori* gastritis with duodenal ulcer. Recent studies have found differences in gastrin-releasing peptide-stimulated acid secretion before and after cure of *H. pylori* infection in *H. pylori* duodenal ulcer and controls[15]. The significance of these observations is unclear as they are reflections of differences in less than maximal doses of the stimulant, and they do not address the differences in parietal cell mass between these groups nor differences in the degree of antral (and/or corpus) damage, *H. pylori* number, etc. that are present. It seems likely that these new observations will ultimately prove to be additional examples of epiphenomena related to differences in the anatomical distribution and degree of *H. pylori* damage. We suspect that acid secretion will ultimately prove to be only a permissive factor.

The fact that duodenal ulcer may also occur in patients with normal gastric acid secretion suggests that other factors are important for the development of this disease. Three major categories of duodenal ulcer disease are now recognized: *H. pylori*-related, NSAID-related, and hypersecretory (e.g. Zollinger-Ellison syndrome)[1]. The most common is duodenal ulcer disease caused by *H. pylori* infection. The tight association between *H. pylori* infection and duodenal ulcer disease has been convincingly established by its almost universal presence in duodenal ulcer disease and by the change in the natural history (cure of the disease) following cure of the infection[1].

Another hypothesis was that the clinical manifestations of *H. pylori* infection seen in various populations were a reflection of the age-of-acquisition of the infection[16]. The hypothesis was that infection in early childhood has led to extensive damage of the gastric corpus and development of atrophic gastritis at an early age. This scenario would lead to reduced acid secretion, thus preventing development of duodenal ulcer. The long duration of chronic atrophic gastritis would also increase the likelihood of the subsequent development of gastric carcinoma[16-18]. This hypothesis was based on the observed differences in frequency of gastric cancer between developing countries (e.g. Peru) and the observation that duodenal ulcer was a 'new Western disease' whose appearance seemed to parallel the suspected change in epidemiology of H. pylori infection in Western societies[1]. Recent studies in developing countries (high prevalence of duodenal ulcer in young adults in developing countries) have suggested that the Peruvian model of early development of atrophic gastritis may not be characteristic of the outcome of H. pylori infection in early childhood[19-22]. These striking differences between the prevalence of duodenal ulcer in different developing countries suggest that local environmental factors (e.g. diet) or differences in the prevalence of virulent H. pylori strains in the population may be more important than previously imagined. The gastric cancer portion of the hypothesis appears to remain valid.

Recent studies have shed light on the interactions between environmental factors and predisposition to duodenal ulcer. For example, a recently completed study of H. pylori infection in 269 pairs of twins (including 36 monozygotic twin pairs reared apart, 64 monozygotic twin pairs reared together, 88 dizygotic twin pairs reared in separate environments and 81 dizygotic twin pairs reared in the same environment) showed a higher concordance rate for H. pylori in monozygotic twin pairs (81%) compared to dizygotic twin pairs (63%)[23]. The correlation coefficient or heritability (relative importance of genetic effects) for monozygotic twins reared apart was 0.66, suggesting that the results of previous twin studies in duodenal ulcer may have actually been surrogates for H. pylori status.

THE ROLE OF THE BACTERIUM

For bacterial pathogens studied to date, the majority of clinically significant disease outbreaks can be traced back to a small number of strains or cell lineages with a bacterial population. For example, specific isolates of E. coli serotype 0157:H7 have been implicated as the aetiological agents of haemorrhagic colitis and haemolytic uraemic syndrome[24]. Staphylococcus aureus isolates responsible for most cases of toxic shock syndrome with a female urogenital focus have been shown to be members of a distinctive cell lineage[25]. Strains of two related cell lineages of Streptococcus pyogenes account for nearly half of all cases of toxic-shock-like syndrome (TSLS) with almost all strains expressing the exotoxin A gene[26].

There are now several studies suggesting that H. pylori isolates from patients with peptic ulcer disease are different from isolates obtained from patients with gastritis alone. Investigations of potential H. pylori virulence factors such as adhesins, mucolytics, phospholipases, motility, and urease have indicated that these phenotypic bacterial factors are universal in all strains. Potential H. pylori virulence factors not present in all strains include the 128K CagA protein (*cagA* gene product) and the vacuolating cytotoxin (*vacA* gene product). Although the 128K CagA protein and the cytotoxin are found in the majority of *H. pylori* isolates tested (on average 63%) they have been observed to be more frequently expressed by clinical isolates associated with peptic ulcer disease than in *H. pylori* isolates obtained from patients with simple gastritis[27–30]. IgG titres (measured by optical density) to a recombinant fragment of the 128K CagA protein were also more frequently observed and significantly higher in patients with duodenal ulcer disease compared to normals, gastritis, or duodenitis[31]. Mucosal IgA recognition of the CagA protein in patients with *H. pylori*-associated ulcer disease were also associated with significantly increased epithelial neutrophil infiltration[32]. Recent studies revealing that epithelial IL-8 production in Cato 3 cells was enhanced by specific *H. pylori* strains expressing the CagA protein are consistent with the observation that strains possessing neutrophil-activating and agglutinating properties were more common in patients with ulcer disease than in patients with gastritis alone[33,34]. The 128K CagA protein and the cytotoxin were discovered by prospective analysis of protein band patterns of *H. pylori* isolates.

Another approach is to use molecular techniques to identify disease-specific differences among isolates. Genotyping studies may be more useful for discriminating among strains from patients with different clinical disorders, as the results are not influenced by differences in phenotypic expression of bacterial virulence factors that are often affected by storage and culture conditions[35]. Molecular epidemiological studies of *H. pylori* isolates by restriction digestion analysis, ribotyping, arbitrary primer analysis, plasmid profiling, and urease gene PCR have been unsuccessful in identifying strains that might be more important in the development of more virulent disease, such as duodenal ulcer disease[36–42]. Until recently the organism has appeared to occur in an almost infinite variety of strains.

Two recent molecular studies suggest that specific strains may be associated with different gastroduodenal disease. DNA–DNA solution hybridization of whole genomic DNA from *H. pylori* strains was utilized to examine differences in strains obtained from patients with simple gastritis and peptic ulcer disease. That study found that, using a probe prepared from whole genomic DNA from an isolate obtained from a patient with duodenal ulcer disease, the mean level of hybridization was high among isolates from duodenal ulcer patients and significantly different from the hybridization level of isolates obtained from subjects with asymptomatic gastritis[43]. Amplification of genomic regions lying between repetitive DNA elements in the *H. pylori* genome by the polymerase chain reaction (rep-PCR) was subsequently used to generate DNA fingerprints of *H. pylori* isolates obtained from individuals with asymptomatic gastritis and from patients with duodenal ulcer disease. Cluster analysis of these DNA fingerprints revealed two major clusters of the strains; one set consisted of isolates from patients with duodenal ulcer disease and the second cluster consisted largely of strains obtained from patients with asymptomatic gastritis. In both studies, isolates from patients with duodenal ulcer disease, while genetically heterogeneous, were more similar to each other and different from isolates obtained from patients with gastritis alone, suggesting the presence of disease-specific strains[44,45]. Specific PCR products in the DNA fingerprints of strains from duodenal ulcer patients may be important in determining virulence of those strains.

The development of probes based on the DNA fragments that differ between *H. pylori* isolates from patients with duodenal ulcer and simple gastritis may allow one prospectively to distinguish disease-specific *H. pylori* strains. Analysis of the clonal nature and genetic diversity of *H. pylori* would generate a system of genetic markers that would permit a rapid, simple, and powerful means to differentiate strains.

If disease-specific *H. pylori* strains can be identified, these may be used as the basis for investigations of interactions examining various physiological and immunological interactions between the host and specific strains, and how this may lead to the different outcomes of *H. pylori* infection. The ability to distinguish clones or specific strains of a bacterial species would be invaluable in testing the hypothesis that a restricted number of strains is associated in a non-random manner to the expression of clinical disease. This type of information will lead to the understanding of factors influencing the organization of the bacterial genome and genetic rearrangements that may occur resulting in virulence loci, and thereby contribute knowledge regarding the evolution of virulence in pathogenic bacteria. Once it is clear that a strain or group of strains is aetiological in the development of a specific disease, these strains may be more intensely examined to identify specific factors by which they influence the development of disease.

SUMMARY

H. pylori infection is the most common cause of duodenal ulcer disease, yet duodenal ulcer is an uncommon outcome of *H. pylori* infection. Possible explanations include differences in the host, in social, dietary or other environmental factors, in the strain of *H. pylori*, or both host and bacterial factors. Host factors may include genetic susceptibility to *H. pylori* infection, excess gastric acid secretion, or both. Potential *H. pylori* virulence factors not present in all strains include the 128K CagA protein (*cagA* gene product) and the vacuolating cytotoxin (*vacA* gene product). Two different molecular techniques have suggested disease-specific differences may exist among *H. pylori* isolates. DNA–DNA hybridization of whole genomic DNA in solution and cluster analysis of rep-PCR genomic DNA fingerprints suggest that isolates from patients with duodenal ulcer disease are different from those obtained from individuals with asymptomatic gastritis. Furthermore, cluster analysis of these rep-PCR DNA fingerprints revealed two major groups of the strains; one set consisted of strains from patients with duodenal ulcer disease and the second cluster consisted largely of strains from individuals with asymptomatic gastritis. These studies suggest that disease-specific cell lineages or strains may exist among *H. pylori* isolates, leading to the various outcomes observed in patients with *H. pylori* infection.

Acknowledgements

This work was supported by the Department of Veterans Affairs and by the generous support of Hilda Schwartz.

References

1. Graham DY, Go MF. *Helicobacter pylori*: current status. Gastroenterology. 1993;105: 279–82.
2. Soll AH. Gastric, duodenal, and stress ulcer. In: Sleisenger M, Fordtran J, editors. Gastrointestinal disease, 5th edn. Philadelphia: WB Saunders; 1993:580–679.
3. McConnell RB. Peptic ulcer: early genetic evidence – families, twins, and markers. In: Rotter JI, Samloff IM, Rimoin DL, editors. The genetics and heterogeneity of common gastrointestinal disorders. New York: Academic Press; 1980:31–41.
4. Gottlieb-Jensen K. Peptic ulcer: genetic and epidemiological aspects based on twin studies. Copenhagen: Munksgaard; 1972.
5. Rotter JI, Sones JQ, Samloff IM *et al.* Duodenal ulcer disease associated with elevated serum pepsinogen I: an inherited autosomal dominant disorder. N Engl J Med. 1979;300: 63–6.
6. McGuigan JE, Trudeau WL. Differences in rates of gastrin release in normal persons and patients with duodenal-ulcer disease. N Engl J Med. 1973;288:64–6.
7. Chittajallu RS, Dorrian CA, Ardill JE, McColl KE. Effect of *Helicobacter pylori* on serum pepsinogen I and plasma gastrin in duodenal ulcer patients. Scand J Gastroenterol. 1992;27:20–4.
8. Chittajallu RS, Dorrian CA, Neithercut WD, Dahill S, McColl KE. Is *Helicobacter pylori* associated hypergastrinaemia due to the bacterium's urease activity or the antral gastritis? Gut. 1991;32:1286–90.
9. Levy S, Dollery CT, Bloom SR *et al. Campylobacter pylori*, duodenal ulcer disease, and gastrin. BMJ. 1989;299:1093–4.
10. Prewett EJ, Smith JT, Nwokolo CU, Hudson M, Sayerr AM, Pounder RE. Eradication of *Helicobacter pylori* abolishes 24-hour hypergastrinaemia: a prospective study in healthy subjects. Aliment Pharmacol Ther. 1991;5:283–90.
11. Graham DY. *Helicobacter pylori*: its epidemiology and its role in duodenal ulcer disease. J Gastroenterol Hepatol. 1991;6:105–13.
12. Dixon MF. *Helicobacter pylori* and peptic ulceration: histopathological aspects. J Gastroenterol Hepatol. 1991;6:125–30.
13. Kekki M, Saukkonen M, Sipponen P, Varis K, Siurala M. Dynamics of chronic gastritis in the remnant after partial gastrectomy for duodenal ulcer. Scand J Gastroenterol. 1980;15:509–12.
14. Meikle DD, Taylor KB, Truelove SC, Whitehead R. Gastritis duodenitis, and circulating levels of gastrin in duodenal ulcer before and after vagotomy. Gut. 1976;17:719–28.
15. El-Omar E, Penman I, Dorrian CA, Ardill JES, McColl KEL. Eradicating *Helicobacter pylori* infection lowers gastrin mediated acid secretion by two thirds in patients with duodenal ulcer. Gut. 1993;34:1060–5.
16. Graham DY. *Helicobacter pylori* in human populations: the present and predictions of the future based on the epidemiology of polio. In: Menge M, Gregor M, Tytgat GNJ, Marshall BJ, McNulty CAM, editors. *Helicobacter pylori* 1990: Proceedings of the Second International Symposium on *Helicobacter pylori*. Berlin: Springer-Verlag; 1991:97–102.
17. Graham DY, Adam E, Klein PD *et al.* Epidemiology of *Campylobacter pylori* infection. Gastroenterol Clin Biol. 1989;13:84–8B.
18. Graham DY, Klein PD, Evans DG *et al. Helicobacter pylori*: epidemiology, relationship to gastric cancer and the role of infants in transmission. Eur J Gastroenterol Hepatol. 1992;4(Suppl.1):S1–6.
19. *Helicobacter pylori* and gastritis in Peruvian patients: relationship to socioeconomic level, age, and sex. The Gastrointestinal Physiology Working Group. Am J Gastroenterol. 1990;85:819–23.

20. Recavarren Arce S, Leön-Barua R, Cok J *et al. Helicobacter pylori* and progressive gastric pathology that predisposes to gastric cancer. Scand J Gastroenterol Suppl. 1991;181:51–7.
21. Burstein M, Monge E, Leön-Barua R *et al.* Low peptic ulcer and high gastric cancer prevalence in a developing country with a high prevalence of infection by *Helicobacter pylori.* J Clin Gastroenterol. 1991;13:154–6.
22. Recavarren Arce S, Leön-Barua R, Cok J *et al.* Low prevalence of gastric metaplasia in the duodenal mucosa in Peru. J Clin Gastroenterol. 1992;15:296–301.
23. Malaty HM, Engstrand L, Pederson N, Graham DY. Is there a genetic influence in *Helicobacter pylori* susceptibility and transmission: the twin study. Am J Gastroenterol. 1992;399:1342(abstract).
24. Whittam TS, Wachsmuth IK, Wilson RA. Genetic evidence of clonal descent of *Escherichia coli* O157:H7 associated with hemorrhagic colitis and hemolytic uremic syndrome. J Infect Dis. 1988;157:1124–33.
25. Musser JM, Hauser AR, Kim MH, Schlievert PM, Nelson K, Selander RK. *Streptococcus pyogenes* causing toxic-shock-like syndrome and other invasive diseases: clonal diversity and pyrogenic exotoxin expression. Proc Natl Acad Sci USA. 1991;88:2668–72.
26. Musser JM, Schlievert PM, Chow AW *et al.* A single clone of *Staphylococcus aureus* causes the majority of cases of toxic shock syndrome. Proc Natl Acad Sci USA. 1990;87:225–9.
27. Figura N, Guglielmetti P, Rossolini A *et al.* Cytotoxin production by *Campylobacter pylori* strains isolated from patients with peptic ulcers and from patients with chronic gastritis only. J Clin Microbiol. 1989;27:225–6.
28. Covacci A, Censini S, Bugnoli M *et al.* Molecular characterization of the 128-kDa immunodominant antigen of *Helicobacter pylori* associated with cytotoxicity and duodenal ulcer. Proc Natl Acad Sci USA. 1993;90:5791–5.
29. Cover TL, Dooley CP, Blaser MJ. Characterization of and human serologic response to proteins in *Helicobacter pylori* broth culture supernatants with vacuolizing cytotoxin activity. Infect Immun. 1990;58:603–10.
30. Tummuru MK, Cover TL, Blaser MJ. Cloning and expression of a high-molecular-mass major antigen of *Helicobacter pylori*: evidence of linkage to cytotoxin production. Infect Immun. 1993;61:1799–809.
31. Xiang Z, Bugnoli M, Rappuoli R, Covacci A, Ponzetto A, Crabtree JE. *Helicobacter pylori*: host responses in peptic ulceration [letter]. Lancet. 1993;341:900–1.
32. Crabtree JE, Figura N, Taylor JD, Bugnoli M, Armellini D, Tompkins DS. Expression of 120 kilodalton protein and cytotoxicity in *Helicobacter pylori*. J Clin Pathol. 1992;45:733–4.
33. Crabtree JE, Taylor JD, Wyatt JI *et al.* Mucosal IgA recognition of *Helicobacter pylori* 120 kDa protein, peptic ulceration, and gastric pathology. Lancet. 1991;338:332–5.
34. Rautelin H, Blomberg B, Fredlund H, Jarnerot G, Danielsson D. Incidence of *Helicobacter pylori* strains activating neutrophils in patients with peptic ulcer disease. Gut. 1993;34:599–603.
35. Versalovic J, Woods CL Jr, Georghiou PR, Hamill RJ, Lupski JR. DNA-based identification and epidemiologic typing of bacterial pathogens. Arch Pathol Lab Med. 1993:in press.
36. Clayton CL, Kleanthous H, Morgan DD, Puckey L, Tabaqchali S. Rapid fingerprinting of *Helicobacter pylori* by polymerase chain reaction and restriction fragment length polymorphism analysis. J Clin Microbiol. 1993;31:1420–5.
37. Langenberg W, Rauws EA, Widjojokusumo A, Tytgat GN, Zanen HC. Identification of *Campylobacter pyloridis* isolates by restriction endonuclease DNA analysis. J Clin Microbiol. 1986;24:414–17.
38. Majewski SI, Goodwin CS. Restriction endonuclease analysis of the genome of *Campylobacter pylori* with a rapid extraction method: evidence for considerable genomic variation. J Infect Dis. 1988;157:465–71.
39. Morgan DD, Owen RJ. Use of DNA restriction endonuclease digest and ribosomal RNA gene probe patterns to fingerprint *Helicobacter pylori* and *Helicobacter mustelae* isolated from human and animal hosts. Mol Cell Probes. 1990;4:321–34.
40. Akopyanz N, Bukanov NO, Westblom TU, Kresovich S, Berg DE. DNA diversity among clinical isolates of *Helicobacter pylori* detected by PCR-based RAPD fingerprinting. Nucl Acids Res. 1992;20:5137–42.
41. Simor AE, Shames B, Drumm B, Sherman P, Low DE, Penner JL. Typing of *Campylobacter*

pylori by bacterial DNA restriction endonuclease analysis and determination of plasmid profile. J Clin Microbiol. 1990;28:83–6.

42. Foxall PA, Hu LT, Mobley HL. Use of polymerase chain reaction-amplified *Helicobacter pylori* urease structural genes for differentiation of isolates. J Clin Microbiol. 1992;30: 739–41.

43. Yoshimura HH, Evans DG, Graham DY. DNA–DNA hybridization demonstrates apparent genetic differences between *Helicobacter pylori* from patients with duodenal ulcer and asymptomatic gastritis. Dig Dis Sci. 1993;38:1128–31.

44. Go MF, Chan KY, Versalovic J, Koeuth T, Graham DY, Lupski JR. DNA fingerprinting of *H. pylori* genomes with repetitive DNA sequence-based PCR (REP-PCR). Gastroenterology. 1993;104:A2401(abstract).

45. Go MF, Tran L, Chan KY, Versalovic J, Kocuth T, Graham DY, Lupski JR. REP-PCR fingerprint analysis reveals gastroduodenal disease-specific clusters of *H. pylori* strains. Am J Gastroenterol. 1993;88:1591.

40
H. pylori and gastric ulcer disease

K. SEPPÄLÄ

INTRODUCTION

It is well known that duodenal ulcer and gastric ulcer are associated with chronic gastritis. *Helicobacter pylori* causes chronic gastritis and its pathogenic role has been confirmed in active chronic gastritis, because after successful eradication therapy of *H. pylori* infection, active granulocytic gastritis disappears rapidly[1]. Eradication of *H. pylori* infection leads to healed or improved chronic gastritis, but this process is slower than has been assumed earlier[2,3].

Many people have *H. pylori* infection, but only a small portion of all infected individuals get peptic ulcer. What really happens in the gastritic stomach before a peptic ulcer has developed is not known. The long-term risk of peptic ulcer was investigated in two studies. Sipponen *et al.*[4] showed that gastritis precedes ulceration. In this 10-year follow-up study of 336 individuals without previous peptic ulcer, with or without gastritis, it was found that, during follow-up, peptic ulcer had developed in one of 133 patients with normal histology but in 29 of 233 (12.4%) with chronic gastritis. The second study was presented in 1993 at the Boston DDW where Cullen *et al.*[5] showed that *H. pylori* infection preceded the development of peptic ulcer. Their results indicated that, during an 18-year follow-up of 407 subjects, peptic ulcer developed in 30 of 157 (19%) serologically *H. pylori*-positive subjects, but only to 11 of 250 (4%) subjects which were originally *H. pylori*-negative.

The aetiology of peptic ulcer is multifactorial and, despite the fact that the therapy is the same, there exist unquestionable differences between duodenal and gastric ulcers. Eradication of *H. pylori* enhances duodenal ulcer healing and greatly reduces the ulcer relapse rate. Recently two reports have shed light on gastric acid output before and after eradication of *H. pylori* infection. Moss and Calam[6] showed that eradication of *H. pylori* significantly decreases basal acid secretion in duodenal ulcer patients. El Omar and co-workers[7] proved that eradication of *H. pylori* lowers gastrin-mediated acid secretion by two-thirds in duodenal ulcer patients. These types of mechanisms have not been studied in *H. pylori*-positive gastric ulcer patients but studies should be done.

The role of *H. pylori* infection in gastric ulcer is less known and less studied than in duodenal ulcer disease. It is known that if chronic gastritis persists a long time, moderate or severe chronic gastritis with intestinal metaplasia and glandular atrophy are common features. Gastritis is shown to be antral dominant in duodenal ulcers, but in gastric ulcer patients there is usually chronic pangastritis with intestinal metaplasia and some grade glandular atrophy in the corpus mucosa[8]. Stomach peptic ulceration occurs in weakened gastric mucosa. We also know that patients with peptic gastric ulcer are, on average, more than 10 years older than patients with duodenal ulcer[8]. Except in the prepyloric area (where the ulcer is more like duodenal ulcer), the peptic gastric ulcers may be located anywhere in the stomach, and occur in border areas of intestinalized gastric areas.

THE FREQUENCY OF *H. PYLORI*-POSITIVE GASTRIC ULCERS

H. pylori infection is not always associated with gastric ulcer. According to Barry Marshall the two main causes of gastric ulcer are *H. pylori* in 70% of cases and NSAID in 30%[10]. The percentage of *H. pylori* infection varies, the range of *H. pylori* infection rates was 59–86% among nine studies consisting of 290 gastric ulcer patients[11]. In some initial studies the biopsies for *H. pylori* were taken only from antrum, and this might have had an effect on the results. For reliable diagnosis of *H. pylori* infection, several biopsies (also from corpus) and other diagnostic methods need to be used. However, if intestinal metaplasia is widespread, false-negative biopsies can occur. There is some earlier evidence that the rate of *H. pylori* infection is low. In the first Finnish study the infection rate was 59% of 33 gastric ulcer patients[12]. A recent study from our hospital showed a 92% infection rate of 170 gastric ulcer cases. In another Finnish study from 10 different hospitals, consisting of 276 gastric ulcer patients, the infection rate was 82% with a range of 55–93% (unpublished results). It is still obvious that, around the world, there are differences in the occurrence of *H. pylori*-positivity in gastric ulcer patients, and this is important to remember.

Today the determination of *H. pylori* infection is mandatory in peptic gastric ulcer. This is necessary because the appropriate therapy can be different, for example, in *H. pylori*-negative and -positive gastric ulcers. We know that in stomach there is a NSAID-induced subgroup of gastric ulcer which is not related to *H. pylori*; but it is often found that NSAID use is common with peptic gastric ulcer patients and, therefore, the role of NSAID in each peptic ulcer can be estimated only after eradication of *H. pylori* in those who are positive[13].

THE TREATMENT OF *H. PYLORI* INFECTION IN GASTRIC ULCER

It is logical to assume that the eradication of *H. pylori* has a positive effect on healing and reduces the relapse rate in gastric ulcer patients, but there are few data available. In a study of 43 individuals with *H. pylori*-positive gastric ulcers, patients were randomized to receive 12 weeks treatment with either cimetidine or cimetidine plus cefixime in the last 2 weeks of therapy[14]. Healing rate was similar in the two groups, but there was a significantly lower recurrence rate at 12 weeks after finishing treatment in the dual-therapy group. Ulcer recurrence was, however, the same in the two groups at 24 weeks. It was also noted that this single therapy was not effective in eradication of *H. pylori*.

Since 1991 there have been only a few studies in which *H. pylori*-positive gastric ulcer patients have been treated with effective eradication therapy. In our study, patients received dual therapy, but later patients have been given other more effective triple or quadruple therapy. The early results of our own Finnish Gastric Ulcer Study Group were presented in abstracts and suggested first, that the eradication of *H. pylori* improves the healing of gastric ulcers[15] and secondly that the relapse rate is significantly lower in the patients having *H. pylori* eradication[16].

Graham *et al.*[17] recently presented their randomized, controlled peptic ulcer study where 109 patients infected with *H. pylori* received either ranitidine or ranitidine plus triple therapy. Successful eradication of *H. pylori* reduced the rate of ulcer recurrence not only in 83 duodenal ulcer patients but also in 26 gastric ulcer patients. Our open *H. pylori*-positive gastritis study included 101 peptic ulcer patients who received triple therapy. In the 12 months follow-up, 13 gastric ulcer patients of a total number of 16 included in the study had no relapses[18].

In the 'German gastric ulcer study' relapse rates during a mean follow-up period of 12 months were 51% in patients who received omeprazole alone, and 35 in patients with triple therapy. Patients were included in the study irrespective of the presence of *H. pylori*, and/or the intake of any ulcerogenic medication such as NSAID, ASA or steroids. Relapses occurred either in patients who remained *H. pylori*-positive or were *H. pylori*-negative before treatment[19]. Börsch and his co-workers have also studied the efficacy of various treatment regimens to eradicate *H. pylori* in *H. pylori*-associated ulcer disease or severe functional dyspepsia. They concluded that omeprazole-enhanced amoxicillin treatment is a simple and effective approach to the eradication of *H. pylori* colonization[20]. They have also followed 50 healed gastric ulcer patients for one year. *H. pylori* eradication (successful in 32 patients) was associated with significant reduction of ulcer recurrences (3.1% versus 55.6%, $p < 0.001$)[21].

THE FOLLOW-UP STUDY OF THE FINNISH GASTRIC ULCER STUDY GROUP

The Finnish Prospective Multicenter Gastric Ulcer Study was carried out to investigate whether eradication of *H. pylori* was an important factor in the healing and in the relapse rate in *H. pylori*-positive gastric ulcers. The trial consisted of 231 *H. pylori*-positive gastric ulcer patients. Patients with gastric ulcers located in corpus or antrum (more than 2 cm from the pyloric

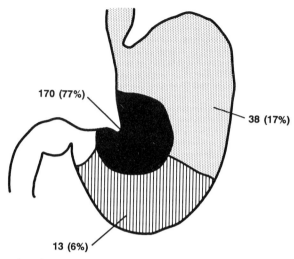

Fig. 1 The location of 221 index ulcers (77% at the angulus, 38% high ulcers or in the greater curvature, 6% in antrum)

ring; ulcer size 5–30 mm) were randomly assigned to three study groups. Group A was given DeNol (240 mg BID) for 8 weeks, together with metronidazole (400 mg TID) or group B DeNol (as in group A) and placebo for the first 10 days. Group C received ranitidine 150 mg BID (for 8 weeks) plus placebo. The outcome in the *H. pylori*-positive or -negative patients was compared by *H. pylori* assessment using endoscopy in weeks 0, 12, 33 and 52.

A total of 231 patients entered, and 203 were available for efficacy analysis. The remaining 28 patients were protocol violations, dropouts or withdrawals.

The great majority of ulcers, 170 (77%) were located at the angulus area of the lesser curvature, 13 (6%) in antrum (at least 2 cm from pylorus) and 38 (17%) high ulcers or in the greater curvature in the corpus (Fig. 1). Two hundred (90.5%) of the patients had peptic ulcer previously, or before admission to the study. Sixty-three (28.5%) of the patients had taken ASA or NSAID (more than once a week). Prior bleeding, or bleeding just before hospital admission, occurred in 36 (15%) of these patients.

The compliance was determined at 4 and 8 weeks when each patient returned his or her allotted medication.

The gastric ulcer status of 203 patients at the 12-week control is presented in Table 1. The results showed that eradication of *H. pylori* significantly ($p < 0.05$) improves the healing of gastric ulcer. The influence of *H. pylori* eradication on the cumulative number of gastric ulcer relapses at the 33- and 52-week control for 159 gastric ulcer patients is presented in Table 2. One-year follow-up results showed that the relapse rate is significantly lower ($p < 0.001$) in the patients having *H. pylori* eradication.

Table 1 The gastric ulcer status of 203 patients at 12-week control

	H. pylori-*positive*		H. pylori-*negative*		
	n	(%)	n	(%)	Total
Ulcer present (left or relapse)	42	(24)	2	(7)*	44
No ulcer	133	(76)	26	(92)	159
Total	175		28		203

*p < 0.05

Table 2 One year follow-up results of 159 gastric ulcer patients comparing the number of cumulative relapses to *H. pylori* status (44 patients with gastric ulcer at 12 weeks excluded)

	H. pylori-*positive*		H. pylori-*negative*		
	n	(%)	n	(%)	Total
Ulcer relapse	63	(47)	0		63
No ulcer relapse	70	(53)	26	(100)*	96
Total	133		26		159

*p < 0.001

THE OPEN TRIPLE THERAPY

Open triple therapy (CBS, metronidazole and amoxicillin) was offered to patients with unhealed ulcers or with ulcer relapse at 12 weeks or later. To date, 94 patients with unhealed gastric ulcers or gastric ulcer relapses have received open triple therapy. The *H. pylori* eradication was successful in 65 patients (69%). Of these, 52 patients with successful eradication have been followed for one year and only one patient (NSAID-user) had an ulcer relapse.

DISCUSSION

The mechanisms causing 'peptic gastric ulcer' are clearly associated with *H. pylori* infection but *H. pylori* gastritis-related changes in antral and corpus physiology may also influence the development of peptic gastric ulcer. Regarding defence mechanisms, the antral mucosa is obviously dissimilar to corpus mucosa. Antral HCO_3 secretion through the mucosa to mucus can be important to prevent damage caused by acid in antrum but less important in corpus. This dissimilarity has been demonstrated in *Necturus* where antrum has a 'leaky' epithelium but corpus mucosa has 'tight' epithelium[22].

The model of receptor-mediated functions in gastric fundic parietal cells has new aspects which are linked with *H. pylori* infection. Mezey and Palkovits[23] have provided evidence for the concept that the locus of the receptors is the inflammatory cells in the lamina propria. In particular, macrophages and plasma cells showed detectable messenger RNA for histamine, muscarinic and gastric receptors, in addition to dopamine receptors. In contrast none of the epithelial cells expressed any of these mRNA. The authors suggested that nitric oxide might mediate the interaction between immune and epithelial cells, and concluded that their results may provide new ideas concerning ulcer pathogenesis. It is known that *H. pylori* infection, among other effects, stimulates gastrin and pepsinogen secretion, activates neutrophils and basophils, and releases oxygen radicals from granulocytes[24]. By causing inflammatory changes, *H. pylori* infection may play a role in acid secretion and in ulcer formation. Because there are different mechanisms behind the development of the two types of peptic ulcers, the inflammation-related changes of gastric functions can be more important in stomach than in duodenum.

Though the mechanism of *H. pylori*-positive gastric ulcer is not clear, it is obvious that successful eradication of *H. pylori* will change the natural history of gastric and duodenal ulcers; that is, the disease is cured, and the risk of ulcer recurrence and complications is virtually eliminated. Eradication of *H. pylori* reduces (and possibly eliminates) recurrent rebleeding in patients who have a bleeding ulcer, as shown by Graham's group[25].

The frequency of *H. pylori* infection in gastric ulcer varies greatly (50–95%). This can be at least partly explained by a diagnostic failure due to intestinal metaplasia and biopsy sampling. If the diagnosis is done with the aid of *H. pylori* culture, histology and serology, the infection rate is shown to be even greater than 90%. Successful *H. pylori* eradication accelerates the healing of not only duodenal, but also gastric cancer. As in duodenal ulcer, the marked reduction in relapse rate of gastric ulcer is solely due to *H. pylori* eradication. This supports the dominant role of *H. pylori* in gastric ulcer disease. The low therapeutic efficacy of our dual therapy (33%) can be explained by a high frequency of metronidazole-resistant *H. pylori* strains in Finland[26]. Better results were obtained with triple (or quadruple) therapy in the study.

Eradication of *H. pylori* can reverse inflammation-related abnormalities in the stomach. It is therefore reasonable to begin long-term prospective *H. pylori* eradication studies to determine the effects upon cancer incidence in high-risk populations from developed countries where the *H. pylori* reinfection rate is low.

In conclusion, all new data demonstrate that *H. pylori* eradication significantly improves gastric ulcer healing and prevents ulcer relapse. Therefore, the eradication therapy is strongly indicated in *H. pylori*-positive gastric ulcer.

SUMMARY

Despite the fact that the frequency of *Helicobacter* infection varies in different parts of the world, the great majority of duodenal and gastric ulcers are associated with *H. pylori*-positive chronic gastritis. Eradication of *H. pylori* enhances duodenal ulcer healing and greatly reduces the ulcer relapse rate. Gastritis is more persistent and severe in gastric ulcer patients than in duodenal ulcer patients; however, it seems that the effect of eradication therapy of *H. pylori* in gastric ulcer is similar. In the randomized, double-blind Finnish Gastric Ulcer Study of 203 *H. pylori*-positive gastric ulcer patients the successful eradication of *H. pylori* infection resulted in both (1) better ulcer healing and (2) a reduced ulcer relapse rate than in *H. pylori*-positive patients, who had unsuccessful eradication or only ranitidine therapy.

These results indicate that in the diagnosis of gastric ulcer one must always consider the association of chronic gastritis with *H. pylori* infection. Complications are a major risk factor in gastric ulcer disease and, therefore, we have to recognize the importance of antibiotics in the therapy of *H. pylori*-positive ulcer patients. The primary treatment can begin with *H. pylori* eradication therapy and H_2-receptor antagonists or proton pump inhibitors.

References

1. Rauws EAJ, Langenberg W, Houthoff HJ, Zanen HC, Tytgat GNJ. *Campylobacter pyloridis*-associated chronic active antral gastritis: a prospective study of its prevalence and the effects of antibacterial and antiulcer treatment. Gastroenterology. 1988;94:229–38.
2. Valle J, Seppälä K, Sipponen P, Kosunen T. Disappearance of gastritis after eradication of *Helicobacter pylori*. A morphometric study. Scand J Gastroenterol. 1991;26:1057–65.
3. Seppälä K, Sipponen P, Kosunen TU. Do changes in gastritis and serum antibodies reflect successful triple therapy in *Helicobacter pylori* infection? 1993; DDW abstract 2367. Gastroenterology. 1993;104(Suppl.):A189.
4. Sipponen P, Varis K, Fräki O *et al.* Cumulative 10-year risk of symptomatic duodenal and gastric ulcer in patients with or without chronic gastritis. Scand J Gastroenterol. 1990;25:966–73.
5. Cullen DJE, Collins BJ, Christiansen KJ *et al.* Long term risk of peptic ulcer disease in people with *Helicobacter pylori* infection – a community based study. 1993; DDW abstract 1861. Gastroenterology. 1993;104(Suppl.):A60.
6. Moss SF, Calam J. Acid secretion and sensitivity to gastrin in patients with duodenal ulcer: effect of eradication of *Helicobacter pylori*. Gut. 1993;34:888–92.
7. El-Omar E, Penman I, Dorrian CA, Ardill JES, McColl KEL. Eradicating *Helicobacter pylori* infection lowers gastrin-mediated acid secretion by two-thirds in duodenal ulcer patients. Gut. 1993;34:1060–5.
8. Sipponen P, Seppälä K, Äärynen M, Helske T, Kettunen P. Chronic gastritis and gastroduodenal ulcer: a case control study on risk of coexisting duodenal or gastric ulcer in patients with gastritis. Gut. 1989;30:922–9.
9. Kekki M, Sipponen P, Siurala M, Laszewicz W. Peptic ulcer and chronic gastritis: their relation to age and sex, and to location of ulcer and gastritis. Gastroenterol Clin Biol. 1990;14:217–23.
10. Marshall BJ. Treatment of *Helicobacter pylori*. In: Marshall BJ, McCallum RW, Ruerrant RL, editors. *Helicobacter pylori* in peptic ulceration and gastritis. Oxford: Blackwell Scientific Publications; 1991:160–86.
11. O'Connor HJ, Axon ATR. *Campylobacter pylori*, gastric ulceration and the post-operative stomach. In: Rathbone BJ, Heatley RV, editors. *Campylobacter pylori* and gastroduodenal disease. Oxford: Blackwell Scientific Publications; 1989:125–38.
12. Niemelä S, Karttunen T, Lehtola J. *Campylobacter*-like organisms in patients with gastric ulcer. Scand J Gastroenterol. 1987;22:487–90.
13. Graham DY. Treatment of peptic ulcers caused by *Helicobacter pylori* (Editorial). N Engl J Med. 1993;328:349–50.
14. Tatsuta M, Ishikawa H, Iishi H, Okuda S, Yokota Y. Reduction of gastric ulcer recurrence after suppression of *Helicobacter pylori* by cefixime. Gut. 1990;31:973–6.
15. Seppälä K, Pikkarainen P, Karvonen A-L, Lehtola J, Gormsen MH, the FGUSG. A double-blind study to compare the efficacy of De-Nol in combination with metronidazole versus De-Nol or ranitidine in combination with methonidazole placebo in the treatment of gastric ulcers. Hepato-Gastroenterology 1991; Abstracts of the European Digestive Disease Week. EDDW abstract No. 175.
16. Seppälä K, Pikkarainen P, Karvonen A-L, Gormsen MH, the FGUSG. The role of

Helicobacter pylori (Hp) eradication in gastric ulcer healing and relapses. 1992; DDW abstract No. 1043. Gastroenterology. 1992;102(Suppl.):A162.

17. Graham DY, Lew GM, Klein PD *et al.* Effect of treatment of *Helicobacter pylori* infection on the long-term recurrence of gastric or duodenal ulcer. Ann Intern Med. 1992;116: 705–8.

18. Seppälä K, Färkkilä M, Nuutinen H *et al.* Triple therapy of *Helicobacter pylori* infection in peptic ulcer. Scand J Gastroenterol. 1992;27:973–6.

19. Bayerdörffer E, Mannes GA, Höchter W *et al.* Antibacterial treatment of gastric ulcers – German Gastric Ulcer Study. 1993; DDW abstract No. 2382. Gastroenterology. 1993;104(Suppl.):A40.

20. Labentz J, Gyenes E, Ruhl GH, Börsch G. Omeprazole plus amoxicillin: efficacy of various treatment regimens to eradicate *Helicobacter pylori*. Am J Gastroenterol. 1993;88:491–5.

21. Labentz J, Börsch G. Role of *H. pylori* in gastric ulcer disease. VII workshop on *Campylobacter, Helicobacter* and related organisms. Brussels Joint Meeting. 1993 (abstract).

22. Kiviluoto T, Mustonen H, Kivilaakso E. The defence mechanisms against intracellular acidosis induced by luminal acid are different in gastric antral and corpus mucosa. DDW, Boston, 1993; abstract No. 1957. Gastroenterology. 1993;104(Suppl.):A119.

23. Mezey E, Palkovits M. Localization of targets for anti-ulcer drugs in cells of the immune system. Science. 1992;258:1662–5.

24. Vaira D, Holton J, Miglioli M, Mule P, Menegatti M, Barbara L. *Helicobacter pylori* and other spiral organisms in gastroduodenal disease. Curr Opinion Gastroenterol. 1992;8: 918–26.

25. Hepps KS, Ramirez FC, Lew GM, Saeed ZA, Graham DY. Treatment of *H. pylori* reduces the rate of rebleeding in complicated peptic ulcer disease. Gastrointest Endosc. 1992;38:234(abstract).

26. Rautelin H, Seppälä K, Renkonen O-V, Vainio U, Kosunen TU. Role of metronidazole resistance in therapy of *Helicobacter pylori* infections. Antimicrob Agents Chemother. 1992;36:163–6.

41
Functional dyspepsia and *H. pylori*: a controversial link

N. J. TALLEY

INTRODUCTION

Dyspepsia can be defined as persistent or recurrent pain or discomfort localized to the upper abdomen, which may or may not be related to meals[1,2]. Dyspepsia accounts for 2–3% of all consultations in general practice, and for 20–40% of all gastrointestinal consultations[3]. A substantial proportion of patients who present for diagnostic evaluation of dyspepsia are not found to have evidence of chronic peptic ulceration, reflux oesophagitis, malignancy, gallstones or the irritable bowel syndrome, and such patients have been labelled as having functional (or non-ulcer) dyspepsia[1,2].

ASSOCIATION OF *H. PYLORI* WITH DYSPEPSIA

The pathogenesis of functional dyspepsia remains uncertain, although abnormalities of visceral perception, motor dysfunction and gastritis or duodenitis have been all considered candidates[1,2]. It is likely that a constellation of factors lead to the development of dyspepsia (Fig. 1); as approximately 50% of patients with functional dyspepsia have *H. pylori* gastritis, it is a reasonable hypothesis that *H. pylori* is one of the component causes, but this is controversial[4–7]. To establish that *H. pylori* is a causal factor requires evidence that this infection is truly associated with functional dyspepsia, that infection precedes the development of symptoms, and that symptoms are abolished by eradication of the infection[5,7]. Unfortunately, the evidence for an aetiological link is equivocal.

H. PYLORI AND ACUTE DYSPEPSIA

Anecdotal evidence suggests that *H. pylori* infection can induce self-limited dyspeptic symptoms. The ingestion experiments of Marshall *et al.*[8] and Morris *et al.*[9] have represented the best-documented examples. While it is

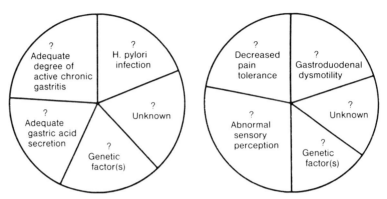

Fig. 1 Hypothetical schema of two groups of sufficient causes for functional dyspepsia. Each sufficient cause comprises by definition a set of minimal events that inevitably produce disease. Note if any component were to be missing (e.g. *H. pylori* in the model on the right), functional dyspepsia would not occur. Also note that functional dyspepsia can occur in the absence of *H. pylori* if other causes are all present (model on the left). From ref. 7, with permission

impossible to exclude factors other than the infection as being related to symptom development, there is general consensus that acute *H. pylori* infection produces a short-lived illness with features that have in the past been attributed to viral gastroenteritis[10]. However, despite the persistence of the infection and development of chronic gastritis, symptoms usually completely resolved in these cases[9,10].

PREVALENCE OF *H. PYLORI* IN FUNCTIONAL DYSPEPSIA COMPARED WITH CONTROLS

Several studies have suggested that *H. pylori* infection is more common in patients with functional dyspepsia than asymptomatic controls, but others have failed to confirm these observations (Table 1)[11-18]. Unfortunately, the control groups utilized in these studies have often been inadequate. For example, comparing outpatients to community controls is not applicable, as referral bias could have resulted in the detection of higher rates of infection in outpatients. Furthermore, some of these studies have not adjusted for confounders such as age, socioeconomic status and ethnicity, which are all strongly linked to the prevalence of *H. pylori* infection[10]. In addition, only one dyspeptic in four sees a physician; the decision to consult is likely to be associated with factors other than symptom status (e.g. psychological distress) that may confound aetiological studies. Thus, studies in outpatients may be misleading.

Population-based studies are less prone to bias and are therefore preferable when examining for true associations. Several population-based studies have examined the relationship between *H. pylori* and chronic dyspepsia. Holtmann *et al.* evaluated 180 blood donors and assessed the relationship between dyspepsia and *H. pylori* infection in this population[19]. It was found that

Table 1 *H. pylori* infection in adult patients with functional dyspepsia and controls

Study/reference	Country	Functional dyspepsia H. pylori-*positive* (%)		Controls H. pylori-*positive* (%)	
		Mean age (*n*)	*Percentage* H. pylori-*positive*	*Mean age* (*n*)	*Percentage* H. pylori-*positive*
Pettross et al.[11]	United States	47 (48)	50	29 (15)	13
Rokkas et al.[12]	United Kingdom	41 (55)	45	40 (15)	13
Rauws et al.[13]	Netherlands	56 (240)	68	38 (34)	21
Lambert et al.[14]	Australia	42 (82)	61	Age-matched	
					25
Strauss et al.[15]	United States	51 (37)	60	45 (24)	25
Inouye et al.[16]	Japan	51 (27)	70	49 (20)	55
Collins et al.[17]	Ireland	36 (20)	56	32 (9)	60
Gutiérrez et al.[18]	Colombia	? (34)	79	? (15)	87

n = Number of patients or controls
? = Unknown

upper gastrointestinal tract symptoms were just as common in those with and without the infection, and adjusting for potential confounders such as age and socioeconomic status did not alter the results. However, blood donors may not be representative of the general population and thus these findings are not conclusive. In a study from Olmsted County, Minnesota, USA, where subjects with dyspepsia and healthy controls were randomly selected from the population and tested for *H. pylori* antibodies, only 18% with dyspepsia were infected compared with 12% of controls (G.R. Locke and N.J. Talley, personal communication). In a rural monastic settlement in southern India, similarly no relationship was found between *H. pylori* infection and the presence of dyspepsia in a random sample of male monks that was examined[20]. Al-Moagel *et al.* evaluated symptoms and *H. pylori* antibody levels in a random population sample from Saudi Arabia; 66% of persons who were asymptomatic and 67% of dyspeptic subjects had *H. pylori* infection[21]. In a cross-sectional study of persons with dyspepsia and controls matched for age and gender who agreed to be endoscoped in a town in northern Norway, *H. pylori* infection was found in 48% with functional dysp~psia and in 36% of controls; the authors concluded that a relationship between *H. pylori* and dyspepsia was dubious[22].

TEMPORAL ASSOCIATION BETWEEN INFECTION AND THE ONSET OF DYSPEPSIA

Evidence that *H. pylori* infection precedes the onset of chronic dyspepsia would strongly suggest that there is a true causal link between these conditions. Parsonnet *et al.* evaluated 341 epidemiologists in a historical cohort study where stored serum samples were tested for *H. pylori* infection. They found that symptoms were experienced similarly by *H. pylori* infected and uninfected subjects, but 11 persons who seroconverted in the interval

Table 2 Symptoms associated with *H. pylori*-positive functional dyspepsia in published studies

Author/reference	Functional dyspepsia (n)	H. pylori- positive (%)	Individual symptom(s) associated with H. pylori*
Marshall and Warren[24]	65	58	'Burping'
Rokkas et al.[12]	55	45	Postprandial bloating
Andersen et al.[25]	33	39	Nil except symptom duration
Deltenre et al.[26]	200	64	'Ulcer-like' symptoms
Tucci et al.[27]	45	60	Epigastric pain or burning more frequent and severe
Börsch et al.[28]	69	52	Flatulence, a *negative* predictor
Sobala et al.[29]	186	41	Nil
Collins et al.[30]	18	50	Nil
Vaira et al.[31]	107	58	Postprandial bloating
Goh et al.[32]	71	56	Nil
Waldron et al.[33]	50	36	Nil
Strauss et al.[15]	37	60	Nil
Kemmer et al.[34]	149	51	Pain relief after food
Schubert et al.[35]	474	36	Nil

*Significant differences between functional dyspepsia patients with and without *H. pylori*

years from being negative to positive for *H. pylori* antibodies were four times more likely to have had upper abdominal symptoms[23]. These results suggest that if symptoms are associated with *H. pylori* infection they are generally self-limited, although the findings remain to be confirmed.

SPECIFIC SYMPTOMS AND SYMPTOM PROFILES IN *H. PYLORI*-POSITIVE FUNCTIONAL DYSPEPSIA COMPARED WITH UNINFECTED PATIENTS

A number of studies[12,16,17,24–35] have attempted to link specific symptoms to patients who have *H. pylori* and functional dyspepsia. Most have failed to find an association (Table 2). In the largest of the studies, for example, Schubert *et al.* evaluated 474 consecutive patients presenting for endoscopy; neither the activity of the gastritis nor the presence of *H. pylori* was associated with pain, nausea, bloating, belching, heartburn, vomiting, flatulence or halitosis[35]. On the other hand, some investigators have found that certain symptoms were more frequent in those with *H. pylori* infection[12,24,27,31,34], but the types of symptoms have been very variable, which probably reflects the presence of unrecognized bias. Unfortunately, individual symptom assessment in most of these studies was undertaken using measures that were not tested for their validity.

Functional dyspepsia is probably a heterogeneous syndrome, and a classification of patients with this disorder has been advanced based on clusters of symptoms[1]. Thus, it has been proposed that one subgroup of patients with functional dyspepsia have symptoms suggestive of peptic ulcer disease (e.g. epigastric pain related to meals, pain at night waking them from sleep) even though no ulcer crater is identifiable, while another subgroup have symptoms suggestive of a gastroduodenal motility disturbance (e.g.

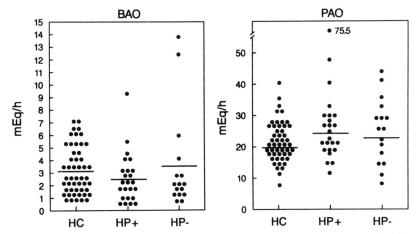

Fig. 2 Basal and peak acid outputs in *H. pylori*-positive and -negative patients with functional dyspepsia. BAO = Basal acid output; PAO = peak acid output; HC = healthy controls; HP = *H. pylori*. Data from ref. 27, with permission

nausea, early satiety, upper abdominal bloating). Although one study found an association between ulcer-like symptoms and *H. pylori* infection[26], other reports have been unable to confirm these findings in outpatients[33] or blood donors[19].

MECHANISMS LINKING *H. PYLORI* AND DYSPEPSIA

There is currently no clear-cut mechanism that could explain how *H. pylori* might induce symptoms in one person and remain a totally asymptomatic infection in another person. Most patients with functional dyspepsia have normal levels of acid secretion, and acid secretion is not different in infected and uninfected patients[27,36] (Fig. 2). There is also no convincing evidence that symptoms correlate with the degree of active gastritis, although conflicting results have been reported[35,37–39].

The possible relationship between *H. pylori* infection and gastric motility remains confusing. While some investigators have detected decreased gastric function in gastritis[40], other studies suggest that *H. pylori* either does not induce motor disturbances[27,41–43] or accelerates gastric motility[44] (Table 3). However, none have carefully evaluated whether motility changes occur in patients following eradication of *H. pylori* and complete healing of the antral gastritis, which is the key experiment.

RANDOMIZED CONTROLLED TRIALS AND SYMPTOM RESOLUTION

Anti-*H. pylori* treatment applied in carefully conducted randomized controlled trials should be able to establish whether or not *H. pylori* infection

Table 3 Gastrointestinal motility in functional dyspepsia and *H. pylori* infection

Study/reference	Abnormality
Delayed	
Moore *et al.*[40]	Postprandial antral hypomotility in chronic gastritis; *H. pylori* not assessed
No difference	
Wegener *et al.*[41]	No significant difference among *H. pylori*-infected and uninfected patients
Barnett *et al.*[42]	Normal gastric emptying in *H. pylori*-infected patients
Tucci *et al.*[27]	Normal gastric emptying in *H. pylori*-infected patients
Pieramico *et al.*[43]	Antral motility not significantly different in *H. pylori*-infected and uninfected patients
Accelerated	
Caldwell *et al.*[44]	Accelerated gastric emptying in *H. pylori*-infected patients

is a cause of dyspepsia. One would predict that, if *H. pylori* was eradicated and gastritis resolved, then symptoms should be substantially reduced on long-term follow-up if *H. pylori* is an important causal factor; it would be most convincing if symptoms were actually abolished entirely (Fig. 1).

A number of trials have tested the effect of suppressing (rather than eradicating) *H. pylori* in functional dyspepsia[14,32,45–54] (Table 4). Unfortunately, all of these studies have suffered from design flaws that make interpretation of the data difficult. Most of the studies have utilized bismuth alone. However, many patients who take bismuth compounds can immediately recognize they are on drug because of the development of black stools and black tongue; therefore, blinding of both patients and investigators is very difficult in such a situation. The development of placebo compounds that can induce black stools may be helpful in future studies[55]. Another problem with all of the trials has been the adequacy with which symptoms have been measured. Some trials have failed to detect statistically significant differences in symptom scores between bismuth and placebo; other studies have found significant results, but the absolute improvement in symptoms has generally been small (Table 4). Adequate long-term follow-up was not undertaken in these studies; therefore it is unclear whether any initial benefit would have persisted with recrudescence of the infection.

Few studies have investigated the effects of eradicating *H. pylori* infection, and here again the results have been conflicting. Talley *et al.* evaluated triple therapy in a randomized, double-blind placebo-controlled trial; although active chronic gastritis resolved, symptoms changed very little, but the trial only included seven patients[56]. Sabbatini *et al.* evaluated 52 patients with functional dyspepsia and antral gastritis[57]. Colloidal bismuth subcitrate with amoxicillin or this regimen plus metronidazole was prescribed in a non-randomized, non-placebo-controlled study. They found that symptoms relapsed in 69% of the patients within 1 year even though most of these patients (72%) continued to be free of *H. pylori* infection after eradication; these authors concluded that any symptomatic improvement in the short term achieved with eradication therapy may not be due to treatment of the *H. pylori* infection itself. Bianchi Porro *et al.* randomized 46 patients to either

Table 4 Published randomized, double-blind, placebo-controlled trials of anti-H. pylori therapy for functional dyspepsia

Author, year/reference	n	Drug regimen	Percentage suppression H. pylori by active therapy	Results (symptom response)*
McNulty et al., 1986[45]	50	BSS/4 weeks	78	Negative
		Erythromycin/2 weeks	7	Negative
Rokkas et al., 1988[46]	52	CBS/8 weeks	83	Positive
Glupczynski et al., 1988[52]	45	Amoxicillin/8 days	91	Negative
Gastroenterology Physiology Working Group, 1988[53]	69	Nitrofurantoin/2 weeks	58	Negative
		Furazolidone/2 weeks	86	Negative
Lambert et al., 1989[14]	82	CBS/4 weeks	59	Positive
Loffeld et al., 1989[47]	50	CBS/4 weeks	30	Negative
Kang et al., 1989[48]	51	CBS/8 weeks	89	Positive
Kazi et al., 1990[49]	52	BSS/3 weeks	77	Positive
Goh et al., 1991[32]	71	CBS/4 weeks	81	Positive
Vaira et al., 1992[50]	80	CBS/4 weeks	67	Positive
Nafeeza et al., 1992[51]	48	CBS/4 weeks	13	Negative
		CBS/4 weeks plus ampicillin/10 days	86	Positive
		Ampicillin/10 days	0	Negative
Marshall et al., 1993[54]	50	BSS/3 weeks	70	Negative
Frazzoni et al., 1993[61]	20	CBS/4 weeks plus metronidazole/10 days	71†	Negative

BSS = bismuth subsalicylate; CBS = colloidal bismuth subcitrate
*Positive symptom response = statistically significant improvement vs. placebo of one (or more) symptoms or the total symptom score
†Eradication

colloidal bismuth alone or colloidal bismuth plus metronidazole; there was no placebo arm. Symptom improvement occurred in 97% of patients and was not related to eradication of *H. pylori*[58]. Holcombe *et al.* randomized 130 northern Nigerian patients to antacid or colloidal bismuth plus amoxicillin[59]. Symptoms were abolished in 28 of 86 patients (33%) who received anti-*H. pylori* treatment compared with 4% on antacid, but symptom improvement failed to correlate with clearance of *H. pylori*; eradication was not assessed[59]. Bamford *et al.* also reported no significant change in symptom scores in 30 *H. pylori*-positive patients after amoxicillin and colloidal bismuth versus placebo[60]. Frazzoni *et al.* randomly assigned 20 patients to either bismuth and metronidazole or placebo; symptom reduction occurred similarly in the active and placebo groups at the end of treatment, and relapse of symptoms after a mean follow-up of 9.7 months did not occur in either group[61].

On the other hand, Patchett *et al.* evaluated 84 patients with functional dyspepsia[62]. They found in a non-randomized, non-placebo-controlled study that the symptom score improved significantly in all patients, regardless of whether *H. pylori* was eradicated or not. However, 1 year after cessation of treatment the symptom score in patients with persistent *H. pylori* infection was higher than in those who remained infection-free[63]. Petrino *et al.* provided triple therapy for 48 patients with functional dyspepsia and *H. pylori* gastritis in a non-randomized non-placebo-controlled study, and found that several symptoms diminished after a 6-month follow-up[64]. While they noted symptomatic improvement in those not successfully eradicated, it was less marked. Pretolani *et al.* evaluated 48 *H. pylori*-positive patients after triple therapy in a randomized non-placebo-controlled study with a follow-up period of 8 months, and reported a decrease in heartburn and belching, but not in other symptoms, after successful eradication[65].

Of concern, most of these eradication studies have been non-placebo-controlled and therefore positive results are almost uninterpretable, as the placebo effect may explain any benefit. The lack of randomization is also worrying because the groups may not have been strictly comparable. Unfortunately, most of the eradication studies have only been published in abstract form to date, and therefore other potential methodological limitations are difficult to assess. More conclusive evidence that eradication of *H. pylori* improves dyspepsia will require careful randomized placebo-controlled trials that preferably employ agents to eradicate the bacteria which themselves do not directly affect the mucosa. Moreover, such studies will require long-term follow-up as the gastritis can take more than 6 months to resolve after successful eradication therapy, and functional dyspepsia is typically a relapsing and remitting disorder[66]. The paucity of adequately designed trials in this area is striking, and better studies are urgently needed.

CONCLUSION

If a patient with functional dyspepsia continues to have complaints despite standard therapy, and if the patient also has *H. pylori* infection, it is unclear whether treatment of the infection will produce any real benefit. There may be a subgroup of patients who do obtain symptom relief with anti-*H. pylori* therapy, but recognition of such a group remains the challenge. While it is tempting to treat the infection in patients with functional dyspepsia, particularly as there are promising new regimens that are less toxic than triple therapy (e.g. omeprazole plus amoxicillin), until it has been more convincingly shown that patients truly benefit, anti-*H. pylori* eradication therapy should usually be reserved for the clinical trial setting.

References

1. Talley NJ, Colin-Jones D, Koch KL, Koch M, Nyrén O, Stanghellini V. Functional dyspepsia: a classification with guidelines for diagnosis and management. Gastroenterol Int. 1991;4:145–60.
2. Talley NJ, Phillips SF. Non-ulcer dyspepsia: potential causes and pathophysiology. Ann Intern Med. 1988;108:865–79.
3. Knill-Jones RP. Geographical differences in the prevalence of dyspepsia. Scand J Gastroenterol. 1991;26(Suppl.182):17–24.
4. Lambert J. The role of *Helicobacter pylori* in nonulcer dyspepsia: a debate – for. Gastroenterol Clin N Am. 1993;22:141–52.
5. Talley NJ. The role of *Helicobacter pylori* in nonulcer dyspepsia: a debate – against. Gastroenterol Clin N Am. 1993;22:153–67.
6. McQuaid KR. Endoscopy-negative dyspepsia. Hold those forceps! J Clin Gastroenterol. 1993;17:97–100.
7. Talley NJ. Is *Helicobacter pylori* a cause of non-ulcer dyspepsia? In: Malfertheiner P, Ditschuneit H, editors. *Helicobacter pylori*, gastritis, and peptic ulcer. Berlin: Springer-Verlag; 1990:361–9.
8. Marshall BJ, Armstrong JA, McGeche DB, Glancy RJ. Attempts to fulfill Koch's postulates for pyloric *Campylobacter*. Med J Aust. 1985;142:436–9.
9. Morris AJ, Ali MR, Nicholson GI, Perez-Perez GI, Blaser MJ. Long-term follow-up of voluntary ingestion of *Helicobacter pylori*. Ann Intern Med. 1991;114:662–3.
10. Talley NJ, Noack KB. The world-wide prevalence of *Helicobacter pylori*: asymptomatic infection and clinical states associated with infection in adults. In: Goodwin CS, Worsley BW, editors. *Helicobacter pylori*: biology and clinical practice. Boca Raton: CRC Press; 1993:63–83.
11. Pettross CW, Appleman MD, Cohen H, Valenzuela JE, Chandrasoma P, Laine LA. Prevalence of *Campylobacter pylori* and association with antral mucosal histology in subjects with and without upper gastrointestinal symptoms. Dig Dis Sci. 1988;33:649–53.
12. Rokkas T, Pursey C, Uzoechina E et al. *Campylobacter pylori* and non-ulcer dyspepsia. Am J Gastroenterol. 1987;82:1149–52.
13. Rauws EA, Langenberg W, Houthoff HJ, Zanes HC, Tytgat GNJ. *Campylobacter pyloridis*-associated chronic active antral gastritis: a prospective study of its prevalence and the effects of antibacterial and antiulcer treatment. Gastroenterology. 1988;94:33–40.
14. Lambert JR, Dunn K, Borromeo M, Korman MG, Hansky J. *Campylobacter pylori* – a role in non-ulcer dyspepsia? Scand J Gastroenterol Suppl. 1989;160:7–13.
15. Strauss RM, Wang TC, Kelsey PB et al. Association of *Helicobacter pylori* infection with dyspeptic symptoms in patients undergoing gastroduodenoscopy. Am J Med. 1990;89:464–9.
16. Inouye H, Yamamoto I, Tanida N et al. *Campylobacter pylori* in Japan: bacteriological feature and prevalence in healthy subjects and patients with gastroduodenal disorders. Gastroenterol Jpn. 1989;24:494–504.
17. Collins JSA, Hamilton PW, Watt PCH, Sloan JM, Love AHG. Superficial gastritis and *Campylobacter pylori* in dyspeptic patients – a quantitative study using computer-linked image analysis. J Pathol. 1989;158:303–10.
18. Gutiérrez D, Sierra F, Gómez MC, Camargo H. *Campylobacter pylori* in chronic environmental gastritis and duodenal ulcer patients. Gastroenterology. 1988;94:A163.

19. Holtmann G, Goebell H, Holtmann M, Talley NJ. Gastrointestinal symptoms in healthy blood donors: pattern of symptoms and *Helicobacter pylori* seroprevalence. Dig Dis Sci. 1994:in press.

20. Katelaris PH, Tippett GHK, Norbu P, Lowe DG, Brennan R, Farthing MJG. Dyspepsia, *Helicobacter pylori*, and peptic ulcer in a randomly selected population in India. Gut. 1992;33:1462–6.

21. Al-Moagel MA, Evans DG, Abdulghani ME *et al.* Prevalence of *Helicobacter* (formerly *Campylobacter*) *pylori* infection in Saudi Arabia, and comparison of those with and without upper gastrointestinal symptoms. Am J Gastroenterol. 1990;85:944–8.

22. Bernersen B, Johnsen R, Bostad L, Straume B, Sommer AI, Burhol PG. Is *Helicobacter pylori* the cause of dyspepsia? BMJ. 1992;304:1276–9.

23. Parsonnett J, Blaser MJ, Perez-Perez GI, Hargrett-Bean N, Tauxe RV. Symptoms and risk factors of *Helicobacter pylori* infection in a cohort of epidemiologists. Gastroenterology. 1992;102:41–6.

24. Marshall BJ, Warren JR. Unidentified curved bacilli in the stomach of patients with gastritis and peptic ulceration. Lancet. 1984;1:1311–15.

25. Andersen LP, Elsborg L, Justesen T. *Campylobacter pylori* in peptic ulcer disease. III. Symptoms and paraclinical and epidemiological findings. Scand J Gastroenterol. 1988;23:344–50.

26. Deltenre M, Nyst J-F, Jonas C, Glupczynski Y, Deprez C, Burette A. Données cliniques, endoscopiques et histologiques chez 1100 patients dont 574 colonisés par *Campylobacter pylori*. Gastroenterol Clin Biol. 1989;13:89–95B.

27. Tucci A, Corinaldesi R, Stanghellini V *et al. Helicobacter pylori* infection and gastric function in patients with chronic idiopathic dyspepsia. Gastroenterology. 1992;103:768–74.

28. Börsch G, Schmidt G, Wegener M *et al. Campylobacter pylori*: prospective analysis of clinical and histological factors associated with colonization of the upper gastrointestinal tract. Eur J Clin Invest. 1988;18:133–8.

29. Sobala GM, Dixon MF, Axon ATR. Symptomatology of *Helicobacter pylori* associated dyspepsia. Eur J Gastroenterol Hepatol. 1990;2:445–9.

30. Collins JSA, Knill-Jones RP, Sloan JM *et al.* A comparison of symptoms between non-ulcer dyspepsia patients positive and negative for *Helicobacter pylori*. Ulster Med. 1991;60:21–7.

31. Vaira D, Holton J, Osborn J *et al.* Endoscopy in dyspeptic patients: Is gastric mucosal biopsy useful? Am J Gastroenterol. 1990;85:701–4.

32. Goh KL, Parasakthi N, Peh SC, Wong NW, Lo YL. *Helicobacter pylori* infection and non-ulcer dyspepsia: the effect of treatment with colloidal bismuth subcitrate. Scand J Gastroenterol. 1991;26:1123–31.

33. Waldron B, Cullen PT, Kumar R *et al.* Evidence for hypomotility in non-ulcer dyspepsia: a prospective multifactorial study. Gut. 1991;32:246–51.

34. Kemmer TP, Dominguez-Münoz JE, Klingel H, Zemmler T, Kuhn K, Malfertheiner P. The association between non-ulcer dyspepsia and *Helicobacter pylori* infection. Eur J Gastroenterol Hepatol. 1993:in press.

35. Schubert TT, Schubert AB, Ma CK. Symptoms, gastritis, and *Helicobacter pylori* in patients referred for endoscopy. Gastrointest Endosc. 1992;38:357–60.

36. Bechi P, Dei R, Amorosi A, Marcuzzo G, Cortesini C. *Helicobacter pylori* and luminal gastric pH. Relationships in nonulcer dyspepsia. Dig Dis Sci. 1992;37:378–84.

37. Toukan AU, Kamal MF, Amr SS, Arnaout MA, Abu-Romiyeh AS. Gastroduodenal inflammation in patients with nonulcer dyspepsia: a controlled endoscopic and morphometric study. Dig Dis Sci. 1985;30:313–20.

38. Czinn SJ, Bertram TA, Murray PD, Yang P. Relationship between gastric inflammatory response and symptoms in patients infected with *Helicobacter pylori*. Scand J Gastroenterol. 1991;26(Suppl. 181):33–7.

39. Tytgat GNJ, Noach LA, Rauws EAJ. Is gastroduodenitis a cause of chronic dyspepsia? Scand J Gastroenterol. Suppl. 1991;182:33–9.

40. Moore SC, Malagelada J-R, Shorter RG, Zinsmeister AR. Interrelationships among gastric mucosal morphology, secretion, and motility in peptic ulcer disease. Dig Dis Sci. 1986;31: 673–84.

41. Wegener M, Börsch G, Schaffstein J, Schulze-Flake C, Mai U, Leverkus F. Are dyspeptic

symptoms in patients with *Campylobacter pylori*-associated type B gastritis linked to delayed gastric emptying? Am J Gastroenterol. 1988;83:737–40.
42. Barnett JL, Behler EM, Appelman HD, Etta GH. *Campylobacter pylori* is not associated with gastroparesis. Dig Dis Sci. 1989;34:1677–80.
43. Pieramico O, Ditschuneit H, Malfertheiner P. Gastrointestinal motility in patients with non-ulcer dyspepsia: a role of *Helicobacter pylori* infection? Am J Gastroenterol. 1983;88: 364–8.
44. Caldwell SH, Valenzeula G, Marshall BJ et al. *Helicobacter pylori* infection and gastric emptying of solids in humans. J Gastrointest Mot. 1992;4:113–17.
45. McNulty CAM, Gearty JC, Crump B et al. *Campylobacter pyloridis* and associated gastritis: investigator blind, placebo controlled trial of bismuth salicylate and erythromycin ethylsuccinate. BMJ. 1986;293:645–49.
46. Rokkas T, Pursey C, Uzoechina E et al. Non-ulcer dyspepsia and short-term De-Nol therapy: a placebo controlled trial with particular reference to the role of *Campylobacter pylori*. Gut. 1988;29:1386–91.
47. Loffeld RJLF, Potters HVJP, Stobberingh E, Flendrig JA, Van Spreeuwel JP, Arends JW. *Campylobacter* associated gastritis in patients with non-ulcer dyspepsia: a double blind placebo controlled trial with colloidal bismuth subcitrate. Gut. 1989;30:1206–12.
48. Kang JY, Tay HH, Wee A, Guan R, Math MV, Yap I. Effect of colloidal bismuth subcitrate on symptoms and gastric histology in non-ulcer dyspepsia: a double blind placebo controlled study. Gut. 1990;31:476–80.
49. Kazi JI, Jafarey NA, Alam SM et al. A placebo controlled trial of bismuth salicylate in *Helicobacter pylori* associated gastritis. JPMA. 1990;40:154–6.
50. Vaira D, Holton J, Ainley C et al. Double blind trial of colloidal bismuth subcitrate versus placebo in *Helicobacter pylori* positive patients with non-ulcer dyspepsia. Ital J Gastroenterol. 1992;24:400–4.
51. Nafeeza MI, Shahimi MM, Kudva MV et al. Evaluation of therapies in the treatment of *Helicobacter pylori* associated non-ulcer dyspepsia. Singapore Med J. 1992;33:570–4.
52. Glupczynski Y, Burette A, Labbe M, Deprez C, DeReuck M, Deltenre M. *Campylobacter pylori*-associated gastritis: a double-blind placebo-controlled trial with amoxycillin. Am J Gastroenterol. 1988;83:365–72.
53. Gastrointestinal Physiology Working Group of Cayetano Heredia and the Johns Hopkins Universities, Morgan D, Kraft W, Bender M, Pearson A. Nitrofurans in the treatment of gastritis associated with *Campylobacter pylori*. Gastroenterology. 1988;95:1178–84.
54. Marshall BJ, Valenzuela JE, McCallum RW et al. Bismuth subsalicylate suppression of *Helicobacter pylori* in nonulcer dyspepsia: a double-blind placebo-controlled trial. Dig Dis Sci. 1993;38:1674–80.
55. Yates S, Barnett C, Peterson WL. Enteric coated charcoal as a means of blinding studies comparing bismuth and H_2-receptor antagonists. Am J Gastroenterol. 1992;87:981–4.
56. Talley NJ, Ormand JE, Carpenter HA, Phillips SF. Triple therapy for *Helicobacter pylori* in nonulcer dyspepsia (letter). Am J Gastroenterol. 1991;86:121–3.
57. Sabbatini F, Castiglione F, Piai G, Daniele B, Sapio E, Mazzacca G. The long-term outcome of dyspeptic patients after *Helicobacter pylori* (Hp) eradication (abstract). Gastroenterology. 1993;104:A182.
58. Bianchi Porro G, Lazzaroni M, Sangaletti O, Bargiggia S. Role of *Helicobacter pylori* in dyspeptic syndrome: Fact or fancy? Gut. 1992;33:S42.
59. Holcombe C, Thom C, Kaluba J, Lucas SB. *Helicobacter pylori* clearance in the treatment of non-ulcer dyspepsia. Aliment Pharmacol Ther. 1992;6:119–23.
60. Bamford KM, Collins JSA, Collins BJ, Hughes DF, Porter KG, Wilson TS. Amoxycillin and colloidal bismuth subcitrate improve associated gastritis but not symptoms in patients with non-ulcer dyspepsia. Klin Wochenschr. 1989;67(Suppl. 18):3.
61. Frazzoni M, Lonardo A, Grisendi A et al. Are routine duodenal and antral biopsies useful in the management of 'functional' dyspepsia? A diagnostic and therapeutic study. J Clin Gastroenterol. 1993;17:101–8.
62. Patchett S, Beattie S, Leen E, Keane C, O'Morain C. Eradicating *Helicobacter pylori* and symptoms of non-ulcer dyspepsia. BMJ. 1991;303:1238–40.
63. O'Morain C. *Helicobacter pylori* and non-ulcer dyspepsia (correspondence). Gastroenterology. 1993;103:341.

64. Petrino R, Di Napoli A, Boero M, Belis D, Bottino P, Chiandussi L. Cure of chronic dyspepsia with eradication of *Helicobacter pylori* (HP) infection. Ital J Gastroenterol. 1991;23(Suppl.):213.
65. Pretolani S, Bonvicini F, Brocchi E *et al.* Non-ulcer dyspepsia: is there any correlation between clinical symptoms and histopathological features? Ital J Gastroenterol. 1991;23(Suppl.):80.
66. Talley NJ. Optimal study design for therapeutic trials in *Helicobacter pylori*-associated nonulcer dyspepsia. In: Menge H, Gregor M, Tytgat GNJ, Marshall BJ, McNulty CAM, editors. *Helicobacter pylori* 1990. Proceedings of the Second International Symposium on *Helicobacter pylori*. Berlin: Springer-Verlag; 1991:252–61.

42
H. pylori and NSAIDs: a meta-analysis on interactions of acute gastroduodenal injury, gastric and duodenal ulcers and upper gastrointestinal symptoms

S. J. O. VELDHUYZEN VAN ZANTEN

INTRODUCTION

Helicobacter pylori is accepted as the cause of antral gastritis and is strongly associated with relapsing duodenal ulcers and to a lesser degree with gastric ulcers[1,2]. Use of non-steroidal anti-inflammatory drugs (NSAIDs) is also conclusively linked to development of gastric ulcers and duodenal ulcers. Since both *H. pylori* infection and NSAID use are highly prevalent the obvious question is whether there is an interaction between these two factors resulting in a change in the frequency with which gastroduodenal pathology occurs. There are three possible scenarios: (1) synergy – an increase in risk, (2) antagonism – a decrease in risk and (3) no interaction – risk unchanged. For clinical practice the important question is, when a patient requires NSAIDs, whether the presence of *H. pylori* infection increases the risk of the development of gastroduodenal pathology, especially gastric ulcer and duodenal ulcer and upper gastrointestinal symptoms.

This systematic overview (meta-analysis) was conducted to address the three most common questions a clinician might ask when a patient requires treatment with NSAIDs. Does presence of *H. pylori* infection increase (1) the risk of acute gastroduodenal injury, (2) the risk of chronic gastroduodenal injury, especially gastric ulcer and duodenal ulcer and (3) occurrence of upper gastrointestinal symptoms?

METHODS

Data sources

A Medline search was conducted going back to 1983, the year *H. pylori* was discovered. The final date of the search was 1 August 1993. The following medical subject headings were used: *Helicobacter pylori* (*Campylobacter pylori* before 1990), NSAIDs, and clinical trial, gastric ulcer, duodenal ulcer or dyspepsia. Searches were limited to articles published in full in the English literature. Studies only published in abstract form were not reviewed. A fully recursive review of retrieved articles was also carried out to identify further studies. Studies had to be prospective, and a minimum sample size of 25 patients was required.

Data extraction

All studies were analysed for data on the following outcome measures: acute gastroduodenal injury, gastric and duodenal ulcer, and upper gastrointestinal symptoms. The quality of each study was assessed on a four-point scale: + + +, high quality, methodologically strong study without important weaknesses; + +, reasonable quality, some weaknesses in study design or study results; +, weak study, with definite shortcomings in design or results; 0 = poor study, a study with serious weaknesses. Also recorded were: the basic study design, sample size, whether an increase in frequency of gastric and duodenal ulcers or dyspeptic symptoms occurred in *H. pylori*-positive compared to *H. pylori*-negative patients taking NSAIDs, and potential problems in the study itself. Although a formal meta-analysis with statistical pooling of the results of individual studies had been planned, this proved impossible due to the marked heterogeneity in design and execution of the studies.

RESULTS

In total 55 studies were identified by the search strategies. Most studies had to be excluded because they were review articles rather than actual clinical trials in which the outcome measures of interest for this study were assessed.

Acute gastroduodenal injury

The study by Lanza *et al.*[3] was the only one that evaluated whether presence or absence of *H. pylori* infection influenced the frequency and severity of acute gastroduodenal injury in 61 normal volunteers who were started on NSAIDs (naproxen 1000 mg or aspirin 3900 mg). The frequency and severity of the acute gastroduodenal injury – mucosal haemorrhage, erosions and ulcers – was assessed by endoscopy 1 week after treatment had been initiated. Twenty-one of the 61 (34%) were *H. pylori*-positive. No significant differences between *H. pylori*-positive and -negative patients, or between naproxen and aspirin users, were detected.

Chronic gastroduodenal injury: gastric and duodenal ulcers

Thirteen studies met the inclusion criteria for assessment of chronic gastro-duodenal injury, especially gastric and duodenal ulcers. Four of these 13 studies had to be excluded: one because it was a retrospective study[4], two because no data were presented to determine the prevalence of ulcers in *H. pylori*-infected versus non-infected patients[5,6] and one because the type of gastroduodenal injury was not described[7]. The results are summarized in Table 1.

It is evident that the quality of the studies was highly variable. Overall there is no convincing evidence that presence of *H. pylori* infection increases the risk of gastric ulcer and/or duodenal ulcer in patients treated with NSAIDs. Studies do agree that histological presence of gastritis is largely determined by the presence of a *H. pylori* infection.

Upper gastrointestinal symptoms

Six studies fulfilled our entry criteria, and these are summarized in Table 2. As can be seen, many studies were rated as having weak designs. The results are summarized in Table 2. Based on these studies there is insufficient evidence that *H. pylori*-positive compared to -negative patients suffer from more dyspeptic symptoms when NSAIDs are used.

DISCUSSION

This systematic overview did not find convincing evidence for an increase in acute gastroduodenal injury, gastric and/or duodenal ulcer or upper gastrointestinal symptoms. This is in agreement with Laine[20], but differs from conclusions reached by others[21,22]. This study is the first meta-analysis in this area, in which the existing literature was systematically reviewed for specific outcome measures.

There are several reasons why the combination of *H. pylori* infection and NSAIDs may lead to a higher frequency of upper gastrointestinal complications. These include effects on gastric acid secretion, change in mucus characteristics, decrease in bicarbonate secretion, alterations of mucosal prostaglandin levels and mucosal blood flow[21,22]. There is no doubt that NSAID-induced ulceration can occur in the absence of histological evidence of *H. pylori* gastritis[23,24]. If there is histological evidence of gastritis in patients who are taking NSAIDs this is usually due to an underlying *Helicobacter pylori* infection[10,13,14,21].

Only one study was identified which looked at the occurrence of acute mucosal injury in healthy volunteers who were started on NSAIDs. No differences were found between *H. pylori*-positive and -negative individuals.

Table 1 Summary of studies with gastric or duodenal ulcer as an outcome measure

Study	Study design	Quality score	Sample size	Patients	H. pylori-positive; n (%)	Gastric and duodenal ulcer	Increased ulcer prevalence H. pylori-positive versus H. pylori-negative NSAID users; n (%)	Comments
Caselli et al.[8]	Cross-sectional cohort	+	185	85 NSAID 100 non-NSAID	26 (31%) 59 (59%)	7 (8%) 11 (11%)	No, 3/26 (12%) versus 4/59 (7%), not statistically significant	Age of patients not given, no H. pylori found in patients on aspirin
Martin et al.[9]	Cross-sectional cohort	+	107	60 dyspepsia 28 controls 19 volunteers	29 Hp$^+$, NSAID$^+$ 31 Hp$^+$, NSAID$^-$ 27 Hp$^-$, NSAID$^+$ 20 Hp$^-$, NSAID$^-$	12 (41%) 14 (45%) 4 (15%) 0 (0%)	No, no figures given	No age-matching, poor definition of control patients, 42% of healthy volunteers were taking NSAID
Shallcross et al.[10]	Cross-sectional cohort	+ + +	430	99 NSAID 331 controls	60 (61%) 191 (58%)	31 (31%) 39 (17%)	No, 23/60 (38%) versus 8/39 (20%), not statistically significant	Presence of gastritis mainly related to presence of H. pylori
Graham et al.[11]	Cross-sectional cohort	+ +	75	75 NSAID	53 (73%)	13 (18%)	No, 11/53 (21%) versus 2/20 (10%) not statistically significant	Mucosal haemorrhage and erosions were more common in H. pylori-negative patients.
Loeb et al.[12]	Cross-sectional cohort	+	50	RA*50 NSAID 61 controls	11 (22%) 15 (25%)	14 (28%) not given	No, data not provided	Presence of gastritis mainly related to presence of H. pylori. Controls did not have endoscopy.
Taha et al.[13]	Cross-sectional cohort	+ +	218	174 NSAID 44 controls	56 (32%) 22 (50%)	68 (39%) 14 (32%)	No, 25/68 (37%) versus 43/106 (41%)	Ulcers more common in NSAID users who had evidence of chemical gastritis

continued

452

Table 1 Continued

Study	Study design	Quality score	Sample size	Patients	H. pylori-positive; n (%)	Gastric and duodenal ulcer	Increased ulcer prevalence H. pylori-positive versus H. pylori-negative NSAID users; n (%)	Comments
Safe et al.[14]	Cross-sectional cohort	+	100	49 NSAID / 51 controls	24 (49%) / 38 (75%)	17 (34%) / 13 (25%)	No, 9/24 (38%) versus 8/25 (32%)	Presence of gastritis mainly related to presence of H. pylori
Hudson et al.[15]	Cross-sectional cohort	++	88	65 NSAID / 23 controls	25 (38%) / 12 (52%)	9 (14%) / 5 (22%)	No, 6/25 (24%) versus 3/40 (8%), not statistically significant	Mucosal prostaglandin levels not decreased in H. pylori-positive NSAID users
Schubert et al.[16]	Cross-sectional cohort	+++	1088	22% NSAID / 48% H. pylori-positive	518 (48%)	Not given for subgroups	No interaction between H. pylori and NSAID by logistic regression	No interaction between H. pylori and NSAID for either gastric or duodenal ulcer

*RA = rheumatoid arthritis

453

Table 2 Summary of studies that have upper gastrointestinal symptoms as an outcome measure

Study	Study design	Quality score	Sample size	Patients	H. pylori-positive, n (%)	Increased symptom severity in H. pylori-positive versus H. pylori-negative NSAID users	Comments
Upadhyay et al.[17]	Cross-sectional cohort	+	52	RA	26 (50%)	Yes, H. pylori-positive patients more dyspeptic symptoms	Poor selection of patients; fourteen patients were seen because of endoscopy
Graham et al.[11]	Cross-sectional cohort	++	75	RA or OA	53 (75%)	No	In separate study no relationship was found between any upper gastrointestinal symptom and H. pylori infection
Jones et al.[18]	Cross-sectional cohort	+	68	68 RA on NSAID or NSAID in the past	29 (43%)	Yes, more dyspeptic symptoms in H. pylori-positive NSAID users	Poor symptom measurement; 48/68 were hospitalized patients; duration NSAID use unclear
Loeb et al.[12]	Cross-sectional cohort	++	50	RA	11 (22%)	No	—
Heresbach et al.[7]	Cross-sectional cohort	+	111	66 NSAID 45 controls	16 (24%) 12 (26%)	No	Only the presence or absence of symptoms was recorded
Gubbins et al.[19]	Cross-sectional cohort	+	132	RA treated with NSAID (77%) and/or gold (78%)	54 (41%)	H. pylori infection had no effect on frequency of NSAID side-effects	Included 78% patients on gold; use of gold did not influence prevalence of H. pylori

RA = rheumatoid arthritis; OA = osteoarthritis

NSAIDs can cause chronic gastroduodenal damage such as mucosal haemorrhage and erosions, but the clinical significance of these abnormalities is uncertain. Evidence to date suggests that *H. pylori* does not increase the prevalence of mucosal haemorrhage or erosions. In fact the study by Graham *et al.* found that mucosal injury was less common in NSAID users who were *H. pylori*-positive compared to non-infected patients[11]. This might be due to the fact that a NSAID-induced decrease in mucosal prostaglandin levels does not occur in *H. pylori*-infected patients[15].

With regard to chronic gastroduodenal injury this study looked specifically at the endpoints gastric ulcer and duodenal ulcer. No evidence for an increased risk of gastric and/or duodenal ulcer was found in chronic NSAID users who were *H. pylori*-positive compared to non-infected patients. However, this conclusion needs to be qualified. All studies were cross-sectional in nature, only providing data on the prevalence of outcome measures at a single time point. In most studies the dose and duration of NSAIDs was not specified. Several studies suffered from suboptimal study design. The sample size of most studies was small, and the power to detect statistically significant differences in the frequency of the outcome measure of interest – gastric and/or duodenal ulcers or dyspeptic symptoms – was therefore low. Some studies showed a somewhat higher number of ulcers in *H. pylori*-positive patients who were NSAID users compared to non-NSAID users, but none of the differences was statistically significant. Using multivariate analysis the large study by Schubert *et al.*[16] found no interaction between *H. pylori* and NSAIDs for an increased risk of gastric or duodenal ulcer formation. Combining the results from all studies there currently is no convincing evidence that the risk of duodenal or gastric ulcer formation is increased in *H. pylori*-positive patients who are started on NSAID therapy. Furthermore, it is also reasonable to assume that, should future studies show that there is an increased risk in the occurrence of gastric or duodenal ulcers, this risk will be low. One study design to answer this question is a trial that randomizes *H. pylori*-positive patients, who require NSAID therapy, to either treatment aimed at eradication of the organism or to no anti-*Helicobacter* treatment *prior* to the institution of the NSAID, to determine whether the subsequent risk of ulcer development is decreased. It remains to be seen whether such a study will ever be undertaken.

Some studies found a lower prevalence of *H. pylori* in NSAID compared to non-NSAID users, but these differences were not statistically significant. Furthermore, these studies did not stratify the data according to age, which is a strong predictor of *H. pylori* infection.

Reliable measurement of upper gastrointestinal symptoms is fraught with difficulties[25,26]. This study found no convincing evidence for an increased prevalence of dyspeptic symptoms in *H. pylori*-positive NSAID users. There was also no difference in the severity of dyspeptic symptoms. However, many studies suffered from poor methodology in the way symptoms and their severity were assessed. The sample size of the studies often was also small.

All studies looked at NSAID users including patients on aspirin. It was noteworthy that no *H. pylori* was found in the patients treated with high-dose aspirin in the Caselli *et al.*[8] study ($n = 7$) and the Iglehart *et al.*[4] study

($n = 4$), although in both studies only histology was used for diagnosis. *In vitro* activity of acetylsalicylic acid against *H. pylori* has been demonstrated[8,27]. Unfortunately, most studies reviewed here did not list which NSAIDs were used, and whether aspirin users were included. This subgroup of NSAID patients could therefore not be further analysed.

Finally, Taha *et al.*[13] raised the possibility that presence of chemical gastritis, defined by foveolar hyperplasia, oedema and presence of muscle fibres in the lamina propria in the absence of chronic inflammatory cells, together with NSAIDs, may lead to an increased risk for ulcer development if *H. pylori* is present. The importance of this finding remains speculative given that in this study the number of non-NSAID users was low, and the fact that chemical gastritis can also be caused by bile reflux[28] in the absence of NSAIDs. In the study by Shallcross *et al.* only one of 60 *H. pylori*-positive NSAID users demonstrated this type of gastritis.

In conclusion the presence or absence of *H. pylori* in patients treated with NSAIDs does not lead to an increased risk in the development of acute gastroduodenal injury, gastric and/or duodenal ulcers or upper gastrointestinal symptoms. However, these conclusions are based on many studies that suffer from suboptimal design. Most studies had small sample sizes, which gave them low statistical power to detect small but statistically significant differences. Nevertheless, it is reasonable to assume that, should there be an increased risk, it probably is small and unlikely to be clinically relevant.

References

1. Veldhuyzen van Zanten SJO, Sherman PM. A systematic overview of *Helicobacter pylori* infection as the cause of gastritis, duodenal ulcer, gastric cancer and non-ulcer dyspepsia: applying the diagnostic criteria to establish causation. Can Med Assoc J. 1994;150:in press.
2. Graham DY, Lew GM, Klein PD *et al.* Effect of treatment of *Helicobacter pylori* infection on the long-term recurrence of gastric or duodenal ulcer. A randomized, controlled study. Ann Intern Med. 1992;116:705–8.
3. Lanza FL, Evans DG, Graham DY. Effect of *Helicobacter pylori* infection on the severity of gastroduodenal mucosa injury after the acute administration of naproxen or aspirin to normal volunteers. Am J Gastroenterol. 1991;86:735–7.
4. Iglehart IW, Edlow DW, Mills L, Morrison SA, Hochberg MC. The presence of *Campylobacter pylori* in NSAID associated gastritis. J Rheumatol. 1989;16:599–603.
5. O'Riordan TG, Tobin A, O'Morain C. *Helicobacter pylori* infection in elderly dyspeptic patients. Age and Aging. 1991;20:189–92.
6. Taha AS, Sturrock RD, Russell RI. *Helicobacter pylori* and peptic ulcers in rheumatoid arthritis patients receiving gold, sulfasalazine and NSAIDs. Am J Gastroenterol. 1992;87:1732–5.
7. Heresbach D, Raoul L, Bretagne JF *et al. Helicobacter pylori*: a risk factor and severity factor of NSAID induced gastropathy. Gut. 1992;33:1608–11.
8. Caselli M, Pezzi R, LaCorte R, Aleotti L, Trevisani L, Stabellini G. *Campylobacter*-like organisms, NSAIDs and gastric lesions in patients with rheumatoid arthritis. Digestion. 1989;44:101–4.
9. Martin DF, Montgomery E, Dobek AS, Patrissi GA, Peura DA. *Campylobacter pylori*, NSAIDs, and smoking: risk factors for peptic ulcer disease. Am J Gastroenterol. 1989;84:1268–72.
10. Shallcross TM, Rathbone BJ, Wyatt JI, Heatley RV. *Helicobacter pylori* associated gastritis and peptic ulceration in patients taking NSAIDs. Aliment Pharmacol Ther. 1990;4:515–22.
11. Graham DY, Lidsky MD, Cox AM *et al.* Long-term NSAID use and *Helicobacter pylori*

infection. Gastroenterology. 1991;100:1653–7.

12. Loeb DS, Talley NJ, Ahlquist DA, Carpenter HA, Zinsmeister AR. Long-term NSAID use and gastroduodenal injury: the role of *Helicobacter pylori*. Gastroenterology. 1992;102: 1899–905.
13. Taha AS, Nakshabendi I, Lee FD, Sturrock RD, Russell RI. Chemical gastritis and *Helicobacter pylori* related gastritis in patients receiving NSAIDs: comparison and correlation with peptic ulceration. J Clin Pathol. 1992;45:135–9.
14. Safe AF, Warren B, Corfield A *et al*. *Helicobacter pylori* infection in elderly people: correlation between histology and serology. Age and Aging. 1993;22:215–20.
15. Hudson N, Balsitis M, Filipowicz F, Hawkey CJ. Effect of *Helicobacter pylori* colonization on gastric mucosal eicosanoid synthesis in patients taking NSAIDs. Gut. 1993;34:748–51.
16. Schubert TT, Bologna SD, Nensey Y, Schubert AB, Mascha EJ, Chan K. Ulcer risk factors: interactions between *Helicobacter pylori* infection, nonsteroidal use and age. Am J Med. 1993;94:413–18.
17. Upadhyay R, Howatson A, McKinlay A, Danesh BJ, Sturrock RD, Russell RI. *Campylobacter pylori* associated gastritis in patients with rheumatoid arthritis taking NSAIDs. Br J Rheumatol. 1988;27:113–16.
18. Jones ST, Claque RB, Eldridge J, Jones DM. Serological evidence of infection with *Helicobacter pylori* may predict gastrointestinal tolerance to NSAID treatment in rheumatoid arthritis. Br J Rheumatol. 1991;30:16–20.
19. Gubbins GP, Schubert T, Attanasio F, Lubetsky M, Perez-Perez GI, Blaser MJ. *Helicobacter pylori* seroprevalence in patients with rheumatoid arthritis: effect of NSAIDs and gold compounds. Am J Med. 1992;93:412–18.
20. Laine L. *Helicobacter pylori*, gastric ulcer, and agents noxious to the gastric mucosa. Gastroenterol Clin N Am. 1993;22:117–25.
21. McCarthy DM. *Helicobacter pylori* infection and gastroduodenal injury by NSAIDs. Scand J Gastroenterol. 1991;26(S187):91–7.
22. Taha AS, Russell RI. *Helicobacter pylori* and NSAIDs: uncomfortable partners in peptic ulcer disease. Gut. 1993;34:580–3.
23. Laine L, Marin-Sorensen M, Weinstein W. NSAID-associated gastric ulcers do not require *Helicobacter pylori* for their development. Am J Gastroenterol. 1992;87:1398–402.
24. Borody TJ, Brandl S, Andrews P, Jankiewicz, Ostapowitz N. *Helicobacter pylori*-negative gastric ulcer. Am J Gastroenterol. 1992;87:1403–6.
25. Veldhuyzen van Zanten SJO, Tytgat KMAJ, Jalali S, Goodacre RL, Hunt RH. Can gastritis symptoms be evaluated in clinical trials? An overview of treatment of gastritis, non-ulcer dyspepsia and *Campylobacter*-associated gastritis. J Clin Gastroenterol. 1989;11:496–501.
26. Veldhuyzen van Zanten SJO, Tytgat KMAJ, Pollak PT *et al*. Can severity of symptoms be used as outcome measures in trials of non-ulcer dyspepsia and *Helicobacter pylori*. J Clin Epidemiol. 1993;46:273–9.
27. Veldhuyzen van Zanten SJO, Goldie J, Hunt RH, Richardson H. The inhibitory effect of salicylate on *Helicobacter pylori*. Ital J Gastroenterol. 1992;23(S2):47–48(abstract).
28. Dixon MF, O'Connor HJ, Axon ATR, King RFJG, Johnston D. Reflux gastritis: distinct histopathological entity. J Clin Pathol. 1986;39:524–30.

Section VIII
Relationship of *H. pylori* gastric carcinogenesis and lymphoma

43
H. pylori and gastric cancer: the significance of the problem

D. FORMAN and P. M. WEBB

INTRODUCTION

The objectives of this chapter are four-fold: first, the evidence associating *Helicobacter pylori* infection with the subsequent development of gastric cancer will be briefly reviewed; second, the magnitude of the association will be assessed; third will be a consideration of the implications of the association on a public health strategy for the prevention of gastric cancer; finally, the implications of the association will be discussed in terms of understanding mechanisms for carcinogenesis in the stomach.

H. PYLORI AND GASTRIC CANCER

Evidence pertaining to the association between *H. pylori* infection and gastric cancer is summarized schematically in Table 1. This has been reviewed in detail elsewhere[1-5]. *H. pylori* infection undoubtedly causes chronic gastritis in the antrum which, given the inability of the host to clear the bacteria, will persist indefinitely, thus giving rise to cellular atrophy and degeneration. By causing gastritis, *H. pylori* can initiate the sequence of events leading to cancer, as outlined in the model proposed by Correa and colleagues[6-8]. Epidemiological studies have shown that there is a geographic association between those areas of the world with high rates of gastric cancer and those

Table 1 Evidence for an association between *H. pylori* and gastric cancer

Evidence	Strength of association
H. pylori causes chronic gastritis	+ + +
Geographic association	+ +
Retrospective studies	+ / −
Prospective studies	+ + +
Intervention studies	Not available

with a high prevalence of *H. pylori* infection[9,10], although there are important exceptions to this general pattern, most notably in Africa[11]. Retrospective studies, in which the prevalence of *H. pylori* infection has been assessed in gastric cancer patients after diagnosis, using either histopathology[12,13] or antibody serology[14–18], and the results compared with prevalence figures for control groups, have given equivocal results. One reason for this might be that by the time gastric cancer has developed, *H. pylori* may no longer be present. The precancerous environment of the stomach, with a high frequency of achlorhydria, severe atrophy and intestinal metaplasia, is known to be prejudicial to *H. pylori* colonization[19,20]; thus a previous infection may have been eliminated.

The most convincing epidemiological evidence in support of an association is that from three prospective studies[21–23]. In these studies, blood was taken from healthy subjects and stored, and *H. pylori* antibody status was later assessed in those who went on to develop gastric cancer. In all three studies, infection was significantly more common in the gastric cancer patients than in appropriately matched control groups. More decisive evidence about the association would be provided by intervention studies in which population groups, randomly assigned to *H. pylori* eradication therapy or placebo (if infected), would be followed up to look at the comparative rates of gastric cancer and/or precancerous lesions. To date no such studies have been reported, although two are in progress in South America.

HOW GREAT IS THE RISK?

If there is a causal relationship between *H. pylori* infection and gastric cancer, the question arises as to how large the risk of gastric cancer is, in those who have been infected. The relative risk estimates from the three prospective studies were 2.8, 3.6, and 6.0, and the pooled estimate was 3.8 (95% confidence interval 2.3–6.2)[2]. Extrapolations from the EUROGAST international correlation study[10] produced an estimated relative risk of 6.0. There is no significant heterogeneity between these values and it has generally been assumed, therefore, that the risk is likely to be in the range of 2.5–6.0. This may, however, be an underestimate. The design of all three prospective studies was such that cancer cases were included irrespective of whether they had provided a blood sample in a period of months, or up to 25 years, prior to diagnosis. Hence, in some individuals, seropositivity was assessed very shortly before diagnosis. Analyses including these latter subjects therefore have the same weakness as the retrospective studies, i.e. cancer cases might be falsely assessed as *H. pylori*-negative. Table 2 shows a combined analysis from the three studies with the time between sample collection and cancer diagnosis divided into 5-year periods[24]. There is a significant trend ($p < 0.05$) towards an increased odds ratio with increasing period of time between the two events, up to 8.7 (95% CI = 2.7–44.7) when seropositivity was assessed 15 years or more before diagnosis. This is consistent with the hypothesis that, for several years before diagnosis, seropositivity may be lost in a proportion of cases. If this is the situation, then an approximately nine-fold relative risk

Table 2 Odds ratios for the association of gastric cancer with H. pylori antibody positivity by time interval between blood sample collection and diagnosis of cancer

Time between sample collection and diagnosis (years)	Cases H. pylori +/−	Controls H. pylori +/−	Matched odds ratio[a]	95% confidence interval
< 5	20/5	34/24	2.13	0.59–8.69
5–9	37/9	46/39	2.28	0.86–6.53
10–14	70/8	58/35	4.37	1.76–12.96
≥ 15	88/10	65/33	8.67	2.66–44.74
Test for trend[b]			$p = 0.049$	

From references 21–23 and unpublished data
[a] Exact odds ratios and 95% confidence intervals
[b] Using conditional logistic regression with time period weighted as 2, 7, 12, 18

as observed in Table 2 after 15 years, might be a more accurate assessment of the strength of the association.

PUBLIC HEALTH IMPLICATIONS

The magnitude of the relative risk has an important influence on the level of attributable risk, i.e. the proportion of cancers that could be avoided if infection did not occur. In a country with a population prevalence of H. pylori infection of 35%, as in many developed countries, a relative risk of 8.7 gives an attributable risk of 73%, whereas a relative risk of 3.8 (the pooled estimate from the three studies) would give an attributable risk of only 50%. If the prevalence of infection were 85%, as in many developing countries, the comparable attributable risks would be 86% and 70% respectively. Table 3 shows the impact of these figures on the worldwide burden of gastric cancer. Of the 327 000 new cases diagnosed annually in the developed world between 162 000 and 238 000 could theoretically be avoided by the eradication of H. pylori. Of the 428 000 diagnoses in the developing world between 301 000 and 371 000 could theoretically be avoided.

The above figures concerning attributable risk present what, at first sight, appears to be an optimistic scenario for the prevention of gastric cancer, which is the second most commonly diagnosed fatal cancer in the world[25]. If H. pylori infection, which can be easily diagnosed and relatively easily treated, has a minimum attributable risk of 50%, then eradication of the infection could result in a substantial saving of life. It is therefore worthwhile considering whether this represents a reasonable objective in terms of public health medicine.

Before discussing the alternative strategies for controlling infection two points need to be emphasized. The first is that there is accumulating evidence for a 'birth cohort effect' of declining H. pylori acquisition in developed countries[26]. In brief, this means that people born in the latter part of this century have a lower likelihood of acquiring the infection than those born earlier. If it is assumed that infection is predominantly acquired in

Table 3 Number of gastric cancers attributable to *H. pylori* infection

	Developed countries	*Developing countries*
New cases per year[a]	327 000	428 000
Estimated prevalence of *H. pylori*	35%	85%
Number of cases attributable to *H. pylori* if:		
RR = 3.8	162 000	301 000
RR = 8.7	238 000	371 000

[a] From Parkin *et al.*[25]

childhood[27,28], then figures showing the increasing prevalence of *H. pylori* infection with age can be interpreted as indicating a declining prevalence in later birth cohorts. This, together with direct studies of the cohort effect[29,30], suggests that in the developed world the prevalence of *H. pylori* infection will decline substantially over the next few decades. This means that any public health programme aiming to reduce the prevalence of *H. pylori* in developed countries would have to be extremely cost-effective in order to achieve more than is already happening without any intervention.

The second point is that, even if one is sceptical about a birth cohort effect for *H. pylori* acquisition, there has been, without doubt, a substantial reduction in gastric cancer rates in the developed world[31]. From the trends evident in young people there is every likelihood that this reduction will continue for several decades. This again poses problems for the cost-effectiveness of any public health strategy designed to prevent the disease. A related consideration is that, as with most solid tumours, gastric cancer is a disease of the elderly. The vast majority of disease diagnosed currently occurs in people over the age of 65 years. It is uncertain whether eradicating or preventing transmission of *H. pylori* in people of this age, who are already likely to have developed precancerous lesions, will reduce their subsequent cancer risk.

There are three possible strategies for preventing gastric cancer through the control of *H. pylori*. One could prevent primary transmission, vaccinate against the organism or eradicate the bacteria in those who are infected. Although there are strong indications that socioeconomic factors early in life, e.g. family size or overcrowding[27,32,33], are the most important risk factors for *H. pylori* acquisition, it is unclear what public health recommendations can currently be made to prevent primary transmission. Pending further research this is not yet a viable strategy. Vaccination is also a long-term prospect, as no vaccine is currently available, and a long development time would be required. In addition, vaccination would be required early in life, whereas gastric cancer occurs in the elderly, so there would be at least a 50-year period (as the vaccinated group aged) before any substantive benefits would materialize.

This leaves the strategy of screening populations to determine who is infected, and treating with antibiotics those who are positive. Although this would theoretically be possible now and, indeed, is the rationale behind the intervention studies referred to above, there would be major problems in implementing such a programme. The most important consideration is that none of the current therapeutic regimens is sufficiently cheap, non-toxic or easily administered as to make it suitable for public health intervention outside controlled trials. Even if an appropriate therapy were available, it would be necessary to establish a screening programme infrastructure in an age group sufficiently old that reinfection after eradication was extremely unlikely, but sufficiently young that eradication would still have a beneficial effect in preventing carcinogenesis. Clearly more research into the natural history of *H. pylori*-associated cancer will be necessary before an optimal screening strategy could be developed. Additional research questions which, if answered, would help improve the efficiency of screening are whether there are specific strains of *H. pylori* associated with gastric cancer, and whether genetic differences in the host affect the pathogenicity of the bacteria. Significant developments, both in basic research and in drug development, are therefore required before this type of approach to the prevention of gastric cancer is likely to be viable. The cost of such a programme will also be an important consideration as, for the reasons mentioned above, it is unlikely to be cost-effective except in high-risk populations. Unfortunately many high-risk populations are in developing countries, and are those least able to afford screening and therapy.

It should be emphasized that these somewhat pessimistic comments about the prevention of gastric cancer apply to public health, population-based initiatives. It is likely that clinicians, especially in primary care, will be increasingly presented with the separate problem of whether to treat *H. pylori* infection in asymptomatic individuals. Here the issues will be slightly different, and the reduction in cancer risk for a specific individual may be a worthwhile objective. However, even this approach needs to be formally evaluated in controlled trials before it can be recommended.

H. PYLORI AND MECHANISMS FOR GASTRIC CARCINOGENESIS

The final section of this chapter is concerned with the question of whether knowledge of the association between *H. pylori* and gastric cancer has had any implications in terms of understanding the mechanisms of carcinogenesis. Prior to the discovery of *H. pylori* it had become generally accepted that dietary factors were the most important aetiological agents for gastric cancer. In particular, diets with high intakes of salt, nitrates and preserved foods, together with low intakes of fruit and vegetables are viewed as representing a high risk. There is indeed substantive epidemiological evidence to support most of these relationships[34,35]. Central to this pathway has been the concept of the endogenous formation of mutagenic and carcinogenic N-nitroso compounds as a result of interactions between dietary compounds in the stomach. *H. pylori* infection fits neatly 'on top of' this process. For N-nitroso compounds to be formed, dietary nitrate has first to be reduced to nitrite. This occurs most readily in conditions of atrophic gastritis when gastric acidity is lost and nitrate-reducing species of bacteria (not *H. pylori*) can colonize the stomach. By causing chronic, and ultimately atrophic, gastritis *H. pylori* could initiate this process, perhaps in a manner similar to salt[1].

Ironically, in doing so it may contribute to its own destruction by allowing competition from other bacterial species within its environmental niche. *H. pylori*-induced gastritis is also associated with suppression of ascorbic acid secretion into the stomach, thereby reducing the concentration of an important inhibitor of the formation of *N*-nitroso compounds[36].

Apart from these mechanisms, *H. pylori* infection may have other consequences of relevance to cancer. The ways in which it chronically impairs host defence mechanisms, both physically and biochemically, disturbs normal cytokine regulation and stimulates the production of toxic oxygen radicals are of direct significance to carcinogenesis. Although these topics are already being studied in relation to other sites of cancer, research on *H. pylori* has initiated investigation into their involvement with gastric cancer. More generally, the concept that an infectious agent might be involved in the aetiology of the disease has not only had an impact on our perception of the basic epidemiology of the disease[37], but has also emphasized the importance of chronic inflammatory agents in cancer. This may be relevant to our understanding of the role of other infections (for example, hepatitis B virus, Epstein-Barr virus, human papilloma viruses or *Schistosoma* species) in other types of cancer[38]. *H. pylori* has therefore, as well as reinforcing aspects of the general model of gastric cancer, produced several shifts in emphasis, and has extended the model in new directions.

SUMMARY

There is a body of consistent evidence supporting the association between *H. pylori* infection and gastric cancer, and it seems likely that the magnitude of this association may be larger than previously indicated. Although this association has profound implications for the prevention of gastric cancer, more research will be required before these can be translated into public health interventions, and they will probably be of most relevance to developing countries. Finally *H. pylori* has brought about substantial modifications in current thinking about the mechanisms that underlie the development of gastric cancer.

References

1. Correa P. Is gastric carcinoma an infectious disease? N Engl J Med. 1991;325(16):1170–1.
2. Forman D. *Helicobacter pylori* infection and gastric carcinogenesis. Eur J Gastroenterol Hepatol. 1992;4(Suppl.2):S31–5.
3. Levine T, Price A. The precancer–cancer sequence. In: Northfield TC, Mendall M, Goggin PM, editors. *Helicobacter pylori* infection. Lancaster: Kluwer; 1993:88–98.
4. Nomura A, Stemmerman GN *Helicobacter pylori* and gastric cancer. J Gastroenterol Hepatol. 1993;8:294–303.
5. Parsonnet J. *Helicobacter pylori* and gastric cancer. Gastroenterol Clin N Am. 1993;22(1): 89–104.
6. Correa P, Haenszel W, Cuello C, Tannenbaum S, Archer M. A model for gastric cancer epidemiology. Lancet. 1975;2:58–60.
7. Correa P. A human model of gastric carcinogenesis. Cancer Res. 1988;48:3354–60.
8. Correa P. Human gastric carcinogenesis: a multistep and multifactorial process – first

American cancer society award lecture on cancer epidemiology and prevention. Cancer Res. 1992;52:6735–40.

9. Forman D, Sitas F, Newell DG et al. Geographic association of Helicobacter pylori antibody prevalence and gastric cancer mortality in rural China. Int J Cancer. 1990;46:608–11.

10. EUROGAST Study Group. An international association between Helicobacter pylori infection and gastric cancer. Lancet. 1993;341:1359–62.

11. Holcombe C. Helicobacter pylori: the African enigma. Gut. 1992;33:429–31.

12. Loffeld RJLF, Willems I, Flendrig JA, Arends JW. Helicobacter pylori and gastric carcinoma. Histopathology. 1990;17:537–41.

13. Farinati F, Valiante F, Germana B et al. Prevalence of Helicobacter pylori infection in patients with precancerous changes and gastric cancer. Eur J Cancer Prev. 1993;2:321–6.

14. Sipponen P, Kosunen TU, Valle J, Riihela M, Seppala K. Helicobacter pylori infection and chronic gastritis in gastric cancer. J Clin Pathol. 1992;45:319–23.

15. Talley NJ, Zinsmeister AR, Weaver A et al. Gastric adenocarcinoma and Helicobacter pylori infection. J Natl Cancer Inst. 1991;83:1734–9.

16. Estevens J, Fidalgo P, Tendeiro T et al. Anti-Helicobacter pylori antibodies prevalence and gastric adenocarcinoma in Portugal: report of a case-control study. Eur J Cancer Prev. 1993;2:377–80.

17. Kuipers EJ, Gracia-Casanova M, Pena AS et al. Helicobacter pylori serology in patients with gastric carcinoma. Scand J Gastroenterol. 1993;28(5):433–7.

18. Hansson L-E, Engstrand L, Nyren O et al. Helicobacter pylori infection: independent risk indicator of gastric adenocarcinoma. Gastroenterology. 1993;105:1098–103.

19. Karnes Jr WE, Samloff IM, Siurala M et al. Positive serum antibody and negative tissue staining for Helicobacter pylori in subjects with atrophic body gastritis. Gastroenterology. 1991;101:167–74.

20. Wyatt JI. Gastritis and its relation to gastric carcinogenesis. Diagnost Pathol. 1991;8(3): 137–48.

21. Forman D, Newell DG, Fullerton F et al. Association between infection with Helicobacter pylori and risk of gastric cancer: evidence from a prospective investigation. BMJ. 1991;302:1302–5.

22. Parsonnet J, Friedman GD, Vandersteen DT et al. Helicobacter pylori infection and risk for gastric cancer. N Engl J Med. 1991;325:1127–31.

23. Nomura A, Stemmermann GN, Chyou P-H, Kato I, Perez-Perez GI, Blaser MJ. Helicobacter pylori infection and gastric carcinoma in a population of Japanese–Americans in Hawaii. N Engl J Med. 1991;325:1132–6.

24. Forman D, Webb P, Parsonnet J. H. pylori and gastric cancer. Lancet. 1994;343:243–4.

25. Parkin DM, Pisani P, Ferlay J. Estimates of the worldwide incidence of eighteen major cancers in 1985. Int J Cancer. 1993;54:594–606.

26. Marshall BJ. Campylobacter pylori: its link to gastritis and peptic ulcer disease. Rev Infect Dis. 1990;12(Suppl.1):S87–93.

27. Mitchell HM, Li YY, Hu PJ et al. Epidemiology of Helicobacter pylori in Southern China: identification of early childhood as the critical period for acquisition. J Infect Dis. 1992;166(1):149–53.

28. Mendall M. Natural history and mode of transmission. In: Northfield T, Mendall M, Goggin P, editors. Helicobacter pylori infection. Lancaster: Kluwer; 1993:21–32.

29. Parsonnet J, Blaser MJ, Perez-Perez GI, Hargrett-Bean N, Tauxe RV. Symptoms and risk factors of Helicobacter pylori infection in a cohort of epidemiologists. Gastroenterology. 1992;102:41–6.

30. Banatvala N, Mayo K, Megraud F, Jennings R, Deeks JJ, Feldman RA. The cohort effect and Helicobacter pylori. J Infect Dis. 1993;168(1):219–21.

31. Munoz N. Descriptive epidemiology of stomach cancer. In: Reed PI, Hill MJ, editors. Gastric carcinogenesis. Amsterdam: Excerpta Medica; 1988:51–69.

32. Galpin OP, Whitaker CJ, Dubiel AJ. Helicobacter pylori infection and overcrowding in childhood. Lancet. 1992;339:619.

33. Mendall MA, Goggin PM, Molineaux N et al. Childhood living conditions and Helicobacter pylori seropositivity in adult life. Lancet. 1992;339:896–7.

34. Howson CP, Hiyama T, Wynder EL. The decline in gastric cancer: epidemiology of an unplanned triumph. Epidemiol Rev. 1986;8:1–27.

35. Forman D. The etiology of gastric cancer. In: O'Neill IK, Chen J, Bartsch H, editors. Relevance to human cancer of *N*-nitroso compounds, tobacco smoke and mycotoxins. Lyon: IARC; 1991:22–32.
36. Mirvish SS, Wallcave L, Eagen M, Shubik P. Ascorbate–nitrite reaction: a possible means of blocking the formation of carcinogenic *N*-nitroso compounds. Science. 1972;177:65–8.
37. Barker DJP, Coggon D, Osmond C, Wickham C. Poor housing in childhood and high rates of stomach cancer in England and Wales. Br J Cancer. 1990;61:575–8.
38. Preston-Martin S, Pike MC, Ross RK, Jones PA, Henderson BE. Increased cell division as a cause of human cancer. Cancer Res. 1990;50:7415–21.

44
The ascorbic acid story

A. T. R. AXON

INTRODUCTION

Scurvy and vitamin C

Scurvy was first described during the crusades of the 13th century, but has been a particular scourge of seamen and explorers. One hundred out of 160 of Vasco de Gama's crew died of scurvy in 1498 when they sailed around the Cape of Good Hope, and a Spanish galleon was found adrift at sea around that time, the entire crew having died of the disease[1]. Admiral Sir Richard Hawkins wrote in 1593: 'that which I have seen most fruitful for this sickness is sower oranges and lemons'. Scurvy continued to exact a terrible toll from sailors and, as late as 1780, 1457 sailors were treated for scurvy in the Haslar Naval Hospital. This observation is surprising in view of the controlled clinical trial undertaken by Captain Lind on 20 May 1747, when 12 patients with scurvy were randomized to a variety of treatments. The results were decisive in favour of oranges and lemons.

The formula of ascorbic acid, shown in Fig. 1, demonstrates the reducing properties of ascorbic acid which is oxidized to dehydroascorbic acid. Both ascorbic acid and dehydroascorbic acid have anti-scorbutic properties, but only ascorbic acid has the reducing properties which may be of importance in cancer prevention.

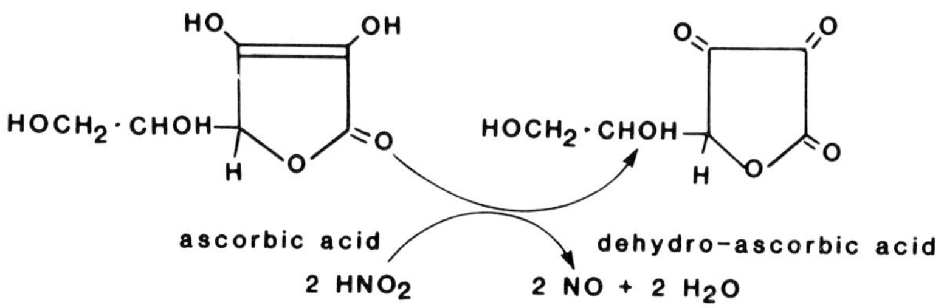

Fig. 1 Oxidation of ascorbic acid to dehydroascorbic acid

Ascorbic acid and gastric juice[2]

The concentration of vitamin C in plasma of normal subjects is variable, ranging between 2 and 135 μg/l[3,4]. Freeman and Hafkesbring in 1951[3] discov-ered that the concentration of vitamin C in the human stomach was sometimes higher than plasma, suggesting an active secretory mechanism. In 1957 Freeman and Hafkesbring[5] found lower gastric juice vitamin C concentrations in peptic ulcer, pernicious anaemia, gastritis and carcinoma of the stomach than in controls, findings confirmed by Singh and Godbole in 1968[6]. Further work in this area has been stimulated by the observation that populations with a high intake of vitamin C-containing foods have a lower incidence of gastric cancer. This association is the most consistent dietary association so far identified[7].

In 1989 three separate papers confirmed the work of Freeman and Hafkesbring demonstrating a concentration gradient of vitamin C between plasma and gastric juice, and showing that the presence of gastritis was associated with a failure of this concentrating mechanism[8-10]. Two of these papers had measured both ascorbic acid and dehydroascorbic acid, and showed ascorbic acid to be much lower in patients with gastritis and virtually absent in those with hypochlorhydria.

The same group studied changes in ascorbic acid secretion following gastric juice stimulation by sham feeding and pentagastric stimulation[4]. The concentration of juice vitamin C in duodenal ulcer did not increase after stimulation, and remained significantly lower than the control group. The prescription of acid-reducing therapy reduced the concentration of gastric ascorbic acid further. When ascorbic acid was incubated with acidic gastric juice it remained stable for 1 h; however, in hypochlorhydric juice no ascorbic acid could be recovered even from samples prepared immediately. The concentration of total vitamin C, however, remained the same, implying that in the hypochlorhydric samples vitamin C had been converted almost immediately to dehydroascorbic acid. Was it the elevation in pH that was responsible for the instability of ascorbic acid? Ascorbic acid incubated with normal acidic acid juice, rendered neutral by the addition of sodium hydroxide, was recovered as effectively as from the original acidic juice. These data suggest that some other factor is present in hypochlorhydric gastric juice which has a destabilizing effect; the changes are not simply a result of the pH difference. It seems likely that oxidants present within the hypochlorhydric gastric juice are responsible for the conversion of ascorbic acid to dehydroascorbic acid.

In summary, it would appear that ascorbic acid is secreted into the stomach at a concentration higher than (and independent of) plasma concentrations. Chronic gastritis interferes with its secretion, reducing both total vitamin C and ascorbic acid concentrations. Hypochlorhydria reduces the concentration of ascorbic acid almost to zero; this is probably mediated by oxidants within the hypochlorhydric gastric juice.

Concentration of ascorbic acid in gastrointestinal tissue

It was recognized as long ago as 1937[11] that dog gastrointestinal mucosa contained high concentrations of vitamin C (duodenal 935 μmol/kg, ileal 869 μmol/kg, colonic 477 μmol/kg stomach fundas, 311 μmol/kg, pyloric mucosa 121 μmol/kg). These levels are approximately 10 times that found in the gastric juice, and this begs the question of whether the secretion into the juice is merely the result of exfoliation of cells into the gastric milieu. This seems unlikely in that the concentration of ascorbic acid in the juice is higher than would be predicted from the degree of cell exfoliation, and would not account for the differences seen between patients with chronic gastritis and normals. Chronic gastritis is associated with a faster cell replication than in normal individuals, and if exfoliation was the mechanism, higher levels of ascorbic acid would be expected in chronic gastritis.

HELICOBACTER PYLORI AND VITAMIN C SECRETION

Helicobacter infection causes a diminution of gastric ascorbic acid secretion. A research worker who had previously performed gastric ascorbic acid secretions on himself contracted *H. pylori* infection[12] and repeated the studies on himself whilst infected. In the initial experiment basal concentrations of ascorbic acid were measured, and the subject was then injected intravenously with ascorbic acid, which led to a rise in ascorbic acid secretion by the stomach. One month after contracting *Helicobacter* infection the concentration of ascorbic acid in the gastric juice was zero both fasting and after the injection. Six months later basal levels of ascorbic acid were still negligible, and there was only a minor increase in gastric juice concentration and ascorbic acid after injection.

The commonest cause of chronic gastritis is *H. pylori* infection, which accounts for the failure of secretion of vitamin C in duodenal ulcer patients, and after successful *Helicobacter* eradication the concentration of ascorbic acid in the gastric juice rises[13].

VITAMIN C AND GASTRIC CANCER

The epidemiological evidence which associates a high intake of vitamin C with a lower incidence of gastric cancer has been alluded to previously. The possible mechanisms whereby vitamin C might protect fall mainly into two areas: the nitrite scavenging effect of the molecule and inactivation of reactive oxygen species. In 1988 O'Connor *et al.*[14] studied the mutagenicity of gastric juice using a bacterial fluctuation assay. Fasting juice was analysed for acidity, ascorbic acid concentration and mutagenicity. Patients were given a week's course of ascorbic acid by mouth and the experiment was repeated. The concentration of vitamin C in the juice increased and the mutagenic activity fell significantly.

THE *N*-NITROSO COMPOUND THEORY

The *N*-nitroso compound theory[15] is based on the observation that many *N*-nitroso compounds are carcinogenic. Under normal circumstances dietary nitrate in the acidic milieu of the stomach is unchanged; however, in hypochlorhydria nitrate-reducing bacteria may colonize the stomach and convert nitrate to nitrite. Nitrite in turn may be metabolized to N-nitroso compounds, either spontaneously in an acidic milieu or by other bacteria. The literature on this subject is confused because N-nitroso compounds are unstable, difficult to measure and there is a wide variety of these compounds, some of which are mutagenic and others which are not. However, it is well documented *in vitro* that ascorbic acid has a nitrite-scavenging effect which not only prevents the formation of N-nitroso compounds but also protects against DNA damage and mutagenicity[16,17]. It does this by scavenging nitrite, as shown in Fig. 1[18]. This blocking action of ascorbate on nitrosation is variable and dependent upon the pH of the milieu and the nature of the amine. The administration of ascorbic acid to animals prevents N-nitroso precursors from causing cancer[18]. Nitrate and proline were given to 10 healthy young adults[19]; this led to the formation of nitroso-proline (a non-carcinogenic compound excreted in the urine); the ingestion of ascorbic acid inhibited nitrate incorporation by 81%.

Although there is some doubt as to the ability of ascorbic acid to deactivate preformed N-nitroso compounds, studies with N-methyl-N-nitroguanidine (MNNG) and dimethylnitrosamine (DMN)[20] have demonstrated that ascorbic acid inhibits mutagenesis. There appears to be a reaction between ascorbate and MNNG that leads eventually to consumption of MNNG, the reaction being enhanced by catalytic amounts of copper(II) and iron(III).

There appear to be at least three ways in which ascorbic acid may be protective where N-nitroso compounds are concerned: (1) the prevention of N-nitroso formation by the scavenging of nitrite; (2) reaction with the N-nitroso compound which leads to its consumption; (3) a non-specific protective effect against mutagenicity.

REACTIVE OXYGEN SPECIES (ROS)

Reactive oxygen species are unstable chemicals which are highly reactive and exist for fractions of a second[21]. They are produced by many biochemical reactions and damage DNA, causing strand breaks, translocations and deletions[22]. Under normal circumstances the body is protected by superoxide dismutase. Irradiation, ischaemia and acute inflammation cause excessive production of ROS which may be responsible for serious damage.

ROS are difficult to study because of their lability; however, they are generated in increased quantity in *H. pylori* infection[23] and their continued overproduction throughout a long period might eventually lead to mutation and eventual carcinoma.

Ascorbic acid scavenges ROS, quenching chemiluminescence in a concentration-dependent fashion[24,25]. This appears to work extracellularly[26] and may therefore have a protective role in preventing ROS damage outside the neutrophil without interfering with the intracellular killing of micro-organisms, which is thought to be mediated at least in part by ROS. In one study ascorbate was the only significant reducing agent for nitroxide, and spin trapping of oxy-radicals was accelerated in cells which were ascorbate depleted; it was inhibited with ascorbate loading[27]. In another experiment hydroxyl radicals (probably the most potent ROS) produced by the radiolysis of water were scavenged by ascorbic acid with the formation of dehydro-ascorbic acid[28].

The role of ROS in gastric cancer is speculative, and direct evidence to show that ascorbic acid is effective within the stomach has yet to be produced. However, this is a further possible mechanism whereby ascorbic acid might protect against the development of gastric cancer.

SUMMARY

Vitamin C exists in two forms: ascorbic acid and dehydroascorbic acid. The change from one to the other is responsible for its anti-oxidant activity. The normal stomach secretes ascorbic acid against a concentration gradient, but this mechanism is abolished by *Helicobacter* infection, and in the hypochlorhydric stomach concentrations of ascorbic acid are negligible. Epidemiological studies suggest that dietary vitamin C is a protective factor against the development of gastric cancer. The diminution of ascorbic acid secretion by *Helicobacter* may represent a risk factor for the development of cancer in patients with chronic gastritis. Possible mechanisms of action include the scavenging of nitrite, thus preventing the formation of N-nitroso compounds; inhibition of the mutagenicity of the preformed N-nitroso compounds; and the scavenging of free oxygen radicals which are over-produced in individuals infected with *H. pylori*. Direct experimental evidence to support these hypotheses is not available, but indirect experimentation has provided circumstantial evidence to suggest that further work in this area is justified.

Acknowledgements

I thank Dr S. S. Mirvish for allowing me to reproduce Fig. 1, and Miss J. Mackintosh for typing the text.

References

1. Harris LJ. Scurvy and vitamin C. In: Vitamins in theory and practice. London: Cambridge University Press; 1935:78–106.
2. Sobala GM. Ascorbic acid in human gastric juice. Cambridge: University of Cambridge; 1993 (dissertation).
3. Freeman JT, Hafkesbring R. Comparative study of ascorbic acid levels in gastric secretion, blood, urine and saliva. Gastroenterology. 1951;18:224–9.
4. Schorah CJ, Sobala GM, Sanderson M, Collis N, Primrose JN. Gastric juice ascorbic acid: effects of disease and implications for gastric carcinogenesis. Am J Clin Nutr. 1991;53: 287S–93S.
5. Freeman JT, Hafkesbring R. Comparative studies of ascorbic acid levels in gastric secretion and blood. III. Gastrointestinal disease. Gastroenterology. 1957;32:878–86.

6. Singh D, Godbole AG. A study of plasma and gastric juice ascorbic acid in peptic ulcer. J Assoc Phys India. 1968;16:833–7.

7. Forman D. Gastric cancer, diet and nitrate exposure. BMJ. 1987;294:528.

8. O'Connor HJ, Schorah CJ, Habibzedah N, Axon ATR, Cockel R. Vitamin C in the human stomach: relation to gastric pH, gastroduodenal disease, and possible sources. Gut. 1989;30:436–42.

9. Sobala GM, Schorah CJ, Sanderson M *et al.* Ascorbic acid in the human stomach. Gastroenterology. 1989;97:357–63.

10. Rathbone BJ, Johnson AW, Wyatt JI, Kelleher J, Heatley RV, Losowsky MS. Ascorbic acid: a factor concentrated in human gastric juice. Clin Sci. 1989;76:237–41.

11. Peters GA, Martin HE. Ascorbic acid in gastric juice. Proc Soc Exp Biol Med. 1937;36: 76–8.

12. Sobala GM, Crabtree JE, Dixon MF *et al.* Acute *Helicobacter pylori* infection: clinical features, local and systemic immune response, gastric mucosal histology, and gastric juice ascorbic acid concentrations. Gut. 1991;32:1415–18.

13. Sobala GM, Schorah CJ, Shires S *et al.* Effect of eradication of *Helicobacter pylori* on gastric juice ascorbic acid concentrations. Gut. 1993;34:1038–41.

14. O'Connor HJ, Habibzedah N, Schorah CJ, Axon ATR, Riley SE, Garner RC. Effect of increased intake of vitamin C on the mutagenic activity of gastric juice and intragastric concentrations of ascorbic acid. Carcinogenesis. 1985;6:11:1675–6.

15. Correa P, Haenszel W, Cuello C, Tannenbaum S, Archer M. A model for gastric cancer epidemiology. Lancet. 1975;2:58–60.

16. Walters CL. Vitamin C and nitrosamine formation. In: Birch GG, Parker KJ, editors. Vitamin C: recent aspects of its physiological and technological importance. London: Applied Science; 1974:78–90.

17. Guttenplan JP. Inhibition by L-ascorbate of bacterial mutagenesis induced by two *N*-nitroso compounds. Nature. 1977;268:368–70.

18. Mirvish SS. Effects of vitamins C and E on *N*-nitroso compound formation, carcinogenesis and cancer. Cancer. 1986;58:1842–50.

19. Wagner DA, Shuker DEG, Bilmanzes C *et al.* Effects of vitamins C and E on endogenous synthesis of *N*-nitrosamino acids in humans: precursor-product studies with [^{15}N] nitrate. Cancer Res. 1985;45:6519–22.

20. Guttenplan JB. Mechanisms of inhibition by ascorbate of microbial mutagenesis induced by *N*-nitroso compounds. Cancer Res. 1978;38:2018–22.

21. Halliwell B. Oxygen radicals: a commonsense look at their nature and medical importance. Med Biol. 1984;62:71–7.

22. Koningsberger JC, Marx JJM, Van Hattum J. Free radicals in gastroenterology. Scand J Gastroenterol. 1988;23(Suppl.154):30–40.

23. Davies GR, Simmonds NJ, Stevens TRJ, Grandison A, Blake DR, Rampton DS. Mucosal reactive oxygen metabolite production in duodenal ulcer disease. Gut. 1992;33:1467–72.

24. Whitehead TP, Thorpe GHG, Maxwell SRJ. Enhanced chemiluminescence assay for antioxidant capacity in biological fluids. Anal Chem Acta. 1992;266:265–77.

25. Dwenger A, Funck M, Lucken B, Scharetzer G, Lehman U. Effect of ascorbic acid on neutrophil functions and hypoxanthine/xanthine oxidase-generated, oxygen-derived radicals. Eur J Clin Chem Clin Biochem. 1992;30:187–91.

26. Anderson R, Lukey PT. A biological role for ascorbate in the selective neutralisation of extracellular phagocyte-derived oxidants. Ann NY Acad Sci. 1987;498:229–47.

27. Mehlhorn RJ. Ascorbate and dehydroascorbic acid-mediated reduction of free radicals in the human erythrocyte. J Bio Chem. 1991;266(5):2724–31.

28. Rose RC. Ascorbic acid metabolism in protection against free radicals: a radiation model. Biochem Biophys Res Commun. 1990;169:430–6.

45
Role of bacterial overgrowth in gastric carcinogenesis

N. D. YEOMANS

The possibility that bacteria in the gastric lumen might be aetiologically important in gastric cancer has been discussed for some years. The sequence of events proposed by Correa *et al.*[1] has attracted the most attention; this is set out in Fig. 1. In essence, Correa *et al.* postulated that the presence of nitrate-reducing bacteria in the gastric lumen leads to the reduction of dietary nitrate to nitrite. This, in turn, has the capacity to nitrosate dietary or endogenously-derived amines and amides to *N*-nitroso compounds (N-NOC) such as nitrosamines and nitrosamides. It is postulated that some of the resulting N-NOC might have carcinogenic potential in humans, since it is known that members of this class (such as *N*-methyl-*N'*-nitro-*N*-nitroso-guanidine and nitrosamides) are powerful direct-acting carcinogens in experi-mental animals[2,3].

The hypothesis has had the advantage of offering an explanation for two known associations with gastric cancer – the associations with pernicious

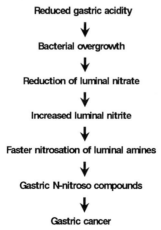

Fig. 1 Diagram of nitrosamine hypothesis proposed by Correa *et al.*[1]

anaemia and with partial gastrectomy – both of which are characterized by elevated bacterial numbers in gastric juice.

However, the search for direct evidence for the Correa hypothesis has produced conflicting results. Despite the good evidence for increased bacterial numbers in conditions such as pernicious anaemia and partial gastrectomy, there is conflicting evidence about whether these conditions increase the rate of formation of N-NOC *in vivo*. The literature on this is reviewed in more detail below.

If bacteria were to play any causal role in gastric carcinogenesis, the mechanism might of course be something other than N-nitrosation. Several studies have recently reported an association between gastric carcinoma and long-term colonization of the gastric mucosa by *Helicobacter pylori*. This may turn out to be the most important connection between gastric bacteria and cancer, and might point to gastritis and chronic inflammation as the major mediators of such an association. The role of *H. pylori* in gastric cancer is dealt with elsewhere in this book, and is not considered further here, except in relation to an alternative hypothesis presented at the end of this review.

BACTERIAL OVERGROWTH IN STOMACH

Gastric juice is normally either sterile or contains only small numbers (up to 10^5/ml) of oropharyngeal-type flora[4-6]. This may be the main reason for the ability to secrete gastric acid conferring some survival value during vertebrate evolution[7,8].

There is an approximate relationship between intragastric pH and the number of organisms in gastric juice, as shown in Fig. 2 which is constructed from pooled data from four studies[4,5,9,10].

In patients who have had acid-lowering surgery, or who have developed atrophic gastritis, bacterial counts in gastric juice are usually higher; sometimes markedly so. In pernicious anaemia the mean bacterial count from several studies was in the range 10^6–10^7 per ml[4,6,9,11]. After partial gastrectomy, or vagotomy and antrectomy, bacterial counts are usually also increased[12-16] – to the order of 10^4/ml. In both atrophic gastritis and the post-resection stomach, the bacterial flora is often qualitatively different from normal. It often consists of a faecal-type flora that contains coliforms and other Gram-negative organisms[9,12,13].

On the other hand, vagotomy without gastric resection has not been clearly implicated in altering gastric flora[10,16,17]. In one study, in which the gastric juice was sampled throughout a 24 h period, the mean pH increased only to 2.2, from a preoperative baseline of 1.7, and bacterial counts did not change significantly[10].

The introduction of effective acid-lowering drugs also provoked concern about possible deleterious increases in bacterial counts. There is reasonable evidence that bacterial counts do increase during therapy. For instance, Ruddell *et al.* found an increase in mean counts of about two logs during 4 weeks of cimetidine therapy[18], and increases have also been found after treatment with ranitidine[19]. A similar increase was reported in a study with

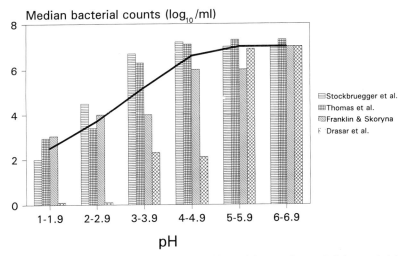

Fig. 2 Relationship between intragastric pH and bacterial counts in gastric juice, pooled from four studies in healthy volunteers and patients with a variety of low acid states: Stockbruegger et al.[9], Thomas et al.[10], Franklin and Skoryna[5], Drasar et al.[4]. Reproduced with permission from Yeomans ND, Lambert JR. Infections of the stomach and duodenum. In: Haubrich WS, Schaffner F, Berk JE, editors. Bockus Gastroenterology, 5th edn. Philadelphia: W.B. Saunders; 1993

the acid-pump inhibitor omeprazole[19]. To date, no long-term consequences of anti-ulcer drugs have been identified, although the total experience does not yet extend beyond about 16 years.

RELATIONSHIP BETWEEN CANCER, ATROPHIC GASTRITIS AND GASTRIC SURGERY

There is now quite a lot of evidence that partial gastrectomy, mostly done for peptic ulcer, increases the likelihood of gastric carcinoma. There is quite a long latent period, and the risk does not seem to increase significantly until 15–20 years have elapsed[20–25]. Even then the relative risk is only about 2–3. On the other hand, the residual area of gastric mucosa is less than in the unoperated stomach, so the risk per unit area may be rather greater than a relative risk of 2–3 implies.

While the association between gastric resection and gastric cancer has been cited as evidence for a role of bacterial overgrowth in carcinogenesis, data from gastric operations in experimental animals raise another possibility. Several studies have shown that gastric resection increases the incidence of gastric tumours induced subsequently by administering a carcinogen[26]. However, if duodenogastric reflux is prevented by creation of a long Roux-en-Y loop, the tumour incidence is markedly reduced[2]. This suggests that some component of the upper intestinal contents, such as pancreatic juice or bile, may be at least as important as bacteria for the cancer risk post-gastrectomy.

Atrophic gastritis in pernicious anaemia is also likely to be premalignant and, as indicated above, this condition is also associated with quite marked bacterial overgrowth. Nevertheless, the increase in cancer incidence in pernicious anaemia may have been overestimated, because of failure to take account of a falling gastric cancer incidence in Western populations in general. One recent study suggested that the relative risk (excluding the risk of ECL cell carcinoids, which were probably included in some earlier studies) may be only about 2^{27}.

NITRITE AND N-NOC PRODUCTION IN PATIENTS WITH BACTERIAL OVERGROWTH

Fuelled particularly by the suggestions that cimetidine might pose a cancer risk, mediated via bacterial overgrowth in the stomach, a large amount of research has been directed at measuring nitrite and N-NOC in low acid states. Most investigators have demonstrated some increase in nitrite concentrations in the gastric juice of patients with partial gastrectomy or atrophic gastritis[9,28]. Similar increases have been found in subjects treated with acid-suppressive drugs[10,19]. There is considerable individual variation, and one explanation may be that only some bacterial strains are capable of reducing nitrate to nitrite[29].

Studies of the formation of *N*-nitroso compounds, however, have given conflicting results. One of the problems has been the specificity and accuracy of the assays for N-NOC. There are many methodological traps, including the non-measurement of volatile compounds and low recoveries of compounds of interest and losses of N-NOC from samples during storage[30-33]. Studies using one of the earliest assays generally found increased concentrations of N-NOC in gastric juice from patients with low acid states and bacterial overgrowth[19,34,35]. However, when an improved assay was used, this relationship was not found[14,36].

Another approach attempting to demonstrate *N*-nitrosation *in vivo* has been to measure the urinary excretion of stable, non-mutagenic nitrocompounds such as nitrosoproline. This is generated by nitrite (from diet or nitrate-reducing bacteria) in the gastric lumen acting on dietary or endogenous proline. Studies using this method have indicated that a substantial part of N-NOC production *in vivo* is due to *chemical* catalysis in acid gastric juice. Hall *et al.* found a *negative* correlation between intragastric pH and *N*-nitrosoproline excretion in pernicious anaemia and post-gastrectomy patients[37]. To highlight the difficulty of interpreting such studies, though, Elder *et al.* found increased excretion of another N-NOC – *N*-nitroso-thiazolidine-4-carboxylic acid – during histamine H_2-antagonist blockade[38]. Thus the findings may differ, not only according to the methods used for analysis, but according to the individual N-NOC being assayed. Given the very large number of potential nitroso compounds that could be generated in the bacterially contaminated stomach, it is hard to be certain that none is important as a mutagenic risk factor.

ROLE OF ASCORBATE AND GASTRITIS IN N-NOC FORMATION

A further level of complexity to the N-NOC story has come from evidence that some antioxidants are natural inhibitors of the formation of nitroso compounds from nitrite. There is some epidemiological evidence that ingestion of fresh fruit and vegetables is protective against gastric carcinoma[39], and this has focused interest on the possible roles of ascorbate and vitamin E. Ingestion of ascorbic acid during the nitrosoproline test produces a sharp fall in N-nitrosoproline excretion[40], and this is made use of to differentiate between the endogenous production of nitrosoproline and the ingested load of preformed nitrosoproline in this test. Ascorbic acid is normally secreted into gastric juice, but its concentration is reduced in patients with chronic gastritis[41]. Thus this observation might identify another contributory mechanism for the increased cancer risk in patients with gastritis.

AN ALTERNATIVE TO THE BACTERIAL OVERGROWTH/N-NOC HYPOTHESIS

The original Correa hypothesis has been attractive for explaining some of the known associations between gastric cancer and gastritis, via the common denominator of low gastric acid and bacterial overgrowth. However, some of the inconsistencies in the evidence, especially to confirm or refute the last step of N-NOC formation, have been referred to above.

The realization that *H. pylori* may be a particularly important risk factor for the intestinal form of gastric carcinoma has added a new dimension to this debate. It is possible that the most important risk factor for developing gastric carcinoma is simply gastritis, whatever its cause. Gastritis is, of course, extreme in pernicious anaemia, with extensive autoimmune attack. Gastritis is also invariant in *H. pylori* infection, and usual in the post-gastrectomy stomach. In the latter situation it is unclear (a) what part is played by the natural progression of the *H. pylori* gastritis that would usually have been an accompaniment of the original ulcer for which the surgery was performed, or (b) how much it is a result of the chemical gastritis that afflicts the partially gastrectomized stomach.

This alternative relationship is set out in Fig. 3. If the neoplastic predisposition is mainly a property of the gastritic mucosa, the reduced acid secretion and bacterial overgrowth may be merely epiphenomena. Nevertheless, we cannot rule out the possibility that N-NOC formation might play a further facilitatory role, if they are indeed produced in the gastritic, low acid-secreting stomach. Indeed Bartsch's group have recently speculated that activated neutrophils and macrophages, by producing nitric oxide and oxyradicals, might produce *endogenous* N-NOC in inflamed gastric mucosae[42].

Another important mutagenic mechanism in gastric mucosa may be simply the increased risk of somatic mutations as a result of continued injury and repair. Cell proliferation has been shown to be substantially increased

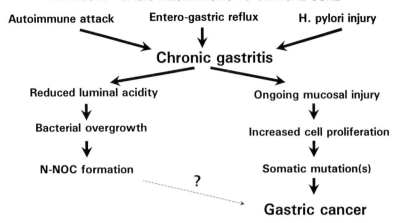

Fig. 3 Putative alternative to the Correa nitrosamine hypothesis of gastric carcinogenesis

in atrophic gastritis and in the postoperative stomach[43,44]. In the former instance the increased labelling index shown by Hansen *et al.*[44] is even more significant when one remembers that the volume of the mucosa is markedly reduced. That is to say, the remaining cells must be cycling even faster than the increased labelling index appears to indicate. Increased cell proliferation is known to be an important promoting mechanism in a variety of experimental cancers. Each cell division has a finite chance of DNA synthetic error, and the more cycles a tissue experiences the greater is the cumulative chance of an oncologically important mutation occurring.

Whether bacterial overgrowth and N-NOC formation is a major mechanism in gastric carcinogenesis, or whether other mechanisms such as mucosal inflammation are more important, may be of some practical importance. In the former case we would have cause to continue to be cautious about inducing a pharmacological achlorhydria and bacterial overgrowth, such as might occur after prolonged high dosage with agents such as omeprazole. If inflammation were found to be more important, there may be an advantage in trying to eradicate a major cause such as *H. pylori* even at the stage of irreversible failure of acid secretion.

Important evidence will come in the future from long-term follow-up of patients in whom *H. pylori* has been eradicated, as well as in patients on long-term, potent antisecretory treatment for conditions such as reflux oesophagitis, in which the confounding factor of gastritis is often absent. The lesson of the post-gastrectomy stomach suggests, though, that we will have to wait patiently for about 20–30 years.

Acknowledgement

This work was supported by a grant from the National Health and Medical Research Council of Australia.

References

1. Correa P, Haenszl W, Cuello C, Tannenbaum S, Archer M. A model for gastric cancer epidemiology. Lancet. 1975;2:58–60.
2. Nishidoi H, Koga S, Kaibara N. Possible role of duodenogastric reflux on the development of remnant gastric carcinoma induced by *N*-methyl-*N'*-nitro-*N*-nitrosoguanidine in rats. J Natl Cancer Inst. 1984;72:1431–5.
3. Tannenbaum SR. *N*-nitroso compounds: a perspective on human exposure. Lancet. 1983;1:629 32.
4. Drasar BS, Shiner M, McLeod GM. Studies on the intestinal flora. I. The bacterial flora of the gastrointestinal tract in healthy and achlorhydric persons. Gastroenterology. 1969;56:71–9.
5. Franklin MA, Skoryna SC. Studies on natural gastric flora. I. Bacterial flora of fasting human subjects. Can Med Assoc J. 1966;95:1349–55.
6. Henning N. Die bakterielle besiedlung des gesunden und des kranken Magens. Archiv Verdaunskr. 1930;47:1–59.
7. Giraud AS, Yeomans ND. Fine structure of the gastric mucosa of a toad, *Bufo marinus*. Cell Tissue Res. 1981;218:663–8.
8. Giraud AS, Yeomans ND. Cell types of the gastric mucosa of a teleost: the river blackfish, *Gadopsis marmoratis*. Aust J Mar Freshwater Res. 1982;33:1103–8.
9. Stockbruegger RW, Cotton PB, Menon GG et al. Pernicious anemia, intragastric bacterial overgrowth, and possible consequences. Scand J Gastroenterol. 1984;199:355–64.
10. Thomas JM, Misiewicz JJ, Cook AR et al. Effects of one year's treatment with ranitidine and of truncal vagotomy on gastric contents. Gut. 1987;28:726–38.
11. Armbrecht U, Bosaeus I, Gillberg R, Seeberg S, Stockbruegger R. Hydrogen (H$_2$) breath test and gastric bacteria in acid-secreting subjects and in achlorhydric and postgastrectomy patients before and after antimicrobial treatment. Scand J Gastroenterol. 1985;20:805–13.
12. Drasar BS, Shiner M. Studies on the small intestinal flora. II. Bacterial flora of the small intestine in patients with gastrointestinal disorders. Gut. 1969;10:812–19.
13. Gray JDA, Shiner M. Influence of gastric pH on gastric and jejunal flora. Gut. 1967;8: 574–81.
14. Keighley MR, Youngs D, Poxon V et al. Intragastric *N*-nitrosation is unlikely to be responsible for gastric carcinoma developing after operations for duodenal ulcer. Gut. 1984;25:238–45.
15. Kyrtopoulos SA, Daskalakis G, Legakis NI et al. Studies in gastric carcinogenesis. ii. Absence of elevated concentrations of *N*-nitroso compounds in the gastric juice of Greek hypochlorhydric individuals. Carcinogenesis. 1985;6:1135–40.
16. Muscroft TJ, Deane SA, Youngs D, Burdon DW, Keighley MR. The microflora of the postoperative stomach. Br J Surg. 1981;68:560–4.
17. Schumpelick V, Schassan HH. Bakteriologie des operierten Magens. Langenbecks Arch Chir. 1980;350:271–9.
18. Ruddell WS, Axon AT, Findlay JM, Bartholomew BA, Hill MJ. Effect of cimetidine on the gastric bacterial flora. Lancet. 1980;1:672–4.
19. Stockbruegger RW, Cotton PB, Eugenides N, Bartholomew BA, Hill M, Walters CL. Intragastric nitrites, nitrosamines, and bacterial overgrowth during cimetidine treatment. Gut. 1982;23:1048–54.
20. Viste A, Bjornestad E, Opheim P et al. Risk of carcinoma following gastric operations for benign disease: a historical cohort study of 3470 patients. Lancet. 1986;2:502–5.
21. Fischer AB. The long-term results following Billroth II resection for duodenal ulcer. Dan Med Bull. 1986;33:319–35.
22. Lundegårdh G, Adami HO, Helmick C, Zack M, Meirik O. Stomach cancer after partial gastrectomy for benign ulcer disease. N Engl J Med. 1988;319:195–200.
23. Arnthorsson G, Tulinius H, Egilsson V, Sigvaldason H, Magnusson B, Thorarinsson H. Gastric cancer after gastrectomy. Int J Cancer. 1988;42:365–7.
24. Caygill CPJ, Hill MJ, Hall CN, Kirkham JS, Northfield TC. Increased risk of cancer at multiple sites after gastric surgery for peptic ulcer. Gut. 1987;28:924–8.
25. Moller H, Toftgaard C. Cancer occurrence in a cohort of patients surgically treated for peptic ulcer. Gut. 1991;32:740–4.

26. Sano C, Kumashiro R, Sarto T, Inokudri K. Promoting effect of partial gastrectomy in carcinogenesis in the remnant stomach of rats after oral administration of *N*-methyl-*N*-nitrosoguanidine. Oncology. 1984;41:124.
27. Brinton LA, Gridley G, Hrubec Z, Houves R, Fraumeni JF. Cancer risk following pernicious anaemia. Br J Cancer. 1989;59:810.
28. Carboni M, Guadagni S, Pistoia MA *et al.* Chronic atrophic gastritis and risk of *N*-nitroso compounds carcinogenesis. Langenbecks Arch Chir. 1988;373:82–90.
29. Leach SA, Thompson M, Hill M. Bacterially catalysed *N*-nitrosation reactions and their relative importance in the human stomach. Carcinogenesis. 1987;8:1907–12.
30. Bavin PM, Darkin DW, Viney NJ. Total nitroso compounds in gastric juice. IARC Sci Publ. 1982;41:337–44.
31. Eisenbrand G, Janzowski C, Pruessmann R. Analytical method for *N*-nitroso compounds. J Chromatogr. 1975;115:602–5.
32. Pignatelli B, Richard I, Bourgade MC, Bartsch H. An improved method for analysis of total *N*-nitroso compounds in gastric juice. IARC Sci Publ. 1987;84:209–15.
33. Smith PRL, Walters CL, Reed PI. The importance of selectivity in the determination of *N*-nitroso compounds as a group. Analyst. 1983;108:895–8.
34. Reed PI, Summers K, Smith PL *et al.* Effect of gastric surgery for benign peptic ulcer and ascorbic acid therapy on concentration of nitrite and *N*-nitroso compounds in gastric juice. IARC Sci Publ. 1984;57:975–9.
35. Reed PI, Smith PL, Haines K, House FR, Walters CL. Effect of cimetidine on gastric juice *N*-nitrosamine concentration. Lancet. 1981;2:553–6.
36. Hall CN, Darkin D, Brimblecombe R, Cook AJ, Kirkham J, Northfield TC. Evaluation of the nitrosamine hypothesis of gastric carcinogenesis in precancerous conditions. Gut. 1986;27:491–8.
37. Hall CN, Kirkham JS, Northfield TC. Urinary *n*-nitrosoproline excretion: a further evaluation of the nitrosamine hypothesis of gastric carcinogenesis in precancerous conditions. Gut. 1987;28:216–20.
38. Elder JB, Burdett K, Smith PL, Walters CL, Reed PI. Effect of H$_2$ blockers on intragastric nitrosation as measured by 24-hour urinary secretion of *N*-nitrosoproline. IARC Sci Publ. 1984;57:969–74.
39. Mirvish SS, Karlowski A, Sams JP, Arnold SD. Studies related to nitrosamide formation: nitrosation in solvents: water and solvent systems, nitrosomethylurea formation in the rat stomach and analysis of a fish product for ureas. IARC Sci Publ. 1978;19:161.
40. Ohshima H, Bartsch H. Quantitative estimation of endogenous nitrosation in humans by monitoring *N*-nitrosoproline excreted in the urine. Cancer Res. 1981;41:3658–62.
41. Rathbone BJ, Johnson AW, Wyatt JI, Kelleher J, Heatley RV, Losowsky MS. Ascorbic acid: a factor concentrated in human gastric juice. Clin Sci. 1989;76:237–41.
42. Bartsch H, Ohshima H, Pignatelli B, Calmels S. Endogenously formed *N*-nitroso compounds and nitrosating agents in human cancer etiology. Pharmacogenetics. 1992;2:272–7.
43. Hansen OH, Svendsen LB. Changes in gastric mucosal cell proliferation after antrectomy or vagotomy in man. Scand J Gastroenterol. 1978;13:947–52.
44. Hansen OH, Johansen A, Larsen JK, Pedersen T, Svendsen LB. Relationship between gastric acid secretion, histopathology, and cell proliferation kinetics in human gastric mucosa. Gastroenterology. 1977;73:453–6.

46
The role of PCR techniques in the epidemiology of *H. pylori* infections

T. TYSKIEWICZ and T. WADSTRÖM

INTRODUCTION

Since the discovery of *Helicobacter pylori* (formerly *Campylobacter pylori*[1]), culture techniques for isolation of this organism from infected gastric tissues have been optimized and a variety of transport media evaluated for isolation of the microbe[2,3]. More recently, *H. pylori* has also been cultured from dental plaques and stool specimens. Altogether these data suggest that a faecal–oral route, as well as an oral–oral route, are important in the spread of these infections in various geographic regions worldwide.

Urease tests on gastric biopsies have become a popular and diagnostic screening test, but culture is still the golden standard[4] to: (1) diagnose *H. pylori* infections to allow antibiotic sensitivity testing for (2) studies of various properties of isolated strains in epidemiological studies and (3) to study routes of infection within families and various population groups[5].

DNA-based approaches for the detection of *H. pylori* have included the use of radiolabelled chromosmal fragments, *in situ* hybridization, and hybridization with oligonucleotides based on 15S rRNA sequences[6], or a protocol for the polymerase chain reaction (PCR) based on DNA sequence analysis of a cryptic fragment cloned from the *H. pylori* genome[7].

A number of PCR protocols have been published within the past few years based on gene sequences for specific *H. pylori* proteins such as the urease A and B subunits, a 26 kDa surface-associated protein[8,9] and optimizing of PCR parameters.

Our findings that a number of patients with PCR-positive gastric biopsies also showed positive saliva samples for *H. pylori* encouraged us to explore more systematically if saliva dental plaque material and stool specimens could be used to diagnose *H. pylori* infections. Parallel with this study we also evaluated various techniques to obtain biopsy material and gastric juices for PCR evaluation, and addressing the problem of contamination of the gastroscopes with problems with false-positive reactions by 'carry-over' from previous patients' examinations[10].

MATERIALS AND METHODS

PCR protocol and handling of patient specimens

Patient specimens, gastric biopsies, gastric juice samples, saliva and dental plaque material were treated as described by Hammar *et al.*[9] and Olson *et al.*[10]. In brief, stool samples were diluted with phosphate buffered saline (1/10 and 1/50) and subjected to PCR. Other samples were treated with magnetic beads (Dynal, Oslo, Norway) coated with an antirabbit *H. pylori* strain CCUG 17874 antibodies and incubated at 20°C for 30 min. Enriched *H. pylori* cells were separated by standard procedure as described for detection of enterotoxigenic *E. coli* in stools[11].

RESULTS

Optimization of PCR parameters

We carefully investigated the specificity and sensitivity of our standard PCR protocol for gastric biopsies and gastric juices before we started to evaluate patient samples obtained by non-invasive methods, saliva, dental plaques and the stool specimens[9,10] (Tables 1 and 2). More recently we added a series of pathogens with follow-up studies after 4–6 months and after treatment with anti-*H. pylori* therapy (T. Tyskiewicz and T. Wadström, in preparation).

Altogether our findings suggest that PCR detected *H. pylori* in dental plaques in a few patients who were culture-negative but PCR-positive on dental plaques and/or saliva samples. However, the results of culture-negative patients with PCR-positive gastric biopsy juice specimen must be interpreted with caution. Several possibilities exist for these results:

1. We detected strains of *H. pylori* with special nutritional requirement (?) not possible to grow on conventional media.
2. The specimen contains non-cultivable forms such as coccoidal forms outnumbering normal spiral organisms (samples should be transported in a special medium below 15°C if transported for more than 4–6 h[12]).
3. Endoscopes were contaminated with *H. pylori* DNA from previous patient investigations.

We specifically investigated the last alternative by investigating disinfected gastroscopes prior to use. We then found that conventional strategies of cleaning were not sufficient to remove precipitated *H. pylori* DNA on the gastroscope surface.

Altogether our data suggest that use of equipment to avoid contamination has to be studied for the future, or specimens should be obtained from aspirates of disposable gastric catheters. The alternative would be to develop standard methods to test for *H. pylori* in stool specimens since saliva or dental plaque may reflect transient oral colonization or contamination of *H. pylori*, but perhaps also various *Helicobacter*-like organisms (HLO) such as

Table 1 PCR nucleic acid amplification of *H. pylori*: some examples (detection of *H. pylori* by PCR)

	Authors/reference
Urease gene	Ho *et al.*, 1991[28]
26 kDa surface protein gene	Hammar *et al.*, 1992[9]
	Olsson *et al.*, 1993[10]
16S RNA	Clayton *et al.*, 1992[24]

Some conclusions
1. PCR will detect as few as 100 organisms in 10-fold dilutions[29] and down to one organism in 16S RNA-based PCR[28].
2. *H. pylori* PCR should not give false-positive results with related *Helicobacter*-like organisms (HLO) such as *H. felis*, *Wollinella* species or *Campylobacter* species.
3. PCR should have the sensitivity of $\geq 93\%$ and a specificity of 100% compared to culture methods as 'golden standard' today *and* histopathology studies.
4. Should work on gastric juice after deacidification.

Our method[9] has a shorter amplification time than other PCR methods for *H. pylori*. Further evaluation of these methods on paraffin-embedded tissue[5] should now be performed. The best method may be most attractive to use in surveys on chronic gastritis, stomach cancer patients' studies

various *Wollinella* species[1] of the oral cavity of normal individuals and patients with parodontitis and other dental disorders.

IMMUNOMAGNETIC BEAD PCR

Magnetic immuno-PCR assays have been developed to detect various intestinal pathogens such as *Salmonella* in stool specimen and in water and food samples. Recently Fluit *et al.*[13,14] reported on this method used to detect as little as one colony-forming unit (c.f.u.) per gram of homogenized food, and tested with beads with a *Listeria* monoclonal antibody.

We have immobilized a rabbit polyclonal antibody on magnetic beads, and investigated with human stool specimens in various dilutions and stool samples (experimentally inoculated with *H. pylori*) cells from young and old cultures with predominating spiral forms and coccoidial forms respectively[15].

Our preliminary findings suggest that this test can be standardized and optimized for semiquantitative determination of *H. pylori* DNA in stool samples. However, several questions remain to be answered, such as the detection sensitivity to be used to discriminate patients infected with *H. pylori* compared to patients transiently passing *H. pylori* from the oral cavity and through the gastric mucin layer. It is likely that this problem can be quite important in those geographic regions where *H. pylori* infections occur at an early age, and we now plan to optimize the magnetic immuno-PCR for studies of spread of *H. pylori* in the environment. Our preliminary data suggest, however, a great variation in surface protein profiles of *H. pylori*, and suggest that beads coated with sera against haemagglutinating and non-haemagglutinating *H. pylori* from various geographic regions should be tested before a standard assay can be recommended[16].

HELICOBACTER CHRONIC GASTRITIS, STOMACH CANCER AND PCR – A FUTURE PERSPECTIVE

The association between *H. pylori* infections in early childhood and the risk of developing chronic gastritis with gastric atrophy and dysplasia will encourage investigators to develop new diagnostic strategies to: (1) detect early infections, (2) follow up eradication of *H. pylori* and study mucosal healing; (3) evaluate the role of *H. pylori* in an 'ageing' stomach in chronic type B gastritis[17,18].

Rapid development of well-standardized sensitive ELISA tests for early detection of *H. pylori* infections in children and young adults have been developed in recent years[19,20]. However, we still lack important knowledge on surface proteins, and antigen variation of strains of different geographic regions of the world to define optimal immunoassays such as ELISA and immunoblot tests.

Optimization of PCR methods in the next year to apply on stool samples will be important, since recent studies showed *H. pylori* from stool samples clearly indicated that patients showed the organism at least during early phases of chronic gastritis. However, it is less clear how these organisms survive in the ageing stomach in late chronic gastritis. It is most likely that the *H. pylori* cell mass will then decline. It is a well-known fact that *H. pylori* cannot grow in a dysplasic or highly differentiated stomach adenocarcinoma, despite the fact that the organism can adhere and colonize on various cancer cell lines[21]. Whether *H. pylori* DNA remain in later stages of chronic gastritis is not known.

We know that treatment of other chronic bacterial infections, such as *Chlamydia* infections of the genital or respiratory tracts, results in a rapid disappearance of degraded DNA detectable by PCR or other ultrasensitive DNA detection methods such as ligase chain reaction (LCR).

The possible role of PCR in studying the relationship of papilloma virus and cervical cancer was reviewed by Melchers *et al.*[22].

The problem of optimizing patient specimen processing for PCR *and* endoscopy contamination has been addressed by investigators using endoscopy diagnosing HIV virus infections in patients with tuberculosis[23]. Future studies should also address the possible role of PCR in detection of non-culturable *H. pylori* that could exist in saliva, faecal samples and in food, as well as in other environments already discussed in an early publication on PCR in the detection of *H. pylori*[24,25].

Van Zwet *et al.*[26] reported that a PCR reaction based on a urease gene sequence was not more sensitive than culture, and discussed various explanations. It was concluded that, in situations where rapid handling of samples for culture is not possible, PCR offers a great advantage. These authors also warned about contamination of negative samples when several gastroscopies are performed in one session. The problem of cleaning gastroscopes is illustrated in our own studies (Table 3). However, in follow-up of patients treated for chronic gastritis to detect slow-growing or resting forms of *H. pylori* in gastric tissues, PCR will probably be an important research tool. In patients with stomach atrophy, *H. pylori* DNA has probably

Table 2   26 kDa protein *H. pylori* PCR

Negative reactions with:
   Campylobacter jejuni (10 strains)
   Wollinella species (8 strains)*
   E. coli, *Klebsiella* sp., *Proteus* sp. (15 strains)
   Bacteroides sp. (10 strains)†

*Two strains weekly positive
†Including *Bacteroides urealyticus*

Table 3   PCR detection of *H. pylori* DNA on gastroscopes after standard cleaning procedures: an example

Laboratory no.	Gastroscope part	PCR reaction
	Upper channel	+
19151	Lower	−
19152	Excision clip (non-sterile)	+
	sterile ring	+
	Gastroscope	
59–62	Gastroscope	+
60		+
61*		−
632*		−
63		+

*After disinfection

Table 4   Detection of *H. pylori* infection in patients with various gastrointestinal symptoms by culture, PCR and serology

Number of patients	21
Culture-positive	12
PCR positive biopsy*	16
gastric juice	16
dental plaque†	18
saliva	15
HP-Serology +	12

*Three biopsies tested per patient. Two strains were isolated from three patients (D. Berg, J. L. Guruge and T. Wadström, in press)
†Three plaque materials were cultured positive

been degraded, but a small amount may be detectable quite late in 'surviving' dormant forms in extracellular matrix or inside a population of subepithelial cells and in dental plaques (Tables 4 and 5).

Most likely magnetic bead-based PCR will become a rapid simple method to detect *H. pylori* in stools in patients with chronic *H. pylori* infections, but maybe not in patients with chronic infections for two or more decades[27].

Acknowledgements

This study was supported by a grant from the Swedish Medical Research Council (16 X 04723) and a grant from the Medical Faculty of Lund and

Table 5 Detection of *H. pylori* in dental plaques from
patients visiting dental clinics in Lund

Patients	23
PCR positive	8/23
Culture positive	1 patient

the Royal Physiographic Society of Lund. The skilful technical assistance of Karin Olsson is much appreciated.

References

1. Goodwin CS, Armstrong JA, Chilvers T *et al.* Transfer of *Campylobacter pylori* and *Campylobacter mustelae* to *Helicobacter* gen. nov. as *Helicobacter pylori* comb. nov. and *Helicobacter mustelae* comb. nov., respectively. Int J Syst Bacteriol. 1989;39:397–405.
2. Krajden S, Fuksa M, Anderson J *et al.* Examination of human stomach biopsies, saliva and dental plaque for *Campylobacter pylori*. J Clin Microbiol. 1989;27:1397–8.
3. Shames B, Krajden S, Fuksa M, Babida C, Penner JL. Evidence for the occurrence of the same strain of *Campylobacter pylori* in the stomach and dental plaque. J Clin Microbiol. 1989;27:2849–50.
4. Westblom TU. Laboratory diagnosis and handling of *Helicobacter pylori*. In Marshall BJ, McCallum RW, Guerrant RL, editors. *Helicobacter pylori* in peptic ulceration and gastritis. Cambridge, MA: Blackwell Scientific Publications; 1991:81–91.
5. McNulty CAM. Detection of *H. pylori* by the biopsy tests. In Rathbone BJ, Heatley RV, editors. *Helicobacter pylori* and gastroduodenal diseases, 2nd edn. Oxford: Blackwell Scientific Publications; 1992:10:58–63.
6. Wetherall BL, McDonald PJ, Johnson AM. Detection of *Campylobacter pylori* DNA by hybridization with non-radioactive probes in comparison with a [35]P-labeled probe. J Med Microbiol. 1988;26:257–63.
7. Vandenberg FM, Zijlmans H, Langenberg W, Rauws E, Schipper M. Detection of *Campylobacter pylori* in stomach tissue by DNA *in situ* hybridisation. J Clin Pathol. 1989;42:995–1000.
8. O'Toole PW, Logan SM, Kostrzynska M, Wadström T, Trust TJ. Isolation, biochemical and molecular analysis of a species-specific protein antigen from the gastric pathogen *Helicobacter pylori*. J Bacteriol. 1991;173:505–13.
9. Hammar M, Tyszkiewicz T, Wadström T, O'Toole PW. Rapid detection of *Helicobacter pylori* in gastric biopsy material by polymerase chain reaction. J Clin Microbiol. 1992;30(1):54–8.
10. Olsson K, Wadström T, Tyszkiewicz T. *Helicobacter pylori* in dental plaques. Lancet. 1993;341:1155–6.
11. Olsvik Ø, Hornes E, Wasteson Y, Lund A. Detection of virulence determinants in enteric *Escherichia coli* using nucleic acid probes and polymerase chain reaction. In Wadström T, *et al.*, eds. Molecular pathogenesis of gastrointestinal infections. New York: Plenum Press; 1991:267–72.
12. Soltesz V, Zeeberg B, Wadström T. Optimal survival of *Helicobacter pylori* under various transport conditions. J Clin Microbiol. 1992;30:1453–6.
13. Fluit AC, Widjojoatmodjo MN, Box ATA, Torensma R, Verhoef J. Rapid detection of *Salmonellae* in poultry with the magnetic immuno-polymerase chain reaction assay. Appl Env Microbiol. 1993;59:1342–6.
14. Fluit AC, Torensma R, Vissmer MJC *et al.* Detection of *Listeria monocytogenes* in cheese with the magnetic immuno-polymerase chain reaction assay. Appl Env Microbiol. 1993;59:1289–93.
15. Mai UEH, Shahamat M, Colwell RR. Survival of *Helicobacter pylori* in the aquatic environment. In Menge H, Gregor M, Tytgat GNJ, Marshall BJ, McNulty CAM, editors. *Helicobacter pylori* 1990: Proceedings of the Second International Symposium on

Helicobacter pylori. Berlin: Springer-Verlag; 1989:91–4.

16. Lelwala Guruge J. Cell surface protein antigens of *Helicobacter pylori* (dissertation), Lund (Sweden). Lund: Lund University Press; 1993.

17. Correa P, Fox J, Fontham E, et al. *Helicobacter pylori* and gastric carcinomas: Serum antibody prevalence in populations with contrasting cancer risks. Cancer. 1993;66:2569–74.

18. Palli D, Decarli A, Cipriani F *et al. Helicobacter pylori* antibodies in areas of Italy at varying gastric cancer risk. Cancer Epid Biomarkers Prev. 1993;2:37–40.

19. Guruge JL, Schalen C, Nilsson I *et al.* Detection of antibodies to *Helicobacter pylori* cell surface antigens. Scand J Infect Dis. 1990;22:457–65.

20. Newell DG, Stacey AR. The serology of *Campylobacter pylori* infections. In: Rathbone BJ, Heatley RV, eds. *Campylobacter pylori* and gastroduodenal disease. Oxford: Blackwell Scientific Publications; 1989:74–82.

21. Wadström T, Ascencio F, Ljungh Å, *et al.* Adhesins of *Helicobacter pylori*. Eur J Gastroenterol. 1993;45(suppl. 2):S12–S15.

22. Melchers WJG, Claas HCJ, Quint WGV. Use of the polymerase chain reaction to study the relationship between human papillomavirus infections and cervical cancer. Eur J Clin Microbiol Infect. Dis. 1991;10(9):714–27.

23. Kennedy DJ, Lewis WP, Barners PF. Yield of bronchoscopy for the diagnosis of tuberculosis in patients with human immunodeficiency virus infection. Chest. 1992;102:1040–4.

24. Clayton CL, Kleanthous H, Coates PJ, Morgan DD, Tabaqchali S. Sensitive detection of *Helicobacter pylori* by using polymerase chain reaction. J Clin Microbiol. 1992;30:192–200.

25. Mapstone NP *et al.* PCR identification of *Helicobacter pylori* in faeces from gastritis patients. Lancet. 1993;341(1):447.

26. Van Zwet AA, Thijs JC, Kooistra-Smid AMD, Schirm J, Snijder JAM. Sensitivity of culture compared with that of polymerase chain reaction for detection of *Helicobacter pylori* from antral biopsy samples. J Clin Microbiol. 1993;31:1918–20.

27. Dixon MF. *Campylobacter pylori* and chronic gastritis. In Rathbone BJ, Heatley RV, editors. *Campylobacter pylori* and 'gastroduodenal disease'. Oxford: Blackwell Scientific Publications; 1989:106–16.

28. Ho S, Hoyle JA, Lewis FA *et al.* Direct polymerase chain reaction test for detection of *Helicobacter pylori* in humans and animals. J Clin Microbiol. 1991;29:2543–9.

29. Valentine JL. PCR for detection of *Helicobacter pylori*. In Persing EDDH, Smith TF, Tenover FC, White TJ, editors. Diagnostic molecular microbiology: principles and application. Washington, DC: American Society of Microbiologists; 1993:282–87.

47
Role of *H. pylori* in atrophic gastritis and intestinal metaplasia

J. LECHAGO

INTRODUCTION

As discussed by Correa and collaborators in this publication (Chapter 35), chronic gastritis can be divided into a non-atrophic and an atrophic variety. The latter, in turn, has been subdivided into several types on the basis of its pathogenesis. In addition to the so-called *chemical gastritis*, associated with either gastroduodenal reflux or with the use of non-steroidal anti-inflammatory drugs (NSAID), two main types of chronic atrophic gastritis have been characterized: *fundic atrophic gastritis*, associated with pernicious anaemia and recognizing an autoimmune aetiology, and *multifocal atrophic gastritis* (MAG), associated with multiple environmental influences and found in areas of the world with a high prevalence of gastric adenocarcinoma[1].

Both MAG and autoimmune gastritis present with intestinal metaplasia as a prominent feature. However, the type of intestinal metaplasia and the eventual evolution of each kind of gastritis are significantly different, as is the possible participation of *Helicobacter pylori* in their pathogenesis. The role of *H. pylori* in atrophic gastritis and intestinal metaplasia will be analysed, reviewing the available evidence for and against, as well as the extent of, such participation. This is not meant to be an exhaustive review, but rather a critical appraisal of some reports selected among the most recent and pertinent contributions to the subject. In the context of such analysis, a number of questions can be raised: (1) Can there be chronic atrophic gastritis and intestinal metaplasia without *H. pylori* infection? (2) Is there a causal relationship between *H. pylori* infection and chronic atrophic gastritis? (3) Does *H. pylori* infection, without participation of other factors, cause intestinal metaplasia and chronic atrophic gastritis? (4) Where do the answers to the preceding questions lead?

CAN THERE BE CHRONIC ATROPHIC GASTRITIS AND INTESTINAL METAPLASIA WITHOUT *H. PYLORI* INFECTION?

There is convincing evidence that the chronic atrophic gastritis of the fundic mucosa associated with pernicious anaemia is not causally related to *H. pylori* infection. Flejou and co-workers[2] reported that only 3/86 (3.5%) patients with pernicious anaemia exhibited the presence of *H. pylori* organisms in the mucosa of the gastric body when examined by light microscopy. They also found that 36% of 44 patients with pernicious anaemia had concomitant antral gastritis, but only 6% of these were infected with *H. pylori*. They speculated that the antral gastritis sometimes accompanying the body gastritis in such pernicious anaemia patients is more likely to be an extension of the primary autoimmune gastritis than to represent a secondary or type B gastritis. This interpretation would appear to be flawed in light of recent information showing that the circulating antibodies found in pernicious anaemia are directed against chief cell pepsinogen and a portion of the proton pump present in the parietal cells of the oxyntic mucosa[3]. Parietal and chief cells are not generally present in the antrum. In another study, Mertz and co-authors[4] reported that only 10% of Finnish subjects with pernicious anaemia had circulating antibodies against *H. pylori* as measured by the ELISA technique. Reinforcing these observations, recent studies carried out by Sipponen and colleagues[5] on a population of Scandinavian patients found abundant *H. pylori* in the gastric mucosa of patients with antral gastritis or pangastritis but, interestingly, none in patients with corpus gastritis and severe atrophy who were also afflicted with pernicious anaemia.

DeLuca argues, at times strenuously, that it is quite plausible that *H. pylori* infection is an aetiological factor in the chronic atrophic gastritis associated with pernicious anaemia[6]. This organism would cause active gastritis of the fundic mucosa, which in turn would result in loss of HCl and intrinsic factor production. He explains away the low incidence of *H. pylori* organisms in such stomachs, or the absence of circulating *H. pylori* antibodies, as the result of self-destruction of *H. pylori* by the achlorhydria resulting from the fundic atrophic gastritis. He further speculates that the normal antrum which is often found in patients with pernicious anaemia is the result of total recovery from the chronic *H. pylori*-associated gastritis once the micro-organism has been eliminated. Such posture not only ignores the current evidence in favour of a familial aetiology for pernicious anaemia[7], but also fails to make sense from an epidemiological point of view. Indeed, if pernicious anaemia were the direct result of *H. pylori* infection, one would expect a high prevalence of pernicious anaemia in geographic areas with a high rate of such infection; yet the opposite seems to be true. Pernicious anaemia is vanishingly rare in most areas of the world where there is a high incidence of *H. pylori* infection, such as Japan, China, and several parts of Latin America. Whereas it is possible that occasional patients with MAG may eventually develop pernicious anaemia because of extreme hypochlor-hydria[8], it seems clear that most patients with pernicious anaemia associated with fundic atrophic gastritis are not infected with *H. pylori*. Therefore, it is safe to assume that chronic atrophic gastritis and intestinal metaplasia may exist in the absence of *H. pylori* infection.

It is of particular interest that the relatively high incidence of gastric adenocarcinoma attributed in the past to patients with pernicious anaemia and atrophic gastritis may, in effect, be a good deal lower when the possibility of concurrent environmental gastritis in these patients is taken into account. Whereas many of the reports attributing a 10% or higher prevalence of gastric adenocarcinoma in pernicious anaemia patients were generated in northern Europe several decades ago[9,10], a more recent study done in the United States failed to confirm such an association[11]. On the basis of this new information, it has been suggested recently that many Scandinavian patients who developed gastric antral adenocarcinomas may have been suffering the consequences of MAG[12]. Indeed, it is possible that pernicious anaemia *per se* may not lead to a significantly higher cancer risk in the current environment of the United States and, probably, of present-day northern Europe.

IS THERE A CAUSAL RELATIONSHIP BETWEEN *H. PYLORI* INFECTION AND CHRONIC ATROPHIC GASTRITIS?

Compelling evidence has been accumulating in favour of a strong causal link between *H. pylori* infection, chronic atrophic gastritis, and gastric carcinoma[13,14]. Craanen and co-workers[15] found in a population of Dutch subjects that intestinal metaplasia was present more often in *H. pylori*-positive patients (33.9%) than in *H. pylori*-negative patients (15.2%); the same group found that type III intestinal metaplasia, the type associated with evolution to gastric adenocarcinoma, was encountered less often in *H. pylori*-infected stomachs as identified by observation of biopsy tissues[16]. This is explained on the basis that *H. pylori* does not easily colonize severely atrophic gastric mucosa containing extensive intestinal metaplasia. Rugge and collaborators[17], in Italy, found that intestinal metaplasia type II and III is present in 65.5% of *H. pylori*-positive patients and in only 25% of *H. pylori*-negative patients, also as determined by observation of gastric biopsy tissues. Fukao and co-workers[18], in Japan, reported that chronic atrophic gastritis was associated with 80–90.6% *H. pylori* antibodies in males and with 79.2–100% in females, as determined by the ELISA technique. Finally, Guarner and collaborators[19] determined that in Chiapas, Mexico, there was a strong association between the presence of *H. pylori* infection as determined by the ELISA method and the presence of gastric atrophy, intestinal metaplasia, gastric mucosal dysplasia, and cancer.

All these findings point to a powerful association between early and intense infection with *H. pylori* and the presence of precancerous lesions of the stomach, namely chronic atrophic gastritis involving antrum and body, and the accompanying intestinal metaplasia. In his dissertation on human gastric carcinogenesis, Correa[20] acknowledged the crucial role of *H. pylori* in initiating the chain of events leading to gastritis, and to the eventual appearance of gastric carcinoma. However, he also sounded a note of caution against regarding *H. pylori* infection as the pivotal determining factor in such a chain of events. He stated that *H. pylori* infection is a contributory, but not sufficient, factor in gastric carcinogenesis. The next section will explore in further detail this controversial subject.

DOES *H. PYLORI*, WITHOUT PARTICIPATION OF OTHER FACTORS, CAUSE INTESTINAL METAPLASIA AND CHRONIC ATROPHIC GASTRITIS?

Whereas *H. pylori* infection is a well-defined and early event in the process leading to the appearance of chronic atrophic gastritis, evidence from different areas of the world indicates that other factors must enter the picture for such an outcome to take place. According to Holcombe[21], in Central Africa, 70–80% of the population have circulating antibodies against *H. pylori* and, in northern Nigeria, 50% of the children under 5 years of age are *H. pylori*-positive. Nonetheless, intestinal metaplasia is present in only 2% of 157 patients with non-ulcer dyspepsia, and gastric adenocarcinoma accounts for less than 2% of all malignancies as a cause of death. In a study conducted by Sierra and collaborators[22] on a population of Costa Rican children, they found that the mountain region of Turrubares, with a high risk for gastric cancer acquisition (84.2 gastric cancers per 100 000 males) has a 65.8% prevalence of IgG antibodies against *H. pylori*, whereas the relatively low-risk coastal region of Hojancha (25.4 gastric cancers per 100 000 males) has a prevalence of 72.4%. It is of particular interest that, when children from these two regions were subjected to the *N*-nitrosoproline test in 12-h urine samples, they demonstrated a significantly higher nitrosation after proline intake in the high-risk areas than in the low-risk areas[23]. These results indicate that children in the high-risk area have a high endogenous nitrosation potential; the reason for this nitrosation potential, however, remains obscure. Finally, in a study by Forman and co-workers[24] in China, although as a whole they found a significant positive correlation between *H. pylori* antibody prevalence and gastric cancer mortality in different counties, they also unveiled a number of remarkable discrepancies. For example, four communities with a 70–98% prevalence of *H. pylori* IgG antibody had a gastric cancer cumulative mortality rate of 10/1000 persons or less. Conversely, six communities displaying a cumulative mortality rate between 32 and 70/1000 persons had a 48–70% prevalence of *H. pylori* IgG antibody.

WHERE DO THE ANSWERS TO THE PRECEDING QUESTIONS LEAD?

The answers to the preceding questions can be summarized as follows: (1) Yes, there can be atrophic gastritis and intestinal metaplasia without the participation of *H. pylori* infection; interestingly, this type of gastritis seems to have a much lower potential for malignant transformation than has been assumed heretofore. (2) It is reasonably well established that there is a direct relationship between the prevalence of *H. pylori* infection and the incidence of chronic atrophic pangastritis with type III intestinal metaplasia, eventually leading to malignant transformation and appearance of gastric adenocarcinoma. (3) In spite of such a direct relationship, *H. pylori* infection is probably not sufficient as the sole causal agent of chronic atrophic gastritis and intestinal metaplasia.

Upon realization that *H. pylori* infection has a causal role in the appearance of chronic atrophic gastritis, there has been a good deal of emphasis on centring the classification of such gastritis around the presence of *H. pylori*[25–27]. It has been suggested that exposure to *H. pylori* infection in adult life results in gastric acid hypersecretion and antral gastritis, both of which combine to result in peptic ulcer disease, particularly duodenal and prepyloric gastric ulcer. Intense exposure to such infection in early childhood, on the other hand, would result in the type of severe pangastritis that leads to atrophy of the gastric mucosa with hypoacidity and eventual development of premalignant lesions[28]. In spite of agreeing with the philosophies spoused by the Sydney classification of gastritis, Sobala and co-workers[27] pointed out that, whereas the presence of *H. pylori* correlated with inflammation, it failed to do so with atrophy in chronic gastritis. They concluded that atrophy and intestinal metaplasia may be initiated by *H. pylori*, but are unaffected by its elimination.

A succession of pathogenetic steps have been suggested in which a simplistic linear progression has been put forth spanning, with some variations, chronic superficial gastritis, chronic active gastritis, chronic atrophic gastritis, gastric dysplasia, and gastric adenocarcinoma[29]. Whereas this progression apparently takes place in a significant number of cases, its uncritical and universal acceptance could dangerously detract from the recognition of those additional environmental factors which are essential for the appearance of premalignant and malignant lesions[30]. Should such linear progression have existed, one would expect that the large cohort of peptic ulcer patients which appeared in the decades of the 1950s and 1960s[31] would currently result in a parallel cohort of gastric carcinoma patients; yet the contrary has happened, since the prevalence of gastric cancer has been declining steadily in the USA during the past two or three decades[32]. Furthermore, in a study by Parsonnet and co-workers[33] in California, it was found that 95% of patients with peptic ulcer disease were seropositive for *H. pylori* antibodies. However, they also found that a history of peptic ulcer disease was negatively associated with the subsequent development of gastric carcinoma (odds ratio 0.2; $p = 0.02$).

What are the practical implications of recognizing the multifactorial nature of the chronic atrophic gastritis associated with the appearance of gastric dysplasia and adenocarcinoma? They are of great importance, as they should prevent gastroenterologists from lumping into one amorphous category of '*H. pylori*-associated gastritis' such disparate conditions as duodenal ulcer-associated chronic active gastritis, demonstrating a negative association with gastric cancer, and multifocal atrophic gastritis, associated with a high risk for gastric carcinoma[30]. The dangers of categorizing gastritis on the basis of aetiology, distribution, and intensity, as is propounded in the Sydney classification[25], are obvious when one examines the fate of patients with environmental gastritis in different settings. In Japan, where gastric adenocarcinoma associated with MAG is very prevalent, the incidence of gastric carcinoma is high but the mortality rate is comparatively low. The Japanese gastroenterologist takes into account the role of environmental factors at play, and patients are placed on a follow-up protocol that enables them to be treated in the early stages of the disease, when it is curable in many cases[34]. In North America, on the other hand, MAG is seldom recognized as such, and patients are customarily treated on a more or less haphazard basis, predicated upon symptomatic relief, until a number of them present with an advanced, generally irretrievable, stage of gastric adenocarcinoma several years later. Because this type of gastritis is not nearly as prevalent in the USA as it is in Japan, massive surveys of the general population are not practical because the low yield would render such strategies non-cost-effective. This situation translates into a significantly higher mortality rate for adenocarcinoma of the stomach in the USA[32]. Of course, this high mortality rate is the composite picture of the diffuse and gastro-oesophageal types of adenocarcinoma, the incidence of which either remains the same or actually increases[32], and the potentially more predictable adenocarcinoma associated with MAG. It has been pointed out that awareness of the existence of such a form of gastritis in a subset of the population of the USA, generally encountered among disadvantaged socioeconomic strata, would make such a survey cost-effective and result in a much improved mortality rate in these patients[35].

In conclusion, the presence of *H. pylori* infection, although very important, is probably not sufficient as the sole causal agent of chronic atrophic gastritis and intestinal metaplasia. Awareness of this fact will help to place into sharper focus the multiplicity of environmental factors that participate in the progression from gastritis to gastric adenocarcinoma. In turn, identification of such factors, and recognition of their morphological manifestations, should eventually result in the improved identification, follow-up and treatment of a subset of patients who are at an increased risk for the acquisition of gastric carcinoma in the developed countries of the West.

References

1. Correa P. Chronic gastritis: a clinico-pathological classification. Am J Gastroenterol. 1988;83:504–9.
2. Flejou J-F, Bahame P, Smith AC, Stockbrugger RW, Rode J, Price AB. Pernicious anaemia and *Campylobacter*-like organisms; is the gastric antrum resistant to colonisation? Gut. 1989;30:60–4.
3. Mardh S, Song Y-H. Characterization of antigenic structures in auto-immune atrophic gastritis with pernicious anaemia. The parietal cell H,K-ATPase and the chief cell pepsinogen are the two major antigens. Acta Physiol Scand. 1989;136:581–7.
4. Mertz HR, Samloff IM, Sjoblom S, Jarvinen H, Sipponen P, Walsh JH. *Helicobacter pylori* seropositivity in pernicious anemia and atrophic gastritis. Gastroenterology. 1991;100:A124(abstract).
5. Sipponen P, Kosunen TU, Valle J, Riihela M, Seppala K. *Helicobacter pylori* infection and chronic gastritis in gastric cancer. J Clin Pathol. 1992;45:319–23.
6. DeLuca VA Jr. Is pernicious anemia caused by *Campylobacter pylori* gastritis? J Clin Gastroenterol. 1989;11:584–5.

7. Kekki M, Siurala M, Varis K, Sipponen P, Sistonen P, Nevanlinna RH. Classification, principles, and genetics of chronic gastritis. Scand J Gastroenterol. 1987;22(Suppl.141): 1–28.

8. Siurala M, Seppala K. Atrophic gastritis as a possible precursor of gastric carcinoma and pernicious anemia. Acta Med Scand. 1960;166:455–74.

9. Mosbech J, Videbaek A. Mortality from and of gastric carcinoma among patients with pernicious anaemia. BMJ. 1950;2:390–4.

10. Sipponen P, Kekki M, Haapakoski J, Ihamaki T, Siurala M. Gastric cancer risk in chronic atrophic gastritis: statistical calculations of cross-sectional data. Int J Cancer. 1985;35:173–7.

11. Schafer LW, Larson DE, Melton LJ III, Higgins JA, Zinsmeister AR. Risk of development of gastric carcinoma in patients with pernicious anemia: a population-based study in Rochester Minnesota. Mayo Clin Proc. 1985;60:444–8.

12. Lechago J, Correa P. Prolonged achlorhydria and gastric neoplasia: is there a causal relationship? Gastroenterology. 1993;104:1554–7.

13. Fox J, Correa P, Taylor N *et al. Campylobacter pylori*-associated gastritis and immune response in a population at increased risk of gastric carcinoma. Am J Gastroenterol. 1989;84:775–81.

14. Correa P, Fox J, Fontham E *et al. Helicobacter pylori* and gastric carcinoma. Serum antibody prevalence in populations with contrasting cancer risks. Cancer. 1990;66: 2569–74.

15. Craanen ME, Dekker W, Blok P, Ferwerda J, Tytgat GNJ. Intestinal metaplasia and *Helicobacter pylori*: an endoscopic bioptic study of the gastric antrum. Gut. 1992;33:16–20.

16. Craanen ME, Blok P, Dekker W, Ferwerda J, Tytgat GNJ. Subtypes of intestinal metaplasia and *Helicobacter pylori*. Gut. 1992;33:597–600.

17. Rugge M, Di Mario F, Cassaro M *et al.* Pathology of the gastric antrum and body associated with *Helicobacter pylori* infection in non-ulcerous patients: is the bacterium a promoter of intestinal metaplasia? Histopathology. 1993;22:9–15.

18. Fukao A, Komatsu S, Tsubono Y *et al. Helicobacter pylori* infection and chronic atrophic gastritis among Japanese blood donors: a cross-sectional study. Cancer Causes and Control. 1993;4:307–12.

19. Guarner J, Mohar A, Parsonnet J, Halperin D. The association of *Helicobacter pylori* with gastric cancer and preneoplastic gastric lesions in Chiapas, Mexico. Cancer. 1993;71: 297–301.

20. Correa P. Human gastric carcinogenesis: a multistep and multifactorial process – First American Cancer Society Award Lecture on Cancer Epidemiology and Prevention. Cancer Res. 1992;52:6735–40.

21. Holcombe C. *Helicobacter pylori*: the African enigma. Gut. 1992;33:429–31.

22. Sierra R, Muñoz N, Peña AS *et al.* Antibodies to *Helicobacter pylori* and pepsinogen levels in children from Costa Rica: comparison of two areas with different risks for stomach cancer. Cancer Epidemiol Biomarkers Prev. 1992;1:449–54.

23. Sierra R, Ohshima H, Muñoz N *et al.* Exposure to *N*-nitrosamines and other risk factors for gastric cancer in Costa Rican children. In: O'Neill IK, Chen J, Bartsch H, editors. Relevance to human cancer of *N*-nitroso compounds, tobacco smoke and mycotoxins. Lyon: IARC; 1991:162–7.

24. Forman D, Sitas F, Newell DG *et al.* Geographic association of *Helicobacter pylori* antibody prevalence and gastric cancer mortality in rural China. Int J Cancer. 1990;46:608–11.

25. Misiewicz JL, Tytgat GNJ, Goodwin CS *et al.* The Sydney System: a new classification of gastritis. Working Party Reports of the 9th World Congress of Gastroenterology. Melbourne: Blackwell Scientific Publications; 1990:1–10.

26. Gastroenterologists in Sydney – Histology and *Helicobacter*. Lancet. 1990;2:779–80.

27. Sobala GM, Axon ATR, Dixon MF. Morphology of chronic antral gastritis: relationship to age, *Helicobacter pylori* status and peptic ulceration. Eur J Gastroenterol Hepatol. 1992;4:825–9.

28. Tytgat GNJ. Does the stomach adapt to *Helicobacter pylori*? Scand J Gastroenterol. 1992;27(Suppl.193):28–32.

29. Antonioli DA. Chronic gastritis: a classification. In: Bayless TM, editor. Current therapy in gastroenterology and liver disease, 4th edn. Philadelphia: Mosby-Year Book; 1994:in press.

30. Correa P, Yardley JH. Grading and classification of chronic gastritis: one American response to the Sydney System. Gastroenterology. 1992;102:355–9.
31. Mendeloff AI. What has been happening to duodenal ulcer? Gastroenterology. 1974;67: 1020–3.
32. Ming S-C. Adenocarcinoma and other malignant epithelial tumors of the stomach. In: Ming S-C, Goldman H, editors. Pathology of the gastrointestinal tract. Philadelphia: Saunders; 1992:584–617.
33. Parsonnet J, Friedman GD, Vandersteen DP *et al. Helicobacter pylori* infection and the risk of gastric carcinoma. N Engl J Med. 1991;3325:1127–31.
34. Hirota T, Ming S-C. Early gastric carcinoma. In: Ming S-C, Goldman H, editors. Pathology of the gastrointestinal tract. Philadelphia: Saunders; 1992:570–83.
35. Lechago J. Premalignant conditions of the stomach. In: Bayless TM, editor. Current therapy in gastroenterology and liver disease, 4th edn. Philadelphia: Mosby-Year Book; 1994:in press.

48
H. pylori-associated gastric lymphoma

M. STOLTE, S. EIDT, E. BAYERDÖRFFER and R. FISCHER

INTRODUCTION

During the course of research into the effects of *Helicobacter pylori* infection, it was established that, among other things, chronic colonization of the gastric mucosa with this organism induced – both in humans and experimental animals – the formation of lymphatic aggregates and lymphoid follicles at the base of the mucosa[1-3]. The normal stomach does not contain mucosa-associated lymphoid tissue (MALT). This new piece of information, namely that acquired MALT in the stomach is a consequence of infection with *H. pylori*, of course, immediately raised the logical follow-on question whether *H. pylori* gastritis might not also be the necessary prerequisite for the development of gastric MALT lymphoma. Initial indications for such a relationship were provided by the epidemiological studies carried out by Parsonnet *et al.*[4]. Shortly afterwards, Wotherspoon *et al.*[5], in a retrospective examination of resected specimens from the stomach containing MALT lymphomas, were able to show that gastric MALT lymphoma is associated with *H. pylori* gastritis in 92% of cases.

Doglioni *et al.*[6] then showed that MALT lymphomas of the stomach are found more frequently in a region densely colonized with *H. pylori* than in one sparsely colonized with the organism.

If the lymphatic aggregates are a consequence of *Helicobacter* infection, it may be logically concluded that *H. pylori* eradication therapy could facilitate the often very difficult diagnostic task of distinguishing between lymphatic aggregates and low-grade MALT lymphoma components in forceps biopsy material: the reactive lymphatic infiltrates would disappear after such treatment, while the lymphoma infiltrates would persist[7]. To our great surprise, however, we also found regression of the low-grade malignant gastric MALT lymphomas.

With the aim of deepening our knowledge about the relationship between *H. pylori* gastritis and gastric MALT lymphomas, we investigated (1) the incidence of *H. pylori* gastritis in MALT lymphoma patients, and (2) the effect of *H. pylori* eradication therapy on MALT lymphomas.

MATERIALS AND METHODS

Incidence of *H. pylori* gastritis in MALT lymphoma patients

A total of 205 surgical specimens containing primary malignant B-cell lymphomas of the MALT type were investigated. The specimens were fixed in 10% formalin, embedded in paraffin, and sections routinely stained with H&E, PAS and Giemsa. The MALT lymphomas were classified into three categories: (1) low-grade malignant lymphomas, (2) high-grade malignant lymphomas with a low-grade component, and (3) high-grade lymphoma with no low-grade component.

The depth of infiltration of the wall of the stomach by the lymphoma was determined in accordance with the UICC classification for gastric carcinoma[8]. In addition, the spread of the lymphoma was determined using the modified Ann Arbor scheme[9]. Only non-nodal lymphomas clearly originating in the stomach were admitted to this study. In 178 cases the gastric mucosa located at a distance of at least 4 cm from the tumour was investigated for the following parameters: infiltration of the lamina propria with lymphocytes, plasma cells and neutrophils; intestinal metaplasia, lymphoid aggregates and lymphoid follicles. An *H. pylori*-associated gastritis was diagnosed when a lymphoplasmacellular infiltrate in combination with neutrophils concentrated around the neck region with infiltration of gastric glands was present; that is, when the gastritis was of the chronic active type. On the basis of these criteria all cases of chronic active gastritis were classified as *H. pylori* gastritis. Since *H. pylori* is known to be difficult, or even impossible, to detect in surgical specimens involving a delay in fixation, the preoperative endoscopic gastric biopsy specimens that had been obtained in 145 of the cases, and were available to us, were investigated for the presence of the pathogen (stain: H&E, Giemsa, PAS, Warthin Starry).

For the statistical analysis, the chi-square test was employed.

Effect of *H. pylori* eradication therapy on MALT lymphomas

In 16 patients with low-grade MALT lymphoma and *H. pylori* gastritis, the effect of *H. pylori* eradication treatment comprising 80 mg omeprazole and 2 g amoxicillin per day[10] over a period of 10 days was studied. A comparison was made between the endoscopic and histological findings prior to treatment and 4 weeks and 3 months after the end of treatment. In some of the patients the follow-up period extended to 6–12 months. After further follow-up and additional endosonographic and histological studies, these preliminary investigations will be reported in more detail elsewhere.

Table 1 Histological classification of 205 gastric MALT lymphomas

Low-grade lymphoma	99
High-grade lymphoma	
with low-grade component	33
without low-grade component	73

Table 2 Depth of infiltration of the gastric MALT lymphomas investigated

pT1	94 (45.9%)
pT2	62 (30.2%)
pT3	41 (20.0%)
pT4	8 (3.9%)

RESULTS

Incidence of *H. pylori* gastritis in MALT lymphoma patients

The histological classification of MALT lymphomas found in the surgical specimens can be seen in Table 1. The depth of penetration of the lesions is shown in Table 2. Investigation of the mucosa at some distance from the tumour showed chronic active gastritis, that is, the typical findings of *H. pylori* gastritis, in 175 of the 178 cases (98.3%). *H. pylori* colonization with chronic active gastritis was found in all the 145 patients who had been biopsied preoperatively. In addition, examination of surgical specimen revealed lymphoid follicles and lymphatic aggregates – i.e. histological changes found almost exclusively in *H. pylori* gastritis – in the antral mucosa in 84.4%, and in the corpus mucosa in 87.3% of the cases.

Effect of *Helicobacter* eradication therapy on MALT lymphomas

In 12 out of 16 patients, endoscopic examination revealed regression of the MALT lymphoma. Histological work-up of the biopsies obtained from these regions of the stomach revealed, at the base of the mucosa, an aglandular lamina propria empty of lymphatic infiltrates. In six of these 12 cases, however, sparse residual lymphoma tissue was to be found.

The patients are being closely followed with endoscopy and biopsy. A final assessment of the effect of this treatment on MALT lymphomas will be possible only 1–2 years after *H. pylori* eradication.

DISCUSSION

Gastric MALT lymphomas originate in the parafollicular zone of lymphoid follicles in the stomach[11,12]. In the normal stomach, of course, no lymphoid follicles are to be found. The development of lymphoid follicles depends on a chronic infection of the gastric mucosa with *H. pylori*[1,2]. It may be logically concluded from these facts that gastric MALT lymphoma can develop only in the stomach in which a prior *H. pylori* infection has led to the acquisition of mucosa-associated lymphatic tissue – in other words, *H. pylori* gastritis with formation of lymphoid follicles is a necessary pre-lymphoma condition.

It is thus not surprising that antibodies against *H. pylori* have been detected in the serum of 90.9% of patients with gastric MALT lymphoma long before the latter developed[4]. This study, however, contained only 11 gastric lymphoma patients. Further evidence in support of a relationship between *H. pylori* gastritis and gastric MALT lymphoma is provided by the study of Wotherspoon *et al.*[5], who were able to detect *H. pylori* in 92% of 110 patients with MALT lymphoma.

The results of our study of surgical specimens and preoperative forceps biopsy material support the findings reported by Wotherspoon *et al.*; our material was found to have an extremely high prevalence (98.3% of the specimens) of chronic active gastritis, the typical picture of *H. pylori*-induced gastritis. In the case of the 145 patients in whom a preoperative biopsy had been done, *H. pylori* colonization with chronic active gastritis was found in 100% of the patients. This rate of *H. pylori* detection in patients with gastric MALT lymphoma is appreciably higher than the *H. pylori* prevalence reported in epidemiological studies conducted in developed countries in adult patients[4,13,14].

The presence of lymphoid follicles and lymphatic aggregates detected at a distance from the MALT lymphoma in the antral and corpus specimens of our patients supports the notion that *H. pylori* gastritis is a pre-lymphoma condition.

With respect to the mechanism of malignant transformation of MALT into MALT lymphoma we can only speculate at present. That chronic infections are capable of triggering lymphoproliferation is already well known in the case of EBV infection[15,16]. However, gastric MALT lymphomas are rare, while *H. pylori* infection is very common. Thus, in the development of MALT lymphomas, in addition to specific strains with a higher immunogenicity, other exogenous factors (e.g. dietary factors, additional viral infections, disorders of immunoregulation) must also be suspected.

Our initial results showing regression of MALT lymphomas following *H. pylori* eradication therapy must, for the present, be interpreted with considerable caution.

When we presented our first six cases showing regression of gastric MALT lymphoma to the German Gastroenterological Congress in 1992, the question naturally arose whether the lymphomas really had been autonomic tumours, or perhaps simply overdiagnosed reactive lymphatic infiltrates. In all of these cases, however, the histological criteria of lymphoepithelial destruction had been demonstrated preoperatively. In the meantime, however, similar observations have been made by the working group in Vienna (B. Dragosics and T. Radaskiewicz, personal communication). In addition, Wotherspoon *et al.*, from the group headed by P. Isaacson in London, has been able to show histological regression of the lymphoma in five out of six patients with low-grade gastric MALT lymphomas[17]. The same group has also demonstrated, on the basis of lymphoma cell cultures, that the growth of cells obtained from low-grade gastric MALT lymphomas in the culture is dependent upon the presence of T lymphocytes and *H. pylori*[18].

These results, too, must, for the present, be considered preliminary and interpreted accordingly. If, however, they can be confirmed, this would represent indisputable proof that *H. pylori* actually does play the determinant role in the development and growth of gastric MALT lymphoma.

SUMMARY

In an attempt to clarify the relationship between *H. pylori* gastritis and MALT lymphoma of the stomach, we investigated (1) the incidence of *H. pylori* gastritis in MALT lymphoma patients, and (2) the effect of *H. pylori* eradication treatment on MALT lymphoma.

Two hundred and five surgical specimens with primary gastric B-cell lymphoma of the MALT type were investigated for the presence of *H. pylori* gastritis. They were classified into low-grade ($n = 93$) and high-grade with ($n = 33$) and without ($n = 73$) a low-grade component. The depth of infiltration of the gastric wall was evaluated in accordance with the UICC classification: pT1 = 94; pT2 = 62, pT3 = 41, pT4 = 8). In 178 cases, mucosa sampled at a distance of more than 4 cm from the tumour was available for evaluation: chronic active *H. pylori* gastritis was detected in 175 of these specimens. Neither tumour diameter, depth of infiltration, nor degree of malignancy had any influence on the prevalence of *H. pylori* gastritis. Lymphoid follicles and lymphoid aggregates known to be present almost exclusively in *H. pylori* gastritis were detected in 84.4% in the antral, and 87.3% in the oxyntic, mucosa. Gastric biopsy material obtained at some distance from the lymphoma in 145 of the surgical patients was investigated. In all of these cases, sections stained with Warthin-Starry revealed colonization with *H. pylori*.

In 16 patients with low-grade MALT lymphoma and *H. pylori* gastritis the effect of *H. pylori* eradication (80 mg omeprazole + 2 g amoxicillin/day for 10 days) was studied. In 12 patients, treatment resulted in extensive regression of low-grade MALT lymphomas, both endoscopically and histologically. Our results support the hypothesis that *H. pylori* induces the development of MALT lymphoma prior to its malignant transformation. Prolonged *H. pylori*-induced inflammation might increase the probability of malignant transformation and proliferation of the lymphoid tissue. This might in part explain why MALT lymphomas have a higher incidence in the stomach than in other organs.

Possible regression of low-grade MALT lymphoma is a further piece of evidence for a pathogenic relationship between *H. pylori* gastritis and these lymphomas.

References

1. Wyatt JI, Rathbone BJ. Immune response of the gastric mucosa to *Campylobacter pylori*. Scand J Gastroenterol. 1988;23(Suppl.142):44–9.

2. Stolte M, Eidt S. Lymphoid follicles of the antral mucosa: immune reaction to *Campylobacter pylori*? J Clin Pathol. 1989;42:1269–71.
3. Krakowka S, Morgan DR, Eaton KA, Radin MJ. Animal models of *Helicobacter pylori* gastritis. In: Menge H, Gregor M, Tytgat GNJ, Marshall BJ, editors. *Helicobacter pylori* 1990. Berlin: Springer; 1991:74–80.
4. Parsonnet J, Vandersteen D, Goates J, Sibley RK, Prittkin J, Chang Y. *Helicobacter pylori* infection in intestinal- and diffuse-type gastric adenocarcinoma. J Natl Cancer Inst. 1991;83:640–3.
5. Wotherspoon AC, Ortiz-Hidalgo C, Falzon MR, Isaacson PG. *Helicobacter pylori*-associated gastritis and primary B-cell gastric lymphoma. Lancet. 1991;338:1175–6.
6. Doglioni C, Wotherspoon AC, Moschini A, De Boni M, Isaacson PG. High incidence of primary gastric lymphoma in northeastern Italy. Lancet. 1992;339:834–5.
7. Stolte M. *Helicobacter pylori* gastritis and gastric MALT-lymphoma. Lancet. 1992;339: 745–6.
8. Hermanek P, Sobin LH, editors. TNM-Klassifikation maligner Tumoren, 4th edn. Berlin: Springer; 1987.
9. Musshoff K, Schmidt-Vollmer H. Prognosis of non-Hodgkin's lymphomas with special emphasis on staging classification. Z Krebsforschung. 1975;83:323–8.
10. Bayerdörffer E, Mannes GA, Sommer A *et al.* Long-term follow-up after eradication of *Helicobacter pylori* with a combination of omeprazole and amoxicillin. Scand J Gastroenterol. 1993;28(Suppl. 196):19–25.
11. Isaacson PG, Spencer J. Malignant lymphoma of mucosa-associated lymphoid tissue. Histopathology. 1987;11:445–62.
12. Isaacson PG, Wotherspoon AC, Diss T, Pan L. Follicular colonization in B-cell lymphoma of mucosa-associated lymphoid tissue. Am J Surg Pathol. 1991;15:819–28.
13. Nomura A, Stemmermann GN, Chyou PH, Kato I, Perez-Perez GI, Blaser MJ. *Helicobacter pylori* infection and gastric carcinoma among Japanese Americans in Hawaii. N Engl J Med. 1991;325:1132–6.
14. Graham DY, Malaty HM, Evans DG, Evans DJ, Klein PD, Adam E. Epidemiology of *Helicobacter pylori* in an asymptomatic population in the United States. Effect of age, race, and socioeconomic status. Gastroenterology. 1991;100:1495–501.
15. Krueger GRF, Papdakis Th, Schaefer HJ. Persistent active Epstein-Barr virus infection and atypical lymphoproliferation. Am J Surg Pathol. 1987;11:972–81.
16. Puerilo T, Tatsumi E, Manolov G *et al.* Epstein-Barr virus as an etiological agent in the pathogenesis of lymphoproliferative and aproliferative diseases in immune deficient patients. Int Rev Exp Pathol. 1985;27:114–82.
17. Wotherspoon AC, Doglioni C, Diss TC *et al.* Regression of primary low grade B-cell gastric lymphoma of mucosa associated lymphoid tissue (MALT) type following eradication of *Helicobacter pylori*. Lancet. 1993;342:575–7.
18. Hussell T, Isaacson PG, Crabtree JE, Spencer J. Cells from low grade B cell gastric lymphomas of mucosa associated lymphoid tissue proliferate in response to *Helicobacter pylori*. Lancet. 1993;342:571–4.

49
Animal models for *Helicobacter*-induced gastric and hepatic cancer

J. G. FOX, K. A. ANDRUTIS and J. YU

GASTRIC CANCER

Although gastric cancer rates have been declining in recent decades, gastric carcinoma remains an important malignancy of the gastrointestinal tract and a significant cause of cancer deaths worldwide[1,2]. Epidemiological studies have shown a wide variation in the incidence of gastric carcinoma in different populations and even within subpopulations of the same geographic area[3,4]. The clearest association occurs between the incidence of gastric cancer and the socioeconomic status of the population[5]. These observations indicate that cultural environmental factors play a major role in the pathogenesis of gastric cancer[6]. The environmental factor usually implicated in the development of gastric cancer is diet; specifically dietary salt, antioxidants (ascorbic acid, β-carotene, vitamin E) and nitrate content[2,6-10].

A multistep model for the development of gastric cancer has been proposed beginning with a state of superficial gastritis progressing to chronic atrophic gastritis, small intestinal metaplasia, colonic metaplasia and ultimately, dysplasia[8] (Fig. 1). Chronic gastritis and atrophy are considered precancerous lesions and the relative risk of gastric cancer is significantly increased in patients with atrophic gastritis[3]. The strong association between *Helicobacter pylori* and chronic atrophic gastritis suggests that *Helicobacter* infection may also play a role in the development of gastric cancer. Evidence supporting this inference shows that *H. pylori* infection causes chronic gastritis; chronic gastritis usually progresses to atrophy and intestinal metaplasia; and atrophy and intestinal metaplasia are associated with an increased risk of gastric cancer[3,4].

H. PYLORI AND GASTRIC CANCER

An increasing number of epidemiological studies reported in the literature beginning in the late 1980s to the present time have concluded that *H. pylori*

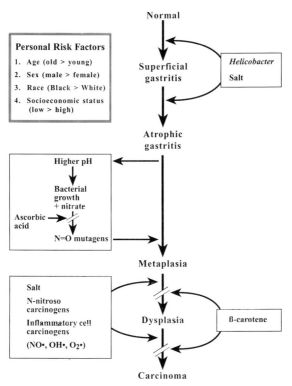

Fig. 1 Proposed cascade of gastric pathological/ecological events in gastric adenocarcinoma (adapted from refs 2 and 8)

is the missing environmental factor in the multifactorial pathogenesis of gastric cancer[3,4,8]. These epidemiological studies have shown that a significant correlation exists between those populations with a high prevalence of *H. pylori* infection and those with a high rate of gastric cancer, and that both variables correlate with socioeconomic status[3,11]. In these populations, *H. pylori* infection is usually contracted at an early age, providing sufficient time for the development of chronic atrophic gastritis, intestinal metaplasia and gastric cancer.

Recently, three prospective and one retrospective case–control epidemiological studies have indicated that *H. pylori* may be involved in approximately 35–60% of gastric cancer cases[12–15] (Table 1). Due to the significant morbidity and mortality associated with gastric cancer, further study of the role of *H. pylori* in the pathogenesis of gastric cancer is required. Animal models have been developed for the study of both gastric carcinogenesis and *Helicobacter* infection. It is our hope that, by combining the significant features of each of these models, we will be able to investigate the effects of *Helicobacter* infection and dietary factors on gastric carcinogenesis.

Table 1 Recent case/control epidemiological studies of *H. pylori* association with gastric cancer

Subjects	No. of cases/controls	Percentage H. pylori-positive by ELISA	Odds ratio	Confidence interval	Reference
Health Maintenance Organization members, California, USA	109 cases gastric cancer 109 controls	84 61	3.6	1.8–7.3 (95%)	Parsonnet et al.[12]
Japanese-American men, Hawaii, USA	109 cases gastric cancer 109 controls	94 76	6.0	2.1–17.3 (95%)	Nomura et al.[13]
Men, England, Wales	29 cases gastric cancer 116 controls	69 47	2.77	1.04–7.97 (95%)	Forman et al.[14]
Mayo Clinic patients, Minnesota, USA	37 cases gastric cancer 252 controls	65 38	2.67	1.01–7.06 (99%)	Talley et al.[15]

ANIMAL MODELS FOR *HELICOBACTER* INFECTION

Several animal models have been described for *Helicobacter* spp.-induced gastric disease. Each of these models has been described in an accompanying chapter (see Chapter 1). Some of these models have particular relevant features which can be used to help answer the question of the potential of *Helicobacter* spp. to induce cancer.

ANIMAL MODELS FOR GASTRIC CANCER

Gastric cancer is an uncommon spontaneous neoplasm of laboratory animal species[16-19]. Spontaneous gastric cancer is most frequently reported in the dog, where it accounts for approximately 1% of all neoplasms. Canine gastric cancer usually originates in the pyloric antrum along the lesser curvature and corresponds to the diffuse histological type. In the past the dog has been used in chemical carcinogenesis studies. These studies are difficult due to the size of the animal, the large amounts of carcinogen required, the extended duration of the studies and the increased costs of obtaining and maintaining dogs. Also, spontaneous gastric cancer has recently been reported in pet ferrets[20,21]. Spontaneous gastric cancer is rare in non-human primates but has been experimentally induced by exposure to petroleum products and oral ingestion of polychlorinated biphenyls and polychlorinated triphenyls.

In rodents, spontaneous forestomach squamous cell carcinomas occur rarely but experimentally they have been associated with parasitic infection, dietary deficiencies and many chemical agents[22-24]. Since forestomach tumours are more analogous to human oesophageal tumours they will not be discussed further. Spontaneous glandular stomach tumours in rodents are very rare, but have been reported to occur more frequently in the Syrian hamster and Strain I mice. Gastric carcinoids occur relatively frequently in aged multi-mammated mice (*Praomys* (*Mastomys*) *natalensis*). Early gastric carcinogenesis studies were hampered by the lack of standardized criteria of induced malignancy. Attempts to reproduce isolated reports of gastric carcinogenesis often failed due to inadequate descriptions of methodology and differing diagnostic criteria used to assess the cancerous process. Factors required of an *in vivo* experimental model for gastric carcinogenesis include a suitable animal species, a characterized chemical or biological agent and an appropriate vehicle or solvent[23].

Several reviews of experimental gastric carcinogenesis have been published[22-24]. The earliest models for gastric adenocarcinoma involved the intramural injection of polycyclic aromatic hydrocarbons[25]. In 1961, *N,N'*-2,7-fluorenylenebisacetamide (2,7-FAA) in feed produced gastric cancer in 10–25% of Buffalo rats after 47 weeks[26]. In 1967, *N*-methyl-*N'*-nitro-*N*-nitrosoguanidine (MNNG) was found to be a more effective carcinogen for the production of gastric cancer in the rat[27]. MNNG administered to rats in drinking water at a concentration of 83 μg/ml produced gastric cancer in 70% of the rats within 12 months. Since that time, MNNG has been the agent of choice in experimental gastric carcinogenesis studies in various species of laboratory animals including the rat, hamster and dog[24]. The mouse is relatively resistant to carcinogenesis of the glandular stomach induced by MNNG. However, in one study, five of 69 Swiss albino mice developed gastric cancer within 54–68 weeks of receiving 100 μg/ml MNNG in the drinking water[28].

MNNG has been recognized and used as a potent mutagen for over 30 years[23,24]. Similar to other alkylnitrosamines, MNNG is converted to the active carcinogen; an unstable alkyldiazo derivative. In acidic conditions MNNG is converted to *N*-methyl-*N'*-nitroguanidine by releasing nitrous acid. In alkaline conditions it is degraded into diazomethane and nitrocyanamide. The ultimate carcinogen is capable of alkylating the purine bases of DNA, RNA and some amino acids leading to subsequent mutation.

MNNG is administered orally either in drinking water or by gavage[24]. In solution, MNNG is heat- and light-labile. Because MNNG is relatively insoluble in water, other vehicles used have included ethanol, DMSO, corn oil and olive oil. Typical drinking water concentrations for the rat range from 30 to 170 μg/ml for 10–12 months with total doses ranging from 400 to 1700 mg. Dogs have received MNNG in the drinking water at similar concentrations and developed gastric cancer from 24 to 36 months. Due to the difficulties in quantitatively measuring dosage and the safety issues involved with human exposure to MNNG in drinking water studies, investigators have also administered MNNG by gavage. Rats have been given single doses of MNNG ranging from 50 to 300 mg/kg. Many other treatment regimens have been combined with MNNG administration to determine their effects on gastric carcinogenesis. Of particular interest are studies that have combined salt, ascorbic acid and antioxidant administration[9,10].

The majority of studies using MNNG as a gastric carcinogen have been applied to the rat model. The susceptibility to MNNG-induced carcinogenesis varies among strains of rats with random-bred Wistar rats most susceptible and inbred Buffalo strain most resistant[24]. We have reviewed a portion of this literature paying particular attention to the age, sex and strain of rat; the dose, vehicle and route of administration of MNNG; the duration of dosing and of the complete study; and the incidence and types of tumours described. Review of this literature shows that MNNG administered by gavage induced predominantly forestomach tumours, while MNNG administered in the drinking water induced predominantly glandular stomach tumours. This observation was recently confirmed in a study which showed that a single intragastric dose of MNNG led to an 80–100% incidence of forestomach tumours and an 8–20% incidence of glandular stomach tumours. Conversely, MNNG in the drinking water led to a 64–100% incidence of glandular stomach tumours and a 0–16% incidence of forestomach tumours. The study also showed that intragastric administration of MNNG produced tumours at a single site, while MNNG in the drinking water induced tumours at multiple sites.

The histopathology of gastric adenocarcinomas produced by MNNG in rats and hamsters ranges from well-differentiated to highly anaplastic and signet ring cell carcinomas[24]. In the stomach, MNNG has also produced squamous cell carcinoma, fibrosarcoma, leimyoma and haemangioma. In the small intestine, MNNG has produced adenocarcinoma, haemangioendothelial sarcoma and fibrosarcoma. Liver and lymph node metastases have been reported. MNNG has also been used for the study of the sequential morphological changes of the glandular stomach of rats during the carcinogenesis process[23,24].

Another widely used chemical carcinogen is N-methyl-N-nitrosourea (MNU)[29]. The action of MNU is similar to that of MNNG, resulting in the methylation of purine residues in DNA, RNA and amino acid residues in proteins. MNU has been administered by various routes to many animal species; it is able to induce a variety of neoplasms dependent on the animal and route of administration. A recent report described the induction of gastric cancer in the mouse treated with MNU[30]. Six-week-old male, BALB/c mice were gavaged with 0.5 mg MNU per mouse (approximately 25 mg/kg) once a week for 10 weeks. Gastrointestinal tumours developed in the forestomach, glandular stomach and duodenum. Most tumours of the glandular stomach were found along the lesser curvature of the pyloric region. Adenomatous hyperplasia was present in 75% of the mice at 20 weeks and 100% of the mice at 40 weeks. Glandular stomach carcinomas were classified into well-differentiated adenocarcinomas, poorly differentiated adenocarcinomas and signet-ring cell carcinomas. The percentage of mice that had developed gastric cancer was 11% (1/9) at 20 weeks, 80% (4/5) at 30 weeks and 100% (4/4) at 40 weeks. Two out of 27 mice also showed evidence of regional lymph node metastasis. MNU-induced gastric carcinogenesis in the mouse appears to closely model human gastric cancer in the development of neoplasms with varying degrees of differentiation and the presence of metastases.

Cellular susceptibility to topical nitrosamine carcinogens is related to both gastric physiology and the cell cycle; postmitotic luminal pyloric epithelial cells receive higher exposure, while the proliferating cells that are more likely to express an initiating event are located deep in the glands where exposure is lower. The overall MNNG-induced mutation rate would thus be expected to be relatively low for normal gastric mucosa in comparison with mucosa in which the more accessible cells are undergoing abnormal proliferation, similar to that observed in *Helicobacter* spp.-associated chronic inflammation occupying the full thickness of the mucosa. The *Helicobacter* spp. infecting gastric mucosa of animals (as well as *H. pylori* in humans) occupy the epithelial surfaces of the neck glands where polymorphonuclear cells migrate from the stroma to the lumen by traversing between the replicating epithelial cells. Bacterial organisms have been previously incriminated as co-carcinogens in experimental animal models of carcinogenesis[31,32]. In these two studies the presence of micro-organisms affected the number of tumours induced by N-nitroso carcinogens. It is tempting, therefore, to suggest that the increased tumour incidence in *Helicobacter*-infected animal models will reflect participation of *Helicobacter* infection in the carcinogenic process.

ANIMAL MODELS FOR *HELICOBACTER*-INDUCED GASTRIC CANCER

To develop animal models for *Helicobacter*-induced gastric cancer we have attempted to combine the significant features of the models for *Helicobacter* infection with features of the models for gastric carcinogenesis. Unfortunately, in terms of animal model development to study pathogenesis, *H. pylori* appears to have a limited host range; this species naturally colonizes human and non-human primates[33]. Experimentally, *H. pylori* will infect gnotobiotic pigs and dogs, but does not infect rodents, lagomorphs, or ferrets[33].

Ferret model

Fortunately, *Helicobacter mustelae*, a natural gastric pathogen of ferrets, has many biochemical, molecular and phenotypic characteristics similar to those of *H. pylori* isolated from the human stomach[34,35]. Recently we described the nearly universal presence of *H. mustelae* in the inflamed mucosa of ferrets and colonization of *H. mustelae* in ferret stomachs shortly after weaning[35]. In addition, Koch's postulates have been fulfilled; that is, oral inoculation of *H. mustelae* into naive ferrets not infected with *H. mustelae* induces a chronic, persistent gastritis similar to that noted in ferrets naturally infected with *H. mustelae*. Ferrets have been proposed as a suitable model to study the pathogenesis and epidemiology of *Helicobacter*-associated chronic gastritis and gastric cancer[36]. The histopathological changes observed closely coincide in topography with the presence of *H. mustelae* (Figure 2). In the oxyntic mucosa, both are limited to the superficial portion (superficial gastritis). In the distal antrum the inflammation occupies the full thickening of the mucosa, the so-called diffuse antral gastritis described in humans. *H. mustelae* are seen at the surface, the pits, and the superficial portion of the glands. In the proximal antrum and the transitional mucosa, the element of focal glandular atrophy and regeneration is added to the lesions described in the distal antrum. This coincides with deep focal *H. mustelae* colonization of groups of antral glands. The pathology of *Helicobacter*-associated gastritis in the ferret model has many similarities with the human disease, and contributes considerably to the interpretation of chronic gastritis in humans. The lesions observed in the distal antrum and the oxyntic mucosa bear a close resemblance to the diffuse antral gastritis observed in humans which, like the ferret model, is usually accompanied by superficial gastritis of the corpus. This is the clinicopathological entity which underlies the duodenal ulcer syndrome[8,36]. The changes observed in the proximal antrum and the transitional zone appear to represent early stages of the multifocal atrophic gastritis of humans, the entity which underlies the gastric ulcer and gastric carcinoma syndromes[8,36]. Moreover, the ferret stomach offers a potentially ideal model because its anatomy, histology and physiology closely resemble those of the human stomach[37]. The structure of the ferret gastric mucosa at the cellular level is remarkably similar to that of humans. Ferrets also secrete gastric acid and proteolytic enzymes under basal conditions.

We have carried out preliminary studies to define the *H. mustelae*-infected ferrets as an animal model of *H. pylori*-associated gastric cancer using MNNG[38]. A study was undertaken to ascertain whether 10 6-month-old female ferrets given a single oral dose of MNNG (50–100 mg/kg) would develop adenocarcinoma of the stomach. Five age-matched unmanipulated control animals were included for comparative purposes. All 15 ferrets were colonized with *H. mustelae*. Mucosal pinch biopsies were obtained endoscopically from the antral and fundal regions of the stomach in both dosed and control animals at 6–12-month intervals. Nine of 10 ferrets dosed with MNNG had gastric adenocarcinoma diagnosed at necropsy (29–55 months after dosing), whereas none of the control ferrets had developed gastric cancer, when examined at an average of 63 months after the initiation of the study (Fig. 3). The one ferret given a total dose of 100 mg/kg developed gastric cancer in 29 months; eight of the nine ferrets given one dose of 50 mg/kg developed cancer. However, all the control animals had mild to moderate gastritis, mostly limited to the antrum with small foci of gland loss. The histological findings in the stomachs of ferrets ~ 26–55 months after being dosed with MNNG indicated invasive adenocarcinoma of the antrum and metastasis to a regional lymph node in one case (Table 2). More frequent and detailed gastric biopsies would have undoubtedly allowed diagnosis of cancer earlier in the course of the cancerous process. The large number of gastric adenocarcinomas in the ferrets in this study may be partially due to *H. mustelae*-associated gastritis present in 100% of the MNNG-treated animals but our results, though suggestive, do not directly implicate *H. mustelae* in MNNG-induced gastric cancer in the ferret. With the recent development of specific pathogen-free ferrets we are now able to address this question. This experiment is under way, and will be described in a future report.

These data suggest that the ferret is an appropriate model to mimic humans for studies involving the role of *H. pylori* in gastric carcinogenesis[38]. This model should also prove extremely useful in further experiments to help delineate co-carcinogenic compounds as well as anticancer mechanism(s) of various dietary substances.

Rodents

Both germ-free rats and germ-free mice can be colonized with *H. felis*[39,40]. Although the rat is the preferred model for gastric carcinogenesis studies, long-term *H. felis* colonization studies in this species have not been performed. This model therefore requires further development before it can be used in carcinogenesis studies with MNNG.

Fortunately, the conventional and specific pathogen-free (SPF) mice can be colonized on a persistent basis with *H. felis*. However, as mentioned previously, studies with MNNG and MNU in the mouse have been limited, and the dosage of the carcinogens needed to consistently produce gastric adenocarcinoma and strain variability to the compounds are largely undetermined. Nevertheless, lesions produced by *H. felis* in the mouse gastric tissue

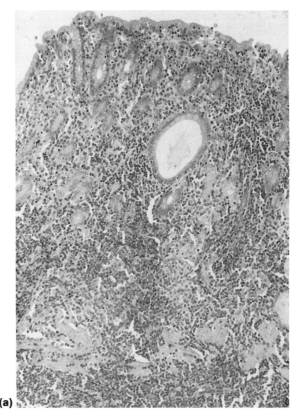

(a)

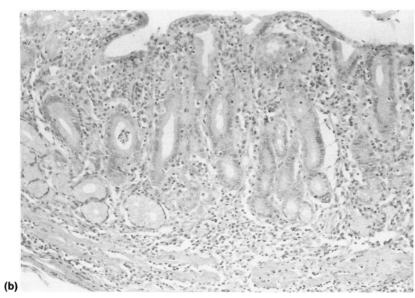

(b)

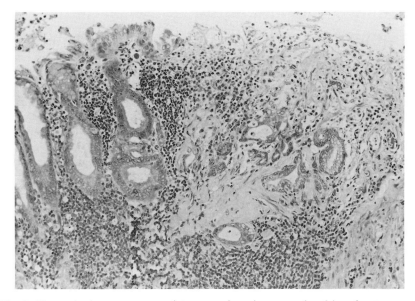

Fig. 3 Desmoplastic response to an intramucosal carcinoma produced in a ferret gavaged with MNNG (H&E × 130)

Table 2 Histological findings in the stomachs of ferrets dosed with MNNG

	Ferret number									
	1	2*	3	4	5	6	7	8	9	10
MAG (multifocal atrophic gastritis)	+	+	+	+	+	+	+	+	+	+
Mucosal ulcers	+				+	+				
Atypical glandular hyperplasia			+					+	+	+
Intramucosal adenocarcinoma		+	+		+	+	+		+	+
Invasive adenocarcinoma	+	+	+	+	+	+	+		+	
Metastatic adenocarcinoma					+					

*Dosed with 100 mg/kg body weight; animal developed clinical and diagnostic features of gastric cancer ∼3 months prior to euthanasia (29 months post-dosing). Eight of nine other ferrets dosed with 50 mg/kg body weight developed gastric tumours[38]

indicate that the model has promise in future experiments. For example, in the first description of *H. felis* gastritis in the germ-free mouse, a moderate degree of glandular epithelial cell hyperplasia was evident at 4 weeks in portions of the gastric mucosa[39]. This was characterized by an overall increase in thickness of the mucosa in areas of inflamed tissue. The changes included lack of epithelial cell maturation and differentiation, increased

Fig. 2 Opposite: Features of multifocal atrophic gastritis (MAG) observed in ferrets: (**a**) demonstrates loss of glands, diffuse lymphocytic infiltration and a cystic gland in the transition zone (H&E × 130); (**b**) shows neck hyperplasia and gland loss (H&E × 260)

Table 3 Inflammation and atrophy in mice colonized with different *Helicobacter* species

| | Conventional mice | | | | | | SPF mice | | | | | |
| | Inflammation | | | Atrophy | | | Inflammation | | | Atrophy | | |
Time*	Con	Hf	Hh	Con	Hf	Hh	Con	Hf	Hh	Con	Hf	Hh
4–8	0	0	0	0	0	0	0	5	0	0	0	0
24–36	0	50	0	0	0	0	0	5	0	0	0	0
40–56	0	40	50	0	10	10	0	8	22	0	0	0
72–76	17	93	67	0	37	25	0	20	41	0	0	0

*Time of colonization in weeks. Hf = *H. felis*, Hh = *H. heilmanii* = *Gastrospirillum*. Inflammation = percentage of animals with significant chronic inflammation. Atrophy = percentage of animals with a significant level of atrophy[42]

basophilia and increased nuclear to cytoplasmic ratio. Also of interest was the enlargement of individual glands and the presence of columnar type epithelium versus cuboidal epithelium. Occasional branching of glands was noted as well as luminal epithelium forming small pseudovillus projections. These lesions persisted for the duration of the study, i.e. 8 weeks[39]. These studies have been extended by documentation of persistent active, chronic gastritis in germ-free mice and SPF mice, infected with *H. felis* for 1 year[41]. Most recently, studies of 72–76-week colonization of conventional and SPF mice have provided additional clues on progression of the lesions in the stomach of infected mice. Conventional mice, infected with either *H. felis* or *H. heilmannii* and also colonized with *H. muridarum* in the lower bowel and stomach, had more significant pathology than the SPF mice which had either *H. felis* or *H. heilmannii* infection only. Indeed, the conventional mice showed significant atrophy and in some cases dysplasia of the glandular element[42] (Table 3).

Of considerable interest was the observation of mucosal-associated lymphoid tissue (MALT) hyperplasia. This may have particular relevance with the recent association of *H. pylori* and MALT lymphoma in humans[43] (see Chapter 48).

Helicobacter hepaticum and liver cancer

An active chronic hepatitis was detected recently in several inbred strains of mice originating from the Frederick Cancer Center barrier-maintained facility. Histologically, the liver lesions advanced with age from a mild focal necrosis with mononuclear cell inflammation to more extensive liver involvement including hepatocytomegaly, bile duct hyperplasia and a peribiliary inflammatory response[44]. Our laboratory has identified this organism associated with the hepatitis by several techniques. Using biochemical, morphological and 16S rRNA sequencing techniques we have determined that the organism seen in silver stains of involved livers of both naturally and experimentally infected mice is a new *Helicobacter* species which we have tentatively named '*H. hepaticum*'[45]. The hepatic lesions were associated with hepatic tumours in A/JCr male mice which normally have a very low

Table 4 *Helicobacter*-associated hepatitis and hepatocellular neoplasms in control A/JCr male mice

Date of sacrifice	Number of mice	Age (weeks)	Hepatitis	Tumours
Jan.–Mar. 1989	48	47 ± 3	0	0
May–July 1989	47	70 ± 6	0	1 (2%)
July 1992	16	54	16 (100%)	1 (6%)
Aug.–Oct. 1992	6	64 ± 3	5 (83%)	3 (50%)
Dec. 1992	12	77	12 (100%)	11 (92%)

All mice were saline-injected controls obtained as weanlings from the FCRDC Animal Production Area and subsequently housed in the same research facility. Mice killed in 1989 were part of a published study[87]. Tumours were diagnosed by histopathological criteria from H&E-stained formalin-fixed sections of nodular liver lesions and were mostly hepatocellular adenomas, except for hepatocellular carcinomas in five animals from the two most recent groups, in which most animals had multiple hepatocellular tumours (modified from ref. 44)

incidence of hepatic tumours (see Table 4). Indeed if this observation is confirmed, it will conclusively prove the direct association of a *Helicobacter* species and induction of cancer.

BIOMARKERS

The gastrointestinal epithelial cells rapidly turn over. In humans the proliferative cell cycle of gastric mucous cells is about 2 days[46]. Many factors such as food intake and growth hormones can affect the proliferation and normal differentiation rates of these epithelial cells[47,48]. Studies indicate that cell proliferation and maturation disturbances are related both to the development and progression of neoplasia[49]. In the preneoplastic stages such as metaplasia of the small and large intestinal types and dysplasia, proliferating epithelial cells differentiate abnormally as they migrate upward to the surface of the gastric mucosa[50]. In the multiple-stage model of gastric cancer, studies by Lipkin and Correa demonstrated that three main features related to risk of developing gastric cancer are an increased rate of cell proliferation, an expansion of the proliferative compartment and a failure of normal maturation in cells[51].

Biomarkers as intermediate end-points of carcinogenesis in chemoprevention trials have been studied extensively during the past 10 years[52]. Premalignant markers have been used to identify and quantitate the proliferating cells in a tissue or compartment. The most widely used technique, historically, for detecting DNA synthesis has been the use of *in vivo* uptake of [^{3}H]thymidine and identification by autoradiography. It provided a great deal of information on both normal and replicating cells, but because it required radiolabel, its use is being supplanted by newer techniques. Current techniques include BrdU labelling and other immunohistochemical. BrdU, a pyrimidine analogue of thymidine, is incorporated into DNA during cell replication and can be detected by an anti-BrdU monoclonal antibody[53]. It has been demonstrated that BrdU is able to selectively label replicating cells in the S phase[54] and is a reliable biomarker for epithelial cell proliferation[55]. Also, the proliferating cell nuclear antigen (PCNA), identified as the DNA polymerase-δ associated protein, was found in the cells of the proliferative compartment of normal gastrointestinal epithelial tissues; it is essential for cellular DNA replication in late G1 phase[56,57].

In the ferret we have obtained preliminary results with PCNA immuno-histochemistry which suggest that the technique may be applicable to ferret gastric tissue. Six *H. mustelae*-infected ferrets ranging in age from 18 to 35 months were used in this study. Mucosal pinch biopsies were obtained from the pylorus and fundus of the stomach at necropsy, fixed in 70% ethanol and then embedded in paraffin and an immunohistochemical staining procedure employed using a monoclonal antibody (PC10). The sections were analysed for microscopidensitometry using an image analysis system consisting of a Hamamatsu monochrome video camera mounted on a Nikon light microscope and coupled to a Macintosh IIcx computer through a data translation video capture board. By viewing at $40 \times$ and analysing areas of $0.0252\,mm^2$, the percentage of pixels was calculated per mm^2 using software (Image 1.2) developed at NIH by Dr Rasband. A minimum of three fields per sample was analysed. PCNA-labelled nuclei were demonstrated by the typical brown stain in the proliferative regions of the gastric mucosal crypts, and foci of positive cells also were found near the apex of the crypt, while the non-replicating cells had normal blue staining of the nuclei. The area of PCNA-stained nuclei was significantly larger in the pylorus (antrum) than in the fundus of the ferret stomach. These results are consistent with the histological changes which are also more severe in the antrum where diffuse inflammation occurs, whereas in the fundus a superficial gastritis only is evident[36]. Similar results using PCNA analysis have been recently observed in *H. pylori*-infected patients when *H. pylori* causes a more severe gastric inflammation in the antrum vs. body of human stomachs[58].

We are also investigating the use of BrdU labelling/staining in the gastric tissue of the ferret and the mouse. We believe that the use of premalignant markers in the animal models of *Helicobacter*-induced gastric carcinogenesis will allow early detection and characterization of the development of GCA in these models.

CHEMOPREVENTION OF GASTRIC CANCER

Vitamin C

Antioxidants, particularly vitamin C and β-carotene, have anticarcinogenic properties based on laboratory data as well as epidemiological evidence. Ascorbic acid scavenges nitrous oxide and makes the compound unavailable for nitrosation in the stomach. Furthermore, recent evidence indicates that many, but not all, patients with *H. pylori* gastritis have lowered ascorbic acid concentrations[59,60]. Other investigators have shown that patients with precancerous lesions of intestinal metaplasia and multifocal atrophic gastritis also have lowered ascorbate and elevated *N*-nitroso compound concentrations[61,62]. To test whether *H. pylori* does indeed impair ascorbic acid secretion into the stomach, animals which need dietary supplementation of vitamin C should ideally be used to mimic vitamin C metabolism in humans. Of the *Helicobacter* animal models presently available, only non-human primates fulfil this criterion, and should prove useful in answering this important question.

β-Carotene

There are convincing data from epidemiological, clinical and animal studies that *β*-carotene also has anticarcinogenic properties[63-67]. Two major hypotheses regarding the chemopreventive effect of *β*-carotene have been proposed. The retinoic acid hypothesis proposes that *β*-carotene exerts its anticancer action by its conversion to retinoids via either central cleavage or excentric cleavage[68,69]. The antioxidant hypothesis postulates that *β*-carotene prevents carcinogenesis by its intrinsic antioxidant property, independent of vitamin A activity[63]. There is currently no universal agreement on which mechanism(s) is (are) most important for the anticancer effect of *β*-carotene.

Numerous prospective and retrospective epidemiological studies over the past decade have reported that a high intake of fresh fruits and green vegetables rich in *β*-carotene and/or an increased serum level of *β*-carotene is/are associated with a reduced risk of gastric carcinoma. Further, several epidemiological studies have demonstrated an inverse association between serum *β*-carotene levels and risk of gastric cancer[70-72]. A cohort study by Haenszel *et al.*[70] showed that serum carotene levels in both sexes were significantly lower in subjects with gastric dysplasia than in those with normal gastric mucosa or less advanced gastric lesions (i.e. chronic atrophic gastritis or intestinal metaplasia of the stomach). The mechanism(s) of how *β*-carotene works as an anticancer agent is (are) uncertain. *β*-Carotene may exert its anticancer action by its conversion into retinoids[68,69], by its intrinsic antioxidant property independent of vitamin A activity[63] or by some other mechanisms such as enhancement of immune function[73] or enhancement of gap junction communication between cells[65]. Previous studies of the relationship between dietary *β*-carotene and cancer are confounded by the rodent models used[74,75]. Rodents do not accumulate appreciable tissue levels of *β*-carotene since they convert practically all *β*-carotene into retinoids in the intestinal mucosa before absorption[76]. Despite poor absorption and low serum and tissue levels of *β*-carotene in rodents, several studies have nevertheless shown a protective effect of dietary *β*-carotene against skin cancer[77,78]. One particular rodent model may have application to *Helicobacter* models and gastric cancer. Rats were dosed with MNNG to induce gastric cancer and were placed on supplemental oral carotenoids[75]. The results suggested that neither *β*-carotene nor canthaxanthin interefered with the development of preneoplastic lesions resulting from the administration of the MNNG, but they clearly inhibited the progression of dysplasia to early and infiltrating carcinomas by more than 50% in the carotenoid-treated groups compared to the non-supplemented control group.

Thus initiation was not affected, but promotion and progression of the precancerous gastric lesions were inhibited. This correlates well with the study by Haenszel *et al.*[70] which indicated (as mentioned above) that of all the micronutrients studied, β-carotene was the one which held the most promise of discriminating between individuals with abnormal and normal gastric mucosa.

β-Carotene metabolism in the ferret

There is limited evidence from animal experiments for β-carotene anticancer activity in chemically-induced cancers[64]. This may be in part due to a lack of an appropriate animal model which mimics human β-carotene absorption and gastrointestinal metabolism. We have recently shown that the domesticated ferret (*Mustela putorius furo*) is an ideal model to mimic human β-carotene absorption and metabolism. In humans, significant conversion of β-carotene to vitamin A takes place in the intestinal mucosa[79]. Approximately 9–17% of oral doses of labelled β-carotene is absorbed via the lymphatic system[80]. About 60–70% of the absorbed radioactivity is found as retinyl esters, whereas 15% remains as intact β-carotene[81]. Ribaya-Mercado *et al.* documented that ferrets absorbed significant amounts of intact dietary β-carotene and accumulated high amounts in various tissues[82,83]. For example, serum β-carotene increased from 0.6 g/dl to 15.3 and 41.5 g/dl after the ferrets were fed 4 or 20 mg of β-carotene/kg body weight daily for 2 weeks. In contrast, serum β-carotene levels in rats remained very low (0.5–0.6 g/dl) despite eating the same doses of β-carotene[82]. Ferret tissues which accumulate large amounts of β-carotene are liver, adrenals, small intestine, stomach and colon after β-carotene feeding[83]. Most recently, an *in vivo* study in ferrets was performed in our laboratory, showing that about 7.5% of the total administered $[^{14}C]\beta$-carotene is taken up by the small intestine after a 4 h intestinal perfusion of a β-carotene micellar solution[84]. The proportion of radioactivity recovered in the lymph collections after a 4 h perfusion was $3.2 + 0.2\%$. Of the total radioactivity in the mesenteric lymph, retinyl esters comprised the major portion (about 63%), whereas about 10% appeared as unchanged β-carotene. The absorption rate for β-carotene into ferret lymph was determined to be 0.054 g/h per 100 cm intestine, whereas the human absorption rate is about 0.038–0.12 g/h per 100 cm intestine, according to the work of Blomstrand and Goodman[80,81].

Not only the absorption but the gastrointestinal metabolism of β-carotene is similar in the human and in ferrets. Several *in vitro* and *in vivo* studies by our group have indicated that retinoic acid is a quantitatively significant metabolite of β-carotene in human and ferret small intestine through an excentric cleavage pathway[85,86]. In an *in vitro* study we demonstrated that significant amounts of retinoic acid are produced when either β-carotene or β-apo-carotenals are incubated with human or ferret intestinal mucosa in the presence of citral, a specific inhibitor for oxidation of retinal to retinoic acid[85]. This similarity in β-carotene absorption and metabolism between humans and ferrets indicates that the ferret is the best laboratory animal model for studying β-carotene absorption, and ideal for studying its possible role in the chemoprevention of *Helicobacter*-associated cancer.

CONCLUSION

By judicious combination of salient features of proven animal models for *Helicobacter* infection and gastric cancer induction by chemicals, useful information will be forthcoming on dissecting the apparent relationship of *Helicobacter* species and cancer. Also the use of predictive biomarkers of early malignancy and development of chemoprevention strategies should enhance our knowledge of mechanisms of bacterial-induced tumorigenesis.

References

1. Rotterdam H, Enterline HT. Pathology of the stomach and duodenum. New York: Springer-Verlag; 1989.
2. Davis GR. Neoplasms of the stomach. In: Sleisenger M, Fordtran JS, editors. Gastrointestinal disease: pathophysiology, diagnosis, management, 4th edn. Philadelphia: WB Saunders; 1989:745–72.
3. Sipponen P. *Helicobacter pylori* infection – a common worldwide environmental risk factor for gastric cancer? Endoscopy. 1992;24:424–7.
4. Sipponen P, Siurala M, Goodwin CS. Histology and ultrastructure of *Helicobacter pylori* infections: gastritis, duodenitis and peptic ulceration and their relevance as precancerous conditions. In: Goodwin CS, Worsley BW, editors. *Helicobacter pylori*: biology and clinical practice. Boca Raton FL: CRC Press; 1993:37–62.
5. Koster T, Vandenbrouke JP. *Helicobacter pylori*: musings from the epidemiological armchair. Epidemiol Infect. 1992;109:81–5.
6. Charnley G, Tannenbaum SR, Correa P. Gastric cancer: an etiologic model. Reprinted from Branbury Report 12: Nitrosamines and human cancer. Cold Spring Harbor Laboratory; 1982.
7. Correa P. Carcinoma of the stomach. Proc Nutr Soc. 1985;44:111–12.
8. Correa P. Human gastric carcinogenesis: a multistep and multifactorial process – First American Cancer Society Award Lecture on Cancer Epidemiology and Prevention. Cancer Res. 1992;52:6735–40.
9. Charnley G, Tannenbaum SR. Flow cytometric analysis of the effect of sodium chloride on gastric cancer risk in the rat. Cancer Res. 1985;45:5608–16.
10. Balansky RM, Blagoeva PM, Mircheva ZI, Stoitchev I, Chernozemski I. The effect of antioxidants on MNNG-induced stomach carcinogenesis in rats. J Cancer Res Clin Oncol. 1986;112:272–5.
11. Mitchell HM. The epidemiology of *Helicobacter pylori* infection and its relation to gastric cancer. In: Goodwin GS, Worsley BW, editors. *Helicobacter pylori*: biology and clinical practice. Boca Raton, FL: CRC Press; 1993:95–114.
12. Parsonnet J, Friedman GD, Vandersteen DP *et al.* Helicobacter pylori infection and the risk of gastric carcinoma. N Engl J Med. 1991;325:1127–31.
13. Nomura A, Stemmermann GN, Chyou PH, Kato I, Perez-Perez GI, Blaser MJ. *Helicobacter pylori* infection and gastric carcinoma among Japanese Americans in Hawaii. N Engl J Med. 1991;325:1132–6.
14. Forman D, Newell DG, Fullerton F *et al.* Association between infection with *Helicobacter pylori* and risk of gastric cancer: evidence from a prospective investigation. BMJ. 1991;302:1302–5.
15. Talley NJ, Zinsmeister AR, Weaver A *et al.* Gastric adenocarcinoma and *Helicobacter pylori* infection. J Natl Cancer Inst. 1991;83:1734–9.
16. Jones TC, Hunt RD. Veterinary pathology. Philadelphia, PA: Lea & Febiger; 1983: 1380–2.

17. Barker IK, Van Dreumel AA. The alimentary system. In: Jubb KVF, Kennedy PC, Palmer N, editors. Pathology of domestic animals, Vol. 2. New York: Academic Press; 1985:1–237.
18. McClure HM, Chapman WL, Hooper BE, Smith FG, Fletcher OJ. The digestive system. In: Benirschke K, Garner FM, Jones TC, editors. Pathology of laboratory animals, Vol. 1. New York: Springer-Verlag; 1978:175–317.
19. Squire RA, Goodman DG, Valerio MG et al. Tumors. In: Benirschke K, Garner FM, Jones TC, editors. Pathology of laboratory animals, Vol. 1. New York: Springer-Verlag; 1978: 1051–283.
20. Rice LE, Stahl SJ, McLeos CG Jr. Pyloric adenocarcinoma in a ferret. J Am Vet Med Assoc. 1992;200:1117–18.
21. Stauber E, Kraft S, Roinette J. Multiple tumors in a ferret. J Sm Exotic Anim Med. 1991;1:87–8.
22. Klein AJ, Palmer WL. Experimental gastric carcinoma: a critical review with comments on the criteria of induced malignancy. J Natl Cancer Inst. 1941;1:559–84.
23. Bralow SP. Experimental gastric carcinogenesis. Digestion. 1972;5:290–310.
24. Sugimura T, Kawachi T. Experimental stomach cancer. Methods Cancer Res. 1973;7: 245–308.
25. Stewart HL, Hare WV. Variations in susceptibility of the fundic and pyloric portions of the glandular stomach of the rat to induction of neoplasia by 20-methylcholanthrene. Acta Un Int Cancer. 1950;176–7.
26. Morris HP, Wagner BP, Ray FE, Snell KC, Stewart HL. Comparative study of cancer and other lesions of rats fed N,N'-2,7-fluorenylenebisacetamide or N-2-fluorenylacetamide. NCI Monogr. 1961;5:1–53.
27. Sugimura T, Fujimura S. Tumor production in glandular stomach of rat by N-methyl-N'-nitro-N-nitrosoguanidine. Nature. 1967;216:943–4.
28. Sigaran MF, Con-Wong R. Production of proliferative lesions in gastric mucosa of albino mice by oral administration of N-methyl-N'-nitro-N-nitrosoguanidine. Gann. 1979;70: 343–52.
29. IARC. N-nitroso-N-methylurea. IARC Monographs on the evaluation of carcinogenic risk of chemicals to man. 1977;227–55.
30. Tatematsu M, Ogawa K, Hoshiya T et al. Induction of adenocarcinomas in the glandular stomach of BALB/c mice treated with N-methyl-N-nitrosourea. Jpn J Cancer Res. 1992;83:915–18.
31. Schreiber H, Nettesheim P, Lijinsky W, Richter CB, Walburg HE Jr. Induction of lung cancer in germfree, specific-pathogen-free, and infected rats by N-methyl-N'-nitro-N-nitrosoguanidine: enhancement by respiratory infection. J Natl Cancer Inst. 1972;49:1107–14.
32. Sumi Y, Miyakawa M. Comparative studies on the production of stomach tumors following the intubation of several doses of N-methyl-N'-nitro-N-nitrosoguanidine in germ-free and conventional newborn rats. Gann. 1981;72:700–4.
33. Fox JG, Lee A. Gastric *Helicobacter* infection in animals: natural and experimental infections. In: Goodwin CS, Worsley BW, editors. *Helicobacter pylori*: biology and clinical practice. Boca Raton, FL: CRC Press; 1993:407–30.
34. Fox JG, Chilvers T, Goodwin S et al. *Campylobacter mustelae*, a new species resulting from the evaluation of *Campylobacter pylori* subsp. *mustelae* to species status. Int J Syst Bacteriol. 1989;39:301–3.
35. Fox JG, Cabot EB, Taylor NS, Laraway R. Gastric colonization by *Campylobacter pylori* subsp. *mustelae* in ferrets. Infect Immun. 1988;56:2994–6.
36. Fox JG, Correa P, Taylor NS et al. *Helicobacter mustelae*-associated gastritis in ferrets: an animal model of *Helicobacter pylori* gastritis in humans. Gastroenterology. 1990;99:352–61.
37. Fox JG. Biology and diseases of the ferret. Philadelphia: Lea & Febiger; 1988.
38. Fox JG, Wishnok JS, Murphy JC, Tannenbaum SR, Correa P. MNNG-induced gastric carcinoma in ferrets infected with *Helicobacter mustelae*. Carcinogenesis. 1993;14:1957–61.
39. Lee A, Fox JG, Otto G, Murphy J. A small animal model of human *Helicobacter pylori* active chronic gastritis. Gastroenterology. 1990;99:1315–23.
40. Fox JG, Lee A, Otto G, Taylor NS, Murphy JC. *Helicobacter felis* gastritis in gnotobiotic rats: an animal model of *Helicobacter pylori* gastritis. Infect Immun. 1991;59:785–91.
41. Fox JG, Blanco M, Murphy JC et al. Local and systemic immune responses in murine *Helicobacter felis* active chronic gastritis. Infect Immun. 1993:2309–15.

42. Lee A, O'Rourke J, Dixon M, Fox JG. *Helicobacter*-induced gastritis: look to the host. Acta Gastro-Enterol Belg. 1993;56(Suppl).
43. Wotherspoon AC, Doglioni C, Diss TC *et al.* Regression of primary low-grade B-cell gastric lymphoma of mucosa-associated lymphoid tissue type after eradication of *Helicobacter pylori*. Lancet. 1993;342:575–7.
44. Ward JM, Fox JG, Anver MR *et al.* Chronic active hepatitis and associated liver tumors in mice caused by a persistent bacterial infection with a novel *Helicobacter* species (submitted for publication).
45. Fox JG, Tulley J, Yan L *et al. Helicobacter hepaticum* sp nov, a microaerophilic bacteria isolated from livers and intestines of mice (submitted for publication).
46. Lipkin M, Bell B, Sherlock P. Cell proliferation kinetics in the gastrointestinal tract of man II. Cell renewal in stomach, ileum, colon and rectum. Gastroenterology. 1964;45:721–9.
47. Riecken EO, Menge H. Nutritive effects of food constituents on the structure and function of the intestine. Acta Hepatogastroenterol. 1977;24:388–99.
48. Leblond CP, Carriere RM. The effect of growth hormone thyroxine on the mitotic rate of the intestinal mucosa of the rat. Endocrinology. 1955;56:261–6.
49. Lipkin M, Higgins P. Biological markers of cell proliferation and differentiation in human gastrointestinal diseases. Adv Cancer Res. 1988;50:1–24.
50. Lipkin M. Biomarkers of increased susceptibility to gastrointestinal cancer: new application to studies of cancer prevention in human subjects. Cancer Res. 1988;48:235–45.
51. Lipkin M, Correa P, Mikol YB *et al.* Proliferative and antigenic modifications in epithelial cells in chronic atrophic gastritis. J Natl Cancer Inst. 1985;75:613–19.
52. Lippman SM, Lee JS, Lotan R *et al.* Biomarkers as intermediate end points in chemoprevention trials. J Natl Cancer Inst. 1990;82:555–60.
53. Gratzner HG. A new reagent for detection of DNA replication. Science. 1982;218:474–5.
54. Dean PN, Dolbeare F, Gratzner H *et al.* Cell-cycle analysis using a monoclonal antibody to BrdU. Cell Tissue Kinet. 1984;17:427.
55. Risio M, Lipkin M, Canelaresi G *et al.* Correlations between rectal mucosa cell proliferation and the clinical and pathological features of nonfamilial neoplasia of the large intestine. Cancer Res. 1991;51:1917–21.
56. Bravo R, Frank R, Blundell PA, Macdonald-Bravo H. Cyclin/PCNA is the auxiliary protein of DNA polymerase-d. Nature. 1987;326:515–20.
57. Sarraf CE, McCormick CSF, Brown GB *et al.* Proliferating cell nuclear antigen immunolocalization in gastrointestinal epithelia. Digestion. 1991;50:85–91.
58. De Koster E, Buset M, *et al.* Influence of HP and gastritis on gastric antrum and corpus mucosal cell proliferation status. Acta Gastroenterol Belg. 1993;56:61.
59. Sobala GM, Pignatelli B, Schorah CJ *et al.* Simultaneous determination of ascorbic acid, nitrite, total nitrosocompounds and bile acids in fasting gastric juice, and gastric mucosal histology: implications for gastric carcinogenesis. Carcinogenesis. 1991;12:193–8.
60. Sobala GM, Schorah CJ, Pignatelli B *et al.* High gastric juice ascorbic acid concentrations in members of a gastric cancer family. Carcinogenesis. 1993;14:291–2.
61. Chen VW, Abu-Elyazeed RR, Zavala DE *et al.* Risk factors of gastric precancerous lesions in a high-risk Columbian population. II. Nitrate and nitrite. Nutr Cancer. 1990;13:67–72.
62. Bartsch H, Ohshima H, Pignatelli B. Inhibitors of endogenous nitrosation. Mechanisms and implications in human cancer prevention. Mutat Res. 1988;202:307–24.
63. Peto R, Doll R *et al.* Can dietary β-carotene materially reduce human cancer rates? Nature. 1981;290:201–8.
64. Krinsky NI. Carotenoids and cancer in animal models. J Nutr. 1989;119:123–6.
65. Zhang L-X, Cooney RV, Bertram JS. Carotenoids enhance gap junctional communication and inhibit lipid peroxidation in C3H/10T1/2 cells: relationship to their cancer chemopreventive action. Carcinogenesis. 1991;12:2109–14.
66. Garewal HS, Meyskens FL, Killen D *et al.* Response of oral leukoplakia to β-carotene. J Clin Oncol. 1990;7:1715–20.
67. Diplock AT. The protective roles of antioxidant nutrients in disease prevention. Backgrounder. 1992;3(1):1–12.
68. Olson JA. Some thoughts on the relationship between vitamin A and cancer. Adv Exp Med Biol. 1986;206:379–98.

521

69. Goodman DS. Overview of current knowledge of metabolism of vitamin A and carotenoids. J Natl Cancer Inst. 1984;73:1375–9.
70. Haenszel W, Correa P, Lopez A *et al.* Serum micronutrient levels in relation to gastric pathology. Int J Cancer. 1985;36:43–8.
71. Gey KG, Brubacher GB, Stahelin HB. Plasma levels of antioxidant vitamins in relation to ischemic heart disease and cancer. Am J Clin Nutr. 1987;45:1368–77.
72. Smith AH, Waller KD. Serum β-carotene in persons with cancer and their immediate families. Am J Epidemiol. 1991;133:661–71.
73. Bendich A. Carotenoids and immune response. J Nutr. 1989;119:112–15.
74. Jones RC, Sugie S, Braley J, Weisburger JH. Dietary β-carotene in rat models of gastrointestinal cancer. J Nutr. 1989;119:509–14.
75. Santamaria L, Bianchi A, Ravetto C *et al.* Prevention of gastric cancer induced by *N*-methyl-*N'*-nitro-nitrosoguanidine in rats fed supplemental carotenoids. J Nutr Growth Cancer. 1987;4:175–81.
76. Crain FD, Lotspeich FJ, Krause F. Biosynthesis of retinoic acid by intestinal enzymes of the rat. J Lipid Res. 1967;8:249–54.
77. Mathews-Roth MM. Antitumor activity of β-carotene canthaxanthin and phytoene. Oncology. 1982;39:33–7.
78. Mathews-Roth MM, Krinsky NI. Carotenoid dose level and protection against UV-B induced skin tumors. Photochem Photobiol. 1985;42:35–8.
79. Gronowska-Senger A, Wolf G. Effect of dietary protein on the enzyme from rat and human intestine which converts β-carotene to retinal. J Nutr. 1970;100:300–8.
80. Goodman DS, Blomstrand R, Werner B *et al.* The intestinal absorption and metabolism of vitamin A and β-carotene in man. J Clin Invest. 1966;45:1615–23.
81. Krinsky NI, Cornwell DG, Oncley JL. The transport of vitamin A and carotenoids in human plasma. Arch Biochem Biophys. 1958;73:233–46.
82. Ribaya-Mercado JD, Holmgren SC, Fox JG, Russell RM. Dietary β-carotene absorption and metabolism in ferrets and rats. J Nutr. 1989;119:665–8.
83. Ribaya-Mercado JD, Fox JG, Rosenblad WD *et al.* β-Carotene, retinol, and retinyl ester concentrations in serum and selected tissues of ferrets fed β-carotene. J Nutr. 1992;122:1898–903.
84. Wang XD, Krinsky NI, Marini RP *et al.* The lymphatic and intestinal absorption of β-carotene in ferret – a useful model for human metabolism. Am J Physiol. 1992;236:G480–6.
85. Wang XD, Tang G, Fox JG *et al.* Enzymatic conversion of β-carotene into β-apo-carotenals and retinoids by human, monkey, ferret, and rat tissues. Arch Biochem Biophys. 1991;285(1):8–16.
86. Wang XD, Krinsky NI, Tang G, Russell RM. Retinoic acid can be produced from excentric cleavage of β-carotene in human intestinal mucosa. Arch Biochem Biophys. 1992;293(2):298–304.
87. Anderson LM, *et al.* Characterization of ethanol's enhancement of tumorigenesis by *N*-nitroso-dimethylamine in mice. Carcinogenesis. 1992;13:2107–11.

50
Flaws in *H. pylori*-related carcinogenesis hypothesis

P. CORREA

INTRODUCTION

Gastric adenocarcinoma, especially the so-called intestinal type, is preceded by a series of morphological alterations of the gastric mucosa. It has been postulated that the following alterations may be sequential in nature: chronic gastritis, atrophy, intestinal metaplasia, dysplasia and invasive carcinomas[1]. It is generally considered that the process is multifactorial, and a hypothesis has been proposed assigning specific aetiological forces to specific points in the chain of causation[2].

Years after the aetiological model was proposed, *Helicobacter pylori* was recognized, and it became clear that this bacterium is the overriding cause of the first step in the cascade of events, namely chronic gastritis. Establishing an aetiological link between an infection initiated decades before the invasive neoplastic outcome becomes a difficult epidemiological challenge. Causality for infectious diseases has ideally been based on the Koch's postulates, namely:

1. The organism must be present in every case of the disease.
2. The organism must be isolated and grown in pure culture.
3. The organism must, when inoculated into a susceptible animal, cause the specific disease.
4. The organism must then be recovered from the animal and identified.

Given today's understanding of the multiple genotypic and phenotypic alterations which eventually lead to neoplasia, it becomes obvious that none of the above postulates can be used to demonstrate a causal relationship between *H. pylori* and gastric adenocarcinoma. The postulates may be very useful to test the causality of acute infectious diseases, but are not applicable to trace the cascade of molecular abnormalities which may have been initiated and stimulated by a bacterial infection, especially when the suspect agent is not in immediate contact with the target molecule, namely gastric epithelial DNA.

On the other hand, Hill's guidelines on causal association may be used to examine the relationship between *H. pylori* and gastric carcinoma[3]. Research in several scientific disciplines has recently contributed information which is relevant to several of the guidelines, and hopefully will continue to contribute new information and allow the development of scientific consensus on the subject. In the following paragraphs examples of scientific information relevant to Hill's guidelines will be discussed.

TEMPORALITY

The cause precedes the effect. Correlation and case–control studies have shown a statistical association between *H. pylori* infection and gastric carcinoma[4-6]. Since in such studies *H. pylori* infection and carcinoma were found at the same time, the temporality issue cannot be resolved. Studies, however, have been conducted in the so-called 'retrospective' or 'historical' cohort fashion. Patients in whom gastric carcinoma was diagnosed, belonged to cohorts whose individuals had previously supplied serum samples which were kept in a freezer for years. Serum antibodies to *H. pylori* were assessed and compared to those of serum samples from individuals of the same cohort who did not develop such tumours[7-9]. All such studies revealed that the risk of developing gastric cancer was significantly higher in subjects previously infected with *H. pylori* than in their non-infected counterparts. These studies, therefore, leave little doubt that the *H. pylori* infection (the presumed cause) was present long before the development of an invasive tumour. A correct temporal relationship between *H. pylori* and gastric carcinoma has therefore been established.

STRENGTH

This parameter is based on the magnitude of the relative risk, which in most studies of analytical epidemiology has been around 2–6. The increase in risk is statistically significant, but not very high. In this situation the role of confounders is more difficult to rule out totally. It is possible that these risks are underestimated because of misclassification and other technical difficulties which may bias the results towards the null. It is also possible that these results reflect the multifactorial nature of gastric carcinogenesis in humans. If several carcinogenic influences are present at the same time, and perhaps interacting positively or negatively, the risk of each factor would represent a fraction of the total complex of causal forces implicated. It would appear then that *H. pylori* may not be the overriding factor in gastric carcinogenesis. Further research is required to establish its possible interaction with other aetiological factors.

DOSE–RESPONSE

Large exposure to the cause is associated with higher rates of the disease. These guidelines are hard to evaluate in the possible *H. pylori*–gastric carcinoma equation. There are no studies demonstrating that a greater bacterial load results in higher cancer rates, although such type of association is not ruled out. Another possible measure of dose–response is the length of the infection, which would imply that exposure to the agent for a longer period of time results in higher cancer rates. It has been shown that high-risk populations acquire the infection during early childhood[10–13]. There are, however, many populations with high prevalence rates of *H. pylori* infection but low gastric cancer mortality rates. Examples of this situation are seen in several continents: in India, South Arabia, Yemen (Asia), Algeria, Ivory Coast, Zaïre (Africa) and the coastal area of Costa Rica (Central America) the infection is either documented or suspected to be present since childhood[13–15]. In spite of these inconsistencies, there is in general a positive correlation between *H. pylori* prevalence and gastric cancer rates[5].

In two populations with high prevalence rates of *H. pylori* infection, namely Okinawa (Japan) and Chiapas (Mexico), a significant, but not large excess in *H. pylori* prevalence has been found in patients with atrophic, as compared to non-atrophic, gastritis[16–18].

Taken together, the above data suggest that a dose–response effect can be found between the length of *H. pylori* infection and the rates of gastric carcinoma. The abundance of inconsistencies, however, strongly suggest that the carcinogenic influences of *H. pylori* are not of an obligatory nature, and could be suppressed in certain populations.

Two explanations could be offered. It may be that inhibitors of carcinogenesis (such as antioxidants) may interfere with the process. Alternatively, it could be that *H. pylori* may facilitate the effect of a carcinogen without itself being a carcinogen. If the only role of *H. pylori* were to increase the rate of cell proliferation[19], in the absence of a carcinogen such hyperproliferation would not be sufficient to increase the rates of gastric carcinoma in epidemic proportions. Such result would suggest a synergistic effect between an infectious agent and a chemical carcinogen, as recently shown for hepato-cellular carcinoma[20].

REVERSIBILITY

Reduction in exposure is associated with lower rates of the disease. This postulate in the case under consideration calls for intervention to reduce the exposure, followed by observation of decreasing rates. Such intervention is obviously not available at the present time. There has been speculation suggesting that the decreasing gastric cancer rates experienced in recent decades may be the result of decreasing prevalence rates of *H. pylori* infection which took place decades before. This inference has been in part reached because, in some populations in which the cancer rates have decreased, the overall prevalence rates of *H. pylori* infection are lower and evidence of the infection is detected later in life than in populations with high rates of gastric cancer. The missing piece in these speculations is information about prevalence rates of *H. pylori* infections 50 or more years previously.

In Japan, mortality rates from gastric cancer have decreased considerably while the present prevalence rates of *H. pylori* infection are high. This inconsistency, however, is less evident when it is considered that the incidence rates in Japan have decreased much less than the mortality rates, suggesting that early diagnosis and treatment have played a major role in preventing deaths from gastric carcinoma.

It thus appears that reversibility in the *H. pylori*–gastric cancer equation has not been demonstrated, even though it may have occurred.

CONSISTENCY

Correlation and case–control studies of the association between *H. pylori* infection and gastric carcinoma have been carried out in many countries. The majority have shown a positive association, but there have been exceptions to the rule, some of them published recently[21]. All published cohort studies, which should carry more weight in the evaluation of causality, have shown a positive association.

Based on the available data, the consistency of the reports favours a causal association, but this is not overwhelming or unanimous.

BIOLOGICAL PLAUSIBILITY

It has been postulated for many decades, but never proven, that chronic infection is a cause of cancer. In the case of chronic gastritis associated with *H. pylori* infection, biological plausibility is suggested by several characteristics of the process: (1) The increased rate of cell proliferation may potentiate carcinogenic influences which by themselves may not be a sufficient cause of neoplastic transformation. (2) The low levels of ascorbic acid in the gastric juice brought about by *H. pylori* infection may interfere with antioxidant and other properties of this vitamin. (3) The inflammatory cells attracted by *H. pylori*, especially macrophages and polymorphonuclear neutrophils, may deliver toxic oxygen radicals which may reach actively dividing epithelial cells, inducing mutations.

Based on the present knowledge, a role of *H. pylori* in gastric carcinogenesis is biologically plausible but far from certain.

CONCLUSION

The available evidence suggests that Hill's guidelines for causal association have been partially met in the case of *H. pylori* infection and gastric carcinoma, as mentioned below.

Temporality: the correct chronological flow of events has been established.
Strength: relative risks of gastric carcinoma are statistically significant but not markedly elevated. This raises questions of possible interactions with other factors.
Dose–response: it has been suggested, but not proven, that the length of the

infection may increase the risk of carcinoma. This is not seen in populations of low socioeconomic standards displaying low gastric cancer risks.
Reversibility: has not been demonstrated.
Consistency: present to a certain degree, with numerous exceptions.
Biological plausibility: present.

A panoramic view of the available evidence is compatible with the idea that *H. pylori* is an incomplete cause of gastric carcinoma. It probably interacts with other factors which, as a group, become a complete carcinogen in certain individuals.

SUMMARY

The available evidence on the possible causal association between *H. pylori* infection and gastric carcinoma was discussed. Such association is not amenable to testing following Koch's postulates, which may be applicable to some infectious diseases. Hill's guidelines of causal association, namely temporality, strength, dose–response, reversibility, consistency and biological plausibility were discussed. It was suggested that *H. pylori* infection may be an incomplete carcinogen which requires interaction with other factors to become a complete carcinogen.

References

1. Correa P, Haenszel W, Cuello C, Tannembaum S, Archer M. A model for gastric cancer epidemiology. Lancet. 1975;2:58.
2. Correa P. Human gastric carcinogenesis: a multistep and multifactorial process. First American Cancer Society Award Lecture on Cancer Epidemiology and Prevention. Cancer Res. 1992;52:6735–40.
3. Hill AB. The environment and disease. Association and causation. Proc R Soc Med. 1965;58:295–300.
4. Forman D, Sitas F, Newell DG. Geographic association of *Helicobacter pylori* antibody prevalence and gastric cancer mortality in rural China. Int J Cancer. 1990;46:608–11.
5. Eurogast Study Group. An international association between *Helicobacter pylori* infection and gastric cancer. Lancet. 1993;341:1359–62.
6. Parsonnet J, Vanderstein D, Goates J, Sibley RK, Pritkin J, Chang Y. *Helicobacter pylori* infection in intestinal and diffuse-type gastric carcinomas. J Natl Cancer Inst. 1991;83:640–3.
7. Nomura A, Stemmermann GN, Chyou PH, Kato I, Perez-Perez G, Blaser MJ. *Helicobacter pylori* infection and gastric carcinoma among Japanese Americans in Hawaii. N Engl J Med. 1991;325:1132–6.
8. Parsonnet J, Friedman GD, Vandusteen DP. *Helicobacter pylori* infection and the risk of gastric carcinoma. N Engl J Med. 1991;325:1127–31.
9. Forman D, Newell DG, Fullerton F. Association between infection with *Helicobacter pylori* and risk of gastric cancer: evidence from a prospective investigation. BMJ. 1991;332:1302–5.
10. Fox J, Correa P, Taylor NJ *et al. Campylobacter pylori*-associated gastritis and immune response in a population at increased risk of gastric carcinoma. Am J Gastroenterol. 1989;84:775–81.
11. Megraud F. Epidemiology of *Helicobacter pylori* infection. Gastroenterol Clin N Am. 1993;22:73–88.
12. Graham D, Adam E, Reddy GT *et al.* Seroepidemiology of *Helicobacter pylori* infection in India. Comparison of developed and developing countries. Dig Dis Sci. 1991;36:1084–8.

13. Sierra R, Muñoz N, Peña S *et al.* Antibodies to *Helicobacter pylori* and pepsinogen levels in children from Costa Rica: comparison of two areas with different risk for stomach cancer. Cancer Epid Biomarkers Prev. 1992;1:449–54.

14. Holcomb C. *Helicobacter pylori*: the African enigma. Gastroenterology. 1992;33:429–31.

15. Shousa S, El Sherif AM, El Guneid A, Murray-Lyon IM. *Helicobacter pylori* and intestinal metaplasia: comparison between British and Yemeni patients. Am J Gastroenterol. 1993;88:1373–6.

16. Fukao M, Imai H, Gey F, Tei Y, Hanoaka T, Sugano K, Watanabe S. *Helicobacter pylori*, dietary factors and atrophic gastritis among Japanese blood donors: a cross-sectional study. Cancer Causes Control. 1993;4:307–12.

17. Tsugane S, Kabuto M, Imai H *et al. Helicobacter pylori*, dietary factors, and atrophic gastritis in five Japanese populations with different gastric cancer mortality. Cancer Causes Control. 1993;4:297–305.

18. Guarner J, Mohar A, Parsonnet J, Halperin D. The association of *Helicobacter pylori* with gastric cancer and preneoplastic lesions in Chiapas, Mexico. Cancer. 1993;71:297–301.

19. Brenes F, Ruiz B, Correa P *et al. Helicobacter pylori* causes hyperproliferation of the gastric epithelium. Pre- and post-eradication indices of proliferating cell nuclear antigen (PCNA). Am J Gastroenterol. 1993;88:1870–5.

20. Qian GS, Ross RK, Yu MC *et al.* A follow-up study of urinary markers of aflatoxin exposure and liver cancer in Shanghai, People's Republic of China. Cancer Epid Biomarkers Prev. (in press).

21. Farinati F, Valiante F, Germana B *et al.* Prevalence of *Helicobacter pylori* infection in patients with precancerous changes and gastric cancer. Eur J Cancer Prev. 1993;321–6.

Section IX
Therapy of *H. pylori* infection

51
Determinants of antimicrobial effectiveness in *H. pylori* gastritis

D. Y. GRAHAM

INTRODUCTION

Helicobacter pylori is a major cause of gastritis. *H. pylori*-associated diseases include: simple gastritis, duodenal ulcer, gastric ulcer, gastric cancer, and primary gastric B-cell lymphoma. Cure of *H. pylori* infection is thought to be desirable because following it the gastritis heals, gastric and duodenal ulcer disease are cured and possibly also are some cases of B-cell lymphoma. In addition, elimination of *H. pylori* from humans should be associated with primary prevention of the *H. pylori* gastritis-associated diseases and their consequences. Unfortunately, *H. pylori* infection has proven difficult to cure[1-4]. Initial studies of *H. pylori* sensitivity showed that *H. pylori* was sensitive to a large number of different antimicrobials[1]. Clinical trials rapidly showed that antimicrobial sensitivity *in vitro* was a poor predictor of *in vivo* effectiveness. After a number of false starts there are now several safe and effective therapies that will cure the infection in the majority of cases[1,5]. To date, no monotherapy is available that consistently yields cure rates of 50% or greater, and poly-antimicrobial therapy is generally required for successful treatment.

The ecological niche for *H. pylori* is the stomach. The organisms reside in gastric mucus both as free-swimming forms and attached to the mucosal surface. In addition, there is evidence for the presence of *H. pylori* within gastric mucosal cells as well as in extra-gastric sites such as dental plaque[6-13]. The gastric environment is very hostile for antimicrobial agents. Attempts to treat infections in the stomach introduced parameters not usually considered when planning antimicrobial therapy in other tissues. Such factors include the physical environment of the stomach with its low pH, active secretion, thick mucus layer, and emptying of contents.

Killing *H. pylori* is not synonymous with cure of the infection; killing is easy, cure has proven to be remarkably difficult[1]. Early studies provided misleading optimism, as it was not recognized that failure to find bacteria immediately after a course of therapy often did not signify cure of the

Table 1 Possible reasons for failure of antimicrobial therapy

Bacterial resistance
Organism not sensitive *in vivo*
Antimicrobial unable to penetrate to site of bacterium
Stationary state (no multiplication)
Presence of binding proteins
Anaerobic environment
Presence of inactivating enzymes
Drug interactions
Patient compliance
Drug distribution and concentration
Duration of therapy

Table 2 Factors that may have major influence on effectiveness of antimicrobial therapy

Formulation (tablet, liquid, colloid, granule, etc.)
Administration in relation to meals
Frequency of drug administration
Dosage of antimicrobial agents
Bismuth salt (e.g. citrate, nitrate, salicylate)
Duration of therapy
Co-therapy to raise pH (e.g. omeprazole)
Administration of mucolytics

infection. Follow-up of patients in whom the infection was thought to be cured showed that the infection had only been suppressed, and rapidly returned to full vigour. Some of the possible reasons for failure of antibiotic therapy are shown in Table 1.

BACTERIAL RESISTANCE AS A CAUSE OF POOR RESPONSE

There are a number of possible causes of apparent or real bacterial resistance to antimicrobials (Table 2). *H. pylori* rapidly develop resistance to many antibiotics, and this has limited the usefulness of a number of potentially effective agents and has necessitated the use of combination therapies. Plasmid-mediated resistance has not yet been demonstrated, but acquired resistance has been demonstrated to a variety of agents and the presence of cross-resistance (e.g. to macrolides) has been strongly suggested.

Development of antibiotic resistance may be, in part, related to the inoculum effect[14]. The inoculum effect is the term used to describe a significant increase in the minimal inhibitory concentration of an antibiotic when the number of organisms inoculated is large. The tremendous number of *H. pylori* organisms in the stomach may help explain development of resistance through the inoculum effect, as it is likely that subpopulations of *H. pylori* with antibiotic resistance are present before the antimicrobial is administered. Bismuth may be an extremely important part of many therapies because of its effect in eliminating or reducing the inoculum effect by decimating the *H. pylori* population with the first few doses. Possibly, only one or two doses of bismuth are all that are required. This has not been tested experimentally.

Another potentially important phenomenon is the biofilm phenomenon. This term denotes the fact that organisms attached to a surface display a significantly increased minimal inhibitory concentration towards antimicrobials. The biofilm phenomenon has been demonstrated with *H. pylori* using tissue culture[15]. Whether it is also present *in vivo* is unknown, but likely.

THE ROLE OF THE STOMACH IN ANTIMICROBIAL EFFECTIVENESS

H. pylori reside 'outside' the body in the same way that gingival and skin bacteria do. In the stomach a form of topical therapy is possible as the relatively small intragastric volume makes it possible to deliver a high concentration of antimicrobial agents directly to the site of infection[16]. Fasting intragastric volume is typically less than 50 ml and postprandially it rarely exceeds 500 ml, allowing small doses of antimicrobial to produce high MIC[2].

Factors that deserve systematic investigation to optimize therapy are shown in Table 2. Formulation of the agent may be extremely important. Capsules tend to be trapped within folds and to release the drug locally, and drugs administered as tablets generally show better intragastric dissolution and distribution[17]. Liquids may provide the best intragastric distribution but may be rapidly emptied from the stomach, and they provide no 'depot effect' as might be present when the contents of capsules or tablets are deposited in gastric mucus[17]. Finally, parenteral administration is both inconvenient and eliminates or reduces any topical effect of a drug. Solubility of the drug is also important, as the solubility of many compounds is markedly reduced in an acidic environment.

Two important considerations in the stomach that can be easily influenced are gastric emptying and acidity. Administration of a drug to the fasting patient may result in the majority of the agent passing into the small intestine before the formulation can either dissolve or disperse. The presence of food delays gastric emptying, is associated with excellent dispersion of an agent, and buffers gastric acid[2,16]. Administration with meals may provide for prolonged residence in the stomach, and the grinding and mixing functions of the stomach ensure wide drug dispersal. The practical aspects of the importance of administration of some drugs with meals is illustrated by the preliminary results obtained with ranitidine–bismuth subcitrate combinations. Both clearance and cure were significantly lower when the bismuth-containing preparation was given fasting compared to when it was given with meals. One potentially negative aspect of administration with meals is that the drug may interact with specific components of the meal and become less available either locally or for absorption. Finally, eating has the beneficial effect of causing desquamation of surface cells and discharge of mucus, which also possibly exposes the organisms to higher concentrations of the agent or may expose a higher percentage of the organisms to the agent[18,19].

Antimicrobial action could possibly be improved by co-therapies with mucolytics or antisecretory drugs. The potential advantages of antisecretory drugs include a decrease in intragastric volume (i.e. increased antimicrobial concentration), increased intragastric pH (possibly increase in effectiveness), as well as a possible direct antimicrobial effect of the antisecretory agent (e.g. proton pump inhibitors).

Low intragastric pH is thought to be a major barrier to effective antimicrobial therapy[1,2,20]. Antibacterial effect is pH-dependent and thus adding a proton pump inhibitor to anti-*H. pylori* regimen is an attractive idea reliably to increase the pH in the stomach. The activity of a number of antimicrobial agents has been tested over the range of pH 5 to 8[21]. Ampicillin was 10-fold more active at neutral pH than at the more acidic pH values. There was only a slight improvement (from 0.5 mg/l at pH 5.5 to 0.12 mg/l at pH 7.5) in the activity of tetracycline. Bismuth and metronidazole were unaffected by the change in pH from 5.5 to 7.5[21,22]. Tetracycline is an acid-stable antimicrobial whose concentration in the gastric mucosa exceeds the MIC90 for *H. pylori* for several hours[22,23]. Adding omeprazole to tetracycline, or to tetracycline and bismuth, produces no benefit in cure rate. Thus, while the combination of omeprazole and another antimicrobial appears attractive, one may not be able to predict the outcome without data from a clinical trial. Why? Substituted benzimidazole proton pump inhibitors, such as lansoprazole and omeprazole, inhibit selectively *H. pylori* growth *in vitro* at a concentration comparable to that of bismuth salts. *In vivo*, therapy with omeprazole is associated with improvement in the severity of the gastritis, suggesting an *in vivo* antibacterial effect. Despite this effect, omeprazole monotherapy does not cure *H. pylori* infection[24-33]. This failure may be related to its inability to reach effective antimicrobial concentration in the stomach after 20–80 mg of omeprazole daily. In the gastric mucosa the concentration of amoxicillin has reached > 322 mg/kg, which is hundreds of times the MIC90 for *H. pylori* at pH 5.5 (0.5 mg/l)[34]. Both bismuth and tetracycline reach an effective concentration level in the gastric mucosa, and thus the failure to achieve a sizeable benefit from the addition of omeprazole to bismuth and tetracycline may mean that the primary effect of omeprazole in enhancing the effectiveness of amoxicillin is related to its effect on pH and not to its inherent antimicrobial activity. Subsequent studies to test this hypothesis might evaluate combinations of omeprazole and bactericidal antibiotics in which a major pH effect on sensitivity is present.

COMPLIANCE AS A FACTOR INFLUENCING ANTIMICROBIAL EFFECTIVENESS

In our experience, failure to take the medications as prescribed is one of the most common reasons for failure[35]. We studied the results of triple therapy in 93 individuals and used stepwise regression analysis to assess which factors were most important in influencing cure rates. Various multi-drug regimens may put a burden on the patient in terms of the number of tablets or capsules required to be taken daily. It is an unproven assumption that fewer dosing

Table 3 Effect of compliance on cure of *H. pylori* infection (eradication rate, percentages)

	Percentage of medicines taken		
Group	All	≥ 60%	< 60%
Duodenal ulcer	90	97	75
Gastric ulcer	91	91	33

Adapted from ref. 35

intervals or shorter duration of therapy will result in better results, and this deserves study. We found that the type of disease (duodenal ulcer, gastric ulcer, or gastritis) did not influence cure rates[35]. The only significant factor was compliance (Table 3). We recommend that, for simplicity, all antimicrobials be given with meals. Experience has shown that a duration of 12–14 days is adequate.

SUMMARY

The ecological niche for *H. pylori* is the stomach, an environment that is very hostile for antimicrobial agents. Factors affecting antimicrobial effectiveness include the physical environment of the stomach with its low pH, active secretion, thick mucus layer which antimicrobials may find difficult to penetrate, as well as frequent emptying of contents which limits the time for antimicrobials to act locally. In addition to the problems encountered in the stomach, bacterial resistance has been a problem limiting the effectiveness of many potentially effective drugs. Although several antimicrobial protocols have been developed, little attention has been given to factors such as the possible importance of drug formulation, administration in relation to meals, or frequency of drug administration. There is considerable current interest in use of antisecretory therapy to possibly enhance antimicrobial effectiveness. Currently, the therapies with the greatest success are those that employ two or three antimicrobials and are administered in multiple dosages/day for 2 weeks.

Acknowledgements

This work was supported by the Department of Veterans Affairs and by the generous support of Hilda Schwartz.

References

1. Börsch GM, Graham DY. *Helicobacter pylori*. In: Collen MJ, Benjamin SB, editors. Pharmacology of peptic ulcer disease. Handbook of experimental pharmacology, Vol. 99. Berlin: Springer-Verlag; 1991:107–48.
2. Graham DY, Börsch GM. The who's and when's of therapy for *Helicobacter pylori*. Am J Gastroenterol. 1990;85:1552–5.

3. Glupczynski Y, Burette A. Drug therapy for *Helicobacter pylori* infection: problems and pitfalls. Am J Gastroenterol. 1990;85:1545–51.
4. Tytgat GN, Noach LA, Rauws EA. *Helicobacter pylori* infection and duodenal ulcer disease. Gastroenterol Clin N Am. 1993;22:127–39.
5. Chiba N, Rao BV, Rademaker JW, Hunt RH. Meta-analysis of the efficacy of antibiotic therapy in eradicating *Helicobacter pylori*. Am J Gastroenterol. 1992;87:1716–27.
6. Bode G, Malfertheiner P, Ditschuneit H. Pathogenetic implications of ultrastructural findings in *Campylobacter pylori*-related gastroduodenal disease. Scand J Gastroenterol. Suppl. 1988;142:25–39.
7. Buck GE, Gourley WK, Lee WK, Subramanyam K, Latimer JM, DiNuzzo AR. Relation of *Campylobacter pyloridis* to gastritis and peptic ulcer. J Infect Dis. 1986;153:664–9.
8. Wyle FA, Tarnawski A, Schulman D, Dabros W. Evidence for gastric mucosal cell invasion by *C. pylori*: an ultrastructural study. J Clin Gastroenterol. 1990;12(Suppl.1):S92–8.
9. Tricottet V, Bruneval P, Vire O *et al. Campylobacter*-like organisms and surface epithelium abnormalities in active, chronic gastritis in humans: an ultrastructural study. Ultrastruct Pathol. 1986;10:113–22.
10. Krajden S, Fuksa M, Anderson J *et al.* Examination of human stomach biopsies, saliva, and dental plaque for *Campylobacter pylori*. J Clin Microbiol. 1989;27:1397–8.
11. Makmudar P, Shah SM, Dhunjibhoy KR, Desai HG. Isolation of *Helicobacter pylori* from dental plaques in healthy volunteers. Indian J Gastroenterol. 1990;9:271–2.
12. Nguyen AM, Engstrand L, Genta RM, Graham DY, El-Zaatari FA. Detection of *Helicobacter pylori* in dental plaque by reverse transcription–polymerase chain reaction. J Clin Microbiol. 1993;31:783–7.
13. Mapstone NP, Lynch DA, Lewis FA *et al.* Identification of *Helicobacter pylori* DNA in the mouths and stomachs of patients with gastritis using PCR. J Clin Pathol. 1993;46:540–3.
14. Brook I. Inoculum effect. Rev Infect Dis. 1989;11:361–8.
15. Megraud F, Trimoulet P, Lamouliatte H, Boyanova L. Bactericidal effect of amoxicillin on *Helicobacter pylori* in an *in vitro* model using epithelial cells. Antimicrob Agents Chemother. 1991;35:869–72.
16. Graham DY, Evans DG. Prevention of diarrhea caused by enterotoxigenic *Escherichia coli*: lessons learned with volunteers. Rev Infect Dis. 1990;12(Suppl.1):S68–72.
17. Graham DY, Smith JL, Bouvet AA. What happens to tablets and capsules in the stomach? Endoscopic comparison of disintegration and dispersion characteristics of two microencapsulated potassium formulations. J Pharm Sci. 1990;79:420–4.
18. Grant R, Grossman MI, Ivy AC. Histological changes in the gastric mucosa during digestion and their relationship to mucosal growth. Gastroenterology. 1953;25:218–31.
19. Willems G. Trophicity of gastric epithelium and its regulation. In: Mignon M, Galmiche J-P, editors. Safe and effective control of acid secretion. Paris: John Libbey Eurotext; 1988:39–50.
20. Hunt RH. Hp and pH: implications for the eradication of *Helicobacter pylori*. Scand J Gastroenterol. Suppl. 1993;196:12–16.
21. Grayson ML, Eliopoulos GM, Ferraro MJ, Moellering RC Jr. Effect of varying pH on the susceptibility of *Campylobacter pylori* to antimicrobial agents. Eur J Clin Microbiol Infect Dis. 1989;8:888–9.
22. Goodwin CS, McNulty CAM. Bacteriological and pharmaceutical basis for the treatment of *Helicobacter pylori* infection. In: Rathbone B, Vealtley V, editors. *Helicobacter pylori* and gastrointestinal disease, 2nd edn. London: Blackwell Scientific Publications. 1992: 224–31.
23. Marshall BJ. Treatment strategies for *Helicobacter pylori* infection. Gastroenterol Clin N Am. 1993;22:183–98.
24. Weil J, Bell GD, Powell K *et al.* Omeprazole and *Helicobacter pylori*: temporary suppression rather than true eradication. Aliment Pharmacol Ther. 1991;5:309–13.
25. Archimandritis A, Tjivras M, Davaris P, Fertakis A. Effect of omeprazole on *H. pylori* after two weeks of treatment. Ital J Gastroenterol. 1991;23:357–8.
26. Hui WM, Lam SK, Ho J *et al.* Effect of omeprazole on duodenal ulcer-associated antral gastritis and *Helicobacter pylori*. Dig Dis Sci. 1991;36:577–82.
27. Rauws EA, Langenberg W, Bosma A, Dankert J, Tytgat GN. Lack of eradication of *Helicobacter pylori* after omeprazole (letter). Lancet. 1991;337:1093.

28. Stolte M, Bethke B. Elimination of *Helicobacter pylori* under treatment with omeprazole. Z Gastroenterol. 1990;28:271–4.
29. Daw MA, Deegan P, Leen E, O'Morain C. Short report: the effect of omeprazole on *Helicobacter pylori* and associated gastritis. Aliment Pharmacol Ther. 1991;5:435–9.
30. Debongnie JC, Delmee M, Mainguet P. *Campylobacter pylori* in gastric, duodenal and jejunal juices and mucosae of patients with duodenal ulcer. Acta Gastroenterol Belg. 1989;52:3–8.
31. Graham DY, Klein PD, Opekun AR *et al. In vivo* susceptibility of *Campylobacter pylori*. Am J Gastroenterol. 1989;84:233–8.
32. Wagner S, Varrentrapp M, Haruma K *et al.* The role of omeprazole (40 mg) in the treatment of gastric *Helicobacter pylori* infection. Z Gastroenterol. 1991;29:595–8.
33. D'Adda T, Bordi C, Lazzaroni M, Bianchi Porro G. Long-term omeprazole monotherapy is ineffective against *Helicobacter pylori* infection [letter]. Am J Gastroenterol. 1992;87:681.
34. McNulty CA, Dent JC, Ford GA, Wilkinson SP. Inhibitory antimicrobial concentrations against *Campylobacter pylori* in gastric mucosa. J Antimicrob Chemother. 1988;22:729–38.
35. Graham DY, Lew GM, Malaty HM *et al.* Factors influencing the eradication of *Helicobacter pylori* with triple therapy. Gastroenterology. 1992;102:493–6.

52
Mucosal antibiotic levels

J. R. LAMBERT and G. ARENA

INTRODUCTION

Helicobacter pylori is a spiral-shaped Gram-negative bacterium causing gastric mucosal infection which results in chronic antral gastritis. Infection is associated with peptic ulcer disease[1,2]. Long-term eradication of *H. pylori* results in resolution of gastritis and a marked decrease in the relapse of peptic ulcer disease. Many studies have shown that *H. pylori* is sensitive *in vitro* to a large range of antibiotics[3,4]; however, regimens to eradicate this organism effectively using oral antimicrobial agents have proven difficult to develop. This chapter reviews some of the important concepts, and our current knowledge of the delivery of antimicrobial agents into the gastroduodenal mucosa.

GASTRIC ENVIRONMENT

H. pylori is situated under and within gastric and duodenal mucus on the surface of epithelial cells, in the intercellular spaces as well as in gastric glands. In this physical environment the pH is 2 near the lumen of the stomach, and is more alkaline at the cell–mucus interface. *H. pylori* is also found in gastric juice, saliva and stool. The gastric environment is not ideal for optimal activity of antimicrobial agents and thus *in vitro* antimicrobial activity would not necessarily predict the *in vivo* effectiveness of antibiotics against *H. pylori*. Thus, eradication of *H. pylori* from the gastric and duodenal mucosa requires a rational understanding of a drug's physicochemical properties and delivery mechanisms into these areas. The physical environment of the stomach – with its peristaltic activity, low luminal pH, active secretions, and a mucus covering layer – have not been considered when planning antimicrobial therapy in the past.

Gastric mucus is a thin layer covering the surface of epithelial cells. It is composed mainly of water (90%) and mucin (10%). The mucins largely consist of glycoproteins arranged in polymeric form consisting of four subunits with disulphide bridges. This forms a water-insoluble gel which is

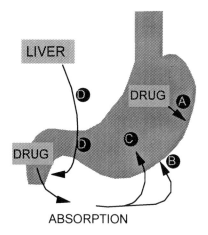

A - LOCAL UPTAKE

B - SYSTEMIC ABSORPTION

C - INTRAGASTRIC SECRETION

D - BILIARY SECRETION (REFLUX)

Fig. 1 Mucosal drug delivery

electronegatively charged and provides a viscous, adhesive layer with lubricant properties.

PRINCIPLES OF *H. PYLORI* THERAPY

The uptake of antimicrobials into gastric mucus and the underlying mucosa may occur via local or systemic absorption and delivery via the blood stream (Fig. 1). Secretion of agents into the gastric lumen and into the biliary system may contribute to drug delivery in a minor way. Bismuth compounds and amoxicillin are taken up into gastric mucosa via the local route. These agents enter the mucus either by a passive process or by mechanisms involving the active participation of components of the membrane. The former is the most common process.

After systemic absorption and delivery into the gastric circulation antimicrobials are then taken up into the gastric mucus from the lamina propria. This may occur via gastric glands or pits from surface epithelial cells. The lack of clinical efficacy of antimicrobials may be caused by the inability to reach *H. pylori* within and below the gastric mucus layer at sufficient bactericidal concentrations either by the local or systemic routes. Agents potentially having a systemic effect include the proton pump inhibitors (omeprazole and lansoprazole) and nitroimidazoles (metronidazole and tinidazole).

With only few exceptions, all antibiotics exhibit activity against *H. pylori in vitro*[3,4] but this *in vitro* susceptibility is not predictive for *in vivo* eradication.

Oral agents effective against *H. pylori* must possess the following properties:

Table 1 Effect of pH on the activity of antimicrobial agents against *H. pylori*

Agent	MIC90 (mg/l)	
	pH 5.5	pH 7.5
Ampicillin	0.5	0.06
Bismuth subcitrate	—	16
Cephalexin	32	2
Ciprofloxacin	2	0.12
Erythromycin	8	0.06
Metronidazole	2	2
Nitrofurantoin	2	1
Penicillin	0.5	0.03
Tetracycline	0.5	0.12

From ref. 6

the agents must be active against *H. pylori in vitro*, including the slow-growing coccal forms, with low susceptibility to acquired resistance. Minimal local and systemic side-effects should occur with administration for 7–14 days. Intragastric activity, which includes rapid dissolution and good dispersion in the stomach, must be seen particularly for the agents known to act by local uptake into gastric mucus. The antimicrobial must be stable and active over a wide pH range, especially at the low pH of the intragastric environment. The biologically active compound of the drug must be of adequate size and charge to allow mucus penetration and entry into the gastric mucosa via the systemic circulation. If the activity of the agent occurs via the systemic route then absorption from the stomach or small intestine is required with delivery into the gastric mucosa. Active secretion back into the gastric lumen may occur with certain drugs.

The pH of gastric juice and of sites within the mucosa may be an important factor that potentially affects drug activity. A wide range of antimicrobial agents are active against *H. pylori* when tested *in vitro* at neutral pH[5]. These include β-lactams, aminoglycosides, macrolides, quinolones, nitrofurans and nitroimidazoles. However, when used alone in clinical trials, eradication of *H. pylori* is rarely successful with monotherapy. The failure of antimicrobials to eradicate *H. pylori* may be caused by a reduced activity in an acid environment with resultant subinhibitory concentrations of antimicrobials in the gastric mucosa. The *in vitro* activity of a number of antibiotics against *H. pylori* over a range of pH 5–8 have been measured and are shown in Table 1. Penicillins and ciprofloxacin were less active at the most acidic pH with nitrofurantoin, tetracycline, metronidazole and bismuth maintaining activity at all pH ranges[6]. Gastric mucosal concentrations have been measured after oral administration of amoxicillin, pivampicillin, ciprofloxacin, erythromycin ethyl succinate suspension and erythromycin stearate with mucosal concentrations above the minimum inhibitory concentration (MIC90) to *H. pylori* at pH 7. However at pH 5.5 the two macrolides attained only subinhibitory levels ranging from 1.2 to 5.2 mg/kg. Arena *et al.*[7] showed a 50% reduction in antral mucosal levels of amoxicillin at pH > 7 following oral ranitidine predosing. Conversely elevated levels of gastric juice and mucosal concentrations of clindamycin occur following parenteral adminis-tration when an H_2-receptor antagonist was co-administered[8,9]. The gastric mucus uptake of bismuth from colloidal bismuth subcitrate is enhanced at a lower pH[10-12].

Since most antimicrobial absorption from the gastrointestinal tract occurs via a passive process, absorption is favoured when the drug is in the non-ionized form. Erythromycin is a basic drug, and when gastric juice pH is low the ionized form develops and this, theoretically, results in destruction and a decreased antimicrobial activity. Amoxicillin and ampicillin are acid-stable and retain good activity at low pH, possibly because of their less ionized state. Both are amphoteric drugs and at acidic pH are present as zwitterions which have a low partition coefficient. This may decrease tissue penetration but increase penetration into mucus, which is 90% water. Thus, the effect of pH is obviously an important factor when choosing effective antimicrobial agents to eradicate H. pylori.

Formulation of the preparation is important in attaining adequate mucosal levels to eradicate H. pylori. The physical properties of the tablet or capsule determine dispersion within the stomach. Gastric mucosal levels of amoxicillin are less after tablet preparation compared with a dissolved tablet[13]. Pivampi-cillin tablets disperse over the gastric mucosa more effectively than do capsules[14]. Eradication studies using colloidal bismuth subcitrate (CBS) have suggested that it is more effective when given as the liquid or chew tablet rather than a swallow tablet[15]. The swallow tablet may incompletely coat the gastric mucosa because of delayed dispersal in the stomach.

The dosing regimen is an important consideration in obtaining sufficient antimicrobial levels. Four hours after a single dose of two CBS tablets there were gastric mucosal concentrations which were subinhibitory, suggesting that more frequent dosing was needed[16,17]. In limited studies it has been observed that four times daily dosage with CBS tablets was more effective than a twice-daily dosage regimen[17].

Gastric mucosal/mucus uptake of a number of agents with activity against H. pylori has been studied. These agents include bismuth compounds, erythromycin, ciprofloxacin, pivampicillin, amoxicillin, metronidazole and clindamycin.

BISMUTH COMPOUNDS

A number of bismuth compounds are in clinical use and include bismuth subsalicylate (BSS), bismuth subgallate, bismuth subnitrate and colloidal bismuth subcitrate (CBS – Denol, Brocades Pharma, Netherlands). In addition ranitidine bismuth citrate and bismuth sucralfate are currently being evaluated. These agents differ markedly in their physical properties, with CBS most soluble in water and BSS relatively insoluble. Table 2 summarizes the studies which have been undertaken evaluating mucosal bismuth levels after oral administration of either BSS or CBS[16,18,19]. Both preparations are uniformly distributed in the gastric mucosa with lower levels in the duodenum. Antral mucosal levels fall rapidly over the first 4 h post-injection.

Table 2 Studies of bismuth compounds into the gastric mucosa

Drug	Reference	Species	Time before biopsy (h)	Antral bismuth (μg/g)
Bismuth subsalicylate	Skoglund and Watters, 1988[18]	Dog	1	320 ± 61
			3	62 ± 14
			6	28 ± 10
Bismuth subsalicylate (Peptobismol 150 mg)	Lambert et al., 1989[19]	Human	1	874 ± 52
			2	34 ± 9
Colloidal bismuth subcitrate	Lambert et al., 1988[16]	Human	1	253 ± 32
			4	22 ± 5
			24	11 ± 2

Bismuth uptake into porcine mucin is optimal at pH < 4, with more than 75% reduction in uptake at higher pH. CBS exists in two commercially available forms – a chew tablet and a swallow tablet. Duodenal ulcer healing is comparable with both preparations; however, H. pylori eradication differs significantly, suggesting differences in local mucosal uptake and efficacy within the gastric mucosa. Systemic pharmacokinetics, including peak plasma concentrations and steady-state levels, differ between the two preparations but do not correlate with the ability to eradicate H. pylori[17,20].

It is also suggested that H. pylori infection reduces the capacity of the gastric mucus to concentrate CBS. This would compromise the attainment of the optimum concentrations of CBS that are necessary for its antibacterial activity[21].

Preliminary studies using bismuth sucralfate have suggested a decreased uptake into pig gastric mucus 1 h after oral ingestion compared with CBS. The fall in mucus bismuth concentrations was greatest with bismuth sucralfate over 3 h post-administration compared with CBS (JR Lambert et al., unpublished observations).

These observations suggest bismuth compounds act locally with uptake into the gastric mucus and mucosa. Differences exist between these compounds with regard to their local pharmacological properties. This conclusion has been supported by the electron microscopic observations showing gastric transmucosal penetration of bismuth particles after oral dosing of human volunteers with CBS but not after BSS[22]. In vivo, CBS is more effective in eradicating H. pylori compared with BSS.

AMOXICILLIN

Amoxicillin is one of the most extensively studied antibiotics. It is locally taken up into the gastric and duodenal mucosa with high concentrations obtained in gastric juice and the mucosa after oral administration (Table 3). Levels attained after oral administration are higher than the MIC90 for H. pylori but fall rapidly in the first 2 h[7,13,23–25]. A significant correlation between concentrations of amoxicillin in gastric juice and mucosa has been

Table 3 Antimicrobial levels in the human gastric mucosa

Drug	Reference	Administration time before biopsy	Antral mucosal levels (μg/g)
Erythromycin, ethylsuccinate (500 mg)	McNulty et al., 1988[5]	85–53 min	2–41
Erythromycin stearate (500 mg)	McNulty et al., 1988[5]	60–42 min	< 1–37
Amoxicillin (500 mg)	McNulty et al., 1988[5]	91–100 min	15– > 322
Pivampicillin (500 mg)	McNulty et al., 1988[5]	120–49 min	48–209
Ciprofloxacin	McNulty et al., 1988[5]	357–84 min	35–1239
Amoxicillin (tablet 1 g)	Cooreman et al., 1990[13]	30 min	0.2 μg/ml
Amoxicillin (liquid 1 g)		30 min	0.65 μg/ml
Amoxicillin (500 mg)	Lambert et al., 1991[23]	60 min (oral)	205
		120 min (oral)	24
		Intravenous	< 0.25
Amoxicillin (500 mg) + ranitidine	Arena et al., 1993[7]	30 min, pH < 5 Gastric juice pH > 7	3.6 ± 0.7 μg/mg protein 1.8 ± 0.3 μg/mg protein
Clindamycin (300 mg)	Dent et al., 1991[8]	30 min	4.5 μg/l juice (no ranitidine)
		Intravenous	6.8 μg/l (ranitidine)

observed[23]. Intravenous administration of amoxicillin results in immeasurable levels in gastric mucosa, suggesting that systemic delivery is not important. The preparation of amoxicillin (tablet vs liquid) and intragastric acidity are important factors in the local uptake of amoxicillin[13]. Elevation of gastric pH results in a diminished uptake of amoxicillin into the gastric mucosa[7].

MACROLIDES

Macrolides are bacteriostatic agents that inhibit bacterial RNA-dependent protein synthesis. *In vitro* they have excellent activity against *H. pylori*. The preparations of erythromycin (ethylsuccinate and stearate) have been measured in the gastric mucosa after oral administration. Levels attained with the stearate form range from 1 to 77 $\mu g/g$ antral mucosa, with many subjects shown to have less than the MIC90 for *H. pylori*[5]. The lack of efficacy can thus be explained by the lower activity of erythromycin in an acidic environment, and the low tissue levels. Secretion of erythromycin across the gastric mucosa of human volunteers after intravenous administration has been reported[24]. Azythromycin, a macrolide with better acid-stability and higher tissue penetration, appears not to be superior to erythromycin.

Another macrolide, clarithromycin, exhibits increased acid-stability in comparison with erythromycin. Its absorption is high, which has resulted in high blood and tissue levels. In humans it is metabolized to 14-hydroxy-clarithromycin, and this derivative is twice as active towards *H. pylori* as the parent compound. Monotherapy with clarithromycin results in low eradication rates, and this is presumably due to insufficient and non-bactericidal concentrations in the gastric mucosa[25]. In addition acquired resistance to clarithromycin has been reported.

CLINDAMYCIN

Clindamycin is a weak base that is stable in low pH and known to concentrate in acidic compartments[26]. It is actively secreted into the gastric lumen after intravenous administration[8,9] with levels in gastric juice up to 4.5 $\mu g/l$. Mucosal levels were enhanced by gastric acid suppression using cimetidine with a five-fold greater concentration at pH 5.0 than at a pH of 2.0 after intramuscular administration to guinea pigs[9]. H_2-receptor antagonists, in spite of lacking *in vitro* activity against *H. pylori*, may be useful therapeutic adjuncts in eradicating this organism by increasing gastric concentrations of antibiotics that behave as weak bases.

NITROIMIDAZOLES

Metronidazole and tinidazole have both been used in combination with CBS or BSS in the eradication of *H. pylori*. Both agents are secreted in saliva, and metronidazole has been shown to be secreted into the gastric lumen after parenteral administration[24]. The use of nitroimidazoles is limited by the development of resistance by strains of *H. pylori*, which lowers the eradication rate even when used in combination with other agents.

TETRACYCLINE

Tetracycline is acid-stable and active at acidic pH. High concentrations are achieved in the gastric mucosa and exceed the MIC for *H. pylori* for several hours. Bismuth and tetracycline administered together may chelate and hence limit absorption. In the case of *H. pylori* infection chelation may be beneficial, potentially resulting in prolonged retention of both drugs in the gastric mucus. Limited data would thus support its role as a gastric luminally active agent.

OTHER ANTIMICROBIALS

The nitrofurans, nitrofurantoin and furazolidone, have *in vitro* activity against *H. pylori*. These agents most likely exert their action as topical agents. Eradication of *H. pylori* with these agents alone is poor, suggesting that inadequate tissue penetration is achieved[27]. The quinolones (ciprofloxacin, nitrofloxacin, ofloxacin) inhibit *H. pylori in vitro*; however, eradication is rarely achieved, as acquired resistance rapidly develops. Ciprofloxacin is secreted in bile at high concentrations with ofloxacin secreted in saliva at concentrations equal to those in serum. Gastric mucosal pharmacokinetics have not been evaluated.

PROTON PUMP INHIBITORS

The gastric proton pump inhibitors – omeprazole, lansoprazole, and pantoprazole – have inhibitory effects against *H. pylori in vitro*[28]. These agents are specifically trapped in the gastric parietal cells. Omeprazole results in suppression of *H. pylori* but long-term eradication does not result. When omeprazole is combined wth amoxicillin or clarithromycin long-term eradication of *H. pylori* occurs in 53–92% of subjects[29-31] depending on the dose and duration of therapy. The mode(s) of action of omeprazole, in its synergy with antimicrobials against *H. pylori*, is unknown. The higher eradication rates achieved with dosing twice daily, along with the *in vitro* activity of proton pump inhibitors against *H. pylori*, suggest that the mode of action is exerted as an antimicrobial agent and not because of its gastric acid suppression. Investigators report MIC90 values in the range of 25–128 mg/l for omeprazole and 6.25–120 mg/l for lansoprazole[28,32]. The antibacterial action of omeprazole has been shown to be dose-dependent and enhanced under acidic conditions[32]. High eradication rates in combination with amoxicillin may be explained by a reduction of the total gastric juice production thus enhancing concentrations of amoxicillin. Lind and colleagues[33] have administered [^{14}C]omeprazole to humans with measurable levels in gastric juice and bile. The low levels found in gastric juice are explained by duodenogastric reflux of bile. These levels in the gastric lumen are low and gastric mucosal levels were not measured in this study.

SYSTEMIC AND MUCOSAL PHARMACOLOGY AND *H. PYLORI* ERADICATION

In spite of the *in vitro* sensitivity of *H. pylori* to a wide range of antimicrobial agents including bismuth compounds and proton pump inhibitors the correlation with *in vivo* eradication is poor. High concentrations of bismuth, amoxicillin, ampicillin, tetracycline, erythromycin and ciprofloxin are obtained in the human gastric mucosa after oral administration; however, eradication of *H. pylori* with these agents as monotherapy is rarely achieved. Several potential explanations exist for the failure of eradication in the context of high mucosal antibiotic levels. Acquired resistance by *H. pylori* to antimicrobial agents including nitroimidazoles, quinolones and macrolides occurs. It is more likely that the antimicrobial agents are present in lower concentrations in colonized areas of the mucosa, particularly in the pits of the gastric glands, in the duodenum and at intercellular junctions. In addition the activity of antimicrobials may be modified by the microenvironment of the gastric epithelium.

Systemic administration of a number of agents has been used in an attempt to eradicate *H. pylori*. This has included imipenem and gentamicin. Levels of antimicrobials observed in gastric mucosa after intravenous administration are low following amoxicillin and imipenem[23,34]. Even though high levels are obtained in plasma with parenteral administration of these agents it cannot be assumed that gastric mucosal uptake will occur.

After the oral administration of CBS no correlation between the systemic pharmacology of bismuth including plasma steady-state levels, maximal plasma concentrations and AUC, and eradication of *H. pylori* has been observed[17].

SUMMARY AND CONCLUSION

The rate of eradication of *H. pylori* using current agents is low unless used in combination. Triple therapy with bismuth compounds, amoxicillin or tetracycline and metronidazole results in eradication rates of up to 92%. Proton pump inhibitors (omeprazole) combined with either amoxicillin or clarithromycin are less effective, although they also have fewer side-effects.

The agents commonly used in *H. pylori* eradication regimens are summarized in Table 4. Our knowledge of the systemic and local gastric mucosal pharmacology/pharmacodynamics of these agents continues to grow. In spite of a poor correlation between systemic and local antimicrobial levels and eradication of *H. pylori* a rational understanding of the factors responsible for drug delivery into the gastroduodenal mucosa is essential. The physicochemical nature of drugs, as well as the gastric environment, must be

Table 4 Summary of pharmacokinetic properties and actions of antimicrobial agents used to treat *H. pylori* infection

Agent	Site of activity	Advantages	Disadvantages
Amoxicillin	? local	no *in vitro* resistance high mucosa levels	*in vitro* activity against *H. pylori* pH-dependent side-effects 5–10%
Tetracycline	? local	no *in vitro* resistance *in vitro* activity not pH-dependent acid-stable high mucosal level cheap	side-effects 1–10%
Metronidazole	local and systemic secretion across gastric mucosa salivary secretion	acid-stable *in vitro* activity not pH-dependent cheap	*in vitro* resistance common side-effects 15–25%
Clarithromycin	?	acid-stable active *in vitro* long half-life	side-effects 1–5%
Erythromycin stearate ethylsuccinate	? systemic secreted in bile and gastric juice	acid-stable active *in vitro*	*in vitro* activity pH-dependent side-effects 10–15% drug active only after absorption
Omeprazole	? systemic	no *in vitro* resistance reported no side-effects gastric mucosal selectivity	expensive
CBS	local	CBS-tablet/liquid best activity against *H. pylori* no major side-effects cheap no *in vitro* resistance high mucosal levels	black mouth/stool
Bismuth subsalicylate	local	less effective cf. CBS *in vivo* highmucosal levels	

547

optimized to ensure effective penetration of active compounds into the gastroduodenal mucus and mucosa. To optimize the use of current agents further research is required more accurately to assess sites of uptake into mucus and mucosa. This will require the use of X-ray diffraction techniques, electron microscopy, atomic absorption spectrometry and radiolabelling studies. Accurate preservation of gastric tissues after sampling is essential to maintain the integrity of structures, particularly the mucus layer. With the further understanding of local action of antimicrobials along with clinical studies it is hoped a rational approach to effective and safe eradication of *H. pylori* can eventually be achieved.

References

1. Tytgat GNJ, Noach LA, Rauws EAJ. *Helicobacter pylori* infection and duodenal ulcer disease. Gastroenterology. Clin N Am. 1993;22:127–39.
2. Graham DY. *Campylobacter pylori* and peptic ulcer disease. Gastroenterology. 1989;96: 615–25.
3. Carley NH, Wadsworth SJ, Starr E, Truat AI, Suh B. *In vitro* susceptibility of *Campylobacter pylori* to quinolones. J Antimicrob Chemother. 1989;24(2):266–7.
4. Lambert JR, Megraud F, Gerbaud G, Courvalin P. Susceptibility of *Campylobacter pylori* to 20 antimicrobial agents. Antimicrob Agents Chemother. 1986;30(5):510–11.
5. McNulty CAM, Dent JC, Ford GA, Wilkinson SP. Inhibitory concentrations against *Campylobacter pylori* in gastric mucosa. J Antimicrob Chemother. 1988;22:729–38.
6. Goodwin CS, McNulty CAM. Bacteriological and pharmacological basis for the treatment of *Helicobacter pylori* infection. In: Rathbone BJ, Heatley RV, editors. *Helicobacter pylori* and gastroduodenal disease, 2nd edn. Oxford: Blackwell Scientific Publications; 1992: 209–16.
7. Arena G, Lambert JR, King RG *et al.* Enhanced amoxycillin uptake into the human gastric mucosa at lower gastric juice pH. Gastroenterology. 1993;104:34.
8. Dent J, Wise R, Boyd E. Mucosal concentration and secretion of clindamycin in the human stomach. J Antimicrob Chemother. 1994 (in press).
9. Westblom TK, Duriex DE. Enhancement of antibiotic concentrations in the gastric mucosa by H2 receptor antagonists. Dig Dis Sci. 1991;36:25–8.
10. Wagstaff AJ, Benfield P, Monk JP. Colloidal bismuth subcitrate. A review of its pharmacodynamic and pharmaco-kinetic properties, and its therapeutic use in peptic ulcer disease. Drugs. 1988;36:132–57.
11. Lee SP. A potential mechanism of action of CBS: diffusion barrier to *Helicobacter pylori*. Scand J Gastroenterol. 1982;17(Suppl.80):17–21.
12. Tasman-Jones C, Maher C, Thomsen L, Lee SP. Mucosal defences and gastroduodenal disease. Digestion. 1987;37(Suppl.2):1–7.
13. Cooreman M, Krausgrill P, Schumacher B, Hengels MJ. Amoxycillin concentrations in antrum, corpus and fundus of the stomach after single oral administration. Klin Wochenschr. 1989;67(Suppl.XVIII):12–13.
14. Hey H, Matzen P, Thorup Anderson J, Didriksen E, Nielsen BA. Gastroscopic and pharmacological study of the disintegration time and absorption of pivampicillin capsules and tablets. Br J Clin Pharmacol. 1979;8:237–42.
15. Lambert JR, Litholis L, Nicholson L, McLean AJ. Bismuth pharmacokinetics following single and multiple dose administration of denol formulations. Hellen J Gastroenterol. 1992;5:A758.
16. Lambert JR, Way DJ, King RG, Eaves ER, Hanksy J. Bismuth pharmacokinetics in the human gastric mucosa. Gastroenterology. 1988;94:A248.
17. Lambert JR, Lin SK, Shembri M, Nicholson L, McLean AJ. Comparison of different preparations of Denol in healing of duodenal ulcer and *Helicobacter pylori* eradication. Hellen J Gastroenterol. 1992;5:190.
18. Skoglund ML, Watters K. Bismuth concentration at site of *Campylobacter* colonization.

Gastroenterology. 1988;94(5):A430.

19. Lambert JR, Way DJ, King RG, Eaves ER. De Nol vs Pepto Bismol – Bismuth pharmacokinetics in the human gastric mucosa. Gastroenterology. 1989;96:A284.

20. Dekker W, Dal Monte PR, Bianchi-Porro G et al. An international multi-clinic study comparing the therapeutic efficacy of colloidal bismuth subcitrate coated tablets with chewing tablets in the treatment of duodenal ulceration. Scand J Gastroenterol. 1986;21(Suppl.122):46–50.

21. Munoz DJB, Tasman-Jones, Pybus J. Effect of Helicobacter pylori infection on the colloidal bismuth subcitrate concentration in gastric mucus. Gut. 1992;33:592–6.

22. Nwokolo CU, Levin JF, Hudson M, Pounder RE. Transmucosal penetration of bismuth particles in the human stomach. Gastroenterology. 1992;102:163–7.

23. Lambert JR, Loncar B, Schembri MA, King R, Turnidge J. Luminal amoxycillin determines gastric mucosal concentrations. Gastroenterology. 1991;100(5):A104.

24. Veldhuyzen van Zanten SJO, Goldie J, Hollingworth J, Siletti C, Richardson H, Hunt RH. Secretion of intravenously administered antibiotics in gastric juice: implication for management of Helicobacter pylori. J Clin Pathol. 1992;45:225–7.

25. Glupczynski Y, Burette A. Drug therapy for Helicobacter pylori infection: problems and pitfalls. Am J Gastroenterol. 1990;85:1545–51.

26. Klempler MS, Styrt B, Alkalinisation of the intralysosomal pH by clindamycin and its effect on neutrophil function. J Antimicrob Chemother. 1983;12(Suppl.c):39–58.

27. Morgan D, Kraft W, Bender M et al. Nitrofurans in the treatment of gastritis associated with Campylobacter pylori: the Gastrointestinal Physiology Working Group of Cayetano Heredia and the Johns Hopkins Universities. Gastroenterology. 1988;95:1178–84.

28. Iwahl T, Satoh H, Nakao M et al. Lansoprazole, a novel benzimidazole proton pump inhibitor, and its related compounds have selective activity against Helicobacter pylori. Antimicrob Agents Chemother. 1991;35:490–6.

29. Lamouliatte H, de Mascarel A, Megraud F et al. Omeprazole improves amoxycillin therapy towards H. pylori associated chronic gastritis. Gastroenterology. 1990;98:A75(abstract).

30. Bayerdorffer E, Mannes GA, Sommer A et al. High dose omeprazole treatment combined with amoxycillin eradicates Helicobacter pylori. Eur J Gastroenterol Hepatol. 1992;4:697–702.

31. Logan RPH, Gummet PA, Hegarthy BT, Walker MM, Baron JH, Misiewicz JJ. Clarithromycin and omeprazole for Helicobacter pylori eradication (letter). Lancet. 1992;340:239.

32. Suerbaum S, Leying H, Klemm K, Opferkuch W. Antibacterial activity of pantoprazole and omeprazole against Helicobacter pylori. Eur J Clin Microb Infect Dis. 1991;10:92–3.

33. Lind T, Andersson T, Skanberg I, Olbe L. Biliary excretion of intravenous ^{14}C omeprazole in humans. Clin Pharm Ther. 1987;42(5):504–8.

34. Sung J, Chung SC, Hoskug S et al. Mucosal pharmacokinetics and pilot study of short course of parenteral imipenem in the eradication of Helicobacter pylori. J Gastroenterol Hepatol. 1994:(in press).

53
H. pylori eradication

G. N. J. TYTGAT and L. A. NOACH

INTRODUCTION

Helicobacter pylori-associated gastroduodenal inflammation is now considered to be the dominant factor in *H. pylori*-associated gastroduodenal ulcer formation. Healing the gastroduodenal mucosa through *H. pylori* eradication leads to a dramatic reduction in gastroduodenal ulcer relapse. Eradication of *H. pylori* proves to be exceptionally difficult. Although the organism is sensitive to many antibiotics *in vitro*, the *in-vivo* eradicating efficacy is often disappointing.

PREREQUISITES FOR CLINICALLY RELEVANT *H. pylori*-ERADICATION SCHEMES

An *H. pylori*-eradication regimen is only clinically relevant and acceptable when an eradication rate of at least 80% can be obtained, without induction of major intolerable clinical or biochemical side-effects and without induction of bacterial resistance[1,2]. None of the antibiotics, given as monotherapy, complies with these requirements. These results were extensively discussed in the first metaanalysis by Chiba *et al.*; they will therefore not be further discussed[3]. Only those combinations of antimicrobials that in the majority of the studies lead to eradication rates of at least 80% will be further analysed. It should be realized that the figure of 80% corresponds, from a microbiological viewpoint, to a minimum value.

CHARACTERISTICS OF CURRENTLY USED ANTI-*H. pylori* ANTIMICROBIALS

H. pylori has been found to be highly susceptible ($MIC_{90} \leq 1$ mg/l) to most antibiotics except nalidixic acid, vancomycin, trimethoprim and sulphonamides. Yet the *in-vivo* efficacy is often surprisingly low. Most investigators consider the topical action as the most important, but the arguments are variable. Especially bismuth, tetracycline, amoxicillin and perhaps furazolidone are considered luminally active agents, whereas metronidazole/tinidazole (in a dose of 20 mg/kg) may have systemic action. A confounding factor for many antibiotics is biliary excretion and subsequent enterogastric reflux, perhaps contributing to topical activity. The minimal inhibitory concentration of antibiotics such as amoxicillin, erythromycin and ciprofloxacin decreases markedly when the intragastric acidity falls and the pH increases from 3.5 to 5.5. Therefore, raising intragastric pH raises the efficacy of several antimicrobials.

Amoxicillin

Amoxicillin (AMO) is the most widely used semisynthetic penicillin. MIC_{90} values of 0.12 mg/l are low; yet monotherapy rarely eradicates the organism. AMO is acid-stable; yet it seems likely that the antibacterial activity of AMO improves when the intragastric pH approaches 7. AMO is absorbed from the stomach and the small intestine. After oral intake the highest concentration is measured after 30 min in antrum biopsy specimens. Whether bactericidal concentrations can be obtained in corpus biopsies is controversial[4-6]. AMO appears to have a largely luminal effect. Parenterally administered AMO reaches inadequate concentrations to achieve MIC values necessary to inhibit *H. pylori* growth. After intravenous administration, AMO is undetectable in gastric juice[5-8]. AMO interferes with the synthesis of peptidoglycans in the cell wall[9]. AMO-resistant organisms appear to be extremely rare[10] and the development of resistance to AMO has not been reported, although occasionally MIC values do appear to rise after therapy (F. Mégraud, personal communication). Side-effects are penicillin allergy, candidiasis and diarrhoea, even pseudomembranous colitis. Up to 10% of the population claims allergy to penicillin. Although no resistance to β-lactam antibiotics has been reported so far, clavulanate, an inhibitor of bacterial β-lactamase added to decrease antimicrobial reasistance (ratio 4/1 w/w), may be added because it has intrinsic anti-*H. pylori* activity and may help in preventing the selection of *H. pylori* strains with decreased AMO sensitivity[11]. However, amoxicillin with clavulanic acid is not superior to AMO alone[12], and carries a risk of substantial hepatotoxicity due to cholestatic jaundice occurring in $\sim 1/100\,000$.

Metronidazole/tinidazole

Metronidazole (MET) is commonly used in *H. pylori*-eradication regimens because of excellent *in-vitro* activity. Average MIC_{90} values are 2.0 mg/l. Nitroimidazoles are actively secreted in gastric juice and in saliva[7,13]. Furthermore MET does not depend on pH for its activity[14]. The half-life of MET is 8–12 h. MET acts as an electron sink accepting electrons from a reduced electron transfer protein, whereby the drug is reduced via its nitro group. The redox potential required for reduction of the nitro group varies from -430 to $-460\,\text{mV}$. Under microaerobic (microaerophilic) conditions *H. pylori* can achieve a redox potential of less than $-430\,\text{mV}$. Resistant strains have lost the ability to achieve a sufficiently low redox potential for the necessary reduction of MET[15]. A mutation in the nitroreductase of the organism is thought to be responsible for the resistance. MET's major disadvantage is the high frequency of primary and secondary or acquired resistance. Unfortunately resistance is defined in different ways: usually resistance is thought to be present when MIC values are equal to or above 8–$32\,\text{mg/l}$. Resistance develops less readily if a second antimicrobial or a bismuth compound is used concurrently. MET resistance has severely limited the usefulness of this drug in triple-therapy regimens, as MET resistance is associated with a marked reduction in eradication rates (see Table 13). This finding suggests that MET may well be critical in the conventional triple-therapy regimens. MET may cause a metallic taste in the mouth, and may induce a furry coat on the tongue. Diarrhoea may occur in 20% of patients.

Bismuth

Colloidal bismuth subcitrate (CBS) is a colloidal suspension at neutral pH but precipitates in an acid environment, yielding crystals of bismuth citrate and bismuth oxychloride (BiOCl), bismuth oxide (Bi_2O_3) and bismuth hydroxide (Bi(OH)$_3$). The bismuth dose is usually calculated as Bi_2O_3. CBS binds to mucus glycoproteins, inhibits pepsin, inhibits acetaldehyde, phospholipases, etc. and stimulates endogenous prostaglandin synthesis.

Bismuth levels rise rapidly in mucosal biopsies, reaching a peak at 30–$60\,\text{min}$ and falling rapidly in the first $4\,\text{h}$ after injection[16]. In antral mucus, MIC values of 2–$16\,\text{mg/l}$ are exceeded only in the first $2\,\text{h}$ after dosing.

CBS has both *in-vitro* and *in-vivo* antimicrobial properties against *H. pylori* (MIC $\leq 25\,\text{mg/l}$) with rapid lysis of the organisms. Bismuth is topically active and readily produces structural degeneration of the organisms near the luminal surface, but not deep in the foveolae. The topical antimicrobial action is largely unknown. Bi^{3+} is a trivalent cation which may bind to sulphydryl groups in proteins. Bismuth accumulates along the bacterial membranes and in the periplasmatic space[17]. *In vitro* this is followed by retraction of the cytoplasmic membrane from the cell wall. CBS also blocks the adherence of *H. pylori* to the gastric epithelial cells[18]. Moreover bismuth inhibits urease and phospholipase and proteolytic activity[19]. CBS probably intercalates in the outer membrane of the organism and may react with enzymes present in the periplasmatic space. CBS is most active against bacteria in the stationary phase[17].

A blood safety margin of 50–$100\,\mu\text{g/l}$ is usually accepted. CBS is the most soluble bismuth salt. Bismuth particles may be absorbed in the stomach[20].

Clarithromycin

Macrolides are bacteriostatic agents that inhibit bacterial RNA-dependent protein synthesis. They bind reversibly to the 50S ribosomal subunits, thereby blocking the translocation reaction of polypeptide chain elongation[21].

Clarithromycin (CLA) or (6-methoxy-erythromycin) and its 14-OH-metabolite has a similar antimicrobial spectrum to erythromycin, but is more acid-stable, is better absorbed, has better tissue penetration and is claimed to have fewer gastrointestinal side-effects.

In vitro the MIC_{90} is 0.03 mg/l (8 times less than for erythromycin). In humans CLA is metabolized to 14-hydroxyclarithromycin. This derivative is twice as active as the parent compound. There is a variable resistance to clarithromycin before therapy and resistance may be induced upon clarithromycin therapy.

Roxithromycine

Roxithromycine (ROX) is a new macrolide, which is more acid-stable and obtains higher tissue levels than erythromycin. ROX has excellent *in-vitro* activity against *H. pylori*.

Tetracycline

Tetracycline hydrochloride (TET) acts by inhibiting protein synthesis. TET binds reversibly to the 30S ribosomal subunits. This process blocks the access of aminoacyl-tRNA to the RNA–ribosome complex preventing bacterial polypeptide synthesis[22].

H. pylori is very sensitive *in vitro* to TET[23], the MIC_{90} varying around 0.12–1.2 mg/l. TET is active at low pH. TET chelates with bismuth, preventing absorption. As both bismuth and TET may be acting topically, this does not seem to be problematic *in vivo*.

Resistance to TET has not yet been reported.

Proton pump inhibitors (PPI)

Omeprazole (OME) and lansoprazole (LAN) have intrinsic *in-vitro* antimicrobial activity[24–26], although the mechanism(s) of action are not entirely clear. In addition, they may improve the antimicrobial activity of acid-sensitive antibiotics by decreasing gastric acidity and perhaps increasing gastric mucosal antibiotic concentrations. Moreover the pK_a of *H. pylori* urease may be affected and low intragastric acidity may favour overgrowth of competing micro-organisms[24–27].

The MIC_{90} for OME is about 50–128 mg/l. For LAN the MIC_{90} is about 6.25 mg/l. It also appears that MIC increase by substitution of position 4 of the pyridine ring by a fluoro-alkoxy group[24].

Activation of the benzimidazoles appears essential for antibacterial action. Acidic conditions greatly increase this activity. The activity at neutral pH appears to parallel the ease with which the benzimidazoles are activated by protons.

Whether the antimicrobial effect of OME is responsible for *H. pylori* eradication is unclear. Some investigators feel that it is unlikely. Monotherapy with OME 40 mg BID merely suppresses but does not eradicate H. pylori[28]. Moreover considering the MIC values, it seems unlikely that effective antibacterial concentrations can be obtained with a dose of 40 mg BID. It is more probable that PPI improve the antimicrobial action of the co-administered antibiotics when the intragastric pH approaches 7.

The bioavailability of AMO does not change during OME therapy[29] but the MIC values of AMO against H. pylori decrease with an increase of pH in the culture medium[30].

A more neutral intragastric pH may promote the activities of most antibiotics and slow down the breakdown of AMO. Moreover a lower volume of gastric juice is associated with a higher AMO concentration in the stomach, and perhaps also an enhanced release of AMO in the gastric lumen. It is also possible that OME induces changes in the microenvironment, promoting AMO penetration to H. pylori.

CAUSES OF ANTIMICROBIAL FAILURE

The discrepancy between the in-vitro and in-vivo antimicrobial efficacy remains largely enigmatic. Many potential causes for failure have been considered in the literature.

H. pylori has a bacterial glycocalyx which appears much thicker in vivo than in vitro[31]. This layer may present a partial barrier to antimicrobials.

H. pylori lying deep in the mucus layer, in the foveolae and occasionally between and within the epithelial cells, may be inaccessible to orally administered antimicrobials. Many antimicrobials are acid-sensitive. Rapid breakdown in the acid gastric milieu will substantially decrease the bioavailability of the drugs.

Acquisition of bacterial resistance is almost certainly significant. Rapid in-vivo resistance formation is seen for various antibiotics: metronidazole, clarithromycin, quinolones (ciprofloxacin, norfloxacin, ofloxazin), etc.

The possibility exists of the formation of sanctuary sites (internalized organisms in epithelial cells?, dormant forms of coccoid forms with different antimicrobial sensitivity?) where the organisms evade the antimicrobial attack, and then later regrow and recolonize the gastric mucosa.

FACTORS AFFECTING H. pylori ERADICATION

Various factors have been studied in relation to H. pylori eradication. Graham et al.[32] have stressed the importance of compliance. Other factors may also be important, as recently presented by Cutler[33] and summarized in Table 1. Unfortunately compliance has been variously defined. Usually tablet counting has been used, but the minimum values for compliance have varied between 60% and 95%. It would appear to be appropriate when at least 80% of the antimicrobial therapy is consumed.

Several studies suggest that the antibiotic efficacy is reduced in smokers

Table 1 Results of multivariate analysis of factors affecting eradication of *H. pylori*[33]

	Odds ratio	95% confidence limits	p-Value
Age	1.10	1.03–1.16	0.002
Gastrointestinal diagnosis (duodenal ulcer/functional dyspepsia versus gastric ulcer)	2.83	1.31–6.13	0.008
Severity chronic antral inflammation	1.35	1.20–12.43	0.02
Compliance	1.67	1.17–23.90	0.03

Table 2 Omeprazole/amoxicillin combination[34]

	Non-smokers		Smokers	
Compliance	n	Percentage H. pylori *eradicated*	n	Percentage H. pylori *eradicated*
Below 90%	37	70	53	38
Above 90%	26	88	9	33

Table 3 Influence of galenical formulation on *H. pylori* eradication[35]

	Clearance of H. pylori	Eradication of H. pylori
AMO/CLAV caps (500/125 mg) × 3 × 21 days OME 20 × 2 × 30 days	7/21 (33.3%)	0/14
AMO/CLAV susp (500/125 mg) × 3 × 21 days OME 20 × 2 × 30 days	10/15 (66.6%)	6/6

versus non-smokers. In Unge's study, *H. pylori* eradication was only 33% in smokers compared to 88% in non-smokers (Table 2)[34]. The mechanisms by which smoking could be inducing resistance to metronidazole are not known. The drug is administered in its inactive form, and has to be reduced to its cytotoxic form by the micro-organism. It has been proposed that metronidazole resistance in *H. pylori* could be due to a decreased ability of strains to achieve a sufficiently low redox potential under microaerobic conditions for the necessary reduction. Smoking may interfere with this redox mechanism, causing a reduction in the transformation of metronidazole into its bioactive metabolite, and may therefore induce resistance of the micro-organism to metronidazole. Another possible explanation for the development of metronidazole resistance in smokers may be that smoking induces higher biotransformation enzyme activity in *H. pylori* strains. An augmented biotransformation enzyme capacity may result in increased and faster metabolism of metronidazole and thus to an increased resistance to the drug.

Some studies have shown galenical formulation to be of importance. An example is the study of Boixeda *et al.* (Table 3) showing that a suspension of AMO/CLAR was superior to corresponding capsules[35].

Table 4 Observed side-effects in 83 patients treated with CBS, tetracycline and metronidazole for 1 week (T1) and 51 patients treated with CBS, amoxicillin and metronidazole for 4 weeks (T3) (percentages)

Side-effects	Regimen T1	Regimen T3
Nausea/vomiting	24	25
Diarrhoea/loose stools	19	19
Antibiotic-related colitis	—	2
Constipation	1	—
Epigastric pain	2	—
Burning oral cavity	6	6
Metallic taste	5	—
Headache/dizziness	10	—
Malaise	6	—
Moniliasis	4	2
Hypersensitivity	5	—

ERADICATION POSSIBILITIES

Tables 5 to 13 summarize the current literature where usually eradication results above 80% were obtained. Those studies with similar antimicrobial combinations where lower eradication rates were obtained are not included. Whenever available the data are also given for MET-sensitive and MET-resistant organisms. It is readily obvious that overall triple therapy with CBS/BSS + MET + TET renders the best eradication results with the lowest degree of variability. The second best is triple therapy with CBS/BIS + MET + AMO. Eradication scores with dual therapy with PPI + AMO or PPI + CLA are somewhat lower.

Advantages of triple therapy

The original triple-therapy schemes (BIS + MET + TET, BIS + MET + AMO) (Tables 5 and 6) provide on balance the highest eradication rates. Few of such studies do not reach the 80% eradication level. These eradication rates appear to be independent from the underlying disease process (gastritis, ulcer disease, etc.).

Disadvantages of triple therapy

Triple therapy has significant compliance problems due to its complex dosing schedule and high incidence of side-effects. In our own studies side-effects were observed in about half the patients (Table 4).

The efficacy of triple therapy with CBS/BSS, MET, AMO or TET, is further undermined by primary or secondary resistance to MET[36,37]. Whenever the data are available, they show a substantial reduction in eradication efficacy in case of MET resistance (Tables 5 and 6). Only in Borody et al.'s study[38] did the influence of MET resistance appear to be insignificant.

Table 5 Eradication of *H. pylori* with triple therapy with tetracycline

Reference no.				n	Eradication (%)	Sensitivity (%)	Resistance (%)
41	CBS 120 × 4 × 28	TET 500 × 4 × 28	MET 200 × 4 × 14	100	94		
42	CBS 120 × 4 × 28	TET 500 × 4 × 28	MET 200 × 4 × 10	39	92		
43	CBS 120 × 4 × 28	TET 500 × 4 × 28	MET 200 × 4 × 10	78	96		
44	CBS 120 × 4 × 28	TET 250 × 4 × 14	MET 200 × 3 × 14	76	91		
45	CBS 120 × 4 × 28	TET 500 × 4 × 10	MET 200 × 4 × 10	100	94		
46	CBS 120 × 4 × 28	TET 500 × 3 × 7	MET 400 × 3 × 7	30	90		
47	CBS 120 × 4 × 28	TET 500 × 3 × 7	MET 400 × 3 × 7	89	84	92	63
48	BSS 1200 × 4 × 21	TET 500 × 4 × 14	MET 250 × 3 × 14	25	88		
49	CBS 120 × 4 × 28	TET 500 × 4 × 14	MET 250 × 4 × 14	23	95		
45	CBS 120 × 4 × 14	TET 500 × 4 × 14	MET 400 × 2 × 14	49	94		
50*	BSS 151 × 5-8 × 14	TET 500 × 4 × 14	MET 250 × 3 × 14	62	89		
51	CBS 120 × 4 × 14	TET 500 × 4 × 14	MET 250 × 4 × 14	130	92		
52	CBS 120 × 5 × 14	TET 250 × 5 × 14	MET 200 × 5 × 14	470		92	87
53	CBS 120 × 4 × 15	TET 250 × 4 × 15	MET 250 × 4 × 15	63		98	
54	BSS 600 × 3 × 14	TET 500 × 3 × 14	MET 400 × 3 × 14	16	94		
55	CBS 120 × 4 × 14	TET 500 × 4 × 14	MET 400 × 3 × 14	19	74	85	50
56	CBS 120 × 4 × 14	TET 500 × 4 × 14	MET 400 × 3 × 14	40	65	91	32
57	CBS 120 × 4 × 15	TET 500 × 4 × 15	MET 500 × 3 × 15	174	92		
58	CBS 120 × 4 × 10	TET 500 × 4 × 15	MET 500 × 3 × 10	38	61	93	38
59	CBS 120 × 6 × 7	TET 250 × 6 × 7	MET 200 × 6 × 7	47	82		
46	CBS 120 × 4 × 7	TET 500 × 4 × 7	MET 400 × 2 × 7	43	91		
60	CBS 120 × 4 × 7	TET 500 × 4 × 7	MET 500 × 3 × 7	81	73	96	38
61							
(a)	CBS 120 × 4 × 7	TET 500 × 4 × 7	MET 400 × 4 × 7	65	94		68
(b)†	CBS 120 × 4 × 7	TET 500 × 4 × 7	MET 400 × 4 × 7	67	98		51

*Combined with RAN 300 × 1 × 28
†Combined with OME 20 × 1 × 28

Table 6 Eradication of *H. pylori* with triple therapy with amoxicillin

Reference no.				n	Eradication (%)	Sensitivity (%)	Resistance (%)
62	CBS 120 × 4 × 28	AMO 375 × 3 × 28	MET 500 × 3 × 14	59	85	93	68
63	CBS 120 × 4 × 28	AMO 250 × 3 × 28	MET 400 × 3 × 28	10	90		
64	BSS 600 × 3 × 28	AMO 750 × 3 × 14	MET 400 × 3 × 14	16	88		
65	BSS 600 × 3 × 28	AMO 750 × 3 × 10	MET 400 × 3 × 10	12	83		
66	CBS 120 × 4 × 10	AMO 500 × 3 × 16	MET 500 × 3 × 10	57	81	97	63
67	CBS 120 × 4 × 14	AMO 500 × 4 × 14	MET 400 × 3 × 14	86	81	91	63
68	BSS 600 × 3 × 14	AMO 500 × 3 × 14	MET 500 × 3 × 14	26	81		
	BSS 600 × 3 × 14	AMO 500 × 3 × 7	MET 500 × 3 × 7	55	80		
69	CBS 120 × 4 × 14	AMO 500 × 4 × 14	MET 250 × 4 × 14	21	95		
70	CBS 120 × 4 × 14	AMO 500 × 3 × 7	MET 400 × 3 × 7	20	90		
68	BSS 600 × 3 × 7	AMO 500 × 3 × 7	MET 500 × 3 × 7	15	90		
71	CBS 120 × 4 × 7	AMO 500 × 4 × 7	MET 400 × 5 × 3	106	72	93	19
72	CBS 240 × 2 × 4	AMO1000 × 2 × 4	MET 250 × 3 × 4	321	91		
73	CBS 120 × 4 × 14	AMO 500 × 4 × 14	MET 500 × 3 × 14	100	84		
74	× 30	AMO	MET	37	87		
75	CBS 120 × 4 × 14	AMO 500 × 3 × 14	MET 500 × 3 × 14	15	95		
	CBS 120 × 4 × 7	AMO 500 × 3 × 7	MET 500 × 3 × 7	17	83		

Advantage of PPI/antibiotic combination

The combination of a proton pump inhibitor (OME, LAN, PAN) plus an appropriate antibiotic (AMO, CLA) provides prompt symptom relief and heals the ulcer, while at the same time eradicating *H. pylori* and effectively curing the disease. Moreover the incidence of side-effects is often limited or negligible.

Disadvantage of PPI/antibiotic combination

A major disadvantage of PPI/antibiotic dual therapy is that eradication rates vary substantially. Indeed many studies do not reach the cut-off level of 80% eradication rate. However, when a BID dosing scheme is used a much more consistent and higher eradication rate is obtained. Moreover, the two German centres reaching the highest eradication rates disagree with respect to the optimal PPI dose. In the study by Bayerdörffer *et al.*[28] there appears to be a dose–response relationship; the higher the OME dose, the higher the eradication rate. In contrast, in the study by Börsch *et al.*[39], increasing the dose of OME above 20 mg × 2 had no further effect on eradication efficacy.

Value of repeat courses

In general AMO resistance does not seem to develop following a failed course of treatment. It therefore seems probable that if a course of OME/AMO therapy fails to eradicate the organism, it is worth repeating the treatment.

Regimens evaluated in metronidazole-resistant patients

Logan *et al.*[40] evaluated 14-day quadruple therapy with OME 40 × 1 × 14 days, AMO 500 mg × 4 × 14 days, CBS 120 mg × 4 × (days 1–7) and ciprofloxacin 750 mg × 2 × (days 7–14) and obtained a 74% eradication.

DISCUSSION

H. pylori eradication dramatically changes the natural history of *H. pylori*-associated gastroduodenal ulcer disease. Elaborate triple therapy regimens (bismuth salt, metronidazole, and tetracycline or amoxicillin) are successful in a high percentage of patients, especially in the absence of primary metronidazole resistance. Yet such treatment regimens are marred by a high incidence of side-effects, are cumbersome, and interfere with compliance. Such combinations lead to side-effects in up to 50% of individuals. These comprise mainly a metallic taste, nausea, diarrhoea, sore mouth and general malaise. There have also been reports of pseudomembranous colitis. The

Table 7 Eradication of *H. pylori* with triple therapy variants

Reference no.				n	Eradication (%)
76	BSS 300 × 4 × 14	TET 500 × 4 × 14	CLA 500 × 3 × 14	29	93

Table 8 Eradication of *H. pylori* with bismuth–imidazole dual therapy

Reference no.			n	Eradication (%)	Sensitivity (%)	Resistance (%)
77	CBS 240 × 2 × 28	MET 400 × 3 × 14 (1–14)	44		86	15
	CBS 240 × 2 × 28	MET 400 × 3 × 14 (15–28)	15		80	
	CBS 240 × 2 × 14	MET 400 × 3 × 14	25		80	
78	BSS	MET			82	18
79	CBS	MET		90		
80	CBS 120 × 4 × 56	TIN 500 × 2 × 10	27	78	91	20
81	CBS 240 × 2 × 28	MET 400 × 3 × 14	43	72	87	
82	CBS 120 × 4 × 28	MET 500 × 3 × 10	21	81		

Table 9 Eradication of *H. pylori* with proton-pump inhibitor–amoxicillin dual therapy

Reference no.			n	Eradication (%)
83	OME 20 × 2 × 14	AMO 500 × 6 × 14	12	92
64	OME 40 × 2 × 14	AMO 750 × 3 × 14	17	82
84	OME 20 × 2 × 14	AMO 500 × 4 × 14	56	82
85	OME 40 × 2 × 10	AMO1000 × 2 × 10	27	82
86	OME 20 × 3 × 14	AMO 500 × 4 × 14	18	83
	OME 20 × 4 × 14	AMO 500 × 4 × 14	20	85
87	OME 40 × 1 × 14	AMO 750 C × 2 × 14	8	63
88	OME 20 × 1 × 28	AMO 500 S × 4 × 28	17	53
89	OME 40 × 1 × 7	AMO 500 S × 4 × 7	31	61
90	OME 20 × 1 × 28	AMO 250 S × 3 × 14	16	31
89	OME 40 × 2 × 7	AMO 500 S × 4 × 7	47	62
91*	OME 40 × 1 × 14	AMO 500 S × 4 × 14	19	74
92	OME 40 × 1 × 14	AMO 500 S × 4 × 14	18	28
64	OME 80 × 1 × 14	AMO 750 C × 3 × 14	17	59
93	OME 40 × 1 × 14	AMO 500 S × 4 × 7	21	29
94	OME 40 × 1 × 28	AMO 750 C × 2 × 14	157	54
95	OME 40 × 1 × 14	AMO 500 × 3 × 14	53	49
96	OME 80 × 1 × 7	AMO 500 S × 4 × 7	13	38
97	OME 20 × 1 × 14	AMO1000 × 2 × 10		37
	OME 20 × 2 × 14	AMO1000 × 2 × 10		60
	OME 40 × 2 × 14	AMO1000 × 2 × 10		70
	OME 60 × 2 × 14	AMO1000 × 2 × 10		85
98	OME 20 × 2 × 14	AMO1000 × 2 × 14	26	92
	OME 40 × 2 × 14	AMO1000 × 2 × 14	21	77
99	OME 20 × 2 × 14	AMO1000 × 2 × 14		85
	OME 40 × 2 × 14	AMO1000 × 2 × 14		79
	OME 40 × 2 × 14	AMO1000 × 3 × 14		82

*MET-resistant patients

complexity of the regimen and the side-effects lead to a reduction in compliance and a lower efficacy. Another problem is metronidazole resistance, with primary resistance being present in 10–20% of cases in the developed world and up to 80% in the developing countries. Triple therapy in patients with resistant organisms is effective in only 30–60% of cases.

A single and comparably effective therapeutic regimen with a low complication rate is a more attractive choice. A 2-week medium–high-dose omeprazole/lansoprazole and amoxicillin 1.5–2 g/day regimen may come closer to the ideal concept of *H. pylori* eradication and ulcer healing pharmacotherapy. Yet this treatment should be universally and equally successful, which it is not at the present time. This treatment regimen is better tolerated by patients since there are fewer side-effects and some studies have suggested that the eradication cut-off value of 80% can be achieved. Further work is needed to confirm these latter results. However, if they are confirmed, this could prove to be the treatment of choice in patients who are not allergic to penicillin.

Patients who fail to respond to each of these regimens should be counselled and advised of the importance of complying with therapy, and then be given the alternative. If patients fail to respond to either regimen, quadruple

Table 10 Eradication of *H. pylori* with proton-pump inhibitor–clarithromycin/roxithromycin dual therapy

Reference no.			n	Eradication (%)	
100	OME 40 × 1 × 14	CLA 500 × 3 × 14	25	80	
101	OME 40 × 1 × 14	CLA 500 × 3 × 14	65	63	
102	OME 40 × 1 × 14	CLA 500 × 3 × 14	26	70	United Kingdom 85
103	OME 20 × 1 × 28	ROX 150 × 2 × 28	17	100	France 56

Table 11 Eradication of *H. pylori* with proton pump inhibitor–antibiotic triple therapy

Reference no.				n	Eradication (%)
104	OME 20 × 1 × 28	AMO 1000 × 3 × 14	MET 500 × 3 × 14	47	94
105	OME 20 × 1 × 28	AMO 1000 × 2 × 15	TIN 1000 × 1 × 10	22	86
106	OME 20 × 1 × 7	CLA 250 × 2 × 7	TIN 500 × 2 × 7	36	100
107	LAN 30 × 1 × 28	ROX 300 × 1 × 14	MET 500 × 2 × 10	17	82
L.G.V. Coelho, personal communication	OME	CBS 120 × 4 ×	TET 250 × 4 × / MET 200 × 3 ×		96
108	OME 20 × 4 × 7	AMO	MET / FUR		80

Table 12 Eradication of *H. pylori* with amoxicillin–imidazole ± H2RA's dual therapy

Reference no.				n	Eradication (%)
66	AMO 500 × 4 × 16	MET 500 × 3 × 10		48	77
2	AMO 750 × 3 × 12	MET 500 × 3 × 12	RAN 300 × 1 × 28	52	89
105	AMO1000 × 2 × 15	TIN 500 × 2 × 10	RAN 300 × 1 × 42	22	81

Table 13 *H. pylori* eradication in metronidazole-sensitive or resistant patients

Reference no.				Days	Total no.	Metronidazole-sensitive (%)	Metronidazole-resistant (%)
60	CBS	AMO	MET	28	44	57	33
47	CBS	AMO	MET	7	78	96	37
71	CBS	TET	MET	7	62	86	54
55	BSS	TET	MET	14	89	92	63
56	CBS	AMO	MET	7	64	93	19
66	CBS	TET	MET	14	19	85	50
73	CBS	TET	MET	16?	40	91	37
67	CBS	AMO	MET	14	57	97	63
80	CBS	AMO	MET	14	100	89	61
77	CBS	AMO	MET	14	86	91	63
66	CBS	TIN		56?	27	91	20
78	CBS	MET		14		86	15
	CBS	TIN				60	
78	BSS	MET		14	44	82	17
51	CBS	TET	MET	14	470	92	87
66	CBS	AMO	MET	14	57	97	63

therapy may be tried, comprising triple therapy plus omeprazole 40 mg BID for a week. This therapy is claimed to have an eradication rate of up to 95%. A further alternative, particularly in patients who have metronidazole-resistant organisms and who are allergic to penicillin, is to use a combination of omeprazole and clarithromycin.

Although the optimal regimen has yet to be identified, combination therapy with a PPI/appropriate antibiotic is likely to become the treatment of choice for eradication of *H. pylori* with a triple or quadruple regimen reserved for failure of the PPI–antibiotic dual therapy.

References

1. Graham DY, Klein PD, Evans DG *et al.* Simple noninvasive method to test efficacy of drugs in the eradication of *Helicobacter pylori* infection: the example of combined bismuth subsalicylate and nitrofurantoin. Am J Gastroenterol. 1991;89:1158–62.
2. Hentschel E, Brandstätter G, Dragosics B *et al.* Effect of raniditine and amoxicillin plus metronidazole on the eradication of *Helicobacter pylori* and the recurrence of duodenal ulcer. N Engl J Med. 1993;328:308–12.
3. Chiba N, Rao BV, Radaemaker JW, Hunt RH. Meta-analysis of the efficacy of antibiotic therapy in eradicating *Helicobacter pylori*. Am J Gastroenterol. 1992;87:1716–27.
4. Lambert JR, Borromeo M, Korman MG, Hansky J. Role of *Campylobacter pyloridis* in non-ulcer dyspepsia. A randomised controlled trial. Gastroenterology. 1987;92:1488.
5. McNulty CAM, Dent JC, Ford GA, Wilkinson SP. Inhibitory antimicrobial concentrations against *Campylobacter pylori* in gastric mucosa. J Antimicrob Chemother. 1988;22:729–38.
6. Cooreman M, Krausgrill P, Schumacher B, Hengels KL. Amoxycillin concentration in antrum, corpus and fundus of the stomach after single oral application. Klin Wochenschr. 1989;67(Suppl. XVIII):12–13.
7. Veldhuyzen van Zanten SJO, Goldie J, Hollingworth J, Siletti C, Richardson H, Hunt RH. Secretion of intravenously administered antibiotics in gastric juice: implications for management of *Helicobacter pylori*. J Clin Pathol. 1992;45:225–7.
8. Hollingworth K, Goldie J, Silletti CF, Li Y, Richardson H, Hunt RH. Gastric secretion of antibiotics used for *Campylobacter pyloridis*. Gut. 1987;28:A1409.
9. Waxman DJ, Strominger JL. Penicillin-binding proteins and the mechanism of action of beta-lactam antibiotics. Annu Rev Biochem. 1983;52:825–69.
10. Famerée D, Ramdani B, Lamy V. Assessment of *Helicobacter pylori*'s sensitivity to tinidazole, amoxycillin and tetracycline among 472 patients. Third Workshop of the *Helicobacter pylori* Study Group. Rev Esp Enf Digest. 1990;78:P219(abstract).
11. Boixeda D, De Rafael L, Cantón R, Sampedro J, de Argila CM, Baquero F. Galenical formulations of amoxicillin/clavulanate and eradication of *Helicobacter pylori* in peptic ulcer patients: preliminary report. Eur J Gastroenterol Hepatol. 1993;4:283–5.
12. Larrey D, Vial T, Micaleff A *et al.* Hepatitis associated with amoxycillin–clavulanic acid combination. Report of 15 cases. Gut. 1992;33:368–71.
13. McNulty CAM. *In vitro* sensitivity of *Helicobacter pylori*. In: Menge H, Gregor M, Tytgat GNJ, Marshall BJ, McNulty CAM, editors. *Helicobacter pylori* 1990. Berlin: Springer-Verlag; 1991:149–54.
14. Grayson ML, Liopoulos E, Ferraro MJ, Moellering RC. Effect of varying pH on the susceptibility of *Campylobacter pylori* to antimicrobial agents. Eur J Clin Microbiol Infect Dis. 1989;8:888–9.
15. Cederbrant G, Kahlmeter G, Ljungh Å. Proposed mechanism for metronidazole resistance in *Helicobacter pylori*. J Antimicrob Chemother. 1992;29:115–20.
16. Lambert JR, Way DJ, King RG, Eaves ER, Hansky J. Bismuth pharmacokinetics in the human gastric mucosa. Gastroenterology. 1988;94:A248.
17. Van der Voort LHM, Van den Bos AP, Kamsteeg H. *In vitro* bactericidal effects of CBS on *Helicobacter pylori*. Rev Esp Enferm Dig. 1990;78(Suppl. 1):103(abstract).
18. Huesca M, Gold B, Sherman P, Lingwood C. Colloidal bismuth subcitrate (CBS) blocks

H. PYLORI ERADICATION

Helicobacter pylori adhesion to glycerolipid receptors. Gastroenterology. 1992;102:A639.
19. Hall DWR. Pharmacology of bismuth containing medicines used to treat Helicobacter pylori infections. Ital J Gastroenterol. 1991;23(Suppl. 2):(abstract).
20. Nwokolo CU, Lewin JF, Hudson M, Pounder RE. Transmucosal penetration of bismuth particles in the human stomach. Gastroenterology. 1992;102:163–7.
21. Yao JDC, Moellering RC Jr. Antibacterial agents. Macrolides. In: Balows A, editor. Manual of clinical microbiology, 5th edn. Washington, DC: American Society for Microbiology; 1991:1074.
22. Yao JDC, Moellering RC Jr. Antibacterial agents. Tetracyclines. In: Balows A, editor. Manual of clinical microbiology, 5th edn. Washington, DC: American Society for Microbiology; 1991:1073.
23. Bayerdörffer E, Ottenjann R. The role of antibiotics in Campylobacter pylori-associated peptic ulcer disease. Scand J Gastroenterol. 1988;23(Suppl. 142):93–100.
24. Iwahi T, Satoh H, Nakao M et al. Lansoprazole, a novel benzimidazole proton pump inhibitor, and its related compounds have selective activity against Helicobacter pylori. Antimicrob Agents Chemother. 1991;35:490–6.
25. Mégraud F, Boyanova L, Lamouliatte H. Activity of lansoprazole against Helicobacter pylori. Lancet. 1991;337:1486 (letter).
26. Suerbaum S, Leying H, Klemm K, Opferkuch W. Antibacteriol activity of pantoprazole and omeprazole against Helicobacter pylori. Eur J Clin Microbiol Infect Dis. 1991;10:92–3 (letter).
27. Bugnoli M, Bayeli PF, Rappuoli R, Pennatini C, Figura N, Crabtree JE. Inhibition of Helicobacter pylori urease by omeprazole. Eur J Gastroenterol Hepatol. 1993;5:683–5.
28. Bayerdörffer E, Mannes GA, Sommer A et al. High dose omeprazole treatment combined with amoxicillin eradicates Helicobacter pylori. Eur J Gastroenterol Hepatol. 1992;4:697–702.
29. Paulsen O, Höglund P, Walder M. No effects of omeprazole-induced hypoacidity on the bioavailability of amoxycillin or bacampicillin. Scand J Infect Dis. 1989;21:219–23.
30. McNulty CAM. Bateriological and pharmacological basis for the treatment of Campylobacter pylori infection. In: Rathbone BJ, Heatley RV, editors. Campylobacter pylori and gastroduodenal disease. Oxford: Blackwell Scientific Publications; 1989:209–16.
31. Wyatt JI, Rathbone BJ, Dixon MF, Heatley RU. Campylobacter pyloridis and acid induced gastric metaplasia in the pathogenesis of duodenitis. J Clin Pathol. 1987;40:841–8.
32. Graham DY, Lew GM, Klein PD et al. Effect of treatment on Helicobacter pylori infection on the long-term recurrence of gastric or duodenal ulcer. A randomized, controlled study. Ann Intern Med. 1992;116:705–8.
33. Cutler AF, Schubert TT. Patient factors affecting Helicobacter pylori eradication with triple therapy. Am J Gastroenterol. 1993;88:505–9.
34. Unge P, Gad A, Eriksson K et al. Amoxicillin added to omeprazole prevents relapse in the treatment of duodenal ulcer patients. Eur J Gastroenterol Hepatol. 1993;5:325–31.
35. Boixeda D, de Rafael L, Cantón R, Sampedro J, de Argila CM, Baquero F. Galenical formulations of amoxicillin/clavulanate and eradication of Helicobacter pylori in peptic ulcer patients: preliminary report. Eur J Gastroenterol Hepatol. 1993;5:283–5.
36. Bell GD, Powell K, Burridge SM et al. Experience with 'triple' anti-Helicobacter pylori eradication therapy: side effects and the importance of testing the pre-treatment bacterial isolate for metronidazole resistance. Aliment Pharmacol Ther. 1992;6:427–35.
37. Noach LA, Langenberg WL, Bertola MA, Dankert J, Tytgat GNJ. Impact of metronidazole resistance on the eradication of Helicobacter pylori. Scand J Infect Dis (submitted for publication).
38. Borody TJ, Brandl S, Andrews P, Ostapowicz N, Jankiewicz E. High efficacy, low dose triple therapy (TT) for Helicobacter pylori (Hp). Gastroenterology. 1993;102:A44.
39. Labenz J, Gyenes E, Rühl GH, Börsch G. Short term therapy with high dose omeprazole and amoxicillin for eradication of Helicobacter pylori. Ital J Gastroenterol. 1991;23(Suppl. 2):109(abstract).
40. Logan RPH, Walker MM, Gummett PA, Karim QN, Baron JH, Misiewicz JJ. The effect of omeprazole (OME) on the dynamics of H. pylori (Hp) infection. IV Workshop Gastroduodenal Pathology and Helicobacter pylori. Ital J Gastroenterol. 1991;23(Suppl. 2):110(abstract).

41. Borody T, Cole P, Noonan S *et al.* Recurrence of duodenal ulcer and *Campylobacter pylori* infection after eradication. Med J Aust. 1989;151:431–5.
42. Borody TJ, George LL, Brandl S *et al. Helicobacter pylori* eradication with doxycyclin–metronidazole–bismuth subcitrate triple therapy. Scand J Gastroenterol. 1992;27:281–4.
43. George LL, Borody TJ, Andrews P *et al.* Cure of duodenal ulcer after eradication of *Helicobacter pylori.* Med J Aust. 1990;153:145–9.
44. Carrick J, Daskalopoulos G, Mitchell H, Lee A. Successful eradication of *H. pylori* infection prevents recurrence of duodenal ulceration. Rev Esp Enferm Dig. 1990;78(Suppl. I):122–3(abstract).
45. Rodionoff P, Hyland L, Ostapowicz N *et al.* Triple therapy for *Helicobacter pylori* (HP) eradication – 1, 2 or 4 weeks? World Congresses of Gastroenterology, 1990. Sydney, Australia (Abstract).
46. Patchett S, Beattie S, Keane C, O'Morain C. Short report: Short-term triple therapy for *H. pylori*-associated duodenal ulcer disease. Aliment Pharmacol Ther. 1992;6:113–17.
47. Xia HX, Daw MA, Sant S, Beattie S, Keane CT, O'Morain CA. Clinical efficacy of triple therapy in *Helicobacter pylori*-associated duodenal ulcer. Eur J Gastroenterol Hepatol. 1993;5:141–4.
48. Truesdale RA, Chamberlain CE, Martin DF, Maydonovitch CL, Peura DA. Long-term follow-up and antibody response to treatment of patients with *Helicobacter pylori.* Gastroenterology. 1990;98:A140.
49. Wang W-M, Chen C-Y, Jan C-M *et al.* Eradication of *Helicobacter pylori* with triple therapy reducing recurrence of duodenal ulcer. 9th Asian Pacific Congress of Gastroenterology, Bangkok, Thailand, 1992: FP-90 (Abstract).
50. Graham DY, Lew GM, Klein PD *et al.* Effect of treatment of *Helicobacter pylori* infection on the long-term recurrence of gastric or duodenal ulcer. A randomized, controlled study. Ann Intern Med. 1992;116:770–1.
51. Borody TJ, Brandl S, Andrews P, Ostapowicz N, Jankiewicz E. High efficacy, low dose triple therapy (TT) for *Helicobacter pylori* (HP). Gastroenterology. 1992;102:A44.
52. Borody T, Andrews P, Brandl S, Devine M. Relevance of *in-vitro* metronidazole resistance to *H. pylori* (HP) eradication and eradication failure. Gastroenterology. 1993;104:A44.
53. Van Zwet AA, Thijs JC, Oom JAJ, Hoogeveen J, Düringshoff BL. Failure to eradicate *Helicobacter pylori* in patients with metronidazole-resistant strains. Eur J Gastroenterol Hepatol. 1993;5:185–6.
54. Labenz J, Gyenes E, Rühl GH, Börsch G. Efficiency of oral triple therapy (BSS/metronidazole/tetracycline) to eradicate HP in DU disease. Ir J Med Sci. 1992;161(Suppl. 10):90 (abstract).
55. Sobala GM, George R, Tomkins D, Finlay J, Manning A. Spontaneous healing of duodenal ulcers after eradication of *H. pylori.* Ir J Med Sci. 1992;161(Suppl. 10):5(abstract).
56. Bell GD, Powell K, Burridge SM *et al.* Experience with 'triple' anti-*Helicobacter pylori* eradication therapy: side-effects and the importance of testing the pre-treatment bacterial isolate for metronidazole resistance. Aliment Pharmacol Ther. 1992;6:427–35.
57. Balatsos V, Delis V, Skandalis N, Archimandritis A. Triple therapy after duodenal ulcer healing with omeprazole or ranitidine eradicates *H. pylori* and prevents ulcer relapses: preliminary results of a year follow up study. Gastroenterology. 1993;104:A37.
58. Burette A, Glupczynski Y, DePrez C, Ramdani B. Two-week combination therapies with tetracycline are less effective than similar regimens with amoxicillin. Acta Gastroenterol Belg. 1993;56:131(abstract).
59. Daskalopoulos G, Carrick J, Lian R, Lee A. Optimising therapy for *H. pylori* gastritis. Ir J Med Sci. 1992;161(Suppl. 10):16(abstract).
60. Noach LA, Bertola MA, Schwartz MP, Rauws EAJ, Tytgat GNJ. Treatment of *Helicobacter pylori* infection. An evaluation of various therapeutic trials. Eur J Gastroenterol Hepatol. 1993(submitted for publication).
61. Hosking SW, Chung SCS, Sung JY *et al.* Duodenal ulcers heal without acid suppression if *Helicobacter pylori* is eradicated – a randomized trial. Gastroenterology. 1993;104:A104.
62. Rauws EAJ, Langenberg W, Houthoff HJ, Zanen HC, Tytgat GNJ. *Campylobacter pyloridis*-associated chronic active antral gastritis. Gastroenterology. 1988;94:33–40.
63. McColl KEL, Fullarton GM, Chittajalu R *et al.* Plasma gastrin, daytime intragastric pH and nocturnal acid output before and at 1 and 7 months after eradication of *Helicobacter*

pylori in duodenal ulcer subjects. Scand J Gastroenterol. 1991;26:339–46.

64. Wagner S, Bleck J, Gebel M, Bär W, Manns M. What treatment is best for gastric *Helicobacter pylori* infection? Ir J Med Sci. 1992;161(Suppl. 10):16(abstract).

65. Wagner S, Varrentrapp M, Haruma K *et al.* The role of omeprazole in the treatment of gastric *Helicobacter pylori* infection. Z Gastroenterol. 1991;29:595–8.

66. Burette A, Glupczynski Y, Deprez C. Evaluation of various multidrug eradication regimens for *Helicobacter pylori*. Eur J Gastroenterol Hepatol. 1992;4:817–23.

67. Rautelin H, Seppälä K, Renkonen OV, Vainio U, Kosunen TU. Role of metronidazole resistance in therapy of *Helicobacter pylori* infections. Antimicrob Agents Chemother. 1992;36:163–6.

68. Börsch G, Mai U, Opferkuch W. Short- and medium-term results of oral triple therapy to eradicate. *C. pylori*. Gastroenterology. 1989;96:A53.

69. Tucci A, Gasperoni S, Stranghellini V *et al.* Comparison of two therapeutic schedules for the treatment of *Helicobacter pylori* infection. Croatian J Gastroenterol Hepatol. 1993;2: 7–10.

70. Lambert JR, Lin SK, Schembri M, Nicholson L, Korman MG. *Helicobacter pylori* therapy randomized study of denol/antibiotic combinations. Rev Esp Enferm Dig. 1990;78(Suppl. 1):115–16(abstract).

71. Logan RPH, Gummett PA, Misiewicz JJ, Karim QN, Walker MM, Baron JH. One week eradication regimen for *Helicobacter pylori*. Lancet. 1991;338:1249–52.

72. Catalano F, Rizzo G, Ayoubi Khajekini MT, Branciforte G, Inserra G, Liberti A. *Helicobacter pylori* positive dyspepsia: results of four days treatment. Ir J Med Sci. 1992;167(Suppl. 10):94A.

73. Seppälä K, Färkkilä M, Nuutinen H *et al.* Triple therapy of *Helicobacter pylori* infection in peptic ulcer. A 12-month follow-up study of 93 patients. Scand J Gastroenterol. 1992;27:973–6.

74. De Bona M, De Boni M, Bellumat A, Doglioni C, Restelli J, Cielo R. Decrease in gastrin, pepsinogen A and C basal serum levels after oral triple therapy (OTT): a marker for *Helicobacter pylori* eradication? Gastroenterology. 1993;104:A63.

75. Chen TS, Tsay SH, Chang FY, Lee SD. Eradication of *Helicobacter pylori* and duodenal ulcer relapse. A comparison of one-week regimen and two-week regimen. Acta Gastro-enterol Belg. 1993;56:132(abstract).

76. Graham DY, Ramirez FC, Lew GM *et al.* Tetracycline, clarithromycin, bismuth: a new effective triple therapy for *Helicobacter pylori* eradication. Gastroenterology. 1993;104:A90.

77. Bell GD, Weil J, Powell K *et al. Helicobacter pylori* treated with combinations of tripotassium dicitrato and metronidazole: efficacy of different treatment regimens and some observations on the emergence of metronidazole resistance. Eur J Gastroenterol Hepatol. 1991;3: 819–22.

78. DeCross AJ, Marshall BJ, McCallum RW. Rationale for metronidazole sensitivity testing (MST) in the treatment of *Helicobacter pylori* infection. Gastroenterology. 1993;104:A65.

79. Marshall BJ, Goodwin CS, Warren JR *et al.* Prospective double-blind trial of duodenal ulcer relapse after eradication of *Campylobacter pylori*. Lancet. 1988;2:1437–41.

80. Goodwin CS, Marshall BJ, Blincow ED, Wilson DH, Blackbourn S, Phillips M. Prevention of nitroimidazole resistance in *Campylobacter pylori* by coadministration of colloidal bismuth subcitrate: clinical and *in vitro* studies. J Clin Pathol. 1988;41:207–210.

81. Weil J, Bell GD, Morden A *et al. Helicobacter pylori* infection treated with a tripotassium dicitrato bismuthate and metronidazole combination. Aliment Pharmacol Ther. 1990;4: 651–7.

82. Peyre S, Bologna E, Stroppiana M, Rizzi R, Bongera M, Sategna-Guidetti C. Eradication rate of *Helicobacter pylori* (HP) with 4 different regimens. Rev Esp Enferm Dig. 1990;78(Suppl. I):107–8(abstract).

83. Adamek RJ, Wegener M, Birkholz S, Opferkuch W, Rühl GH, Wedmann B. Modified combined omeprazole/amoxicillin therapy regimen for eradication of *H. pylori* – a pilot study. Ir J Med Sci. 1992;161(Suppl. 10):90(abstract).

84. Labenz J, Gyenes E, Rühl GH, Börsch G. Zweiwöchige Amoxycillin/Omeprazole-Therapie zur *Helicobacter pylori*-Eradication. Klin Wochenschr. 1992;69:P37(abstract).

85. Bayerdörffer E, Mannes GA, Sommer A *et al.* High dose omeprazole treatment combined with amoxicillin eradicates *Helicobacter pylori*. Eur J Gastroenterol Hepatol. 1992;4:

697–702.

86. Rokkas T, Mavrogeorgis A, Liatsos C, Rallis E, Kalogeropoulos N. Evaluation of the combination of omeprazole and amoxycillin in eradicating *H. pylori* and preventing relapses in duodenal ulcer patients. Proceedings Digestive Disease Week, Barcelona, 1993, A-99.

87. Unge P, Gad A, Gnarpe H, Olsson J. Does omeprazole improve antimicrobial therapy directed towards gastric *Campylobacter* in patients with antral gastritis? A pilot study. Scand J Gastroenterol. 1989;24(Suppl. 167):49–54.

88. Lamouliatte H, De Mascarel A, Megraud F *et al.* Omeprazole improves amoxicillin therapy towards *Helicobacter pylori* associated chronic gastritis. Gastroenterology. 1990;98:A75.

89. Labenz J, Gyenes F, Rühl GH, Börsch G. Amoxicillin–omeprazole treatment for eradication of *Helicobacter pylori*. Eur J Gastroenterol Hepatol. 1991;39(Suppl. 1):S10(abstract).

90. Bell GD, Powell K, Weil J *et al.* Experience with omeprazole in combination with either amoxicillin or colloidal bismuth subcitrate in patients with metronidazole resistant *Helicobacter pylori*. Eur J Gastroenterol Hepatol. 1991;3:923–6.

91. Logan RPH, Gummett PA, Karim QN. A treatment regimen for metronidazole resistant *Helicobacter pylori* (MRHP). Ital J Gastroenterol. 1991;23(Suppl. 2):110(abstract).

92. Logan RPH, Rubio MA, Gummett PA *et al.* Omeprazole and amoxicillin suspension for *Helicobacter pylori*. Ir J Med Sci. 1992;161(Suppl. 10):16(abstract).

93. Labenz J, Gyenes E, Rühl GH, Börsch G. Pretreatment with omeprazole endangers the efficiency of amoxicillin/omeprazole treatment to eradicate HP. Ir J Med Sci. 1992;161 (Suppl. 10):15(abstract).

94. Unge P, Eriksson K, Bergman B *et al.* Omeprazole and amoxicillin in patients with duodenal ulcer: *Helicobacter pylori* eradication and remission of ulcers and symptoms during a 6-month follow-up. A double-blind comparative study. Gastroenterology. 1992;102:A183.

95. Bell GD, Powell KU, Bunidge SM *et al.* Short report: Omeprazole + antibiotic combinations for the eradication of metronidazole-resistant *Helicobacter pylori*. Aliment Pharmacol Ther. 1992;6:751–8.

96. Collins R, Beattie S, O'Morain C. High dose omeprazole plus amoxicillin in the treatment of acute duodenal ulcer. Ir J Med Sci. 1992;161(Suppl. 10):96.

97. Mannes GA, Bayerdörffer E, Hele C, Ruckdeschel G, Stolte M. An increasing dose of omeprazole combined with amoxicillin increases the eradication rate of *Helicobacter pylori*. Proceedings Digestive Disease Week, Barcelona, 1993, A-100.

98. Labenz J, Rühl GH, Bertrams J, Börsch G. Amoxicillin plus omeprazole for eradication of *Helicobacter pylori* in gastric ulcer disease. Proceedings Digestive Disease Week, Barcelona, 1993, A-99.

99. Labenz J, Rühl GH, Bertrams J, Börsch G. Amoxicillin plus omeprazole for eradication of *Helicobacter pylori* in duodenal ulcer disease. Proceedings Digestive Disease Week, Barcelona, 1993, A-96.

100. Logan RPH, Gummett PA, Hegarthy BT, Walker MM, Baron JH, Misiewicz JJ. Clarithromycin and omeprazole for *Helicobacter pylori*. Lancet. 1992;340:239(letter).

101. Schaufelberger HD, Logan RPH, Gummet PA. The effect of patients compliance on *Helicobacter*. Proceedings Digestive Disease Week, Barcelona, 1993, A-104.

102. Greaves RG, Cayla R, Mendelson MG. Omeprazole versus clarithromycin and omeprazole for eradication of Hp. Proceedings Digestive Disease Week, Barcelona, 1993, A-101.

103. Marzio L, Cellini L, Grossi L, Di Girolamo A, De Leonardis T, Alameddine M. Treatment of *Helicobacter pylori* infection with an association of omeprazole and roxydromycine: a study *in vivo* and *in vitro*. Ital J Gastroenterol. 1991;23(Suppl. 2):111(abstract).

104. Fiocca R, Villani L, Luinetti O *et al. Helicobacter pylori* (HP) eradication and sequential clearance of inflammation in duodenal ulcer patients treated with omeprazole and antibiotics. Ir J Med Sci. 1992;161(Suppl. 10):93–4(abstract).

105. Lamouliatte H, Bernard PH, Cayla F, Megraud F, De Mascarel A, Quinton A. Controlled study of omeprazole–amoxicillin–tinidazole vs ranitidine–amoxicillin–tinidazole in *Helicobacter pylori* associated duodenal ulcers (DU). Final and long-term tresults. Gastroenterology. 1992;102:A106.

106. Bazzoli F, Zagari RM, Fossi S. Efficacy and tolerability of a short term low dose.

Gastroenterology. 1993;109:A40.
107. Van Ganse E, Burette A, Glupczynski Y, Deprez C. Lansoprazole plus roxithromycin and metronidazole for eradication of *H. pylori*: results of a pilot study. Proceedings Digestive Disease Week, Barcelona, 1993, A-102.
108. Coelho LGV, Passos MCF, Chansson Y *et al.* One week US $12.00 therapy heals duodenal ulcer and eradicates *H. pylori*. Ir J Med Sci. 1992;161(Suppl. 10):3(abstract).

54
H. pylori resistance to antibiotics

F. MÉGRAUD

INTRODUCTION

Eradication of *Helicobacter pylori* has become a major goal for gastroenterologists since it was proved that eradication can alter the natural history of peptic ulcer and possibly gastric cancers.

However, there are two principal reasons why this goal is difficult to achieve: one is the resistance of *H. pylori* strains to antimicrobial agents, and the other is the 'resistance' of the patients, through their lack of compliance to the drug regimens.

In this chapter the specific questions related to resistance of *H. pylori* to antibiotics will be reviewed.

DEFINITIONS

The susceptibility of a bacterial isolate to an antimicrobial agent is determined by the minimal inhibitory concentration (MIC), i.e. the lowest concentration of the compound which is able to prevent the outgrowth of a standard inoculum of the bacteria. As a general definition, an organism is considered to be susceptible to a compound if its MIC is at most one-fourth of the obtainable peak serum level of the drug[1]. Despite the fact that the peak serum level is not relevant for the eradication of *H. pylori*, and that there are not enough data to set up specific criteria for *H. pylori*, we shall accept the definition as it is.

However, one must keep in mind that because of the special ecological niche and because of the pharmacological properties of the drugs, an agent to which *H. pylori* is susceptible *in vitro* may not be effective *in vivo*.

Resistance to an antimicrobial agent is defined as the inverse of susceptibility Resistance of strains can be divided into two categories.

1. Natural resistance to the agent, i.e. all the isolates of the bacterial species considered are resistant and have always been resistant; and the species is excluded from the antimicrobial spectrum of the agent. This is also described as the intrinsic resistance of the bacterial species, and is mostly

Table 1 Antimicrobial agents concerned by the natural resistance of *Helicobacter pylori*

Glycopeptides: vancomycin
Sulphamides
2,4-diaminopyridine: trimethoprim
First-generation quinolones*
β-lactams: cefsulodin* (only)
Polymyxins*
Antifungal compounds*

*Some strains may be susceptible

due to a barrier to penetration of the compound. The list of agents to which *H. pylori* is naturally resistant is presented in Table 1.
2. Acquired resistance, i.e. strains of the bacterial species are usually susceptible but some may become resistant by different genetic mechanisms: mutation in a chromosomal gene or infection by a plasmid.

With respect to *H. pylori*, at this stage there is no argument proving that acquired resistance is due to infection by a plasmid or any other kind of gene acquisition. Acquired resistance is most likely due to mutations as in *Mycobacterium tuberculosis*.

There is also the concept of 'pharmacological' resistance for those *H. pylori* strains susceptible *in vitro* but resistant *in vivo* to a given antibiotic. This *in vivo* resistance is essentially due to the inability of the agent to achieve a sufficient concentration at the site of the infection.

METHODS OF DETECTION[2]

A strain will be classified as resistant according to its MIC level.

Reference technique for determining MIC

The reference technique is the determination of MIC in agar. A standard inoculum of *H. pylori* is distributed on several plates containing a progressive concentration of the compound to be tested. After 3 days' incubation the plates are observed, and the MIC (being the smallest concentration with no growth) is expressed in μg/ml or mg/l. This technique is not adapted to routine procedures but to testing a series of strains.

However, the different variables of this technique, in particular the inoculum size, the duration of incubation and the medium, have not been evaluated specifically for *H. pylori*.

The determination of MIC in broth is not adapted to *H. pylori* because of the difficulty in growing the organism under such conditions.

Techniques used routinely to determine MIC

For routine testing, diagnostic laboratories often use an agar diffusion method according to the Kirby–Bauer protocol. Small circles of filter paper (discs) containing standard quantities of the agents are placed on a plate previously inoculated with a standard inoculum of the bacteria. After an incubation of 2–3 days the diameter of the inhibition zone is recorded. This method has been calibrated by using the reference method for MIC. However, because of the slow growth of *H. pylori*, this method is not completely satisfactory.

A new system named the Epsilometer test (E test), which is a variant of the disc method, has been found to be of great interest in measuring the MIC of various agents for *H. pylori*. A plastic strip containing a predefined, continuous and exponential antibiotic gradient on one side and a graded continuous MIC scale that covers 15 two-fold dilutions on the opposite side is placed at the surface of an appropriate agar plate inoculated with bacteria in the same way as for a disc diffusion test. After incubation, the interaction of the antimicrobial agent gradient and the bacterial inoculum tested results in an elliptic inhibition zone. The MIC is read at the intersection of the inhibition zone with the graded scale printed on the strip.

When using this method, a very good correlation with the reference technique was found[3–6]. This method is less affected by the size of the inoculum, or by the duration of incubation. It is reliable and simple enough to be used routinely. It has even been claimed to be better than the agar dilution test[6].

Since no particular enzyme or gene responsible for *H. pylori* resistance has yet been identified there are no detection methods based on the study of these elements.

ACQUIRED RESISTANCE OF *H. PYLORI* TO ANTIBIOTICS

Acquired resistance has been described in four groups of antimicrobial agents: nitroimidazoles, macrolides, fluoroquinolones and rifamycins. The particularity of this resistance is that it concerns all the compounds within a group of antibiotics. For example, when an *H. pylori* strain is resistant to metronidazole it is also resistant to tinidazole and ornidazole. The same is true for the other groups of antibiotics.

Resistance to nitroimidazoles

Nitroimidazoles have the property of being secreted into the stomach[7]. Their MIC is relatively high, but the compound is not influenced by pH, in contrast to most of the other groups of antimicrobial agents[8]. They were among the first drugs to be used in an attempt to eradicate *H. pylori*.

Rate of resistance

A case of resistance, defined as an MIC $> 8 \, \text{mg/l}$, was first described in Australia by Goodwin *et al.*[9], and this phenomenon has subsequently been reported worldwide.

The first point which must be considered is the primary resistance

Table 2 Primary resistance of *H. pylori* to nitroimidazole compounds observed in various countries worldwide

	No. of strains tested	Percentage resistance	Method	Reference
Europe: specific reports				
Belgium	206	27	Breakpoint method	10
Finland	559	26	Disc diffusion test	11
France	97	41.2	E test	12
Ireland	189	27.5	Agar dilution test	13
The Netherlands	140	6.4	Disc diffusion test	14
European Study	443	27.5	E test	15
Belgium	54	24		
Finland	50	34		
France	23	25		
Greece	39	49		
Ireland	35	20		
Italy	25	24		
Portugal	50	26		
Spain	15	7		
Sweden	50	14		
The Netherlands	33	38		
UK	44	20		
	25	26		
America				
USA	25	24	Agar dilution test	16
Australia	100	17	Agar dilution test	9
Asia				
Malaysia	37	10.8	Disc diffusion test	17
Bangladeshi–UK community	22	95	Disc diffusion test	18b
Africa				
Zaïre	32	84	Breakpoint test	10
Burkina Faso	35	77	E test	18

supposedly linked to previous contact of the *H. pylori* strain with nitroimidazoles during treatment for another infection unrelated to *H. pylori*, and the resistance secondary to a treatment regimen aimed at eradicating *H. pylori*.

Primary resistance. A comparative analysis gives a rough idea of the situation even though it may suffer from the lack of standardization of tests and from the short series usually reported (Table 2).

There is no country where this resistance has not been reported. In North America and Australia the resistance rate is around 20%, while in Europe it is closer to 30%, with great variation observed between countries both in the specific reports as well as in a multicentre study using the same methodology (7–49% resistance)[15]. The results can be explained by the type of patients recruited. Women are more likely to harbour resistant strains than men: 34.7% vs 23.9% in the European multicentre study ($p < 0.05$), but statistical significance was reached only in the age group 20–39 years ($p < 0.01$). The same results were also reported in studies in Ireland and the Netherlands. This is probably linked to the fact that, in Europe, women are more likely to have received nitroimidazole for gynaecological infections.

In Africa the rate of resistance is considerably higher, in the range of 80–

Table 3 Secondary resistance of *H. pylori* to nitroimidazole compounds

Author (ref.)	No. of patients	Percentage resistant after treatment	Compounds used
Single drug therapy			
Goodwin et al.[9]	27	70	Tinidazole 10 days
Hirschl et al.[19]	9	89	Metronidazole 4 weeks
Patey et al.[20]	4	50	Metronidazole 3 weeks
Dual or triple therapy			
Goodwin et al.[9]	20	10	CBS–tinidazole 10 days
Burette et al.[21]	36	6	Amoxicillin–metronidazole 10 days
	106	35	Amoxicillin-tinidazole 4–8 days
	15	40	CBS–tinidazole 8 days
	50	36	Amoxicillin–CBS–tinidazole 4 days
	37	50	Tetracycline–CBS–tinidazole 4 days
	30	3	Amoxicillin–CBS–metronidazole 10 days

CBS = Colloidal bismuth citrate

90%. This can also be explained by previous treatment for parasitic diseases (amoebiasis, giardiasis) which occur frequently in these countries.

Among European patients, if the ethnic origin is considered, differences are observed. In a French study there was a marked difference between the rate of *H. pylori* resistance for the strains isolated from local subjects (11.5%) versus those isolated from patients coming from developing countries, mainly Africa (42.5%). In the European multicentre study, natives from northern European countries had a lower rate of *H. pylori* resistance (20.5%) compared to those from European Mediterranean countries (33%), or North African and other non-Caucasian subjects (40%).

In summary, resistance is related to previous nitroimidazole use, and varies dramatically from one population to another, indicating the need for careful monitoring.

Secondary resistance.   When a nitroimidazole compound is used as the only antimicrobial agent to treat *H. pylori* infection, the strains are most likely to become resistant in all cases by the end of treatment (Table 3).

When the nitroimidazole compound is given in association with another antimicrobial agent during a sufficient period of time (> 10 days), the rate of acquired resistance decreases to < 10%. If a third antimicrobial agent is used for a minimum of 10 days, the rate of acquired resistance is close to zero.

In vitro, it is very easy to select 'mutants' resistant to nitroimidazoles by using Szybalski gradients[22]. They appear at subinhibitory concentrations. So it is conceivable that *in vivo*, and when using combination therapy, such conditions occur if there is a lack of compliance by the patient. By exposing the bacteria to concentrations 4–8 times the MIC value, Haas *et al.* obtained resistant 'mutants' at a frequency of 10^{-5} to 10^{-6} organisms[23].

Mechanism of resistance

There are two mechanisms of acquiring resistance, plasmid-mediated resistance and mutational resistance. The latter is the most likely mechanism because the presence of plasmids in *H. pylori* has never correlated with metronidazole resistance[24], and because mutational resistance is the usual mechanism with nitroimidazole compounds.

The mechanism of action of nitroimidazoles against anaerobic organisms is known in some detail. They target the bacterial DNA which will be oxidized, causing strand breaks, helix destabilization and subsequent cell death[25].

The compound penetrates into the cell by passive diffusion which is enhanced by the rate of intracellular reduction and will be subsequently reduced.

The result is an imidazole radical and a nitrite ion, NO_2^-. If reduction occurs in the presence of oxygen, the damage is limited because oxygen will remove the electron from NO_3 re-forming the original drug (futile cycling). The mechanism of action in *H. pylori* has not been studied, and may eventually be found to be different; so the mechanism of resistance is not known[26].

An interesting observation was made by Cederbrant *et al.*, who observed that when strains resistant to metronidazole were incubated anaerobically during a transitory period of 2–12 h, they became susceptible. They proposed that these strains had a decreased ability to achieve a sufficiently low redox potential under microaerobic conditions for the reduction of metronidazole[27].

Resistance to macrolides and lincosamides

Macrolides are divided into three groups of compounds according to the number of carbon atoms present in the lactone ring[28]. Those with 14 carbons are erythromycin, roxithromycin, clarithromycin, dirithromycin, flurithromycin and oleandomycin. Only one compound forms the class name azalide with 15 carbons: azithromycin. Compounds with 16 carbons include spiramycin, josamycin, miocamycin and rokitamycin. Lincosamides are closely related, and include lincomycin and clindamycin.

Resistance affects all the compounds within the group.

Since it has been shown that clarithromycin is able to eradicate *H. pylori*[29], there is a renewed interest for macrolides in treating *H. pylori* infection. These compounds have the ability to achieve a high concentration in the mucus and to concentrate intracellularly[30]. Their *in vitro* activity is greatly influenced by pH.

Rate of resistance

Primary resistance. The rate of resistance is, in all cases, much lower than for nitroimidazoles. Resistance is probably linked to the use of macrolides for respiratory tract infections. In the UK, for example, where these drugs are not widely used, resistance is seldom found. This is not the case in France

Table 4 Resistance of *H. pylori* to macrolides

Primary resistance

	No. of strains tested	Percentage resistance	Method	Reference
Europe				
France	97	9.3	E test	12
Belgium	18	11	Agar dilution method	31
The Netherlands	68	3	Disc diffusion	32
Switzerland	11	0	Disc diffusion	33
Africa				
Burkina Faso	35	14	E test	17
America				
USA	37	11	Agar dilution method	34
Australia	108	1.9	Disc diffusion	34

Secondary resistance

Author (Ref.)	No. of patients	Percentage resistance after treatment	Compounds used
Burette *et al.*[31]	16	19	Omeprazole + clarithromycin 14 days
Peterson *et al.*[34]	33	21	Clarithromycin 14 days
Noach *et al.*[32]	19	47	Clarithromycin 14 days
Fried *et al.*[33]	11	9	Ranitidine + clarithromycin 14 days

where a macrolide (josamycin) has been used extensively for the past 10 years. Although no resistant strains were found in our first survey in 1984–85, the rate is now 9%[12]. In Belgium it was found to be 11%[31], in the Netherlands 3%[32], in Switzerland 0%[33], and in the USA it was 11%[34] (Table 4). Among *H. pylori* strains collected in Western Africa the resistance rate was 14%[18].

Secondary resistance. Glupczynski and Burette were the first to report acquired resistance to a macrolide, in 1990. In a pilot study with azithromycin administered alone, none of the patients' stain was eradicated, while strains resistant to macrolides were recovered from nine out of 12 patients and were subsequently recovered from the patients for many months thereafter[36]. The same authors also observed resistance when roxithromycin was administered to patients with omeprazole[37]. Concomitant administration of metronidazole prevented the acquisition of resistance to roxithromycin but not to metronidazole[38].

In studies carried out in Belgium and the USA, using clarithromycin alone or with omeprazole, the rate of acquired resistance to macrolides was 19%[31] and 21%[34], respectively.

It is not clear if clindamycin is able to induce such resistance. In a study by Westblom *et al.*, using clindamycin and BSS, one out of four post-treatment strains was resistant[39]. Because of this limitation it is important to monitor *H. pylori* susceptibility to macrolides in order to determine whether or not these compounds can be used as single antimicrobial agents in eradication regimes.

In vitro the selection of *H. pylori* 'mutants' resistant to macrolides is also possible, but at a lower frequency than for the nitroimidazoles[23].

Mechanism of resistance

Macrolides interact at the ribosomal level to block protein synthesis. Bacterial ribosomes classically become resistant to macrolides by methylation of specific adenine residues.

No studies have been performed which provide an insight into the mechanism of resistance to macrolides in *H. pylori*. It is most likely that this resistance results from a mutation rather than from a plasmid-mediated origin.

Resistance to macrolides by *Campylobacter jejuni* has been extensively studied by Yan and Taylor[40]. They confirmed that erythromycin binds to the 50S ribosomal subunit and inhibits protein synthesis, but the probable mutation in a gene encoding a ribosomal protein has yet to be found. However, unlike macrolide resistance in *H. pylori*[23], it has not been possible to select spontaneous mutants of *C. jejuni* by plating on a medium containing low concentrations of erythromycin.

Resistance to fluoroquinolones

The second-generation quinolones, the fluoroquinolones, are composed of norfloxacin, ofloxacin, pefloxacin, enoxacin, cripofloxacin, lomefloxacine, sparfloxacin and other molecules still in development. The MICs of ciprofloxacin and sparfloxacin are the lowest. These components also accumulate in the gastric mucosa and their activity is very much pH-dependent. There is also a cross-resistance within this group of molecules.

Rate of resistance

Primary resistance. The rate of resistance by *H. pylori* to fluoroquinolones is still very low; less than 1% in all the countries where it has been tested[41]. This is probably related to the fact that these expensive drugs have not been widely used, but reserved for serious illnesses in contrast to the macrolides.

Secondary resistance. The first report of acquired resistance by *H. pylori* during a fluoroquinolone treatment (ofloxacin) in monotherapy was made by Glupczynski *et al.* in 1987[42]. Other reports followed involving ciprofloxacin and norfloxacin[19,43-45].

Resistance occurred in 70–100% of the post-treatment isolates with a 16–64-fold increase in the MIC value of the fluoroquinolone tested. Resistance to fluoroquinolones by *H. pylori* persisted as a stable feature after repeated subculture of the strain, as well as *in vivo*. *In vitro* the frequency of mutation is lower than that observed with macrolides and nitroimidazoles (10^{-8} to 10^{-9})[23].

Mechanisms of resistance

The exact mechanism of *H. pylori* resistance to fluoroquinolones is not known. However, the observations made, as well as the usual target of these drugs, indicate that it probably involves a modification of the bacterial DNA gyrase, and that it is a consequence of a chromosomal mutation rather than a plasmid-mediated process.

Resistance to rifamycins

There are two compounds in this group of antibiotics: rifampicin and rifaximin. Rifaximin is a non-absorbable molecule of potential interest in the treatment of *H. pylori* as a topical agent[46].

Frequency of resistance

No primary resistance to rifamycins has been reported, probably because these compounds are also not widespread. Hirschl reported the acquisition of resistance in three out of eight patients after treatment with rifampicin as monotherapy[19].

Mechanism of resistance

There is no information on the mechanism of resistance, which is probably chromosomally mediated.

Resistance to streptomycin and kanamycin

Kanamycin is part of the aminoglycoside group of antibiotics, and there is no report of its use to treat *H. pylori*. Streptomycin-resistant mutants have been obtained *in vitro* by culture on media containing subinhibitory concentrations of this antibiotic. Resistance to kanamycin has never been observed in wild isolates. *In vitro* Ferrero *et al.* achieved expression of the kanamycin resistance gene (aph3'-III) in *H. pylori* after electrotransformation while constructing isogenic urease-negative mutants[47].

Other agents

No resistance has yet been reported by *H. pylori* to β-lactams (except one strain reported resistant to cefixime, but no details were given[48]), aminoglycosides (except kanamycin and streptomycin), tetracyclines, chloramphenicol, nitrofuranes or bismuth salts.

IN VIVO RESISTANCE

Despite their good activity *in vitro*, most the above agents do not eradicate *H. pylori in vivo*. This can be explained by the inadequate pharmacological properties of these drugs in relation to the particular niche in which *H. pylori* is located, and not by bacterial resistance with the exception of the examples discussed.

To be effective the agent must: be active at an acidic pH, penetrate the gastric mucus, penetrate intracellularly, reach sequestered niches in the stomach such as the cardia, and be bactericidal.

THERAPEUTIC IMPLICATIONS OF THE OCCURRENCE OF RESISTANCE

Since bacterial resistance is a major determinant in the failure of therapy aimed at eradicating *H. pylori*, it must be taken into account in the control of the infection.

As for any other infectious disease where resistance to the drug may occur, it is necessary to test the susceptibility of the strain before treatment and to culture the organism. In case of treatment failure it is also necessary to test the susceptibility to determine if the organism has acquired resistance. Before obtaining the result it is possible to use a probabilistic approach; for example, in Africa metronidazole should not be used, nor should it be taken by immigrants from these countries living in Europe. After the antibiotic spectrum of activity is known, an adaptation of the treatment will be made if necessary.

The impact of resistance on the outcome of treatment is especially evident for metronidazole (Table 5). With dual therapies a very low eradication rate is obtained if the strain is metronidazole-resistant (0–25%). In contrast, the results are satisfactory for metronidazole-susceptible strains.

The standard triple therapy administered for more than 7 days gave an eradication rate consistently higher than 90%. Metronidazole resistance was overcome in 40–60% of the strains according to the study. Preliminary data also indicate that clarithromycin-resistant strains cannot be eradicated by this agent[55].

A second consequence is that compounds known to induce acquired resistance should not be used as a single antimicrobial agent, but always in combined therapy. This approach has been used successfully for years to treat infection by *Mycobacterium tuberculosis*, for which the same mechanisms of resistance (chromosomal mutations) occur. If mutation to resistance cannot be prevented, the selection of treatments may be critical. The principle of combined therapy dates back to Ehrlich in the first trials with chemotherapy. It has a simple rationale: if one bacterial cell in 10^6 mutates to be resistant to drug A, and one in 10^7 to drug B which lacks cross-resistance, only one in 10^{13} will develop both mutations, i.e. a very exceptional event. This is highlighted in Table 3, for *H. pylori* in relation to metronidazole treatment. If the treatment regimen is administered for more than 10 days, the selection of resistant strains to metronidazole decreases to 10% or less.

Table 5 Impact of nitroimidazole resistance on the outcome of eradication regimens

Author (ref.)	Regimen	Eradication (Metro^S)		Eradication (Metro^R)	
Double therapy					
Goodwin et al.[9]	CBS-Tini 10 days	20/22	(90.9%)	1/5	(20%)
Burette et al.[21]	Amox-Tini 8 days	28/41	(68%)	0/13	
	Amox-Metro 10 days	34/36	(94%)	3/12	(25%)
De Cross et al.[16]	BSS-Metro 10 days		(81.6%)		(16.7%)
Triple therapy with bismuth <7 days					
Burette et al.[21]	CBS-Amox-Tini 4 days	30/50	(60%)	0/15	
	CBS-Tetra-Tini 4 days	17/37	(46%)	0/12	
Triple therapy with bismuth >7 days					
Burette et al.[21]	CBS-Amox-Metro 10 days	29/30	(97%)	17/27	(63%)
Noach et al.[49]	CBS-Tetra-Metro 7 days	47/49	(96%)	11/29	(38%)
Bell et al.[50]	CBS-Amox-Metro 14 days	19/21	(90%)	6/19	(31.6%)
Rautelin et al.[51]	CBS-Amox-Metro 14 days		(91%)		(63%)
Lian et al.[35]	CBS-Tetra-Metro 14 days	51/57	(86.4%)	6/14	(42.9%)
Logan et al.[52]	CBS-Amox-Metro 7 days	40/43	(93%)	4/21	(19%)
Triple therapy with antisecretory agents					
Lamouliatte et al.[53]	Ome or Rani + Amox + Tini 14 days	34/41	(83%)	2/12	(16.6%)
Hentschel et al.[54]	Rani + Amox + Metro 12 days	44/46	(95%)	2/5	(40%)

CBS: colloidal bismuth subcitrate; BSS: bismuth subsalicylate; Metro: metronidazole; Tini: tinidazole; Amox: amoxicillin; Tetra: tetracycline; Rani: ranitidine; Ome: omeprazole; S = susceptible; R = resistant

FUTURE OF RESISTANCE IN *H. PYLORI*

To date, acquired resistance by *H. pylori* has most usually and probably concerned only mutational resistance at the chromosomal level. However, there is no assurance that plasmid-mediated resistance will never occur. This is of special concern for β-lactam antibiotics and especially amoxicillin which is currently the drug of choice for *H. pylori*.

After the introduction of benzylpenicillin in the UK the frequency of resistance by *Staphylococcus aureus* increased from virtually nothing to 60% within 6 years and is now 90% worldwide. *Haemophilus influenzae* and *Neisseria gonorrhoeae* resistance to β-lactams also occurred, but began later and has not developed to the same magnitude. Nevertheless, there are still bacteria which are continuously exposed to β-lactams such as *Streptococcus pyogenes* and *Neisseria meningitidis* which are still susceptible to penicillin G.

H. pylori has also been exposed to β-lactams, especially amoxicillin, for the past 20 years, and still appears to be highly susceptible, so that the probability of such resistance, while possible, seems improbable. The reason may be linked to the fact that *H. pylori* colonizes as the only resident in an isolated niche, which obviously does not favour exchanges with other organisms. Nevertheless, the recent finding that *H. pylori* can be cultured from faeces[56] may 'alter' this situation, especially if the bacterium is demonstrated to multiply in faeces rather than simply to survive.

Besides the hypothesis plasmid-mediated resistance to β-lactams, it may be more likely that the susceptibility of *H. pylori* to β-lactams will decrease in the future in the same way as for *Streptococcus pneumoniae*. For this bacterium, resistance is not plasmid-mediated but can be transferred by transformation and the penicillin-binding proteins are involved. Strains with decreased susceptibility to amoxicillin have already been found, but the mechanism has not been investigated.

CONCLUSION

Because of the unique niche colonized by *H. pylori*, it has been difficult to find the appropriate drug combination to eradicate the organism. This goal is now being approached but, at the same time, resistance to some of the major antibiotics currently in use is being discovered frequently. This is yet another hurdle on the way to eradicating this bacterium; but was the case different for other bacteria?

References

1. Davis DB. Chemotherapy. In: Davis BD, Dulbecco R, Eisen HN *et al.*, editors. Micriobiology, 4th edn. Philadelphia: Lippincott; 1990:201–8.
2. Mégraud F. *Helicobacter pylori*. In: Courvalin P, Goldstein F, Philippon A, Sirot J, editors. L'Antibiogramme, 2nd edn. Paris: MPC-Vidéom; 1994(in press).
3. Glupczynski Y, Labbé M, Hansen W *et al.* Evaluation of the E test for quantitative antimicrobial susceptibility testing of *Helicobacter pylori*. J Clin Microbiol. 1991;29: 2072–5.
4. Cederbrant G, Kahlmeter G, Ljungh A. The E test for antimicrobial susceptibility testing of *Helicobacter pylori*. J Antimicrob Chemother. 1993;31:65–71.
5. Knapp CC, Ludwig MD, Washington JA. *In vitro* activity of metronidazole against *Helicobacter pylori* as determined by agar dilution and agar diffusion. Antimicrob Agents Chemother. 1991;35:1230–1.
6. Hirschl AM, Hirschl MM, Rotter ML. Comparison of three methods for the determination of the sensitivity of *Helicobacter pylori* to metronidazole. J Antimicrob Chemother. 1993;32:45–9.
7. Veldhuyzen Van Zanten SJ, Goldie J, Hollingsworth J *et al.* Secretion of intravenously administered antibiotics in gastric juice: implications for management of *Helicobacter pylori*. J Clin Pathol. 1992;45:225–7.
8. McNulty CA, Dent J, Ford GA *et al.* Inhibitory antimicrobial concentrations against *Campylobacter pylori* in gastric mucosa. J Antimicrob Chemother. 1988;22:729–38.
9. Goodwin CS, Marshall BJ, Blincow ED *et al.* Prevention of nitroimidazole resistance in *Campylobacter pylori* by coadministration of colloidal bismuth subcitrate: clinical and in vitro studies. J Clin Pathol. 1988;41:207–10.
10. Glupczynski Y, Burette A, De Koster E *et al.* Metronidazole resistance in *Helicobacter pylori*. Lancet. 1990;335:976–7.
11. Rautelin H, Seppala K, Renkonen OV *et al.* Role of metronidazole resistance in therapy of *Helicobacter pylori* infections. Antimicrob Agents Chemother. 1992;36:163–6.
12. Cayla R, Lamouliatte HC, Brugmann D *et al.* Pretreatment resistances of *Helicobacter pylori* to metronidazole and macrolides. Acta Gastroenterol Belg. 1994;56(Suppl.):65.
13. Xia HX, Daw MA, Beattie S *et al.* Prevalence of metronidazole-resistant *Helicobacter pylori* in dyspeptic patients. Ir J Med Sci. 1993;162:91–4.
14. Becx MC, Janssen AJ, Clasener HA *et al.* Metronidazole resistant *Helicobacter pylori*. Lancet. 1990;335:539–40.
15. Glupczynski Y and a European Multicentre Study Group on Antibiotic Susceptibility of *Helicobacter pylori*. Results of a multicentre European survey in 1991 of metronidazole

resistance in *Helicobacter pylori*. Eur J Clin Microbiol Infect Dis. 1992;11:777–81.

16. De Cross AJ, Marshall BJ, McCallum RW *et al.* Metronidazole susceptibility testing for *Helicobacter pylori*: comparison of disk, broth, and agar dilution methods and their clinical relevance. J Clin Microbiol. 1993;31:1971–4.
17. Parasakthi N, Goh KL. Metronidazole resistance among *Helicobacter pylori* strains in Malaysia. Am J Gastroenterol. 1992;87:808.
18. Willemin B, Camou C, Rochereau A *et al. Helicobacter pylori* in Africa. Is there an African enigma? Acta Gastroenterol Belg. 1994;56(Suppl.):93.
18b. Banatvala N, Davies GR, Abdi Y *et al.* 95% metronidazole resistance in *Helicobacter pylori* infection in a UK Asian community. Gastroenterology. 1993;104:37.
19. Hirschl AM, Hentschel E, Schütze K *et al.* The efficacy of antimicrobial treatment in *Campylobacter pylori*-associated gastritis and duodenal ulcer. Scand J Gastroenterol. 1988;23(Suppl.142):76–81.
20. Patey O, Chaplain C, Dublanchet A *et al.* Failure of treatment with metronidazole for *Campylobacter pylori* infection. In: Mégraud F, Lamouliatte H, editors. Gastroduodenal pathology and *Campylobacter pylori* ICS 847. Amsterdam: Elsevier; 1993:629–32.
21. Burette A, Glupczynski Y, De Prez C. Evaluation of various multi-drug eradication regimens for *Helicobacter pylori*. Eur J Gastroenterol Hepatol. 1992;4:817–23.
22. Szybalski W, Bryson V. Genetic studies on microbial cross resistance to toxic agents. I. Cross resistance of *Escherichia coli* to fifteen antibiotics. J Bacteriol. 1952;64:489–99.
23. Haas CE, Nix DE, Schentag JJ. *In vitro* selection of resistant *Helicobacter pylori*. Antimicrob Agents Chemother. 1990;34:1637–41.
24. Kisters V, Glupczynski Y, Van Naelten C *et al.* Analysis of plasmid DNA in *Helicobacter pylori*: clinical and epidemiological correlations. Rev Esp Infect Dig. 1990;78(Suppl.1):20–1.
25. Edwards DI. Nitroimidazole drugs – action and resistance mechanisms. I. Mechanisms of action. J Antimicrob Chemother. 1993;31:9–20.
26. Edwards DI. Nitroimidazole drugs – action and resistance mechanisms. II. Mechanisms of resistance. J Antimicrob Chemother. 1993;31:201–10.
27. Cederbrant G, Kahlmeter G, Ljungh A. Proposed mechanism for metronidazole resistance in *Helicobacter pylori*. J Antimicrob Chemother. 1992;29:115–20.
28. Mazzei T, Mini E, Novelli A *et al.* Chemistry and mode of action of macrolides. J Antimicrob Chemother. 1993;31(Suppl. C):1–9.
29. Graham DY, Opekum AR, Klein PD. Clarithromycin for the eradication of *Helicobacter pylori*. J Clin Gastroenterol. 1993;16:292–4.
30. Harrison JD, Jones JA, Morris DC. Azithromycin levels in plasma and gastric tissue, juice and mucus. Eur J Microbiol Infect Dis. 1991;10:862–4.
31. Burette A, Glupczynski Y, Deprez C *et al.* Omeprazole alone or in combination with clarithromycin for eradication of *Helicobacter pylori*: results of a randomized double-blind controlled study. Gastroenterology. 1993;104:49.
32. Noach LA, Bosma NB, Tytgat GNJ. Clarithromycin resistance and *Helicobacter pylori* infection. European United Gastroenterology Week, Barcelona 1993:A103.
33. Fried R, Beglinger C, Green R *et al.* Clarithromycin in combination with ranitidine for eradication of *Helicobacter pylori* from the gastric mucosa of patients with a history of non-ulcer dyspepsia. European United Gastroenterology Week, Barcelona 1993:A103.
34. Peterson WL and the Clarithromycin–*Helicobacter pylori* study group. Clarithromycin as monotherapy for eradication of *Helicobacter pylori*. Am J Gastroenterol. 1992;87:1274.
35. Lian JX, Carrick J, Daskalopoulos G. Metronidazole resistance significantly affects eradication of *Helicobacter pylori* infection. Gastroenterology. 1993;104:133.
36. Glupczynski Y, Burette A. Failure of azythromycin to eradicate *Campylobacter pylori* from the stomach because of acquired resistance during treatment. Am J Gastroenterol. 1990;85:98–9.
37. Glupczynski Y, Burette A. Drug therapy for *Helicobacter pylori* infection: problems and pitfalls. Am J Gastroenterol. 1990;85:1545–51.
38. Van Ganse E, Burette A, Glupczynski Y *et al.* Lansoprazole plus roxithromycin and metronidazole for eradication of *Helicobacter pylori*: results of a pilot study. European United Gastroenterology Week, Barcelona 1993:A102.
39. Westblom TU, Madan E, Subik MA. Double-blind randomized trial of bismuth subsalicylate

and clindamycin for treatment of *Helicobacter pylori* infection. Scand J Gastroenterol. 1992;27:249–52.

40. Taylor DE. Antimicrobial resistance of *Campylobacter jejuni* and *Campylobacter coli* to tetracycline, chloramphenicol and erythromycin. In: Nachamkin I, Blaser MK, Tompkins LS, editors. *Campylobacter jejuni*, current status and future trends. Washington, DC: ASM; 1992:74–86.

41. Westblom TU, Unge P. Drug resistance of *Helicobacter pylori*: memorandum from a meeting at the Sixth International Workshop on *Campylobacter, Helicobacter*, and related organisms. J Infect Dis. 1992;165:974–5.

42. Glupczynski Y, Labbé M, Burette A *et al.* Treatment failure of ofloxacin in *Campylobacter pyloridis* infection. Lancet. 1987;i:1096.

43. Stone JW, Wise R, Donovan IA *et al.* Failure of ciprofloxacin to eradicate *Campylobacter pylori* from the stomach. J Antimicrob Chemother. 1988;22:92–3.

44. Mertens JCC, Dekker W, Ligtvoet EEJ *et al.* Treatment failure of norfloxacin against *Campylobacter pylori* and chronic gastritis in patients with non-ulcerative dyspepsia. Antimicrob Agents Chemother. 1989;33:256–7.

45. Canton R, de Rafael L, Boixeda D *et al. In vivo* acquired resistance to fluoroquinolones in *Helicobacter pylori* during therapy with ciprofloxacin alone or ciprofloxacin plus amoxicillin clavulanate. In: Pajares JM, Pena AS, Malfertheiner P, editors. *Helicobacter pylori* and gastroduodenal pathology. Berlin: Springer; 1993:305–11.

46. Mégraud F, Bouffant F, Camou-Juncas C. *In vitro* susceptibility of *Helicobacter pylori* to rifaximin. Eur J Clin Microbiol Infect Dis. 1994;in press.

47. Ferrero RL, Cussac V, Courcoux P *et al.* Construction of isogenic urease-negative mutants of *Helicobacter pylori* by allelic exchange. J Bacteriol. 1992;174:4212–17.

48. Loo VG, Sherman P, Matlow AG. *Helicobacter pylori* infection in a pediatric population: *in vitro* susceptibilities to omeprazole and eight antimicrobial agents. Antimicrob Agents Chemother. 1992;36:1133–5.

49. Noach LA, Bosma NB, Tytgat GNJ. CBS and clarithromycin: alternative therapy for *Helicobacter pylori* infection in patients with metronidazole resistant strains? United European Gastroenterology Week, Barcelona 1993: A102.

50. Bell GD, Powell K, Burridge SM *et al.* Experience with triple anti-*Helicobacter pylori* eradication therapy: side effects and the importance of testing the pre-treatment bacterial isolate for metronidazole resistance. Aliment Pharmacol Ther. 1992;6:427–35.

51. Rautelin H, Kosunen TU, Seppala K. Eradicating *Helicobacter pylori*. Lancet. 1992;339:55.

52. Logan RPH, Gummett PA, Misiewicz JJ *et al.* One week eradication regimen for *Helicobacter pylori*. Lancet. 1991;338:1249–52.

53. Lamouliatte H, Brugmänn D, Cayla R, Bernard PH, Mégraud F, Quinton A. Metronidazole resistance in *Helicobacter pylori* associated duodenal ulcers. Ir J Med Sci. 1992;161(Suppl. 10):52.

54. Hentschel E, Brandstätter G, Dragosirs B *et al.* Effect of ranitidine and amoxicillin plus metronidazole on the eradication of *Helicobacter pylori* and the recurrence of duodenal ulcer. N Engl J Med. 1993;328:308–12.

55. Greaves RG, Cayla R, Mendelson MG *et al.* Omeprazole vs clarithromycin and omeprazole for eradication of *Helicobacter pylori*. European United Gastroenterology Week, Barcelona 1993:A101.

56. Thomas JE, Gibson GR, Darboc MK *et al.* Isolation of *Helicobacter pylori* from human faeces. Lancet. 1992;340:1194–5.

55
The role of acid suppression in the treatment of *H. pylori* infection

R. H. HUNT

THE RELATIVE ROLE OF ACID AND *H. PYLORI* IN ULCER DISEASE

Treatment to eradicate *H. pylori* infection has proved especially difficult, with many different antibiotics investigated either alone, or in combination with other antibiotics or bismuth compounds. Trials of antisecretory therapy plus bismuth and two antibiotics have shown an acceleration of duodenal ulcer healing rates and very high *H. pylori* eradication rates[1]. More recently therapeutic combinations employing acid suppression obtained with the proton pump inhibitors omeprazole and lansoprazole and one or more antibiotics (usually amoxicillin) have attracted increasing attention.

An *H. pylori* eradication therapy, which combines an antisecretory agent and antibiotic, is logical for patients with duodenal ulcer, since they have either normal or increased gastric acid secretion and an increased parietal cell mass contributing to the hypersecretion of gastric acid. Furthermore, antisecretory drugs have achieved widespread acceptance for their rapid symptom relief and fast duodenal ulcer healing. In this regard the proton pump inhibitors are significantly better than the H_2-receptor antagonists[2], making them a logical first choice for therapy.

The relationship between *Helicobacter* infection, gastric acid secretion and gastrin release is very complex[3,4]. *H. pylori* colonizes the antrum of the stomach, facilitated by its urease and motility, which is aided by the spiral structure of the organism and the multiple flagella. Urease, together with a spectrum of bacterial products, leads to: weakening of the mucus bicarbonate layer; damage to surface epithelial cells; the release of cytokines with an associated inflammatory response, which results in further damage to mucosal cells; and effects on the regulatory mechanism involving the release of somatostatin and gastrin with a consequent effect on gastric acid secretion and gastric motility. Over time these effects, together with the trophic effect of a persistently raised plasma gastrin, may lead to an increase in the parietal cell mass and hypersecretion of gastric acid, with the subsequent development of gastric metaplasia in the duodenal cap. These areas of gastric metaplasia then become colonized with *H. pylori* from the gastric antrum, leading to further inflammation in the duodenal cap. Inflamed gastric metaplasia in the duodenal cap, with altered sialomucin production, and the already compromised junctional mucosa, weakens the normally well orchestrated and buttressed mucosal defences. With ongoing normal or increased acid secretion and peptic activity, mucosal damage and ulceration can occur.

The exact effects of *H. pylori* on gastric secretory mechanisms in the pathogenesis of duodenal ulcer remain to be more clearly defined[4]. However, gastric acid secretion is still of paramount importance in the pathogenesis of duodenal ulcer disease, and it is clear that the mucosal damage, inflammation and gastric metaplasia in the duodenal cap predispose to ulceration in the presence of normal or increased acid secretion.

H. PYLORI AND INTRAGASTRIC ACIDITY

H. pylori does not thrive in an environment of profound hypoacidity, and is not seen in patients with achlorhydria as occurs with chronic atrophic gastritis and in patients with pernicious anaemia. Moreover, in patients taking omeprazole it was observed that the organism seemed to disappear from the gastric antrum, with an accompanying improvement in antral gastritis, and migrate to the fundus where the gastritis increased[5].

H. pylori colonizes the stomach at the interface of the mucus/bicarbonate layer and surface epithelial cells where the pH is between 6 and 7. *In vitro* studies show that the organism will replicate in the presence of urea down to a pH of 4.3 and survive without replication to a pH of 2.3 (Goldie *et al.*, unpublished observations). Furthermore, it does not like to grow in a pH in excess of 7. Thus, when acid secretion is effectively suppressed, the minimal H^+ in the lumen of the stomach results in little or no back-diffusion of acid across the mucus bicarbonate layer. The pH of the mucous/submucous environment rises because of the continuing bacterial urease activity, and becomes alkaline due to unbuffered ammonia. Thus, it is probable that *H. pylori* can tolerate this alkaline pH for only a short period of time. This has potentially important implications, because treatment with antisecretory drugs in doses and regimens which can raise pH close to neutrality might make it more difficult for *H. pylori* to survive.

COMBINATION THERAPY WITH ANTISECRETORY DRUGS AND *H. PYLORI* ERADICATION REGIMENS

Early trials combining acid suppression treatment with *H. pylori* eradication regimens studied a quadruple treatment with ranitidine 150 mg BID and triple therapy with bismuth five or eight tablets/day, metronidazole 750 mg/day and tetracycline 2 g/day[1]. This study showed higher duodenal ulcer healing rates when *H. pylori* eradication was combined with acid suppression than when ranitidine was given alone: 37% and 18% after 2 weeks and 74% and 53%

at 4 weeks, respectively. These ulcer healing rates rose to 96% and 80% after 12 weeks. However, this study did not report ulcer healing when triple therapy was given alone. A further study, conducted in 155 duodenal ulcer patients in Hong Kong[6], showed that ulcer healing with omeprazole could be further accelerated when classical triple therapy with bismuth 120 mg, metronidazole 400 mg and tetracycline 500 mg, all given QID for 2 weeks, was prescribed in addition to omeprazole. Duodenal ulcer healing at 4 weeks was significantly higher at 95% with the four-drug combination when compared with omeprazole alone at 79%[6]. Eradication of *H. pylori* was reported in 95% of those on the four-drug regimen compared with 4% on omeprazole alone. More recently, Hentschel *et al.*[7] combined ranitidine 300 mg HS for 6 or 10 weeks with metronidazole 500 mg and amoxicillin 750 g TID for the first 12 days. These investigators observed a duodenal ulcer healing rate of 92% at 6 weeks and 98% at 10 weeks with the three-drug combination therapy, in contrast to 75% and 94% respectively with ranitidine alone, and *H. pylori* eradication rates were 89% and 2% respectively. There was also a highly significant reduction in ulcer recurrence at 1 year with 8% recurrence following the combination therapy and 86% recurrence after ranitidine alone. However, for those patients who were *H. pylori*-negative after treatment ulcer recurrence was 2%.

Several studies which have examined *H. pylori* eradication with omeprazole and amoxicillin in combination have reported a considerable variation in the results. Bell *et al.*[8] treated 16 patients giving omeprazole 20 mg in the evening in combination with amoxicillin syrup 250 mg TID and recorded an eradication rate of 31.3%. However, omeprazole given in the evening has a lesser effect on suppressing intragastric acidity and for a much shorter duration of the 24-hour period than when given in the morning[9]. Unge *et al.*[10], in a large Scandinavian multicentre study, achieved a 54% eradication rate with omeprazole 40 mg and amoxicillin 750 mg BID. In this study amoxicillin was not started until after the first 2 weeks of the treatment. In the Labenz *et al.* study[11] one group showed a lower eradication rate in patients pretreated with omeprazole before amoxicillin treatment was started. This was also the case in the Unge *et al.* study, and may provide one explanation as to why the omeprazole/amoxicillin combination achieved only 54% eradication in their study. Bayerdorffer and colleagues[12] reported an eradication rate of 82% after 10 days omeprazole 40 mg BID and amoxicillin 1 g BID with further omeprazole 20 mg daily given for a total treatment course of 6 weeks, compared to 0% eradication after a comparable dose regimen of omeprazole alone. Moreover, in this study the 9-month duodenal ulcer recurrence rates were 0% in those who were treated with the combination regime versus 48% in those treated with omeprazole alone. In open studies reported by Labenz *et al.*[13], 1 week of treatment with omeprazole 40 mg BID and amoxicillin 500 mg BID resulted in only a 61.7% eradication. However, omeprazole 20 mg BID and amoxicillin 500 mg QID for 2 weeks in 62 patients resulted in an eradication rate of 82.8%.

In addition to these studies, there are numerous abstracts which report that combination therapy with omeprazole and amoxicillin can effectively eradicate *H. pylori* infection[14] and several conclusions can be drawn from these reports. As has been shown by Axon[15] the BID regimes of omeprazole seem necessary, but the exact dose and timing are yet to be defined. It appears that amoxicillin should be given in a dose of not less than 500 mg TID. Furthermore, at least two studies[4,10] suggest that treatment should be started with amoxicillin and omeprazole simultaneously, and continued for not less than 2 weeks.

Inhibition of acid secretion by omeprazole given twice a day in combination with amoxicillin has achieved eradication rates as high as those seen with triple therapy. These results are better than those reported in a meta-analysis of triple therapy with colloidal bismuth, metronidazole and amoxicillin at 73%, but less than with colloidal bismuth metronidazole and tetracycline at 93%[16]. Moreover, triple therapy is associated with problems of compliance and significant side-effects which are seen in more than 30% of patients, and these can include: dizziness, headache, nausea, diarrhoea, antibiotic-related colitis, drug hypersensitivity, metallic taste, sore mouth and tongue, paraesthesiae, and resistance to metronidazole.

WHAT CAN BE LEARNT ABOUT DOSE AND DURATION OF TREATMENT?

A critical review of the literature indicates that combination therapy with omeprazole and amoxicillin can effectively eradicate *H. pylori* infection, and several conclusions can be drawn from the existing reports. Our findings support the conclusions of Axon[15] that BID regimes of omeprazole provide better rates of eradication at 84% than single daily doses unless these doses exceed 40 mg UID, and that 2 weeks treatment is significantly better than 1 week[14]. Moreover, the results of studies of omeprazole combined with two antibiotics show an eradication rate of 83%, which does not further increase the therapeutic gain over the BID regimens. However, these studies have so far been undertaken with single daily doses of omeprazole rather than the more effective BID regimens. There are a few small studies with lansoprazole which have been published in abstract. These have studied only a single daily dose of lansoprazole 30 mg in combination with amoxicillin or clarithromycin, and show eradication rates between 72% and 78%. The results of studies which employ a BID dose of lansoprazole are eagerly awaited.

It has been suggested that doses of omeprazole need be not higher than 20 mg BID since there was no apparent therapeutic gain with 40 mg BID or higher in the studies reported by Labenz *et al.*[13]. While this conclusion is supported by our own studies[14] and that of Axon[15] it is dependent on knowing the target pH needed for optimal therapeutic efficacy of the proton pump inhibitor/antibiotic combinations, and this has not yet been determined.

Since the plasma half-lives of omeprazole, lansoprazole and pantoprazole are short and of the order of 1 h it is difficult to obtain achlorhydria with these drugs. Indeed, with a single morning dose of omeprazole 20 mg the pH is above 3 for an aggregate time of between 16 and 18 h, and with a single morning dose of omeprazole 60 mg the pH is above 3 for about 22 h[18]. When omeprazole 20 mg is given in the evening the pH is above 3 for only about 9 of the 24 h. This may explain the poor results of *H. pylori* eradication in the study reported by Bell *et al.* in 1991[8] (see above) when omeprazole was given in a single dose of 20 mg in the evening. Thus, the timing, magnitude and frequency of the dose of a proton pump inhibitor are likely to be important. If the target intragastric pH required for optimal synergy of the combinations is close to neutrality it is possible that a TID dose of the proton pump inhibitor would be more effective than either an UID or BID dose regimen.

Furthermore, the antibiotics need to be given in BID or even TID doses. Amoxicillin must be given in a dose of not less than 500 mg TID, and reviews which considered the duration of treatment[14,15] indicate that therapy should be started with amoxicillin and omeprazole simultaneously, and continued for a minimum of 2 weeks.

WHAT HYPOTHESES EXIST IN SUPPORT OF THE SYNERGISTIC EFFECTS OF THESE TWO TREATMENTS?

Both omeprazole and the newer proton pump inhibitor, lansoprazole, are effective against *H. pylori in vitro* at an MIC50 between 12.5 and 50 μg/l[19,20]. This effect can be enhanced by the substitution of a fluoro-alkoxy group at position 4 of the pyridine ring, and several acid conversion metabolites of lansopazole have been shown to be 3–4-fold more potent than the parent compound[21]. More recently Nagata *et al.*[22], and Kuhler *et al.*[23] have shown that both lansoprazole and omeprazole are potent inhibitors of *H. pylori* urease. This *in vitro* effect is three to four times more potent than the effect of acetohydroxamic acid, which is a well-characterized inhibitor of bacterial urease. The *in vitro* inhibition of *H. pylori* urease by lansoprazole and omeprazole is thought to result from covalent binding by these substituted benzimidazoles to sulphydryl groups in the urease molecule. At this time it is not known whether this effect is acting on intracellular urease or that expressed on the bacterial cell membrane.

It has been shown recently that the three proton pump inhibitors, omeprazole, lansoprazole and pantoprazole, all bind to an ATPase of the 'p' type on the membrane of live *H. pylori*[24]. This enzyme is rarely found in bacteria and is more usually found as an ATPase of eukaryotic cell membranes. All three drugs showed a strong inhibitory activity for this ATPase when studied in an acid environemnt of pH 4.0, but not at a neutral pH of 7.3.

However, it is more difficult to understand whether any of these *in vitro* effects might occur *in vivo*, since *H. pylori* colonizes the mucus–bicarbonate layer, overlying gastric epithelium in the stomach and duodenal mucosa, favouring a pH range from about 2.6 to 6.8. Omeprazole and lansoprazole are prodrugs formulated as granules which are enterically coated and encapsulated to protect them from acid activation in the stomach soon after ingestion and before reaching the upper small intestine, where they are released and absorbed. The substituted benzimidazoles are weak bases, and are therefore concentrated in the highly acidic secretory canaliculi of the parietal cell at a pH close to 1. This is a hostile environment in which *H. pylori* are seldom seen. In the secretory canaliculus omeprazole and lansoprazole are activated to the sulphenamide, which binds covalently to the proton pump to inhibit acid secretion. These sulphenamides are rapidly degraded as pH rises, and probably would not be found in the mucus–bicarbonate layer. Thus, it is hard to explain how the *in vitro* finding of inhibition of *H. pylori* by metabolites of lansoprazole or omeprazole can occur *in vivo*. However, at the high and more frequent BID dosing used in *H. pylori* eradication combinations, it is conceivable that the pH in the stomach rises to levels comparable to those seen in the upper small intestine. This would make it theoretically possible for release of the native drug in the stomach, thus providing some direct topical effect.

Other factors may also play a prominent role in the efficacy of proton pump inhibitor–antibiotic combinations. Most antibiotics, including amoxicillin, are acid-labile and will be protected from the harsh intragastric environment by raising the gastric juice pH[20,21]. For example there is a 10-fold decrease in the MIC50 for both ampicillin and clarithromycin when the pH is raised from 5.5 to 7.0[25]. In addition to this effect the PPI markedly inhibit gastric juice volume, thus increasing the concentration of antibiotics in gastric juice.

By controlling meal-stimulated acid secretion, the proton pump inhibitors provide more effective, prolonged and predictable control of acid secretion throughout the 24-h period than the H_2-receptor antagonists.

Omeprazole 20 mg daily raises the intragastric pH above 3 for 16–18 h of the day and omeprazole 60 mg for 22 h out of the 24-h day[18], and it is probable that lansoprazole and pantoprazole provide similar suppression in equipotent doses. However, analyses reporting higher pH thresholds have seldom been reported. Omeprazole 20 mg, 40 mg or 60 mg given once daily in the morning provided 11.31, 13.05, 13.36 h above pH 6.0, and 5.05, 5.10 and 6.50 h above pH 7.0, respectively[17]. These combined observations may explain, in part, the differences seen in clinical trials of *H. pylori* eradication to date. The intragastric acidity profile of the higher and more frequent doses of omeprazole, lansoprazole or pantoprazole used in the antibiotic combinations with amoxicillin described above have not yet been reported. Moreover, it is not yet known what the optimal target pH profile should be to protect amoxicillin from acid degradation, although it has been suggested that a dose of omeprazole 40 mg daily is sufficient to permit amoxicillin to reach the optimal concentration and activity in the gastric mucosa[17]. However, this conclusion assumes that the effect of omeprazole is solely one of increasing the availability of amoxicillin, the relevance of which has been questioned by the recent observation that there is an increased uptake of amoxicillin into the human gastric mucosa at lower gastric juice pH[26].

There are probably several other physiological consequences of the effective control of intragastric acidity by proton pump inhibitors which might play an important role in the efficacy of the proton pump inhibitor/antibiotic combinations. *H. pylori*-specific immunoglobulins are secreted across the gastric mucosa and are rapidly degraded by the proteolytic activity of gastric juice[27]. Raising intragastric pH to the levels obtained with the proton pump inhibitors markedly inhibits peptic activity[28], and this reduction in proteolytic activity probably leads to a prolonged half-life and higher concentrations of *H. pylori*-specific immunoglobulin in gastric juice.

Several other host resistance factors are critical to eradicating *mucosal* infections. In histological specimens from throughout the gastrointestinal tract it can be seen that there is neutrophil migration across the gastrointestinal mucosa during any inflammation. In the chronic active gastritis which occurs with *H. pylori* infection neutrophils are seen migrating across the gastric mucosa into the mucus–bicarbonate layer[29]. Effective neutrophil function is necessary for bacterial killing, and this is highly pH-dependent since this process requires the production of oxygen intermediates, active Fc component recognition and function in addition to phagocytosis. All these functions are likely to be inhibited when the pH within the mucus–bicarbonate layer falls much below pH 6.8. In humans, studies have shown that the pH gradient across the mucus–bicarbonate layer becomes more acidic during *H. pylori* infection[30]. As a further indication that acidification is detrimental to neutrophil function, there is evidence that bacterially derived succinic acid can inhibit neutrophil function by lowering intracellular pH[31].

WHAT ARE THE pH TARGETS OF THE PPI AND ANTIBIOTIC COMBINATIONS?

If the target intragastric pH required for optimal synergy of the combinations is close to neutrality it is possible that a TID dose would be more effective than either a UID or BID dose regimen. Until the results of 24-h intragastric pH studies are published it is not possible to predict with any degree of certainty what the best doses of the proton pump inhibitors should be.

CONCLUSIONS

The results of combination treatment with proton pump inhibitors and amoxicillin reported by many authors are very exciting, and promise a significant advance in an area where therapy has been recognized to be difficult. At this time there are numerous abstracts reporting small studies. Should these results be confirmed by larger studies, the PPI–antibiotic combination promises the convenience of treatment for duodenal ulcer which provides the most rapid symptom relief with fast and predictably high healing rates, combined with the chance of a cure of the infection, by eradicating *H. pylori* infection, in more than three-quarters of those treated.

Much work still needs to be done to determine the optimal combinations, frequency and magnitude of the doses of these combinations and the exact mechanisms by which eradication of *H. pylori* is achieved. Until such time as the results of such studies become available, the gastroenterologist has an alternative to triple therapy which provides greater convenience, promises better compliance and fewer side-effects, and which has been endorsed as a treatment regime by an international working party at the recent First United European Congress of Gastroenterology, held in Athens in September 1992[32]. However, it would be unwise to advocate the widespread use of eradication treatment in primary care until the best combinations and dose regimens have been determined and their synergistic mechanism of action better understood.

References

1. Graham DY, Lew GM, Evans DG *et al*. Effect of triple therapy (antibiotics plus bismuth) on duodenal ulcer healing. Ann Intern Med. 1991;115(4):266–9.
2. Morgan DG, Burget DW, Howden CW *et al*. Rates of duodenal ulcer (DU) healing by drug classes: a meta-analysis. Gastroenterology. 1993;104(4):A150.
3. Rangachari PK. *Helicobacter pylori* and hypergastrinaemia: the quisling option. Scand J Gastroenterol. 1991;187(Suppl.26):85–90.
4. Rademaker JW, Hunt RH. *H. pylori* and gastric acid secretion: the ulcer link? Scand J Gastroenterol. 1991;187(Suppl.26):71–7.
5. Unge P, Gad A, Gnarpe H *et al*. Does omeprazole improve antimicrobial therapy directed towards gastric *Campylobacter pylori* in patients with antral gastritis? Scand J Gastroenterol. 1989;167(Suppl.24):49–54.
6. Hosking SW, Ling TKW, Yung MY *et al*. Randomized controlled trial of short term treatment to eradicate *Helicobacter pylori* in patients with duodenal ulcer. BMJ. 1992;306:502–4.
7. Hentschel E, Brandstatter G, Dragosics B *et al*. Effect of ranitidine and amoxicillin plus metronidazole on the eradication of *Helicobacter pylori* and the recurrence of duodenal ulcer. N Engl J Med. 1993;328(5):308–12.
8. Bell GD, Powell K, Weil J *et al*. Experience with omeprazole in combination with either amoxicillin or colloidal bismuth subcitrate in patients with metronidazole-resistant *Helicobacter pylori*. Eur J Gastroenterol Hepatol. 1991;3:923–6.
9. Chiverton SG, Howden CW, Burget DW, Hunt RH. Omeprazole (20 mg) daily given in the morning or evening: a comparison of effects on gastric acidity, and plasma gastrin and omeprazole concentration. Aliment Pharmacol Ther. 1992;6:103–11.
10. Unge P, Gad A, Eriksson K *et al*. Amoxicillin added to omeprazole prevents relapse in the treatment of DU patients. Eur J Gastroenterol Hepatol. 1993;5(5):325–31.
11. Labenz J, Gyenes E, Ruhl GH, Borsch G. Omeprazole plus amoxicillin: efficacy of various treatment regimens to eradicate *Helicobacter pylori*. Am J Gastroenterol. 1993;88:491–5.
12. Bayerdorffer E, Mannes GA, Sommer A *et al*. High dose omeprazole treatment combined with amoxicillin eradicates *Helicobacter pylori*. Eur J Gastroenterol Hepatol. 1992;4: 697–702.
13. Labenz J, Gyenes E, Ruhl GH, Borsch G. Efficacy of omeprazole and amoxicillin to eradicate Hp. Am J Gastroenterol. 1992;87:A115.
14. Mohamed H, Chiba N, Wilkinson J, Hunt RH. Eradication of *Helicobacter pylori* (Hp): a meta-analysis. Gastroenterology. 1994;106(5):in press.
15. Axon ATR. The role of omeprazole and antibiotic combinations in the eradication of *Helicobacter pylori*. Scand J Gastroenterol. 1993:in press.
16. Chiba N, Rao BV, Rademaker JW, Hunt RH. Meta-analysis of the efficacy of antibiotic therapy in eradicating *Helicobacter pylori*. Am J Gastronterol. 1992;87(12):1716–27.
17. Savarino V, Mela GS, Zentilin P, Vigneri S, Celle G. Acid inhibition and amoxicillin activity against *Helicobacter pylori*. Am J Gastroenterol. 1993;11:1975–6.
18. Burget DW, Chiverton SC, Hunt RH. Is there an optimal degree of acid suppression for healing of duodenal ulcers? Gastroenterology. 1990;99:345–51.
19. Iwahi T, Satoh H, Nakao M. Lansoprazole, a novel benzimidazole proton pump inhibitor, and its related compounds have selective activity against *Helicobacter pylori*. Antimicrob Agents Chemother. 1991;35(3):490–6.
20. Mainguet P, Delmee M, Debongnie JP. Omeprazole, *Campylobacter pylori*, and duodenal ulcer. Lancet. 1989;2:389–90.

21. Van Zanten SJO, Goldie J, Hollingsworth J, Siletti C, Richardson H, Hunt RH. Secretion of intravenously administered antibiotics in gastric juice: implications for management of *Helicobacter pylori*. J Clin Pathol. 1992;45:225–7.
22. Nagata K, Satoh H, Iwahi T, Shimoyama T, Tamura T. Potent inhibitory action of the gastric proton pump inhibitor lansoprazole against urease activity of *Helicobacter pylori*: unique action selective for *H. pylori* cells. Antimicrob Agents Chemother. 1993;37:769–44.
23. Kuhler T, Fryklund J, Bergman N-A, Weilitz J, Larson H. Omeprazole and analogues inhibit urea-dependent ammonia production by *Helicobacter pylori*. Acta Gastroenterol Belg. 1993;56:137.
24. Mauch F, Bode G, Malfertheiner P. Identification and characterization of an ATPase system of *Helicobacter pylori* and effect of proton pump inhibitors. Am J Gastroenterol. 1993;88:1801–2.
25. McNulty CA, Dent JC, Ford GA, Wilkinson SP. Inhibitory antimicrobial concentrations against *Campylobacter pylori* in gastric mucosa. J Antimicrob Chemother. 1988;22:729–38.
26. Arena G, Lambert JR, King RG *et al.* Enhanced amoxicillin uptake into the human gastric mucosa at lower gastric juice pH. Gastroenterology. 1993;104:A34.
27. Rademaker JW, Zettel L, Jacobson K, Chiba N, Ernst PB, Hunt RH. Gastric juice immunoglobulins – immunophysiological interaction in *Helicobacter pylori* infection. Gastroenterology. 1993;104:A176.
28. Dent J, Hunt RH, Modlin I, Peura D, Soll AH. Acid-related diseases: clinical science and implications for management (Submitted for publication).
29. Terada S, Negayama K, Kawanishi K. Neutrophil migration into the mucous layer in *Helicobacter pylori* associated gastritis. Eur J Gastroenterol Hepatol. 1993;5(Suppl.1): S45–9.
30. Beardshall K, Adamson D, Gill J, Unwin R, Calam J. *Helicobacter pylori* raises the pH in the juxtaepithelial region of the mucus layer of the gastric antrum and body. Gastroenterology. 1991;32:A569.
31. Rotstein ORD, Nasmith PE, Grinstein S. The bacteroides by-product succinic acid inhibits neutrophil respiratory burst by reducing intracellular pH. Infect Immun. 1987;55:864–70.
32. Scrip. New *H. pylori* therapy recommendations. Scrip. 1992;1760:22.

56
Prospects for vaccination against *H. pylori* infection

B. J. UNDERDOWN

INTRODUCTION

The development of effective immunization strategies to prevent or control *Helicobacter pylori* infection in humans has received increasing attention in the past few years[1-3]. Exploration of this approach seems particularly worthwhile, since there is no evidence, to date, that indicates currently available antimicrobial treatment protects individuals from reinfection. Moreover, the possible emergence of antibiotic-resistant strains of *H. pylori* lends attractiveness to the immune approach.

Success in developing an effective vaccine hinges on a number of key strategies. Of primary importance is the demonstration that immunological memory can be established at the site of infection and/or disease. Animal models are often important in assisting investigators to identify the type of immunity required and the 'protective' antigens that can elicit appropriate immunity. However, as useful as animal models are, they often do not completely mimic the human infection and/or disease. In this regard, current animal models require establishment of infection with several doses of relatively large inocula of *Helicobacter*, which suggests that a permissive host model may not yet have been found. In addition to the important steps which lead to proof of concept, there are many regulatory steps which must be passed before a vaccine, shown previously to be efficacious in animals, is licensed. This latter step to establish efficacy requires substantial investment in clinical trials. Thus, time lines are often quite long even after protection has been demonstrated in the animal model.

IMMUNOLOGICAL MEMORY AND MUCOSAL IMMUNITY

Despite some initial uncertainty in the late 1960s and early 1970s, there seems little doubt that immunological memory can be generated at mucosal sites such as the intestine. For example, individuals who survive clinical cholera rarely become reinfected with the same serotype of *Vibrio cholera*[4] and live oral polio vaccine effectively eliminated the carrier state in immunized populations[5]. In contrast, one of the outstanding features of *H. pylori* infection, from the immunological perspective, is the chronicity of infection in a high proportion of the human population which increases with time. Indeed, there is very little evidence of acquired immunity to this infection in humans. Unfortunately, the stomach has not been well characterized immunologically, and the extent to which immunological memory can be generated in the stomach is unknown.

Most of our current knowledge concerning mucosal immune responses comes from studies in the intestine. Induction of immune responses takes place initially within specialized lymphoid aggregates which occur intermittently along the bowel such as the visually identifiable Peyer's patches[6]. M cells which overlie the Peyer's patches[7] are thought to be highly active in delivering luminal antigens to the lymphoid cellular machinery, which is highly committed to IgA antibody production[8]. Once the immune response is generated, effector cells, including antibody-producing cells as well as T and B memory cells, migrate via the lymphatic circulation and blood to the lamina propria of the intestine, as well as to other mucosal sites[8]. Induction of such mucosal immune responses appears to occur readily with live replicating organisms, many of which appear to be taken up selectively by M cells overlying Peyer's patches[7]. Non-living particulate antigens also appear to be taken up selectively by M cells, which explains current efforts to develop microparticle-based systems for effective antigen delivery via oral immunization. In contrast, soluble antigen does not seem to be effective in inducing primary immune responses when delivered orally, and can under certain conditions induce systemic unresponsiveness[10]. However, once primed by a particular living or non-living immunogen, soluble antigen, delivered orally, can evoke a secondary mucosal and systemic immune response[11].

The stomach, viewed from this paradigm, may be immunologically deficient, since an analogous M cell/lymphoid apparatus has not been described at this site. On the other hand, memory in the stomach could potentially be generated either by antigen which traverses the gastric epithelium directly, or by antigen which has left the stomach and has been taken up by the M cells of the small intestine. Clearly, more work needs to be undertaken to understand the regulation of the immune response in the stomach.

Setting aside the possibility that the stomach may not be as robust as some other mucosal sites in generating protective immunity, *H. pylori* itself may have characteristics which enable it to suppress local immune responses, as has been reported for organisms which inhabit the intestine, such as *H. polygyrus*[12]. Alternatively, *H. pylori* may have the capacity to drive the host's immune response preferentially into a non-protective pathway such as has been decribed for some infectious agents[13]. Apparent failure to generate effective mucosal immunity to *H. pylori* stands in sharp contrast to the clear evidence that a number of immune and inflammatory effector elements are activated in *H. pylori* infection. This includes the synthesis of IgA and IgG antibody, as well as the recruitment of lymphocytes and polymorphonuclear leukocytes to the site of infection[14]. It is possible that in spite of the clear evidence that an active immune response is generated in *H. pylori*-infected hosts, the manner in which such responses are induced may promote responses which are not protective. It is possible that soluble *H. pylori* antigens taken up by mucosal epithelium mediate systemic unresponsiveness to critical *H. pylori* antigens.

It should also be noted that failure to eliminate a primary infection of *H. pylori* does not necessarily imply that acquisition of immunity cannot be achieved. In the case of murine giardiasis some strains of mice which are unable to eliminate a primary infection have been demonstrated to resist a secondary challenge (following elimination of *Giardia muris* with metronidazole)[15,16]. Whether immunity to a secondary challenge exists in human *H. pylori* infection could be studied directly by treating a group of infected human hosts, and comparing the rate at which such hosts reacquire the infection in comparison to a group of appropriately matched non-infected subjects treated in a similar fashion. Knowledge that, under certain conditions, immunity can be established to *H. pylori* may be important in designing a vaccine development programme. Without a sound knowledge of the basis for the chronicity of infection, and the extent to which infected hosts can generate potentially protective responses, vaccine development will be attenuated.

WHAT IMMUNE RESPONSES COULD BE PROTECTIVE AGAINST *H. PYLORI*?

H. pylori is primarily an extracellular infection. While some organisms clearly adhere to mucus-secreting cells of the gastric mucosal epithelium, many organisms can be observed in the mucous layer. As a general rule, immunity to extracellular infections is thought to be mediated primarily by antibody and at the mucosae, by secretory IgA antibody, in particular. IgA antibody is thought to protect the host by combining with bacteria to reduce their motility and ability to adhere specifically to mucosal epithelial cells[17]. More recently, Mazanac and colleagues have presented evidence that indicates that IgA antibody may also exert its antimicrobial function within epithelial cells[18]. Given its location it is difficult, but not impossible, to imagine other immune effector elements such as Fcα-bearing monocytes[19], eosinophils[20] and neutrophils[21] being active in the lumen of the stomach, let alone the small intestine. Unfortunately, the available data indicate that serum and secretory antibody exists in most infected hosts. Thus, we could postulate that either the quantity or quality (affinity, isotype) of the antibody produced is insufficient to generate a protective response.

With respect to other effector elements, there are insufficient data to assess the role which cytotoxic lymphocytes (CTL), intraepithelial lymphocytes (IEL) or CD4-mediated cellular immunity might play. Adoptive transfer studies, in which cells are taken from immune hosts and injected into naive hosts, could be used to identify relevant protective elements, provided that a suitable animal model for such studies could be established.

THE ANIMAL MODELS

Most vaccine development programmes begin with animal experiments to verify the immunogenicity of the vaccine antigens chosen for study. Ideally, the animal species chosen should not only be useful for immunogenicity studies, but should serve as a host for infection, so that the effectiveness of various immunization strategies offering protective responses can be assessed.

The current models for *Helicobacter* infection in animals (see Chapter 00 in this volume) offer much opportunity for study of immunogenicity studies, as well as studies which assess protection, but these models may fall short in a number of characteristics. Chief among these is the fact that multiple relatively large doses ($\sim 10^8$ of organisms) are used to establish infection, and under these conditions prominent virulence factors such as urease may be overaccentuated compared to the infection in natural hosts. For example, it seems clear that, in both the rodent and porcine models, urease appears critical. In pigs, urease-deficient *H. pylori* failed to induce gastritis[22], and in the mouse model immunization with *H. pylori* urease protected mice from challenge with *H. felis*[3]. In contrast, humans infected with *H. pylori* generate substantial amounts of serum and secretory antibody to urease and, despite this, become chronically infected. The apparent paradox created by these contradictory findings might be explained in a number of ways. For example, it is possible that, in the case of *H. pylori*, natural infection of humans may occur via a small number of organisms which establish in an ecological niche such as the mouth where urease may not be critical[21].

CURRENT DATA CONCERNING IMMUNIZATION

Recent experiments by several groups indicate that mice immunized intra-gastrically with a sonicate of whole *H. felis* or recombinant *H. pylori* urease are rendered resistant to a challenge infection in the mouse *H. felis* model[1-3]. The immunization protocol included the use of the mucosal adjuvant cholera toxin (10 μg/mouse) to promote the synthesis of IgA antibodies. Unfortunately, challenge was relatively soon after the last immunizing dose, and the effectiveness of this strategy in inducing immunological memory needs to be clarified.

A number of other protective antigens are possible candidate antigens. Flagellar proteins[23] which promote bacterial motility and adhesins[24] which promote bacterial attachment to the gastric epithelium are prime candidates for evaluation. An additional approach focused on the inflammation-promoting properties of *H. pylori* would involve evaluation of chemotaxins[25] as possible protective antigens. The complexity of this infection suggests that a single antigen is unlikely to be sufficient. For example, satisfactory immunity to *Vibrio cholera* requires both antitoxin and antibacterial immunity[26]. Seen in this light a genetically engineered *H. pylori*, modified to eliminate molecules that promote inflammation, would be of interest. Such a recombinant organism might produce self-limiting infections instead of chronic infections observed, and may with subsequent attenuation be the best route to

Table 1 Strategies for immunization via mucosal surfaces

Replicating particles	Non-replicating particles	Receptor-targeted
Salmonella	Iscoms	CTX-CTB
E. coli	Liposomes	Adhesins
BCG	Microparticles	Antireceptor antibodies
Adenovirus		
Vaccinia virus		
Polio virus		

producing a protective vaccine. A subunit approach, on the other hand, is likely to require an effective delivery system. Some of those currently available are listed in Table 1. Live attenuated recombinant systems[27,28] have the advantage of employing some replication potential and using the natural attachment factors of the recombinant vector. To be useful, such vectors must be highly attenuated to avoid complications in immunocompromised hosts, as well as residual pathology in normal hosts. Inert particulate systems such as Iscoms[29], polylactide–glycolide particles[30] and liposomes[31] have been proposed as a means of protecting vaccine antigens from the hostile environment of the gastrointestinal tract and delivery of antigen to M cells. Cholera toxin has been shown to be a highly potent adjuvant when administered orally, mixed with the antigen or as a toxin–antigen conjugate[32]. Unfortunately, the difficulties in receiving approval for a cholera toxin-containing oral vaccine seem formidable, and the B subunit of cholera toxin is much less effective than the toxin[33]. Other molecular targeting systems such as anti-MHC II antibody coupled to antigen[34] may be effective under certain circumstances when administered orally (Estrada et al., submitted).

WHAT RESPONSES ARE DESIRED TO PRODUCE AN EFFECTIVE VACCINE?

The simplest objective from a conceptual level would be to convert H. pylori infection from a chronic to a self-limiting infection. Sterile immunity, in other words, may not be the desired objective. From this perspective, identification of those factors (both host and microbial) which promote inflammation may be crucial, since it is possible that promotion of an inflammatory response is critical to H. pylori in establishing itself and growing to high levels in the chronically infected hosts. Attenuation of the early inflammatory response may allow IgA antibody (the most likely candidate effector) to promote elimination of the organism. An analysis of the cytokine response early in infection might assist in the identification of T cell responses which promote ineffective immune responses. This, in turn, might generate approaches in which vaccine vehicles incorporate specific immunomodulatory molecules to direct the immune response along a protective path, rather than along a disease-promoting path.

SOME LOGISTICS OF VACCINE DEVELOPMENT

Given the relatively slow acquisition of *H. pylori* (approximately 1–2% per year), a clinical trial to determine the outcome in a human population immunized with a test vaccine might take considerably longer than most vaccine trials with other human infectious diseases. Moreover, it is not immediately apparent which of the multitude of strategies currently under development for mucosal immunization would be effective.

SUMMARY

Recent work indicates that, in experimental animals, immunization may protect against *Helicobacter* infection. The steps which need to be taken to bring this to humans are many. A greater understanding of the role that inflammation plays in promoting chronic infection in human hosts may be key to identifying molecules which should be inhibited in any vaccine strategy. Currently, many delivery systems for oral vaccine delivery are under development. Few of these have come to market. Undoubtedly, the general problem of mucosal vaccination must be solved before an effective *H. pylori* vaccine becomes available.

References

1. Chen M, Lee A, Hazell S. Immunisation against gastric *Helicobacter* infection in a mouse/*Helicobacter felis* model. Lancet. 1992;339:1120–1.
2. Czinn SJ, Nedrud JG. Oral immunization against *Helicobacter pylori*. Infect Immun. 1991;59:2359–62.
3. Davin C, Blum AL, Corthesy-Theulaz I *et al. H. pylori* urease elicits protection against *H. felis* infection in mice. Gastroenterology. 1993;104:A1035.
4. Holmgren J, Svennerholm AM. Cholera and the immune response. Prog Allergy. 1983;33:106–19.
5. Ogra PL, Karzon DT, Righthand F, MacGillivray M. Immunoglobulin response in serum and secretion after immunization with live and inactivated polio vaccine and natural infection. N Engl J Med. 1968;279:893–900.
6. McGhee JR, Mestsecky J, Dertzbaugh MT, Eldridge JH, Hirasawa M, Kiyono H. The mucosal immune system: from fundamental concepts to vaccine development. Vaccine. 1992;10:75–88.
7. Sanderson IR, Walker WA. Uptake and transport of macromolecules by the intestine: possible role in clinical disorders (an update). Gastroenterology. 1993;104:622–39.
8. Craig SW, Cebra JJ. Peyer's patches: an enriched source of precursors for IgA-producing immunocytes in the rabbit. J Exp Med. 1971;134:188–200.
9. McDermott MR, Bienenstock J. Evidence for a common mucosal immunologic system. I. Migration of B immunoblasts into intestinal, respiratory, and genital tissues. J Immunol. 1979;122:1892–8.
10. Bruce MG, Ferguson A. Oral tolerance to ovalbumin in mice: studies of chemically modified and 'biologically filtered' antigen. Immunology. 1986;57:627–30.
11. Dunkley ML, Husband AJ, Underdown BJ. Cognate T cell help in the induction of IgA responses *in vivo*. Immunology. 1990;71:16–19.
12. Dehlawi MS, Wakeland D, Behnke JM. Suppression of mucosal mastocytosis by infection with the intestinal nematode *Nematospiroides dubius*. Parasite Immunol. 1987;9:187–94.
13. Pearce EJ, Caspar P, Grzych JM, Lewis FA, Sher A. Downregulation of Th1 cytokine production accompanies induction of Th2 responses by a parasitic helminth. *Schistosoma*

mansoni. J Exp Med. 1991;173:159–62.

14. Marshall BJ, Warren JR. Unidentified curved bacilli in the stomach of patients with gastritis and peptic ulceration. Lancet. 1984;1:1311–15.
15. Underdown BJ, Roberts-Thompson IC, Anders RF, Mitchell GF. Giardiasis in mice: studies on the characteristics of chronic infection in C3H/H3 mice. J Immunol. 1981;126:669–72.
16. Skea D, Underdown BJ. Acquired resistance to *Giardia muris* in X-linked immunodeficient (Xid) mice. Infect Immun. 1991;59:1733–8.
17. Underdown BJ, Schiff JM. Immunoglobulin A: strategic defence initiative at the mucosal surface. Annu Rev Immunol. 1986;4:389–417.
18. Mazanec MB, Kaetzel CS, Lamm ME, Fletcher D, Nedrud JG. Intracellular neutralization of virus by immunoglobulin A antibodies. Proc Natl Acad Sci USA. 1992;89:6901–5.
19. Monteiro RC, Cooper MD, Kubagawa H. Molecular heterogeneity of Fcα receptors detected by receptor-specific monoclonal antibodies. J Immunol. 1992;148:1764–70.
20. Abu-Ghazaleh RI, Fujisawa T, Mestecky J, Kyle RA, Gleich CJ. IgA-induced eosinophil degranulation. J Immunol. 1989;142:2393–400.
21. Hostoffer RW, Krukovets I, Berger M. Increased FcαR expression and IgA-mediated function on neutropils induced by chemoattractants. J Immunol. 1993;150:4532–40.
22. Eaton KA, Morgan DR, Brooks CL, Krakowka S. Essential role of urease in the pathogenesis of gastritis induced by *Helicobacter pylori* cytotoxin. Infect Immun. 1991;59:1264–70.
23. Suerbaum S, Josenhans C, Labigne A. Cloning and genetic characterization of the *Helicobacter pylori* and *Helicobacter mustelae* flaB flagellin genes and construction of *H. pylori* flaA- and flaB-negative mutants by electroporation-mediated allelic exchange. J Bacteriol. 1993;174:3278–88.
24. Clyne M, Drumm B. Adherence of *Helicobacter pylori* to primary human gastrointestinal cells. Infect Immun. 1993;61:4052–7.
25. Kozol R, McCurdy B, Czanko R. A neutrophil chemotactic factor present in *H. pylori* but absent in *H. mustelae.* Dig Dis Sci. 1993;38:137–41.
26. Holmgren J, Svennerholm A-M. Bacterial enteric infections and vaccine development. Gastroenterol Clin N Am. 1992;21:283–302.
27. Prevec L. Adenoviruses as expression vectors and recombinant vaccines. Trends Biotechnol. 1990;8:85–7.
28. Schodel F. Prospects for oral vaccination using recombinant bacteria expressing viral epitopes. Adv Vir Res. 1993;41:409–46.
29. Mowat AM, Donachie AM. Iscoms – a novel strategy for mucosal immunization? Immunol Today. 1991;12:383–5.
30. Eldridge JH, Meulbroek JA, Staas JK, Tice TR, Gilley RM. Vaccine-containing biodegradable microspheres specifically enter the gut-associated lymphoid tissue following oral administration and induce a disseminated mucosal immune response. Adv Exp Med Biol. 1990;251:191–202.
31. Jackson S, Mestecky J, Childers NK, Michalek SM. Liposomes containing anti-idiotypic antibodies: an oral vaccine to induce protective secretory immune responses specific for pathogens of mucosal surfaces. Infect Immun. 1990;58:1932–6.
32. Elson CO, Ealding W. Generalized systemic and mucosal immunity in mice after mucosal stimulation with cholera toxin. J Immunol. 1984;132:2736–41.
33. Lycke NY. Cholera toxin promotes B cell isotype switching by two different mechanisms. J Immunol. 1993;150:4810–21.
34. Carayanniotis G, Barber BH. Adjuvant-free IgG responses induced with antigen coupled to antibodies against class II MHC. Nature. 1987;327:59–61.

Index

INDEX